EDITION

6

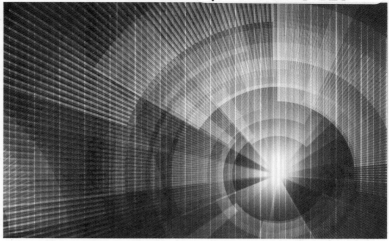

Perspectives on Nursing Theory

EDITED BY

PAMELA G. REED, RN, PhD, FAAN
Professor
The University of Arizona
College of Nursing
Tucson, Arizona

NELMA B. CRAWFORD SHEARER, RN, PhD
Associate Professor and Co-Director
Hartford Center of Geriatric Nursing Excellence
College of Nursing & Health Innovation
Arizona State University
Phoenix, Arizona

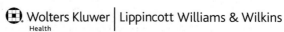
Wolters Kluwer | Lippincott Williams & Wilkins
Health
Philadelphia · Baltimore · New York · London
Buenos Aires · Hong Kong · Sydney · Tokyo

Acquisitions Editor: Carrie Brandon
Product Manager: Helen Kogut
Editorial Assistant: Jacalyn Clay
Design Coordinator: Joan Wendt
Illustration Coordinator: Brett MacNaughton
Manufacturing Coordinator: Karin Duffield
Prepress Vendor: SPi Global

6th edition

9 8 7 6 5 4 3 2 1

Printed in China

Library of Congress Cataloging-in-Publication Data
Perspectives on nursing theory / edited by Pamela G. Reed, Nelma B. Crawford, Shearer. —6th ed.
   p. ; cm.
  Nursing theory
  Anthology of previously published articles.
  Includes bibliographical references and index.
  ISBN 978-1-60913-748-9 (alk. paper)
  1. Nursing—Philosophy. 2. Nursing models. I. Reed, Pamela G., 1952– II. Shearer, Nelma B. Crawford, 1950– III.
Title: Nursing theory.
  [DNLM: 1. Nursing Theory—Collected Works. 2. Philosophy, Nursing—Collected Works. WY 86]
  RT84.5.P47 2011
  610.7301—dc23

2011015851

CCS0811

About the Editors

Pamela G. Reed is a metatheoretician and Professor at the University of Arizona College of Nursing in Tucson, where she also served as Associate Dean for Academic Affairs for 7 years. She is a three-time graduate of Wayne State University in Detroit, receiving a BSN, an MSN (with a double major in child–adolescent psychiatric mental health nursing and teaching), and a PhD with a major in nursing (focused on life span development and aging) in 1982. Dr. Reed pioneered research into spirituality and well-being with her doctoral research with terminally ill patients. She also developed a theory of self-transcendence and two widely used research instruments, the *Spiritual Perspective Scale* and the *Self-Transcendence Scale*. Her publications and funded research reflect a dual focus: spirituality and other facilitators of well-being in life-limiting illness, and nursing metatheory and knowledge development. Dr. Reed also enjoys time with her family, reading, classical music, swimming, and hiking in the mountains and canyons of Arizona.

Nelma B. Crawford Shearer is a researcher and Associate Professor and Co-Director of the Hartford Center of Geriatric Nursing Excellence at Arizona State University. She earned a BS from South Dakota State University, an MEd from the University of Missouri-St. Louis, an MS from Southern Illinois University in Edwardsville, and a PhD from the University of Arizona. She teaches theoretical foundations of nursing at the graduate and doctoral levels. She is an American Nurses Foundation scholar and a John A. Hartford Foundation Institute of Geriatric Nursing Research scholar. Dr. Shearer has developed a research and theory-based intervention to promote health empowerment in older adults. Her work has been continuously funded, with the most recent support from the National Institute of Nursing Research to test her *health empowerment intervention* with homebound older adults. She and her husband Jim have been married 37 years, have two children, and reside in Tempe, Arizona, where she enjoys her family, entertaining friends, antiquing, gardening, and going for long bike rides.

W e dedicate this book to students and teachers who value nursing knowledge and who enjoy participating in its development and application to enhance human health and well-being.

Pamela G. Reed

Nelma B. Crawford Shearer

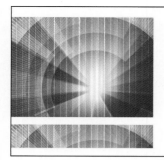

Reviewers

Margaret W. Bultas, RN, MSN, CPNP-PC
Assistant Professor
Goldfarb School of Nursing at Barnes Jewish College
St. Louis, Missouri

Judith J. Chodil, RN, PhD
Professor Emeritus
California State University Dominguez Hills
Carson, California

Mary Ann Dailey, RN, PhD
Chairperson, Department of Nursing
Kutztown University of Pennsylvania
Kutztown, Pennsylvania

Susan Sweat Gunby, RN, PhD
Dean and Professor
Georgia Baptist College of Nursing of Mercer University
Atlanta, Georgia

Barbara J. Guthrie, RN, PhD, FAAN
Associate Professor and Associate Dean for
Academic Affairs
Yale School of Nursing
New Haven, Connecticut

Carolyn A. Phillips, RN, PhD
Associate Professor
School of Nursing and Graduate School of
Biomedical Sciences
University of Texas Medical Branch
Galveston, Texas

Mary Pickett, RN, PhD
Associate Professor
Villanova University
College of Nursing
Villanova, Pennsylvania

Reviewers

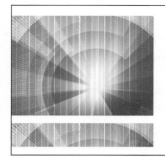

Preface

Purpose of the Book

Theoretical thinking is the purview of all nurses who participate in knowledge development. Theory enhances the effectiveness and status of a discipline. Disciplines and professions are characterized by specialized knowledge and autonomous practitioners who lead in the production and use of their knowledge. Scholars from healthcare disciplines increasingly are recognizing the value of theory in the quality of inquiry in, for example, gerontology, social work, health promotion, and nutritional science. They are revving up attention to theory to achieve a level of sophistication already found in nursing. This book reveals nursing's rich repertoire of theoretical perspectives and tools for knowledge building. A review of the unit introductions shows the breadth and diversity of nursing perspectives on theory.

The book is designed to provide a comprehensive overview of the important discussions taking place regarding the structures, methods, and processes of knowledge building in nursing. The chapters are straightforward in presenting material relevant to graduate level students, teachers, researchers, and practitioners. Theory touches the work of nurses in many ways, whether they are applying, evaluating, generating, or modifying theory through their practice and research.

The Meanings of Theory

The term, *theory*, holds special meanings across disciplines, from the humanities to the sciences. In nursing, theory has a flexible and broadened meaning. Historically, *nursing theory* referred primarily to the classic conceptual models, which are useful in clarifying our disciplinary perspectives about human beings, their health and environment, and nursing care. Nursing has evolved to embrace theories of different types and levels of abstraction, as well as broader philosophical perspectives about science, knowledge, and reality. These theoretical elements are as significant as formal empirical inquiry in developing knowledge and generating evidence. They merit careful study, reflection, and evaluation.

Nursing contexts are imbued with the *theoretical*, that is, the philosophies, values, frameworks, concepts, and perceptions that surface in human encounters. *Theory-informed* means reflecting on and explicating these conceptual elements that reside within nursing care and research. Contemporary customs of praxis, reflective practice, evidence-based practice, and research translation all are enhanced by theory. Theory connects the conceptual to the concrete, and connects abstraction to action to generate relevant knowledge for nursing situations.

Structure of the Book

This book is an anthology of classic and contemporary peer-reviewed articles that address various theoretical and philosophical perspectives on knowledge development in research and practice. Of the 52 chapters, almost half (21) are new with the remaining 31 chapters, retained from the 5th edition, deemed seminal readings. This 6th edition continues in the same spirit as previous editions, revising the framework to include new units and modify existing units, and refreshing the text with new articles that reflect the changes in theoretical thinking while preserving classic writings. Biographical information and personal commentaries by chapter authors orient readers to the gist of each chapter. Unit Overviews and Discussion Questions developed by the editors clarify the metatheoretical context of each unit and challenge readers to relate the content to their own situation. Together, the 52 chapters orient readers to 21st century thought while maintaining a vital connection to the history of nursing theory.

Organization of the Chapters

The chapters are organized topically into nine units that represent important domains of nursing metatheory concerning knowledge development in research and practice. The units will help readers clarify foundations for their own scholarly inquiry—foundations to support their *substantive* focus as well as *methodological* and *ethical* approaches in their research and practice inquiry. A diversity of philosophical views and theoretical tools is presented. The units are not mutually exclusive, but they represent clusters of articles that present key ideas for each metatheoretical domain.

- Unit 1: Structures of Nursing Knowledge Development
- Unit 2: The Inseparability of Theory and Practice
- Unit 3: Theory and Knowledge Translation
- Unit 4: Philosophies of Nursing Science in Research
- Unit 5: Epistemology and Evidence in Practice
- Unit 6: Tools for Theory Development
- Unit 7: Characteristics and Criteria of Nursing Theories
- Unit 8: Philosophies of Nursing Practice
- Unit 9: Future Directions for Nursing Theory

This new edition is intended to not only inform scholars and future scholars of nursing but to be used as a catalyst for continued thinking about the what, how, and why of knowledge development in nursing. May these chapters be read more than once for the dialogue and enthusiasm they can generate about nursing knowledge and one's role in its evolution.

Pamela G. Reed
Nelma B. Crawford Shearer

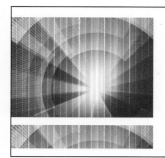

Acknowledgments

Many people have contributed to making this book a success for nursing. We first thank the contributors whose timeless ideas and insights about nursing are recorded between the covers of this book. Their articles comprise the chapters of this book and, together, provide a comprehensive set of perspectives about our discipline that are relevant to nursing knowledge.

We thank our students, past-present-future, who helped inspire the purpose for creating this book. It is our hope that these chapters will facilitate students' learning about the metatheoretical foundations of our discipline.

We appreciate everyone at Wolters Kluwer Health | Lippincott Williams & Wilkins for their dedicated work in transforming ideas about nursing metatheory into a portable package for students and faculty. We especially thank Barbara Corbin, former Project Manager and Karen Ettinger, current Project Manager, O'Donnell & Associates (OD&A), who supported and expertly guided us through all of the details and deadlines to make this project a success. We also must acknowledge Helen Kogut, Product Manager, for her sustained guidance and support. We also appreciate G. Biju Kumar, Project Manager at SPi Global. We extend thanks to Carrie Brandon, Executive Acquisition Editor, and our special appreciation to Jacalyn Clay, Editorial Assistant, at Wolters Kluwer Health | Lippincott Williams & Wilkins for their essential roles in producing another innovative edition of this book.

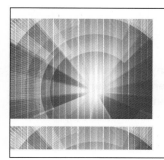

Contents

UNIT 1

Structures of Nursing Knowledge Development

CHAPTER 1

Nursing Theory and Practice: Connecting the Dots   2

Jo-Ann Marrs
Lois W. Lowry

CHAPTER 2

Yes, Virginia, Nursing Does Have Laws   10

Pamela B. Webber

CHAPTER 3

Philosophy, Science, Theory: Interrelationships and Implications for Nursing Research   17

Mary Cipriano Silva

CHAPTER 4

On Nursing Theories and Evidence   23

Jacqueline Fawcett
Jean Watson
Betty Neuman
Patricia H. Walker
Joyce J. Fitzpatrick

CHAPTER 5

Integration of Nursing Theory and Nursing Ethics   30

Michael Yeo

CHAPTER 6

A Treatise on Nursing Knowledge Development for the 21st Century: Beyond Postmodernism   37

Pamela G. Reed

UNIT 2

The Inseparability of Theory and Practice

CHAPTER 7

Toward Compassionate Action: Pragmatism and the Inseparability of Theory/Practice   48

Gweneth Hartrick Doane
Colleen Varcoe

CHAPTER 8

The Practitioner as Theorist   56

Rosemary Ellis

CHAPTER 9

"Lest We Forget": An Issue Concerning the Doctorate in Nursing Practice (DNP)   62

Ann L. Whall

CHAPTER 10

The Link Between Nursing Discourses and Nurses' Silence: Implications for a Knowledge-Based Discourse for Nursing Practice   64

Connie J. Canam

CHAPTER 11

Transcending the Limits of Method: Cultivating Creativity in Nursing   73

Gweneth A. Hartrick

UNIT 3 Theory and Knowledge Translation

CHAPTER 12
Knowledge Translation in Everyday Nursing: From Evidence-Based to Injury-Based Practice   82
Gweneth Hartrick Doane
Colleen Varcoe

CHAPTER 13
Nursing Theory as a Guide to Practice   93
William K. Cody

CHAPTER 14
The Situation-Specific Theory of Pain Experience for Asian American Cancer Patients   101
Eun-Ok Im

CHAPTER 15
Theory and Knowledge Translation: Setting Some Coordinates   111
Jo Rycroft-Malone

CHAPTER 16
Unitary Appreciative Inquiry: Evolution and Refinement   121
W. Richard Cowling III
Elizabeth Repede

UNIT 4 Philosophies of Nursing Science in Research

CHAPTER 17
Complex Critical Realism: Tenets and Application in Nursing Research   134
Alexander M. Clark
Sue L. Lissel
Caroline Davis

CHAPTER 18
Bridging the Gulf Between Science and Action: The "New Fuzzies" of Neopragmatism   145
Catherine A. Warms
Carole A. Schroeder

CHAPTER 19
An Analysis of Changing Trends in Philosophies of Science on Nursing Theory Development and Testing   153
Mary Cipriano Silva
Daniel Rothbart

CHAPTER 20
The Advocate-Analyst Dialectic in Critical and Postcolonial Feminist Research: Reconciling Tensions Around Scientific Integrity   162
Sheryl Reimer-Kirkham
Joan M. Anderson

CHAPTER 21
Validity and Validation in the Making in the Context of Qualitative Research   171
Mirka Koro-Ljungberg

CHAPTER 22
The Cocreating Environment: A Nexus Between Classical Chinese and Current Nursing Philosophies   178
Joan E. Dodgson

CHAPTER 23
Scientific Inquiry in Nursing: A Model for a New Age   185
Holly A. DeGroot

UNIT 5 Epistemology and Evidence in Practice

CHAPTER 24
Fundamental Patterns of Knowing in Nursing   200
Barbara A. Carper

CHAPTER 25
Patterns of Knowing: Review, Critique, and Update   207
Jill White

CHAPTER 26

Mediating the Meaning of Evidence Through Epistemological Diversity 217
Denise Tarlier

CHAPTER 27

Nursing Epistemology: Traditions, Insights, Questions 227
Phyllis R. Schultz
Afaf I. Meleis

CHAPTER 28

Fundamental Patterns of Knowing in Nursing: The Challenge of Evidence-Based Practice 235
Sam Porter

CHAPTER 29

Knowledge Development and Evidence-Based Practice: Insights and Opportunities from a Postcolonial Feminist Perspective for Transformative Nursing Practice 244
Sheryl Reimer-Kirkham
Jennifer L. Baumbusch
Annette S. H. Schultz
Joan M. Anderson

CHAPTER 30

The Use of Postcolonialism in the Nursing Domain: Colonial Patronage, Conversion, and Resistance 257
Dave Holmes
Bernard Roy
Amélie Perron

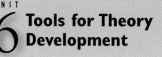

UNIT 6

Tools for Theory Development

CHAPTER 31

Concept Analysis: Examining the State of the Science 266
Judith E. Hupcey
Janice Penrod

CHAPTER 32

Rethinking Concept Analysis 274
Mark Risjord

CHAPTER 33

Levels of Theoretical Thinking in Nursing 282
Patricia A. Higgins
Shirley M. Moore

CHAPTER 34

Development of Situation-Specific Theories: An Integrative Approach 289
Eun-Ok Im

CHAPTER 35

Middle Range Theory: Spinning Research and Practice to Create Knowledge for the New Millennium 301
Patricia Liehr
Mary Jane Smith

UNIT 7

Characteristics and Criteria of Nursing Theories

CHAPTER 36

Theories: Components, Development, Evaluation 312
Margaret E. Hardy

CHAPTER 37

From Practice to Midrange Theory and Back Again: Beck's Theory of Postpartum Depression 321
Gerri C. Lasiuk
Linda M. Ferguson

CHAPTER 38

Theoretical Substruction Illustrated by the Theory of Learned Resourcefulness 329
Abir K. Bekhet
Jaclene A. Zauszniewski

CHAPTER 39
A Theory of Theories: A Position Paper 336
James Dickoff
Patricia James

CHAPTER 40
Perspectives on Nursing Theory 343
Margaret E. Hardy

CHAPTER 41
Criteria for Evaluation of Theory 352
Jacqueline Fawcett

CHAPTER 42
Parse's Criteria for Evaluation of
Theory With a Comparison of
Fawcett's and Parse's Approaches 358
Rosemarie Rizzo Parse

UNIT
8 Philosophies of Nursing
Practice

CHAPTER 43
The Focus of the Discipline Revisited 362
Margaret A. Newman
Marlaine C. Smith
Margaret Dexheimer Pharris
Dorothy A. Jones

CHAPTER 44
An Ontological View of Advanced
Practice Nursing 372
Cynthia Arslanian-Engoren
Frank D. Hicks
Ann L. Whall
Donna L. Algase

CHAPTER 45
Nursing: The Ontology of the Discipline 378
Pamela G. Reed

CHAPTER 46
The Power of Wholeness,
Consciousness, and Caring: A Dialogue
on Nursing Science, Art, and Healing 383
W. Richard Cowling, III
Marlaine C. Smith
Jean Watson

CHAPTER 47
A Multiparadigm Approach
to Nursing 392
Joan C. Engebretson

UNIT
9 Future Directions for
Nursing Theory

CHAPTER 48
A Central Unifying Focus for
the Discipline: Facilitating Humanization,
Meaning, Choice, Quality of Life,
and Healing in Living and Dying 402
Danny G. Willis
Pamela J. Grace
Callista L. Roy

CHAPTER 49
Nursing Reformation: Historical
Reflections and Philosophic
Foundations 413
Pamela G. Reed

CHAPTER 50
Historical Voices of Resistance:
Crossing Boundaries to Praxis
Through Documentary Filmmaking
for the Public 419
Paula N. Kagan

CHAPTER 51
Unity of Knowledge in the Advancement
of Nursing Knowledge 430
Karen K. Giuliano
Lynda Tyer-Viola
Ruth Palan Lopez

CHAPTER 52
A Practice Discipline That's Here
and Now 437
Merian C. Litchfield
Helga Jónsdóttir

Author Index 449
Subject Index 452

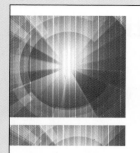

Structures of Nursing Knowledge Development

This section is designed as a mini-symposium on metatheory to introduce readers to basic definitions, components, issues, and terminology in theory, philosophy, and knowledge development. The chapters weave the reader through various metatheoretical dimensions and structures of nursing knowledge to inform as well as provoke discussions about the meaning and relevance of theory for nurses.

Topics in this unit include the following: 1) approaches to linking the conceptual and empirical, linking theory and practice; 2) a new typology of knowledge and the possibility of laws of nursing; 3) an expanded framework of nursing theories based upon some of the most prevalent patterns of knowing, beyond the usual empirical pattern; 4) the ways that nursing theories and nursing ethics can inform and transform each other; and 5) a philosophy of nursing science for the 21st century that integrates the best from modernism and postmodernism.

These core issues about theory endure while their applications may change as the context of nursing evolves over time. These chapters (and actually all graduate level coursework) address topics that are best understood when chapters are not only read,

but *reread* and followed by classroom or online discussions. Through discussions and rereading, students can translate theory into insights that enhance their daily practices in research and caregiving.

QUESTIONS FOR DISCUSSION

- Reflecting on your own work, identify a practical or easily observable event that interests you. What have you read or what ideas do you have that might explain how or why this event occurs, or how it may be linked to other events? In doing this, you begin to think theoretically, by making connections between the empirical (observable) and the conceptual (hunches and ideas).

- Are there any established or broadly accepted ideas in practice or research that you think could be called "laws of nursing"?

- What are differences among the following components of nursing knowledge: philosophy, science, and theory?

- How might ethics influence theory? How can nursing theories influence what we define as ethical?

Nursing Theory and Practice: Connecting the Dots

JO-ANN MARRS, EdD, MSN, MS, BS
LOIS W. LOWRY, RN, DNSc

The authors propose connecting the dots among theory, practice, and research by adopting an expanded conceptual-theoretical-empirical structure of nursing knowledge and matrix process to guide the placement of nursing knowledge in a contextual whole. An overview of the theoretical journey of nursing knowledge development is contrasted with the journey from practice resulting in a theory-practice disconnect. Both approaches are united to present an integrated view of the dimensions of the knowledge development of nursing as a professional discipline.

Much as a young child struggles to connect the dots on a picture in an activity book, nursing has been trying to connect the dots between nursing theory, research, and practice. It is the hypothesis of the authors that *the picture* is about to be completed, but that the pattern of the dots has been somewhat divergent and scattered among nurse theorists, researchers, and practitioners as they have each taken different approaches in completing the holistic picture of nursing knowledge. Some have traveled inductively and others, deductively. Both are about to meet in the middle in order to *connect the dots* for a holistic view of nursing. The journey to completion will focus on a matrix that can provide a logical process for practitioners and theoreticians to access the state of the nursing knowledge development.

We propose an approach that combines an expanded conceptual-theoretical-empirical (CTE) structure of knowledge development and a process for adding to, revising, and moving about within the field of nursing knowledge. Fawcett's (2000) five-level hierarchical structure of nursing knowledge, now referred to as a holarchy (Fawcett, 2005) provides the *what* of nursing knowledge to be included within the field. We propose that practice theory be explicitly added to the present structure. The essence of practice theory is a focus on a limited number of variables, a desired goal, and specific actions necessary to achieve the goal. At present, practice theories are included in the level of mid-range theory at a low middle-range level. This is confusing and does not add clarity to the CTE structure. In our proposal, theories that meet the criteria of practice theory will be explicitly designated in the CTE structure.

The *how* of adding to, refining, or revising the CTE structure is an adaptation of a matrix process used to promote learning and change within organizations (Shibley, 2001). The five-step matrix proposed here guides the process for considering contributions to the hierarchy of nursing knowledge. Setting forth a vision is the first step. Our vision is to establish a clearinghouse in which all contributions to nursing knowledge will be registered and analyzed. The second step is the development of a cognitive infrastructure or mental model to guide placement of nursing knowledge within the clearinghouse in a way that connections between theories and action can be demonstrated. The third step in the process, the systemic structure, is the plan for operationalization. The fourth and fifth steps are key to success of the matrix process, that is, the identification of events and an analysis of patterns among the contributions to new nursing knowledge so that theoretical linkages are identified.

Prior to a detailed discussion of the expanded CTE structure and the matrix process, a brief historical overview of the development of nursing knowledge through deductive and inductive means is provided as the backdrop for understanding the respective contributions to nursing knowledge of each type of thinking. We will begin our discussion through the theoretical lens.

Theoretical Overview

Our theoretical journey has taken the discipline of nursing through various stages and milestones. In the beginning, Florence Nightingale focused on patient care and hygiene to enhance healing, which gave

ABOUT THE AUTHORS

JO-ANN MARRS was born in Linz, Austria. She graduated from St. Mary's School of Nursing in Knoxville, TN, with a diploma in nursing. She received a BS, an MS in education, an MSN in nursing, and her EdD from the University of Tennessee. She received a post master's certificate in Family Nurse Practitioner from Pittsburg State University in Pittsburg, KS. Dr. Marrs also holds a Legal Nurse Consultant Certificate. She led a national effort to implement background checks for nursing programs and has written articles and spoken on the subject. She is interested in educational research and in obesity in children. As an administrator, she has developed numerous degree programs and has taught nursing since 1972. She is a Professor and Clinical Coordinator for the Regents Online Degree Program at East Tennessee State University. She likes to do arts and crafts and garden.

LOIS W. LOWRY is Professor Emerita at East Tennessee State University. She received her BSN degree from Cornell University-New York Hospital School of Nursing in 1955, achieved her MN from the University of Florida in 1977 with a double major in maternal–infant health and psychiatric/mental health, and earned her DNS in educational administration from the University of Pennsylvania in 1987. Her research areas included studies in patient satisfaction with prenatal care, spirituality and aging, and the development of critical thinking in baccalaureate nursing students. Dr. Lowry's interest in nursing theory began with her first course in her doctoral program, taught by Dr. Jacqueline Fawcett, who sparked her desire to contribute to theoretical knowledge development. She is a charter member of Neuman Systems Model (NSM) Trustees, Inc., and continues to write, consult, and lecture about the NSM in practice, education, and research. Dr. Lowry is married to Dr. Robert L. Lowry, a Presbyterian minister, and has 5 children and 12 grandchildren. Her hobbies are hiking, camping, swimming, and singing.

nursing its mission and focus. Throughout the first half of the 20th century nursing practice was based on principles and traditions through an apprenticeship form of education. By midcentury the emphasis was that of nursing as a service requiring a strong scientific base that was acquired within university settings. As our nurse leaders shared their ideas about the essences and empirics of nursing, they spoke out about the need for theory to guide the practice of nursing. They reminded us that theory is the goal of scientific work and is essential to the development of any profession (Chinn & Kramer, 1999; Meleis, 1997). Thus, through the second half of the 20th century, nursing made rapid progress toward the development of theoretical knowledge; first, through the application of theories borrowed from other disciplines, followed by the creation of grand theories and conceptual models. Much of the early theory development was based on the ideal of nursing, or what ought-to-be nursing practice (Barnum, 1990). However, the conceptual models for education and practice contributed to defining a unique nursing perspective that was useful in practice settings. Each model's description of the nursing process encouraged reflective problem-solving and showed nurses the connection between nursing models and practice (Chinn & Kramer, 1999). In addition, the identification of the dominant phenomena within the field of nursing

knowledge, the metaparadigm, asserted the distinct domain of the discipline of nursing (Fawcett, 1996).

At one time, nursing was greatly influenced by the writings of Dickoff and James (1968) who advocated a model of *practice-oriented theory* including four levels of theorizing: factor-isolating, factor-relating, situation-relating, and situation-producing. Since nursing is a practice discipline, it is logical that situation-producing theory be given the greatest consideration because it will guide actions that have an impact on reality (Walker & Avant, 2005). Other pioneers of nursing theory supported the necessity of building theoretical knowledge from the study of nursing actions for the goal of providing better nursing care (Ellis, 1968; Jacox, 1974; McCarthy, 1972).

Given the importance of practice theory, it is interesting that there was little growth of this level of theory. A reason posited for the lack of growth was its practical nature, thus, it was not very exciting (Walker & Avant, 2005). It may be thought of as *common sense* or too time and place bound to be considered theory. Practitioners may not be aware that the assessing, planning, prioritizing, and decision-making that engages them while caring for their clients reflects processes necessary in theoretical thinking. Practice theory is based on the assumption that the practitioner has the cognitive skills necessary to be able to discriminate among several patients with the same symptoms, and would take the action that is most effective in each case. With a thorough education in nursing theory, and the opportunity to engage in theory-based practice over time, practitioners can be expected to contribute to nursing theory development. Nurses learn to practice nursing very well by studying nursing theories intensely. Problem-solving at the midrange and practice levels must be aligned with the whole gestalt of philosophy, theory, and method in order to advance the body of knowledge which is nursing (Cody, 2003). Practitioners' attention to and appreciation of theory is more likely to be caught when theoretical knowledge focuses on specific nursing phenomena from practice.

However, the abstract nature of theory has created a schism between nurse theorists, nurse scientists, and practitioners. Nurse theorists emphasize the *knowing* that is based on philosophies and theories of nursing. On the other hand, practicing nurses focus on the *doing* and often deny that theories are useful to them in their everyday work. Yet all professional nurses are urged to build bridges between knowing and doing.

The complexity of nursing practice requires the efforts of practitioners who encounter phenomena and theorists/researchers who discover new relationships among concepts. It is the position of the writers that the advancement of nursing knowledge only occurs when discipline-specific research is conducted. If practice theory is to gain acceptance, it must demonstrate the hierarchical connection between midrange and grand theories; which in turn, stem from the philosophy of nursing science, paradigms, and worldviews of nursing. Often, the knowledge and skill sought at the practice level follows the requirements for licensure and expectations of corporate employers or are just practical solutions to nursing problems (Cody, 2003).

Utilizing a multitude of methods for knowledge development, including inductive approaches, could enhance the progress of nursing knowledge development as long as connections to theoretical knowledge are made explicit. Other disciplines, such as sociology and psychology, have developed theory from observing reality. What has been the pathway of practitioners in nursing who have attempted to connect the dots inductively?

Practice Overview

From the practitioner's point of view, the development of nursing knowledge has somewhat mirrored that of the development of medicine. This is particularly noticeable when one examines the inductive development of practice theory with the development of medicine. In ancient Greece the Hippocratic School of ancient Greece classified disease using the concept of *humors* rather than supernatural or magical forces. By 1893, the International Classification of Diseases and Causes of Death was being used by medicine to categorize illness. Other nomenclature systems used in medicine include the Standard Diagnostic and Statistical Manual of Mental Disorders; International Classification of Injuries, Disabilities, and Handicaps; Standard Nomenclature of Disease and Operations; Systematized Nomenclature of Pathology; and Systematized Nomenclature of Medicine (Gordon, 1998).

Historically, nursing also used these medical classifications to organize its knowledge, since these were the only concepts available to use until the mid-20th century. As nursing research increased, there was an interest in classification systems for coding studies. The best known system is that of the North American Nursing Diagnosis Association (NANDA; Gordon, 1998). NANDA is recognized as one of the pioneer organizations in the development of a classification system for nursing practice. Several nurse theorists, including Roy, King, Newman, and others, joined their efforts and presented an organizing framework for nursing diagnoses called Patterns of Unitary Man (Humans) to the NANDA and Taxonomy Committee in 1977. While there was much controversy over this as a framework, and some theorists (Roy, Parse, and others) disagreed with the paniculate nature of the diagnostic system, in 1984, this framework was renamed Human Response Patterns and was accepted in 1986. This consists of the patterns of choosing, communicating, exchanging, feeling, knowing, moving, perceiving, relating, and valuing. The nursing diagnoses were intended to provide a conceptual model for interpreting a set of observations which would be firmly grounded in studies of the phenomenon. An inductive approach was used initially by NANDA to identify these concepts within the medical model frame of reference. Up to this point, research was minimal and literature about the concepts negligible. With an inductive methodology that NANDA leaders used, diagnostic concepts were formed from a set of empirical indicators (signs/symptoms), arising from practice observations. Further studies led to the identification of contributing factors that came to be the focus of nursing interventions. NANDA's (2001) latest work, *Nursing Diagnoses: Definitions and Classifications (2001-2002)*, features a new multiaxial framework that organizes the diagnoses into domains according to Gordon's functional health patterns (NANDA, 2001). These formulations, however, were not connected to existing theories and models. Likewise, as nursing followed medicine in developing nursing diagnoses, nurses used medical treatments and the patient's ability to carry out physicians' orders as a high priority in the traditional typology of nursing interventions. Eventually, following the format of nursing diagnoses, and nursing clinical judgment development, nurses began to name nurse-initiated interventions in textbooks.

Since 1987, research to develop a vocabulary and nursing intervention classification system (NIC) has been conducted at the University of Iowa by Bulechek and McCloskey (1992). The nursing intervention classification (NIC) research team identified a set of nursing intervention concepts through content analysis of the literature and linked them to NANDA diagnoses and to nursing outcomes classification (NOC). The research team identified three types of interventions. They are defined as "any direct care treatment that a nurse performs on behalf of a client. These treatments include nurse-initiated treatments resulting from nursing diagnoses, physician-initiated treatments resulting from medical diagnoses, and performance of the daily essential functions for the client [who] cannot do these" (Bulechek & McCloskey, 1992, p. 21).

Since 1998, there have been biennial NANDA-NIC-NOC conferences to help to link these three systems. Outcomes are linked to the problem (nursing diagnosis) in a diagnostic statement. Interventions are linked to the related or contributing factors. Diagnosis-intervention linkages (McCloskey & Bulechek, 1996) assume that a nursing diagnosis is being used as a contributing factor for another nursing diagnosis and that the classification is similar to a dictionary of terms. These three taxonomies are becoming the standard for nursing practice because they provide the content focus for nursing process and serve to identify and communicate the unique function of nursing. Thus the taxonomies provide a standardized vocabulary to clarify nursing's role to other healthcare professionals and patients. A caution is in order, however, for taxonomies represent the realities of nurses who developed them, but not necessarily the majority of nurses who care for patients (Meleis, 1997). More important, the nursing process and classification systems are not based on theoretical underpinnings and do not allow nurses to connect the dots in the CTE structural hierarchy without further research.

The current emphasis on evidence or outcomes-based practice in nursing is another example of the tendency to follow the lead of medicine. Evidence-based medical practice originated as the gold standard for integrating individual clinical expertise with the best available clinical evidence from clinical research studies, particularly clinical trials. It has been suggested that the roots of evidence-based practice can be traced as far back as the 3rd century B.C. Whatever the origin, it appears that nursing has once again adopted a process utilized by medicine to guide nursing practice, rather than building upon our unique nursing knowledge. The trend toward evidence-based practice and its focus on outcomes as the end results of care, linked to diagnoses and interventions, does not support a theoretical link. Rather this approach is fostered by institutions and typically reinforces and supports the medical model, without concern for connections to the structural hierarchy of nursing knowledge.

Conceptual-Theoretical-Empirical Structures

Whereas the historical developments have claimed to further the advancement of nursing knowledge, there continues to be a *disconnect* among the works of theorists, researchers, and practitioners. Is there a way to unite the approaches in thinking so that theorists, researchers, and practitioners can embrace an integrated view of the dimensions of our professional discipline and the activities associated with those dimensions? These authors believe that this is possible through enhancing the development of our existing CTE systems of knowledge. Fawcett (2000) posited a five-level hierarchical structure of nursing knowledge based upon levels of abstraction. This heuristic device places the metaparadigm of nursing at the highest level of abstraction, the philosophies of nursing science just below the metaparadigm, and the conceptual models of nursing at the third level. Below the conceptual models are theories and the lowest level of abstraction is represented by empirical indicators. Each of these levels is well-defined and described in the literature (Fawcett), so will not be further explicated here.

These authors propose that the CTE hierarchy be expanded to explicitly place additional elements into the structure that have guided scholars in their thinking and practitioners in their practice as the discipline has expanded its roles. Table 1-1 displays the proposed hierarchy. Table 1-2 provides the definitions for each component in the hierarchy. Note that grand theories are placed just below conceptual models, indicating that they are derived from conceptual models, such as Newman's (1994) theory of health as expanding consciousness and Parse's (1998) human becoming theory, both of which were sparked by Rogers' (1970) science of unitary human beings. Middle-range theories are located somewhat below grand theories on the hierarchy because they are made up of fewer concepts and propositions. These theories are written at a more concrete level of abstraction so that they can assist in interpreting behaviors, situations, and events. They can be applied to practice situations and can be tested through research methodologies. Some midrange theories are derived from nursing conceptual models, such as Orem's (2001) theories of self-care, self-care deficit, and nursing systems, and Neuman's (2002) theory of prevention as intervention. Other midrange theories identify other disciplines as their source, such as social support (Norbeck, 1981); or nursing

TABLE 1-1	**Expanded Hierarchy of Nursing Knowledge**
Components	**Level of Abstraction**
Metaparadigm	Most abstract
Philosophies	
Conceptual models	
Grand theories	
Middle-range theories	
Practice theories	
(situation-producing, situation-relating, factor-relating, factor-isolating)	
Empirical indicators	Most concrete
(standards for practice, assessment formats, classification taxonomies, intervention protocols, evaluation criteria)	

observations and taxonomies as sources of their generation, like the Omaha Classification System for community health nursing (Martin & Scheet, 1992). The literature has indicated that the level of abstraction attributed to mid-range theories is quite broad. Thus, Liehr and Smith (1999) have categorized midrange to include high-middle, middle and low middle, depending on scope and level of abstraction. Their categorization tends to add confusion rather than clarity to the CTE hierarchy. Rather, we suggest explicit placement of

TABLE 1-2	**Definitions of Conceptual-Theoretical-Empirical Components**	
Component	**Definition**	**Example**
Metaparadigm	Global concepts that identify the phenomena of the discipline	Person, environment, health, nursing
Philosophies	Ontological and epistemological claims about values and beliefs of the discipline	Totality and simultaneity paradigms
Conceptual models	Set of abstract concepts and their propositional statements that address the metaparadigm concepts	Neuman systems model, Orem's self-care framework, Rogers' science of unitary human beings
Grand theories	Set of fewer abstract concepts and propositional statements that are broad in scope and derived from conceptual models	Newman's theory of health as expanding consciousness, Parse's theory of human becoming, Watson's theory of human caring
Middle-range theories	Limited number of concepts and propositions written at a more specific level	Mishel's uncertainty in illness, Norbeck's model for social support, Swanson's theory of caring
Practice theories (practice-oriented focus, predictive focus)	One or two variables and their propositional connection stated in prescriptive terms or predictive terms and related to a specific situation	Huth and Moore's theory of acute pain management
Empirical indicators	Real world proxy for midrange or practice theory concept	Instruments, protocols

practice theory below the midrange level to include those theories that focus on a narrow view of reality and may be considered as low middle-range; for example, the theory of balance between analgesia and side effects (Good & Moore, 1996) and the theory of acute pain management in infants and children (Huth & Moore, 1998).

Practice theories may be as simple as a single concept that is operationalized, and may be linked to a special population or situation. Practice theories can evolve deductively from a midrange or grand theory (Newman, 1994), or may be inductively formulated from a specific situation, as demonstrated by Im and Meleis (1999) who brought theoretical understanding to a delimited clinical situation. It is important, however, that practice theories be aligned with the whole gestalt of philosophy of nursing science, theory, and method in order to advance the body of knowledge of nursing (Cody, 2003). Within our expanded CTE structure, the four levels of theory proposed by Dickoff and James (1968) are situated below practice theory. Finally, at the lowest and most concrete level of the hierarchy are the empirical indicators. Empirical indicators are directly connected to midrange and/ or practice theories by means of operational definitions for each theory concept that is being generated or tested. Empirical indicators are the tools, instruments, and procedures that the researcher uses to test midrange or practice theories. Likewise, empirical indicators can be the protocols or clinical procedures that a practitioner will use to direct nursing actions in a precise manner (Fawcett, 2000). In our hierarchy, standards for practice, assessment formats, classification taxonomies, intervention protocols, and evaluation criteria are given as examples of empirical indicators from the practice arena. Each of these must be connected to the more abstract elements of the hierarchical structure (philosophies, conceptual models, or grand theories) to be considered as contributions to the development of nursing knowledge. A caution is in order here. Many protocols, taxonomies, critical pathways, and other such systems are created and required by corporate employers with no intent to develop nursing knowledge. This has contributed to confusion for practicing nurses, and the opinion that theory is unnecessary for practice.

Strategies for Implementation

A matrix provides a logical map to guide the process for connecting the dots. The matrix includes five 5 parts: vision, a mental model, systemic structures, patterns, and events. The matrix process (Figure 1-1) illustrates the interaction among the parts. *Vision*

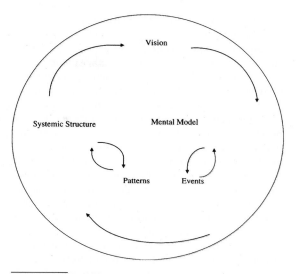

Figure 1-1 *Process Matrix.*

suggests the creation of a clearinghouse that contains the field of nursing knowledge. This clearinghouse will be centrally located so that there will be global access at all times. Contributors to nursing knowledge can go to the clearinghouse to explore the state of the science in nursing at any hour of the day or night, for the purpose of finding gaps and areas for further study. For example, an online site could be created or incorporated into an existing site, such as the Sigma Theta Tau International online library, and will contain references to theories and research studies that currently represent the field of knowledge in nursing.

The *mental model* that stems from the vision can be illustrated as a sea of dots within a frame. Each dot represents a separate piece of nursing research or theoretical knowledge. The expanded CTE hierarchy (Table 1-1) adds the basic structure to guide placement of a new dot. Further delineation within the structure will be necessary to complete the picture of the connected dots. For example, major categories will be identified, such as focus areas in practice, education, and administration. Each major category will be further subdivided by more defining attributes; for example, the practice focus may include adult issues, women's health issues, children's health, and others. Each of these will be further divided by settings, age and type of subject (individual, group, or community), wellness or illness issues, and so forth. The subdivisions can be more and more specific as new pieces of research are completed or theoretical statements tested. Each contribution will be placed in the appropriate location within the frame. To illustrate, suppose researchers wish to explore the concept of *uncertainty in illness* and find that this concept is located within the major category of midrange theory. Many studies are found that demonstrate *uncertainty* with Caucasian female subjects, but none with African American. Thus, the researchers would recognize the gap and plan their study to enhance the knowledge of that theory under the subconcept of ethnicity. The mental model of the clearinghouse is useful in illustrating where there is a gap and new knowledge is needed. On the other hand, if a knowledge contribution is presented and there is no visible connection to any existing knowledge, the dot representing that piece would be placed near the periphery of the frame as an outlier. Outliers would not be discarded for they may represent a new breakthrough in knowledge, or an idea whose time has not yet come. Inclusion within the frame is a reference point for further exploration of ways to connect to existing theoretical knowledge.

The mental model, which is the cognitive infrastructure for the clearinghouse, points to the *systemic structure*. This part of the process provides the specifics of operation and implementation of the clearinghouse. Some person or persons (called archivists) will be responsible for the ongoing operation. As new submissions of knowledge from researchers, theorists, and practitioners are received, the archivist will analyze them for best fit within the field of knowledge. Questions like, "Is this piece of work supportive of other work in the field, or an expansion of an idea in the field?" or "Does this work not connect to any theoretical underpinnings?" will guide the analysis. The archivist will respond to the contributors, informing them of the links to theoretical knowledge in the field, or the lack thereof. The archivist will work in collaboration with an advisory board composed of experts in the field of research and theory who will assess the theoretical adequacy of the contribution and make recommendations about placement.

Two critical pieces of this matrix process are *patterns* and *events*. They are located within the figure between the mental model and systemic structure, and the arrows in both directions represent processes of reflection and action taken by the advisory board and archivists. Events are situations or discrete happenings that occur independently of one another, such as a specific research study. The experts will evaluate each event and compare to other events in the frame to discern patterns that will guide placement within the frame. The observation and assessment of patterns is a critical step within the process. Experts will consider, "Does this contribution of knowledge enhance the field of nursing knowledge?" "Is this an outlier or a disconnect?" Including these two steps in the process enables one to learn to tolerate complexity and contradictions. If the contribution is theoretically sound, then we can expand the vision and add more information to the mental model and specificity to the CTE structure.

For example, Newman (1994) proposed a research as praxis methodology that stems from her theory of health as expanding consciousness. This dot of knowledge would be connected to the grand theory. On the other hand, the NANDA classification system originated from observing a need in practice (mental process) to doing something about it (systemic system) without reflection (events and patterns). Thus, the end result was the creation of an unwanted condition and a theoretical disconnect.

Conclusion

We propose the expanded CTE structure and matrix process as a means of connecting the dots for nurse theorists, researchers, and practitioners. The time is right to close the theory-practice gap. Many have expressed concern about the continued existence and advancement of the discipline of nursing, unless the theorists, researchers, and practitioners integrate their thinking (Cody, 2003; Fawcett, 2000). Nursing discipline-specific CTE systems provide an alternative to the institutional model of practice, in which standardized plans and rules and regulations are primary. Nurses who use nursing models and theories provide an alternative base for nursing practice from a theoretical perspective. Then nurses will talk nursing, think nursing, and do nursing.

The contributions of nurse theorists and researchers who advanced nursing knowledge through theoretical thinking are well-documented and accepted by the nursing community; whereas, the inductive contributions of practitioners are often not accepted as examples of theoretical thinking. Nurse scholars are encouraged to openly consider all contributions of nurses, challenging those that are not theoretically sound to clarify linkages to existing nursing theoretical knowledge. The creation of a clearinghouse to register and evaluate contributions for theoretical adequacy would serve to connect the dots in a way that respects both the contributions of theoretical scholars and practitioners, so that bridges will be built and nursing knowledge advanced. We invite the readers to respond to our proposal.

REFERENCES

Barnum, B. J. S. (1990). *Nursing theory: Analysis, application, evaluation* (3rd ed.). Glenview, IL: Scott Foresman/Little, Brown.

Bulechek, G., & McCloskey, J. (1992). *Nursing interventions: Essential nursing treatments*. Philadelphia: Saunders.

Chinn, P. L., & Kramer, M. K. (1999). *Theory and nursing* (5th ed). St. Louis, MO: Mosby.

Cody, W. K. (2003). Nursing theory as a guide to practice. *Nursing Science Quarterly, 16*, 225–231.

Dickoff, J., & James, P. (1968). A theory of theories: A position paper. *Nursing Research, 17*, 197–203.

Ellis, R. (1968). Characteristics of significant theories. *Nursing Research, 17*, 217–222.

Fawcett, J. (1996). On the requirements for a metaparadigm: An invitation to dialogue. *Nursing Science Quarterly, 9*, 94–97.

Fawcett, J. (2000). *Analysis and evaluation of contemporary nursing knowledge.* Philadelphia: F. A. Davis.

Fawcett, J. (2005). *Contemporary nursing knowledge* (2nd ed.). Philadelphia: F. A. Davis.

Good, M., & Moore, S. M. (1996). Clinical practice guidelines as a new source of middle-range theory: Focus on acute pain. *Nursing Outlook, 44*, 74–79.

Gordon, M. (1998, September 30). Nursing nomenclature and classification system development. *Online Journal of Issues in Nursing, 3* (2). Retrieved October 15, 2005, from http://www.nursingworld.org/ojin/tpc7/tpc7_l.htm

Huth, M. M., & Moore, S. M. (1998). Prescriptive theory of acute pain management in infants and children. *Journal of Society of Pediatric Nurses, 3*, 23–32.

Im, E., & Meleis, A. I. (1999). Situation-specific theories: Philosophical roots, properties, and approach. *Advances in Nursing Science*, 22(2), 11–24.

Jacox, A. K. (1974). Theory construction in nursing: An overview. *Nursing Research, 23*(1), 4–13.

Liehr, P., & Smith, M. J. (1999). Middle range theory: Spinning research and practice to create knowledge for the new millennium. *Advances in Nursing Science, 21*(4), 81–91.

Martin, L. S., & Scheet, N. J. (1992). *The Omaha system: Applications for community health nursing.* Philadelphia: Saunders.

McCarthy, R. T. (1972). A practice theory of nursing care. *Nursing Research, 21*, 406–410.

McCloskey, J. C., & Bulechek, G. M. (1996). *Nursing intervention classification (NIC)* (2nd ed.). St. Louis, MO: Mosby.

Meleis, A. I. (1997). *Theoretical nursing: Development and progress* (3rd ed.). Philadelphia: Lippincott.

North American Nursing Diagnosis Association. (2001). *Nursing diagnosis: Definitions and classification, 2001–2002.* Philadelphia: Author.

Neuman, B., & Fawcett, J. (2002). *The Neuman systems model* (4th ed.). Upper Saddle River, NJ: Prentice Hall.

Newman, M. A. (1994). *Health as expanding consciousness* (2nd ed.). New York: National League for Nursing.

Norbeck. J. S. (1981). Social support: A model for clinical research and application. *Advances in Nursing Science, 3* (4), 43–59.

Orem, D. E. (2001). *Nursing: Concepts of practice* (6th ed.). St. Louis, MO: Mosby.

Parse, R. R. (1998). *The human becoming school of thought: A perspective for nurses and other health professionals.* Thousand Oaks, CA: Sage.

Rogers, M. E. (1970). An *introduction to the theoretical basis of nursing.* Philadelphia: F. A. Davis.

Shibley, J. J. (2001). *A primer on systems thinking and organizational learning.* Portland, OR: Portland Learning Organization Group.

Walker, L. O., & Avant, K. C. (2005). *Strategies for theory construction in nursing* (4th ed.). Upper Saddle River, NJ: Pearson Prentice Hall.

THE AUTHORS COMMENT | Nursing Theory and Practice: Connecting the Dots

This work arose from our concern about the disconnect between theory and practice. Theoreticians develop their thinking deductively, whereas practitioners use an inductive approach. We hope to integrate both approaches into a meaningful whole that will advance the development of nursing knowledge. Our idea combines the structure of nursing knowledge with a process for adding to, revising, and identifying new contributions to knowledge in a uniform way. We invite readers to respond to our proposal.

JO-ANN MARRS
LOIS W. LOWRY

Yes, Virginia, Nursing Does Have Laws

PAMELA B. WEBBER, PhD, APRN, BC, FNP

In this article the author explores the possibility of the emergence of nursing laws as a natural consequence of the maturation and evolution of selected areas of nursing knowledge. To support this proposition, the evolution of social and scientific laws and their meanings are discussed. In addition, the roles that empirical validation and logical adequacy play in epistemological development, including the development of discipline-specific laws, are explored. Two areas of nursing knowledge in which laws may be emerging, as well as the foundation of these laws, are identified. **Key words:** *nursing laws, nursing science, nursing theory*

In 1897, when New York Sun columnist Francis Pharcellus Church (1897/2007) penned the now famous editorial titled "Yes, Virginia, There Is a Santa Claus," he succeeded not only in touching hearts, but also in helping people begin to view tradition differently, and to recognize a different truth that moves beyond the obvious. Looking beyond tradition and the obvious is also characteristic of nursing's century-long journey into scholarship and knowledge development. In seeking to understand and move the profession forward, academics have debated phenomena such as technical and professional education preparation; theory-based practice and practice-based theory; philosophies, models, and theories; and empiricism and phenomenology.

Another phenomenon has evolved that will no doubt stimulate similar discourse. This phenomenon is the possibility of the emergence of nursing laws. These are not the laws of jurisprudence governing nursing practice that are traditionally associated with individual state practice acts, but are instead, laws associated with the natural maturation and evolution of selected areas of essential nursing knowledge. Although the idea of nursing laws may sound farfetched or neomodernistic, it is the next logical step in the evolution of nursing knowledge. Unfortunately, recognizing, naming, and framing nursing laws may be as foreign to us now as discipline-specific theory was to practicing nurses in the mid-1900s.

Evolution of Meanings of Law

To understand the emergence of nursing laws, one must first understand the diverse meanings of the word law. Hermeneutically, we know and understand that meanings of words evolve over time according to the nature, needs, and sophistication of society and subsets within society (Johnson & Webber, 2005). The term *law* evolved from the old Norse term *lag* and the old English term *lagu*, both of which mean *to be laid down or firmly affixed* (Jewel & Abate, 2001). The term quickly became associated with social and cultural rules of behavior as seen in the early Greek and Roman civilizations. During Biblical times the term law was used to describe the first five books of the Old Testament. These five books, which were also called the Pentateuch or Torah, established very specific rules governing religious behavior of the early Jews. By the time of the Renaissance, which occurred between the 12th and 16th centuries, the definition and use of laws had expanded to include social, political, and scientific contexts. Social and political laws focused on expanded rules for human behavior, whereas scientific laws emerged that established rules associated with the occurrence of phenomena in nature.

By the end of the 16th century, the desire for discovery had prompted the initiation of a scientific revolution. Whereas scientists prior to this revolution used logic and philosophical or Aristotelian analysis to explore natural phenomena, scientists and other authors during the scientific revolution moved toward measurement and numerical analysis (Kuhn, 1970). This approach resulted in the nature, or the perception of the nature, of science becoming mechanical and empirical (Veltman, n.d.). A byproduct of this empirical focus is that scientists of the time began using mathematical and empirical evidence as criteria for forming scientific laws, an approach that persists today. Scientific discovery focused on quantification through experimentation as the primary method for examining phenomena and forming associated facts, principles, and laws.

ABOUT THE AUTHOR

PAMELA BAYLISS WEBBER earned an ASN at Shenandoah University, a BSN, an MSN, and a PhD at George Mason University and completed the postgraduate FNP program at the University of Virginia. Pam is a Professor in the Division of Nursing at Shenandoah University. She is an accomplished educator and, in May 2000, was honored by the Virginia Nurses Association and the Virginia Nurses Foundation as one of 50 Pioneer Nurses in the state of Virginia for the century. In 2001, Pam was featured as an outstanding nursing faculty in *Nursing and Health Care Perspectives*. In addition, she has published numerous articles in the areas of nursing education, theory, research, and reasoning, including the 2010, 3rd edition of *Introduction to Theory and Reasoning in Nursing*, which she co-authored with Dr. Betty Johnson. Pam has been an invited speaker for numerous regional, national, and international nursing organizations for over 30 years. She has been married to a great guy (Jeff) for 31 years, has three wonderful adult children (Michael, Sarah, and Cindy), an adorable 1-year-old grandson (Jacey), and an old, but lovable, mutt named Molly. Pam and her family live in Winchester, which is in the northern Shenandoah Valley of Virginia.

Experimentation, by its nature, involves quantification and predictability. These concepts also emerged as essential characteristics of scientific laws and play an essential role in advancing specific areas of knowledge to the status of a law. Hempel (1965) defined a general law as "a statement of universal conditional form which is capable of being confirmed or disconfirmed by suitable empirical findings" (p. 231). He also indicated that laws serve the purpose of connecting events to patterns that form a basis for both prediction and explanation (p. 232). Explanation that supports predictability also supports reliability of the information being used, which is essential in science. The association of empiricism, explanation, predictability, and reliability significantly influenced nursing's journey into scholarship since the profession's foundation is, in part, built on science and nursing's early research foundation was quantitatively based.

Empirical Validation

Concurrent with the development of scientific laws was the emergence of a *mania for measurement* or the, at times, frenzied requirement for empirical validation of theory, facts, principles, and laws, which was considered an essential feature of early modern science (Koyrè, 1939/1978; Veltman, n. d.). Today, the idea that a law must have empirical evidence supporting 100% predictability is still widely accepted (Hempel, 1965; Hickman, 2002; Polifroni, 1999). According to Hickman (2002) scientific laws "predict the results of given experiments 100% of the time. Laws compose the basis of most of the natural sciences. As nursing is a human science, the rigor and objectivity of the laboratory are both impossible and inappropriate to duplicate" (p. 5). The requirement for empirical testing with 100% predictability in defining a law furthered the separation between social and scientific laws, since social laws or rules of social behavior involve more than empirical validation (Bird, 2004; Kuhn, 1970).

By the mid-20th century scientists, theorists, and educators began questioning the adequacy of empirical validation and the accuracy of 100% predictability as the primary criterion for forming scientific laws. In 1959, Scriven, at the annual meeting of the American Association for the Advancement of Science, proffered that laws of science, with few exceptions, are inaccurate and, at best, only approximations of the truth, with a limited range of applicability (Swartz, 2006). This notion was supported by the work of Glanz (1997) and others who demonstrated that Einstein's long-standing laws of physics do not allow 100% predictability, especially when considering the constancy of the speed of light and black holes. Furthermore, Katz and Katz (1995), medical researchers, said that although science provides a beautiful picture of the natural world and insight into disease, it can also lead to error. They argued that the understanding of science is imperfect and that scientific laws are assailable. Katz and Katz based their argument on the fact that modern clinical research trials commonly reveal inconsistencies in scientific laws, and that these inconsistencies represent a reality that disagrees with the previously demanded predictability of science. In conjunction with this observation, Katz and Katz questioned whether these inconsistencies reflect imperfections in the ability to interpret the law or the illusory nature of the laws themselves (Katz & Katz, 1995).

Of particular importance to the changing nature of scientific laws are the major premises behind chaos and complexity theories, which assert that the existence of infinitesimal known and unknown variables, with known and unknown levels of interaction and significance in almost all phenomena, makes 100% predictability unlikely, even in the best science (Johnson & Webber, 2005). Do these variables minimize the need to strive for empirical evidence to support laws that provide underpinnings of a particular body of knowledge? Of course not, but it does suggest two things. The first is that laws, even scientific laws, like theory, evolve, and secondly it keeps us mindful that empirical predictability is no longer the sole defining characteristic of a law, which opens the possibility of the emergence of new types of laws, or, at minimum, a redefining of the term law.

Logical Adequacy

If empirical evidence and 100% predictability are no longer the defining characteristics of a law, is it possible that laws may emerge from behavior-based disciplines, such as nursing, is supported only in part by empirical science? This is, perhaps, one of the most significant questions nursing scholars need to ask in this century. If the answer is "yes," it represents an epistemological landmark that may result in a paradigm shift for the discipline. Kuhn (1970), author of *The Structure of Scientific Revolutions*, stated that all epistemological crises begin with a blurring paradigm, followed by the consequent loosening of rules, and the eventual emergence of a new paradigm, along with vigorous discourse over its acceptance. Kuhn's view is supported by Bird (2004) who indicated that revolutionary new paradigms are derived from the failure of existing paradigms to resolve certain questions. Nursing has selected areas of knowledge where the traditional descriptors of facts, principles, scientific laws, theories, and philosophies do not adequately describe the occurring phenomena.

So how do we evaluate these areas to determine if they are significant enough to become nursing's first discipline-specific laws? The most likely choice is through determination of logical adequacy. Simply stated, logical adequacy is a method of explaining and validating theory, facts, principles, and laws that may include, but go beyond, empirical testing. Logical adequacy, like empirical predictability, has gone through periods of revolution. Hempel (1965) indicated that scientific explanation offered through logical adequacy needed to contain at least one law of nature, logical consequences, and be either empirically based or empirically testable. However, Kuhn (1970) and Bird (2004) indicated that science is more than a group of empirical outcomes and that scientists do not make their judgments as a result of consciously or unconsciously following rules, empirical or otherwise. Kuhn (1970) further indicated that values play

an important role in guiding scientist's judgments. Kuhn's interpretation allows for a broader definition of logical adequacy and expands the criteria by which knowledge can be evaluated and put forth as facts, principles, theories, and laws. Collectively, the broader definition of logical adequacy involves, in varying degrees of influence, truth, order, precision, coherence, comprehensiveness, reasonable predictability and reliability, values, consequences, and hermeneutic interpretation and reinterpretation (Bird, 2004; Kuhn, 1970; Polifroni, 1999; Silva, 2004).

Understandably, societal laws, and their subsets, have evolved more frequently through logical adequacy than as a consequence of empirical testing and 100% predictability. Empirical evidence, when available, certainly plays a role in the development of laws guiding the individual and collective behavior of society and its subsets; however, empirical evidence is not as decisive a factor in societal or behavioral law as it is in science. Nursing is an example of a societal subset in which logically adequate laws that guide selected aspects of behavior and practice may have begun to emerge.

Redefining Laws

The vast majority of nursing phenomena are a mix of quantitative and qualitative variables, thus the profession will inherently require integration of both. Does this mean that the profession will never be able to develop nursing laws? No it does not. However, it does suggest that the traditional definition of law needs to be expanded to encompass the evolution of knowledge associated with these combined phenomena. It further suggests a need to be more representative of the current reality, and to be capable of providing relevant, safe, and effective rules of behavior to guide nursing practice. Im and Chee (2003) indicated that exploration and validation of phenomena containing empirical and qualitative characteristics require the use of fuzzy logic or reasoning that respects the benefits of both and recognizes the gray areas where they merge. In other words, paradigms may need blurring, rules may need loosening, and discourse must be initiated.

When advancing selected knowledge to the status of law, the profession certainly needs to utilize the elements of logical adequacy; however, any rule of behavior significant enough to be advanced to the status of law and capable of influencing and guiding global nursing practice should also demonstrate:

- *Teleologia*, a Latin word meaning *end goal* (Jewel & Abate, 2001). In the formation of any law, the goal is to guide behavior toward a goal inherently imbedded in the law itself. Any nursing law must have a clear and concise goal, consistent with the intent of safe and effective nursing care.

- *Practical applicability or implementable usefulness.* Guidelines and rules that meet the criteria for logical adequacy, but do not consistently guide behavior or demonstrate longitudinal achievement of desired outcomes, are incapable of being evaluated and, as a result, are not sustainable as laws. Any law with practical application must guide behavior to achieve a desired goal or, at least, indicate what not to do.

- *Universality or applicability to all human beings.* Global acknowledgment of the desirability and applicability of the goal and premise of a proposed law is necessary to achieve the intent of the law, and ultimately to guide global nursing practice.

Transition Thinking

No doubt some would argue that it is not necessary to elevate selected areas of nursing knowledge to the position of laws or that nursing knowledge is simply not capable of producing laws. Perhaps it is the traditional understanding of theory and knowledge development that prevents nurses from embracing the idea. The word *theory* originated from the Greek word *theoria*, which means to speculate. This speculative origin inherently raises questions regarding validity and reliability of theory. However, like the word *law*, the meaning of *theory* has evolved over time to mean organized information intended to explain and guide (Jewel & Abate, 2001). Organized information begins as speculative theory (concepts, propositions, hypotheses), and over time is evaluated in terms of empirical testing and/or logical adequacy for its ability to explain and guide. Theory that is affirmed as a consequence of this process moves to the status of established theory and is used as a valid and reliable tool for answering questions, solving problems, explaining phenomena,

and generating new speculative theory. Established theory and the facts, principles, and laws that emerge from it, are taught in every required course in nursing. The evolution of the meaning of theory is apparent when nurses say they understand the *theory* behind a particular phenomenon or skill and when nurse educators say they teach *theory-based* classes. Nurse educators are using theory in the established, as opposed to the speculative sense. Articulation of the duality of speculative and established theory helps students, nurses, and faculty differentiate and operationalize the knowledge typology, which in turn allows them to see and understand the interrelationships among theory, research, practice, and reasoning (Johnson & Webber, 2005) (refer to Figure 2-1). Ultimately, this typology facilitates understanding of the progressive intricacies of interaction among the components of knowledge, especially with regard to how and where laws may emerge. Silva (2004), when discussing components of theory, made the link that is perhaps most significant to this point of view, by indicating that facts, principles, and laws do not constitute theory unless they are interrelated and have relevance to a common problem or issue. If a common problem, issue, or other teleological activity is significant enough to force evolution of guiding facts and principles from theory, and if the demands for logical adequacy, practical applicability, and universality have been met, the profession should consider the elevation of that information to the status of law.

Examples of Nursing Laws

While nursing currently has no discipline-specific laws, selected areas of nursing knowledge do meet the revised criteria for formation of laws. Perhaps the most prominent of these areas is self-care. Self-care, as a theoretical concept, first entered mainstream nursing in 1971 with the publication of Orem's *Concepts of Practice*, which challenged the health-related wisdom of *doing for* patients and redirected nurses

Expanded Knowledge
Facts, Principles, Laws emerge ← → Established Theory
Established Theory formulated
Research conducted, critiqued, and replicated and/or
Determine Logical Adequacy
External (confounding) **Variables** and **Assumptions** identified
Research questions formed ← → Speculative Theory
Propositions/Internal variables identified
Concepts identified
Ideas/Questions generated about the phenomenon
Phenomena observed in practice

R E A S O N I N G

Figure 2-1 *Knowledge typology.*

toward the more therapeutic approach of facilitating patients to *care for self* whenever and however possible. Nurses balked at the atypical language and complexity of the theory itself; however, they embraced the logic of self-care as therapeutic. Over time, nurses ceased focusing on doing for patients such as, feeding, bathing, and turning who could perform these activities themselves and began directing their care toward helping individuals, families, groups, and communities maximize their ability to meet their own self-care needs. An essential assumption in self-care is that when necessary, nurses will fulfill care requirements of individuals until such time as the individuals or other care providers, such as family members, can assume that responsibility. Orem's (1971) *Concepts of Practice* is now in its sixth edition and has expanded to include three separate theories. These theories have undergone extensive global research that has supported the benefits of self-care. This support also is evidenced by the International Orem Society for Nursing Science and Scholarship (http://www.scdnt.com/newsl/newsl.html) and by the journal dedicated to publishing self-care research, Self-Care and Dependent Care Journal.

The vast majority of nurses, both past and present, do not practice the promotion of self-care as Orem packaged it; they have extrapolated the facts and principles from this theory that were most valuable, specifically those associated with the promotion of the therapeutic benefits of self-care, and repeatedly and successfully integrated them into diverse practice settings. The elevation of the value of self-care beyond the constraints of some of the individual subconcepts and propositions within Orem's original theories

made it easier to integrate self-care in nursing practice throughout the world. Today, nursing's focus on helping people care for themselves is evident from the bedside to the global community and has gained both national and international momentum (Department of Health and Human Services, 1995; Holmes & Gastaldo, 2002; National Health Service, 2006). In 2002, when discussing nursing's role in government and public policy, Holmes and Gastaldo, highlighted the role nursing played in bringing the importance of self-care and self-responsibility to the forefront of socially responsible policy. In addition, promotion of self-care is a primary focus in Great Britain's National Health Service (National Health Service, 2006). In 2003, Sigma Theta Tau convened a conference in Sorrento, Italy, to discuss how nurses in southern Europe and the Mediterranean could best contribute to the health of communities in the new millennium. The result, in part, called for encouraging self-care through partnerships among nurses, individuals, families, and communities.

Elevating promotion of self-care to the status of a law would clearly focus the profession on a globally desirable goal, increase practical awareness, and guide students, nurses, and faculty in the delivery of care. This intentionality could also positively influence healthcare effectiveness and costs on a long-term basis. These approaches have the potential to make a significant difference in the health and well-being of global society. Nursing's goal of promoting self-care meets the criteria for logical adequacy, teleologia, practical applicability, and universality; as a result, promotion of self-care constitutes one of nursing's first laws. Figure 2-2 provides the pathway demonstrating the evolution of this law.

Expanded Knowledge: Promotion of the maximum level of self-care possible is therapeutically desirable and a goal of nursing.
Facts, Principles, and Laws Emerge:
- **Law:** Effective nursing care promotes the highest level of self-care possible for individuals, families, groups, communities, and global society.
- **Principle:** Nurses meet self-care needs and/or assists individuals, families, groups, and communities in meeting self-care needs.
- **Fact:** Individuals, families, groups, and communities have varying ability to meet self-care needs.
Established Theory is Formed, Developed, and Tested:
- A theory of self-care
- Self-care deficit theory of nursing
- A theory of nursing systems
External/Confounding Variables and Assumptions:
- Self-care is necessary to maintain physical and mental wellbeing
- Human beings want to care for self
Proposition: Nurses provide care for or assist individuals, families, groups, and communities achieve the maximum level of self-care possible.
Concepts:
- Self-care
- Human beings with self-care needs
- Nurses
Ideas/Questions: Nurses provide care for those who cannot care for themselves and/or assist those who can until such time as they become independent
Observed Phenomenon: Human beings function better and are happier when they can care for themselves; however, human beings vary in their capacity to care for self because of ability, illness, age, and education.

Figure 2-2 *Pathway to the law of self-care.*

Expanded Knowledge: Promotion of culturally congruent care is desirable and therapeutic and a goal of nursing care

Facts, Principles, and Laws Emerge:
- **Law:** Effective nursing care integrates cultural values and beliefs of diverse individuals, families, groups, communities, and global society.
- **Principle:** Diverse cultures have specific values and beliefs that influence health and health care.
- **Fact:** Individuals, families, groups, and communities belong to different cultures and/or subcultures that influence their values and beliefs related to health and well being.

Established Theory is Formed (Developed and Tested)
- Culture Care Diversity and Universality Theory

External/Confounding Variables/Assumptions:
- Level of cultural awareness
- Desire to provide culturally congruent care
- Value of cultural diversity

Proposition: Effective nurses provide culturally congruent care.

Concepts:
- Cultural Uniqueness
- Effective nursing care

Ideas/Questions : Effective nurses provide culturally congruent care.

Observed Phenomenon: Every individual belongs to a culture and/or subculture that has unique beliefs and values that influence health, well-being and the delivery of nursing care.

Figure 2-3 *Pathway to the law of culturally congruent care.*

THE LAW OF SELF-CARE: Effective nursing care promotes the highest level of self-care possible for individuals, families, groups, communities, and global society.

Another nursing law that may be emerging is that of culturally congruent care. This concept entered mainstream nursing in 1985 with the articulation of Leininger's culture care theory. Leininger's (1985) theory, which has been expanded several times, brought into focus the profession's need to recognize, value, and consistently integrate the unique needs of the culturally diverse. Unfortunately, like self-care theory, culture care theory was burdened with atypical language and complexity that made it difficult for nurses to utilize in its original form. As with most theory, however, nurses extracted the most valuable facts and principles associated with the theory and embedded them in their practice, nursing textbooks, classroom lectures, and clinical experiences. Delivery of culturally congruent care in this era of rapid globalization has emerged as more than just a focus within nursing care. It has become fundamental to nursing behavior in the 21st century and beyond (Murphy, 2006). This change is evidenced by the development of the Transcultural Nursing Society (www.tcen.org), an international organization whose mission is to advance culturally congruent nursing care. Nursing's goal of promoting culturally congruent care meets the criteria for logical adequacy, teleologia, practical applicability, and universality, and as a result, promotion of culturally congruent care constitutes another law of nursing. Figure 2-3 provides a sample pathway demonstrating how this law evolved.

THE LAW OF CULTURALLY CONGRUENT CARE: Effective nursing care integrates cultural values and beliefs of diverse individuals, families, groups, communities, and global society.

Have the concepts of self-care and culturally congruent care matured to the point that they provide rules of behavior that guide all of nursing practice and have global applicability? Have they matured beyond simple facts and principles, and if so, do they constitute nursing's first laws? If students in schools of nursing or nurses within the profession are not integrating self-care and culturally congruent care into their daily practice, should they be? Should the profession let these and other emerging laws establish the direction for all of nursing practice on a global scale? These questions, over the next few decades, will no doubt stimulate needed and valuable discourse regarding nursing's knowledge development. From this author's perspective, nursing needs these laws to provide clear and unprecedented direction for effective global nursing practice and to crystallize professional intent in a time of dramatic change. So, yes, Virginia, nursing does have laws. If we can recognize them, keep a clear vision regarding how and when they evolve, and then facilitate their development, then the best is yet to come.

REFERENCES

Bird, A. (2004). Thomas Kuhn. *Stanford encyclopedia of philosophy.* Retrieved October 10, 2006, from http://plato stanford.edu/entries/thomas-kuhn/

Church, P. (2007) Yes, Virginia, there is a Santa Claus. Retrieved September 22, 2007, from *http://www.newseum.org/yesvirginia/* (Original work published 1897).

Department of Health and Human Services. (1995). *The informed consumer: Self-care, self-help, and selecting health care.* Retrieved September 5, 2006, from http://www.health.gov/nhic/Partnerships/1995/inform.htm

Glanz, J. (1997). Visions of black holes. *Science, 275,* 476–478.

Hempel, C. G. (1965). *Aspects of scientific explanation.* New York: Macmillan.

Hickman, J. S. (2002). An introduction to nursing theory. In J. B. George (Ed.), *Nursing theories: The base for professional nursing practice* (5th ed., pp. 1-20). Upper Saddle River, NJ: Prentice Hall.

Holmes, D., & Gastaldo, D. (2002). Nursing as a means of governmentality. *Journal of Advanced Nursing, 38,* 557–565.

Im, E., & Chee, W. (2003). Fuzzy logic and nursing. *Nursing Philosophy,* 4(1), 53–60.

Jewel, E. J., & Abate, F. (Eds.). (2001). *The new Oxford American dictionary.* New York: Oxford University Press.

Johnson, B., & Webber, P. (2005). *Introduction to theory and reasoning in nursing.* Philadelphia: Lippincott Williams & Wilkins.

Katz, A. M., & Katz, P. B. (1995). Emergence of scientific explanations of nature in ancient Greece: The only scientific discovery? *Circulation, 92,* 637–645.

Koyrè, A. (1978) *Galileo studies* (J. Mepham, Trans.). Atlantic Highlands, NJ: Humanities. (Original work published 1939)

Kuhn, T. (1970). *The structure of scientific revolutions.* Chicago: University of Chicago Press.

Leininger, M. M. (1985). Transcultural care diversity and universality: A theory for nursing. *Nursing & Health Care, 6,* 209–212.

Murphy, S. (2006). Mapping the literature of transcultural nursing. *Journal of the Medical Library Association, 94*(2), E143–E151.

National Health Service. (2006). *Self-care.* Retrieved July 31, 2006, from http://www.dh.gov.uk/PolicyAndGuidance/OrganisationPolicy/SelfCare/fs/en

Orem, D. (1971). *Nursing: Concepts and practice.* New York: McGraw-Hill.

Polifroni, E. C. (1999). Explanation in science. In E. C. Polifroni & M. Welch (Eds.), *Perspectives on philosophy of science: A historical and contemporary anthology* (p. 149–153). Philadelphia: Lippincott.

Sigma Theta Tau International. (2003). *Preferred future for nursing professionals.* Retrieved September 5, 2006, from www.nursingsociety.org/programs/Arista_SouthernEurope.doc

Silva, M. C. (2004). Philosophy, science, theory: Interrelationships and implications for nursing research. In P. G. Reed, N. C. Shearer, & L. H. Nicoll (Eds.), *Perspective on nursing theory* (4th ed. pp. 3–9). Philadelphia: Lippincott Williams & Wilkins.

Swartz, N. (2006). Laws of nature. *The Internet encyclopedia of philosophy.* Retrieved August 20, 2006, from http://www.iep.utm.edu/l/lawofnat.htm

Veltman, K. H. (n. d.). *The emergence of scientific literature and quantification 1520–1560.* Retrieved July 17, 2006, from www.sumscorp.com/articles/art14.htm

THE AUTHOR COMMENTS | Yes, Virginia, Nursing Does Have Laws

I have been blessed during my career to have many inspiring education mentors who nurtured a strong Socratic tendency to ask questions and challenge contemporary thought, especially in nursing education, theory, research, and reasoning. Among these long-time mentors are Dr. Mary Cipriano Silva, whose body of work with nursing science and ethics provided a solid foundation for adductive and abductive inquiry; Dr. Em Olivia Bevis, whose body of work, passion for nursing education, and skill at swimming upstream provided a road map for turning the tide of mainstream nursing education; and, last but not least, my star students who demanded and participated in the synthesis of the concepts and relationships that culminated in this article.

I am convinced that one of the reasons many of nursing's global challenges never seem to get resolved is the lack of a clear professional intent. We have used the theoretical and research work of the last 100 years to help us clarify the 'how to' of our work, and, if we look closely enough, some of it also helps crystallize the 'where to' or overarching intent of our work. This 'where to' has emerged in the form of epistemological laws, which, for the first time in history, offers nursing education and service a specific road map and destination, as well as accountability for the trip. This clarity of focus has the potential to lead to the creation of a new paradigm not just for nursing, but for a healthcare system that is also looking for 'where to'.

PAMELA B. WEBBER

3

Philosophy, Science, Theory: Interrelationships and Implications for Nursing Research

MARY CIPRIANO SILVA, RN, PhD, FAAN

If nurse researchers are to study the structure of nursing knowledge, they must first understand the relationships among philosophy, science, and theory. Although many articles have spoken to the nature of theory or science in nursing (Andreoli & Thompson, 1977; Hardy, 1974; Jacox, 1974; Leininger, 1968; Walker, 1971), few have examined the links between them and fewer yet have examined the role of philosophy in the deriving of nursing knowledge. To bridge this gap, I would like to present an overview of the relationships among philosophy, science, and theory, and then describe some implications for the conduct of nursing research.

Relationships Between Philosophy and Science

Although in western civilization the precise origin of what we call pure knowledge is difficult to trace, most scholars agree that significant advancements occurred during the great Age of Greece (500 B.C. to 300 B.C.). During this time those ideals commonly associated with western civilization—freedom, optimism, secularism, rationalism, and high regard for the dignity and worth of the individual—were developed (Burns, 1955, p. 163).

Greek learning formed a single entry called philosophy and, even into the nineteenth century, this term was used to designate man's total knowledge. To designate all knowledge as philosophy was possible because our body of knowledge was relatively small and no real distinctions were made between different kinds of knowledge.

The Industrial Revolution, however, dramatically altered man's perception about the structuring of knowledge. The Darwinian hypothesis of natural selection, cell and germ theories, revolutionary discoveries about energy and matter, and the advent of psychoanalysis were but a few contributors to the knowledge explosion. No longer was philosophy considered adequate to answer questions about natural phenomena, and science divorced itself from it. New disciplines were formed—embryology, cytology, immunology, anesthesiology, to name a few—each asking their own questions and seeking their own answers.

This specialization, however, created a new problem: Although each discipline revealed unique and enlightening aspects of man, the ultimate questions about his nature and purpose went unanswered. Science had taken man apart but had not put him back together. Once again philosophy was sought out—this time to unify scientific findings so that man as a holistic being might emerge. This is in keeping with Kneller's (1971, p. 3) view of the philosopher as one whose work begins before and after the scientist has done his job.

The philosopher is concerned with such matters as the purpose of human life, the nature of being and reality, and the theory and limits of knowledge. Questions the philosopher might ask are "Is man inherently good or evil?", "Is truth absolute or relative?", "What does 'knowing' mean?". His approach to understanding reality is characterized by formulating sets of assumptions and beliefs derived from his own personal experience and his contemplation of it in relation to the studied experiences of others (Association for Supervision and Curriculum Development [ASCD] Commission on Instructional Theory, 1968, p. 2). Intuition, introspection, and reasoning are some of his methodologies.

The scientist, on the other hand, is primarily concerned with causality. Cause and effect, in one way or another, are central to his goal of deriving scientific laws (Labovitz and Hagedorn, 1976, p. 3). Questions the scientist might ask are "Does treatment X, and only treatment X, cause Y?", or "What is the relationship between X and Y?" His approach to understanding reality is characterized by tentativeness, verifiability, observation, and experience. Reality becomes interpretable to him through such mechanisms as hypothesis-testing, operational definitions, and experiments. The scientists' position is summarized by Kerlinger (1973): "If an explanation cannot be formulated in the form of a testable hypothesis, then it can be considered to be a metaphysical explanation and thus not amenable to scientific investigation. As such, it is dismissed by the scientist as being of no interest" (p. 25).

ABOUT THE AUTHOR

MARY CIPRIANO SILVA was born and raised in the small town of Ravenna, OH. She earned a BSN and an MS from Ohio State University and a PhD from the University of Maryland. She also undertook postdoctoral study at Georgetown University in healthcare ethics. The focus of her scholarship and key contributions to nursing has been in philosophy, metatheory, and healthcare ethics. She is a Professor Emerita of Nursing at George Mason University, Fairfax, VA. When not working, she attends foreign films, the Shakespeare Theatre, and fine and performing arts events.

However, despite different focuses and methodologies, the philosopher and scientist share the common goal of increasing mankind's knowledge.

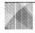

Relationships Between Science and Theory

Before analyzing the relationships between science and theory, let us first briefly review some characteristics of science as a system, based on principles of Van Laer (1963, pp. 8–19):

1. **Science must show a certain coherence.** Science must constitute a coherent whole of interrelated facts, principles, laws, and theories which are appropriately ordered. An explication of unrelated data, no matter how valuable, does not constitute a science.

2. **Science is concerned with definite fields of knowledge.** Man is no longer able to know all things. Consequently, he must specialize so that he might know one field, or an aspect of it, well.

3. **Science is preferably expressed in universal statements.** Science ultimately is concerned with commonalities of properties that transcend the specific; science seeks to discover the universal characteristics of phenomena under investigation. Its goal is to reduce data to their most fundamental common denominator.

4. **The statements of science must be true or probably true.** What constitutes truth is a vexing epistemological question. One may suggest, however, that scientific statements are true if they express the nature of things as they are. But man, being finite, frequently does not know the true nature of things. And so it is to the scientist we often turn to help us find reality in a systematic, scholarly, and trustworthy way. His job, according to Scheffler (1965), is "not to judge the truth infallibly, but to estimate the truth responsibly" (p. 54).

5. **The statements of science must be logically ordered.** One does not draw conclusions before stating hypotheses. Science is usually best served through careful observance of scientific methods such as the deductive-inductive or analytic-synthetic method.

6. **Science must explain its investigations and arguments.** Scientists have a responsibility not only to report their research findings, but as importantly, to explain the arguments and demonstrations which led them to their conclusions.

The above six principles certainly are not the exclusive domain of science. Many of them apply equally as well to philosophy or theory, once again underscoring the ebb and flow of relationships among philosophy, science, and theory.

We again see these relationships when we ask the question, "What is the aim of science? "Typical responses are that science aims to describe, understand, predict, control, or explain phenomena. But Kerlinger (1973) offers a different perspective: "The basic aim of science is theory" (p. 8).

But what are the components of theory and how do they relate to science? There is no easy answer, no one correct response. Basic philosophical differences exist among scientists regarding the constructional processes composing science and theory. These differences stem from varying philosophical orientations—realism, idealism, pragmatism, and others—each with its own interpretation of reality.

To complicate the situation further, the many terms used to define theory can be bewildering. For example, words such as propositions, assertions, axioms, postulates and maxims, to name a few, are sometimes used interchangeably, at other times with different meanings. When one looks carefully, however, some common denominators of theory emerge. They are set, postulates, definitions, and hypotheses. Let us now briefly examine how each contributes to theory, and consequently, to science.

1. **Set.** Set is a well-defined collection of objects or elements. Facts, principles, and laws do not, in and

of themselves, constitute theory. However, when a scientist selects particular facts, principles and laws from the universal set (ie, from the set of all elements under discussion) because of their interrelationships and relevance to the problem under investigation, he fulfills the requirements of set needed for theory development.

2. **Postulates.** The central core of a theory consists of its postulates. These are statements of general truth that serve as essential premises for whatever is being investigated. Postulates are usually stated as generalizations which are consistent with scientific evidence related to one's research problem. They form the essential presuppositions from which hypotheses are deduced and tested. Rogers (1970, pp. 46–47), for example, in developing her theoretical basis of nursing, identified four essential postulates about man. These postulates speak to man's wholeness, fluidity, sense of pattern and organization, and sentience.

3. **Definitions.** Definitions of terms are important for communication among scholars. Terms can be defined as primitive, theoretical, and key (ASCD Commission on Instructional Theory, 1968, pp. 10–12). Primitive terms are those which cannot be defined by specifying operations or by referring to other operationally defined terms. They represent entities which one can only intuitively experience. Purpose and need are examples of primitive terms. Theoretical terms are those which cannot be defined by pointing to particular operations, but which can be defined by their relationship to other terms which are operationally defined. Motivation is an example of a theoretical term. Key terms are those which can and must be operationally defined so that hypotheses under study can be tested. Learning is an example of a key term when it is essential to a hypothesis and can be operationally defined by use of valid and reliable instruments. Key terms are essential for replication research and theory verification.

4. **Hypotheses.** Hypotheses are predictions which have been deduced from a set of postulates and which state the relationship between two or more variables. They imply that the relationship between these variables can be observed and tested. This is no small matter, but one that is crucial in bridging theory and science. For if we cannot observe what we study, we cannot measure it. If we cannot measure it, we do not know whether or not it contributes to theory. If we do not know its impact on theory, we cannot know its potential contribution to science. Nurses are becoming more aware of these relationships. In a study of priorities in clinical nursing research, the highest priority in regard to "impact upon patient welfare"

was given to items concerned with determining reliable and valid indicators of quality nursing care (Lindeman, 1975).

Because well stated hypotheses are based on observation of fact which permit them to be "proven" or "disproven," they are powerful instruments of science. Through systematic and rigorous testing of hypotheses, phenomena are explained and, depending on the amount of verifiable evidence, these phenomena have predictive ability, first as theory, then principles and laws (Weinland, 1975, p. 31). Through the power of hypotheses, mankind's knowledge is increased, or at the very least in the case of disproven hypotheses, his ignorance is reduced.

If we now synthesize the above four common denominators of theory, we arrive at a workable definition: Theory refers to a set of related statements (most commonly, **postulates** and **definitions**) which have been derived from scientific data and from which plausible **hypotheses** can be deduced, tested, and verified. If verified, theory becomes part of the body of science from which other sets of postulates can be derived. The process of theory building, therefore, involves the formulation and testing of hypotheses which have been deduced from a set of statements derived from scientific knowledge and philosophical beliefs.

 ## Implications for Nursing Research

When the research process is examined by studying the relationships among philosophy, science, and theory, one arrives at perspectives different from traditional viewpoints about the derivation and significance of nursing knowledge. These perspectives are discussed below:

1. **Ultimately, all nursing theory and research is derived from or leads to philosophy.**
   Traditionally, one is led to believe that nursing research begins with theory. I believe it begins and ends with philosophy and this awareness enhances one's perspective about the research process.

   If one examines the four main branches of philosophy—logic, epistemology, metaphysics, and ethics—one begins to see the links between them and the process of nursing research. Through logic, researchers are able to establish the validity of various thoughts and the correctness of their reasoning. Germane to the research process is the ability to establish logical relationships between theory selection and problem identification, problem identification and hypothesis testing, hypothesis testing and derivation of valid conclusions.

Epistemology, the study of the theory of knowledge, is also crucial to the process of nursing research. For is not the aim of research to discover, expand, or reaffirm knowledge? Yet, what constitutes knowledge is no simple matter. Inherent in the concept of knowledge are conditions of truth, secure belief, and evidence (Scheffler, 1965, p. 21). The truth condition claims that if one "knows" something to be true, he must be judged not to be in error. The belief condition stipulates if one "knows" something to be true, he also believes it to be true. The evidence condition states that one evaluates knowledge against all adequate standards of evidence at a particular time. Although nurse researchers have recognized the evidence condition of knowledge, they seemingly have paid less attention to the truth and belief conditions. By identifying and applying the contributions of epistemology to nursing, nurse researchers can gain further insights into the research process.

Metaphysics studies the most general concepts used in ordinary life and science by examining the internal structure of the language used in various disciplines (Harré, 1972, p. 30). Of particular interest to the nurse researcher is an examination of the concept of causality. Questions the researcher might ask include: Is causality a necessary condition of objective experience? Can causality be demonstrated empirically? What are acceptable scientific criteria for the establishment of causality?

Finally, the study of ethics comes to grips with moral principles and values. Although all researchers are, I hope, familiar with the ethical requirements of informed consent and protection of the rights of human subjects, some, perhaps, have not considered other pertinent concepts. For example, what are ethical implications inherent in the nature of the research problem? What ethical considerations do advancements in science and technology present? What are the ethics involved in collaborative research and the reporting of research? To whom are researchers ultimately accountable? Although the "pure" scientist may argue that the use to which knowledge is put is not his business, I believe research cannot be conceived apart from its moral implications.

2. **Philosophical introspection and intuition are legitimate methods of scientific inquiry.** Historically and traditionally, nurses have been indoctrinated into a singular approach to the derivation of nursing knowledge—the scientific method. As early as the 1930s, scientific criteria were used to evaluate procedural demonstrations (Gortner & Nahm, 1977). In the 1960s, McCain (1965) stressed nursing by assessment, not intuition.

This stress on the scientific method continues strongly today. For example, Riehl and Roy (1974, p. 293), among others, express disapproval about nursing actions based on intuition. Gortner (1974) suggests that the logic of science is closed to intuition. In addition, many graduate nursing students have been indoctrinated into a methodology of nursing research which excludes anything but strict adherence to the scientific method.

The time has come to question this singular approach to the study of nursing knowledge. The time has come to value truths arrived at by intuition and introspection as much as those arrived at by scientific experimentation. For, in fact, the scientist has no greater claim to truth than does the theoretician or the philosopher. Yet, nurse scholars seem hesitant to acknowledge intuition and introspection as valid methods of acquiring knowledge.

However, what we scorn, others praise. Burner (1977; p. 56, p. 67), for example, tells us that the development of intuitive thinking is an objective of many highly regarded teachers and is considered to be a valuable asset in science. Intuition is not knowledge arrived at out of nothing; rather, it is knowledge arrived at by a deep grasp of a subject, although one may not be able to articulate the process by which a conclusion is reached. The derived knowledge may not always be correct, but neither is knowledge arrived at with all the advantages of the scientific method. The large numbers of unsubstantiated hypotheses support this assertion.

In addition, knowledge gained through introspection cannot be overlooked as it constitutes one of the major approaches to the derivation of knowledge—rationalism. The prime example, of course, is mathematics where truth is deduced from reasoning and not contingent on observation or experience. According to Scheffler (1965), mathematicians conduct no experiments, surveys, or statistics, yet "they arrive at the firmest of all truths, incapable of being overthrown by experience" (p. 3).

The point to be made here is that we must keep our minds open to all potential avenues which lead to advancement of nursing knowledge. We must be careful not to impose our value judgments about the research process on others if, in the end, we narrow their thinking and undermine their creativity. For example, during the conduct of my dissertation, although never explicitly stated, it was inferred time and again that the experimental research design with its emphasis on causality is superior to all other types of research. Descriptive, historical, and other valuable types of research were quietly but steadfastly refuted.

3. **Nursing knowledge arrived at by the scientific method too often sacrifices meaningfulness for rigor.** Although rigorous research designs are praiseworthy, if not used judiciously, they can impede rather than enhance the research process. Too much rigor can (and often does) lead to trivial research problems with the logical outcome of trivial research results. The same is true of definition of terms and statistics. One can meticulously operationally define the independent and dependent variables in one's hypotheses, but if these definitions are so narrow that they have little or no meaning for nursing practice, what is the point? In terms of statistics, one can find statistically significant differences among groups (if they exist) if a large enough sample is used. However, for practical purposes, the differences may be so small as to be negligible. Such statistics can be impeccably and rigorously applied, yet offer little to the advancement of nursing knowledge and, at best, be misleading.

Although one expects sufficient rigorism of design so that there is confidence in the results, the pursuit and worship of rigorism and experimentation for their own sake—as at times seems the case—needs questioning. Cook and LaFleur (1975, p. 2) maintain that experimentation (with its implications for rigorism) as an exclusive method of obtaining knowledge is becoming a dead end as too little meaningful behavior can be understood by this method alone.

How can this situation be improved? As previously noted, researchers can begin to examine other ways to derive nursing knowledge. This does not necessarily mean that we give up a method we believe in, only that we open our minds to other approaches. Most of us, for example, have traditionally considered probability theory as the basis for accepting or rejecting hypotheses. Yet, Frank (1957, pp. 327–331) discusses another option: logical probability. Instead of reducing probability statements to statements about relative frequencies, one uses inductive logic to arrive at the probable truth or falsity of the data. The statements of inductive logic are purely logical and say nothing about physical facts; that is, they are not statements that are derived from observations. The basic premise is as follows: The inductive probability of a hypothesis **h** on the basis of a certain evidence **e** is high; or stated in another way, the evidence **e** confirms to a high degree the hypothesis **h**. Although the precise logical formulations derived to arrive at the above premise are beyond the scope of this paper, the possibilities of validating hypotheses in nontraditional ways are interesting to ponder.

In summary, when nurse researchers examine the total philosophy-science-theory triad, they develop a more holistic and less traditional approach to the possibilities of deriving nursing knowledge. They are more open to contributions of other disciplines and less likely to see the research process as though through a glass darkly.

REFERENCES

Andreoli, K. G., & Thompson, C. E. (1977). The nature of science in nursing. *Image, 9*, 32–37.

Association for Supervision and Curriculum Development Commission on Instructional Theory (ASCD). (1968). *Criteria for theories of instruction*. Washington, DC: National Education Association.

Bruner, J. (1977). *The process of education*. London: Harvard University Press (Originally published 1960).

Burns, E. M. (1955). *Western civilization: Their history and their culture* (4th ed.). New York: W. W. Norton.

Cook, D. R., & LaFleur, N. K. (1975). *A guide to educational research* (2nd ed.). Boston: Allyn and Bacon.

Frank, P. (1957). *Philosophy of science: The link between science and philosophy*. Englewood Cliffs, NJ: Prentice-Hall.

Gortner, S. R. (1974). Scientific accountability in nursing. *Nursing Outlook, 22*, 764–768.

Gortner, S. R., & Nahm, H. (1977). An overview of nursing research in the United States. *Nursing Research, 26*, 10–33.

Hardy, M. E. (1974). Theories: Components, development, evaluation. *Nursing Research, 23*, 100–107.

Harré, R. (1972). *The philosophies of science: An introductory survey*. London: Oxford University Press.

Jacox, A. (1974). Theory construction in nursing: An overview. *Nursing Research, 23*, 4–13.

Kerlinger, F. N. (1973). *Foundations of behavioral research* (2nd ed.). New York: Holt, Rinehart, and Winston.

Kneller, G. F. (1971). *Introduction to the philosophy of education* (2nd ed.). New York: John Wiley & Sons.

Labovitz, S., & Hagedorn, R. (1976). *Introduction to social research* (2nd ed.). New York: McGraw-Hill.

Leininger, M. (1968). Conference on the nature of science and nursing: Introductory comments. *Nursing Research, 17*, 484–486.

Lindeman, C. A. (1975). Delphi survey of priorities in clinical nursing research. *Nursing Research, 24*, 434–441.

McCain, R. F. (1965). Nursing by assessment—not intuition. *American Journal of Nursing, 65*, 82–84.

Riehl, J. P., & Roy, C. (1974). *Conceptual models for nursing practice*. New York: Appleton-Century-Crofts.

Rogers, M. E. (1970). *An introduction to the theoretical basis of nursing*. Philadelphia: F. A. Davis.

Scheffler, I. (1965). *Conditions of knowledge: An introduction to epistemology and education*. Glenview, IL: Scott, Foresman.

Van Laer, P. H. (1963). *Philosophy of science: An introduction to some general aspects of science* (2nd ed.). Pittsburgh: Duquesne University Press.

Walker, L. O. (1971). Toward a clearer understanding of the concept of nursing theory. *Nursing Research, 20*, 428–435.

Weinland, J. D. (1975). *How to think straight*. Totowa, NJ: Littlefield, Adams (Originally published 1963).

THE AUTHOR COMMENTS | Philosophy, Science, Theory: Interrelationships and Implications for Nursing Research

My inspiration for this article came from a long-standing interest in philosophy and the need I saw to bridge the gap between philosophy, science, and theory. In addition, when this article was written, the strong emphasis on empirical research offended my integrative and intuitive nature. The three implications for nursing research contained in this article continue to be important to the development, testing, and evaluation of nursing theory in the 21st century.

MARY C. SILVA

CHAPTER 4

On Nursing Theories and Evidence

JACQUELINE FAWCETT, PhD, FAAN

JEAN WATSON, RN, PhD, AHN, BC, FAAN

BETTY NEUMAN, RN, PhD, FAAN

PATRICIA H. WALKER, RN, PhD, FAAN

JOYCE J. FITZPATRICK, RN, PhD, MBA, FAAN

Purpose: To expand the understanding of what constitutes evidence for theory-guided, evidence-based nursing practice from a narrow focus on empirics to a more comprehensive focus on diverse patterns of knowing. *Organizing Construct:* Carper's four fundamental patterns of knowing in nursing—empirical, ethical, personal, and aesthetic—are required for nursing practice. A different mode of inquiry is required to develop knowledge about and evidence for each pattern. *Conclusions:* Theory, inquiry, and evidence are inextricably linked. Each pattern of knowing can be considered a type of theory, and the modes of inquiry appropriate to the generation and testing of each type of theory provide diverse sources of data for evidence-based nursing practice. Different kinds of nursing theories provide different lenses for critiquing and interpreting the different kinds of evidence essential for theory-guided, evidence-based holistic nursing practice.

Evidence-based practice is in the forefront of many contemporary discussions of nursing research and nursing practice. Indeed, the term "seems to be the up-and-coming buzzword for the decade" (Ingersoll, 2000, p. 151). The current call for evidence-based nursing practice has set the debate in a conventional, atheoretical, medically dominated, empirical model of evidence, which threatens the foundation of nursing's disciplinary perspective on theory-guided practice (Walker & Redmond, 1999). More specifically, as Ingersoll (2000) pointed out, almost all discussions of evidence-based practice are focused on the primacy of the randomized clinical trial as the only legitimate source of evidence. Furthermore, most discussions of evidence-based practice treat evidence as an atheoretical entity, which only widens the theory-practice gap (Upton, 1999). Moreover, although multiple patterns of knowing in nursing have been acknowledged at least since the publication of Carper's work in 1978, nurses have ignored this disciplinary perspective and reverted to a medical perspective of evidence when discussing evidence-based nursing practice.

The purpose of this paper is to invite readers to join in a dialogue about what constitutes the evidence for theory-guided, evidence-based nursing practice. We are initiating the dialogue by offering a comprehensive description of theoretical evidence that encompasses diverse patterns of knowing in nursing. We advance the argument that each pattern of knowing can be considered a type of theory and

that the different forms of inquiry used to develop the diverse kinds of theories yield different kinds of evidence, all of which are needed for evidence-based nursing practice.

On Nursing Theories

Diverse patterns of knowing were identified by Carper (1978), who expanded the historical view of nursing as an art and a science in her classic paper, "Fundamental Patterns of Knowing in Nursing." She identified four ways or patterns of knowing in nursing: empirics, ethics, personal, and aesthetics. Carper's work is significant in that it "not only highlighted the centrality of empirically derived theoretical knowledge, but [also] recognized with equal importance and weight, knowledge gained through clinical practice" (Stein, Corte, Colling, & Whall, 1998, p. 43). Chinn and Kramer (1999) expanded Carper's work by identifying processes associated with each pattern of knowing. Their work has enhanced understanding of each pattern of knowing and has brought Carper's ideas to the attention of a wide audience of nurses.

The pattern of empirical knowing (Table 4-1) encompasses publicly verifiable, factual descriptions, explanations, and predictions based on subjective or objective group data. In other words, empirical knowing is about "averages." This pattern of knowing, which constitutes the science of nursing, is well

ABOUT THE AUTHORS

JACQUELINE FAWCETT received her Bachelor of Science degree from Boston University in 1964; her master's in Parent–Child Nursing from New York University in 1970; and her PhD in nursing, also from New York University, in 1976. Dr. Fawcett currently is a professor, College of Nursing and Health Sciences, University of Massachusetts, Boston. She is a Professor Emerita at the University of Pennsylvania. Starting with her dissertation, Dr. Fawcett conducted a program of research dealing with wives' and husbands' pregnancy-related experiences that was derived from Martha Rogers' conceptual system. Subsequently, she undertook a program of research dealing with responses to caesarean birth derived from the Roy Adaptation Model of Nursing. A third program of research, also derived from the Roy Adaptation Model, focuses on function during normal life transitions and serious illness. Dr. Fawcett is perhaps best known for her metatheoretical work, including many journal articles and several books. Since 1996, Dr. Fawcett has lived in the midcoast region of Maine with her husband John and a now-tame feral cat, Lydia Dasher. She and her husband own Fawcett's Art, Antiques, and Toy Museum. She swims laps and walks on a treadmill at a fitness center for exercise and relaxation and sails on a windjammer off the Maine coast during the summer.

JEAN WATSON is a Distinguished Professor of Nursing and holds the Murchinson-Scolville Chair in Caring Science at the University of Colorado Health Sciences Center (HSC). She is the founder of the original Center for Human Caring and previously served as the Dean of the University of Colorado HSC School of Nursing. She is a past President of the National League for Nursing. Born in West Virginia, July 21, 1940, Dr. Watson earned undergraduate and graduate degrees in nursing and psychiatric-mental health nursing and holds her PhD in educational psychology and counseling. Dr. Watson is known for her theoretical work on the art and science of human caring. She is the founder of the Watson Caring Science Institute. Her latest books and articles address empirical measurements of caring and new postmodern philosophies of caring and healing that bridge paradigms and point toward transformative models for the 21st century. Dr. Watson is the recipient of many awards and honors, including an international Kellogg Fellowship in Australia, a Fulbright Research Award in Sweden, five honorary doctoral degrees, the National League for Nursing's Martha E. Rogers Award, New York University's Distinguished Nurse Scholar Award, and the Fetzer Institute's Norman Cousins Award. Her hobbies include international travel, skiing, hiking, biking, and writing.

BETTY M. NEUMAN was born September 11, 1924, on a 100-acre farm near Lowell, OH. She received her nursing diploma in 1947 from what is now the Akron General Hospital and her BSN in 1957 and MS (major in mental health and community health) in 1966, both from University of California, Los Angeles. In 1985, she obtained her PhD degree in Clinical Psychology from the Pacific Western University School of Psychology in Los Angeles. Her most significant contribution is her theoretical model, the Neuman Systems Model, first published in 1972. Despite its widespread significance and application, Dr. Neuman regards her model as a work in progress. Her model has helped enhance the scientific perspective and basis of nursing and provides theoretic grounding for nursing education, research, and practice throughout the world. Dr. Neuman's hobbies include participating in the holistic health movement through her own primary prevention health regimen of walking and weight training. She is also a licensed real estate agent and continues to travel internationally for consultations and speaking engagements.

PATRICIA H. WALKER is the Vice President for Nursing Policy and Professor in the Graduate School of Nursing at the Uniformed Services University of the Health Sciences in Bethesda, MD. Born in Kansas, she graduated with a BSN from the University of Kansas and subsequently received her master's and doctorate degrees from the University of Mississippi. Dr. Walker is a recognized scholar who has continually tried to integrate education, practice, and research through faculty practice and practice-based research. She influenced the development of faculty practices as a business and nationally focused many of her presentations and publications on the link between practice and research, particularly cost and quality outcomes research. Her focus on outcomes is exemplified through the promotion of cost and quality outcomes research linked to the practice environment and her leadership with faculties nationally and internationally for competency-based education. For recreation and fulfillment outside nursing, she plays golf, plays the piano, and enjoys creative cooking.

JOYCE J. FITZPATRICK is the Elizabeth Brooks Ford Professor of Nursing, Case Western Reserve University, Frances Payne Bolton School of Nursing, where she served as the Dean from 1982 to1997. Her educational background includes a BSN from Georgetown University, an MS from The Ohio State University (psychiatric nursing), a PhD from New York University, an MBA from Case Western Reserve University, and an honorary doctorate (Doctor of Humane Letters) from Georgetown University. She has a strong and continuing interest in nursing science development, including both theory and research. She is the author of more than 275 scholarly publications and author/editor of more than 35 books (having won the *American Journal of Nursing* Book of the Year award 20 times in the past 25 years), Editor of the *Annual Review of Nursing Research* series, and Editor of the journal that she launched in 1989, *Applied Nursing Research.*

established in nursing epistemology and methods. Empirical knowing is generated and tested by means of empirical research. The next section of this paper extends the common focus on empirics as the primary focus of evidence, and offers a new lens for considering theory-guided evidence and diverse ways of knowing that can and should be integrated into nurses' evidence-based practice initiatives.

TABLE 4-1   Patterns of Knowing: Types of Nursing Theories, Modes of Inquiry, and Evidence

Pattern of Knowing: Type of Nursing Theory	Description	Mode of Inquiry	Examples of Evidence
Empirics	Publicly verifiable, factual descriptions, explanations, or predictions based on subjective or objective group data; the science of nursing	Empirical research	Scientific data
Ethics	Descriptions of moral obligations, moral and nonmoral values, and desired ends; the ethics of nursing	Identification, analysis, and clarification of beliefs and values; dialogue about and justification of beliefs and values	Standards of practice, codes of ethics, philosophies of nursing
Personal	Expressions of the quality and authenticity of the interpersonal process between each nurse and each patient; the interpersonal relationships of nursing	Opening, centering, thinking, listening, and reflecting	Autobiographical stories
Aesthetics	Expressions of the nurse's perception of what is significant in an individual patient's behavior; the art and act of nursing	Envisioning possibilities, rehearsing nursing art and acts	Aesthetic criticism and works of art

Diverse Patterns of Knowing

In contrast to empirics, the other patterns of knowing are less established, but they are of increasing interest for the discipline of nursing in particular and for science in general. Ethical knowing, personal knowing, and aesthetic knowing are required for moral, humane, and personalized nursing practice (Stein et al., 1998). The pattern of ethical knowing (Table 4-1) encompasses descriptions of moral obligations, moral and nonmoral values, and desired ends. Ethical knowing, which constitutes the ethics of nursing, is generated by means of ethical inquiries that are focused on identification and analysis of the beliefs and values held by individuals and groups and the clarification of those beliefs and values. Ethical knowing is tested by means of ethical inquiries that focus on dialogue about beliefs and values and establishing justification for those beliefs and values.

The pattern of personal knowing refers to the quality and authenticity of the interpersonal process between each nurse and each patient (Table 4-1). This pattern is concerned with the knowing, encountering, and actualizing of the authentic self; it is focused on how nurses come to know how to be authentic in relationships with patients, and how nurses come to know how to express their concern and caring for other people. Personal knowing is not "knowing one's self" but rather knowing how to be authentic with others, knowing one's own "personal style" of "being with" another person. Personal knowing is what is meant by "therapeutic nurse-patient relationships." Personal knowing is developed by means of opening and centering the self to thinking about how one is or can be authentic, by listening to responses from others, and by reflecting on those thoughts and responses.

The pattern of aesthetic knowing shows the nurse's perception of what is significant in the individual patient's behavior (Table 4-1). Thus, this pattern is focused on particulars rather than universals. Aesthetic knowing also addresses the "artful" performance of manual and technical skills. Aesthetic knowing is developed by envisioning possibilities and rehearsing the art and acts of nursing, with emphasis on developing appreciation of aesthetic meanings in practice and inspiration for developing the art of nursing.

Carper (1978) and Chinn and Kramer (1999) pointed out that each pattern of knowing is an essential component of the integrated knowledge base for professional practice, and that no one pattern of knowing should be used in isolation from the others. Carper (1978) maintained that "Nursing … depends on the scientific knowledge of human behavior in health and in illness, the aesthetic perception of significant human experiences, a personal understanding of the unique individuality of the self and the capacity to make choices within concrete situations involving particular moral judgments" (p. 22). Elaborating, Chinn and Kramer (1999) pointed out the danger of using any one pattern exclusively. They said:

> When knowledge within any one pattern is not critically examined and integrated with the whole of knowing, distortion instead of understanding is produced. Failure to develop knowledge integrated within all of the patterns of knowing leads to uncritical acceptance, narrow interpretation, and partial utilization of knowledge. We call this "the patterns gone wild." When this occurs, the patterns are used in isolation from one another, and the potential for synthesis of the whole is lost. (p. 12)

The current emphasis on empirical knowing as the only basis for evidence-based nursing practice is an outstanding example of a "pattern gone wild."

Patterns of Knowing as Theories

The question arises as to whether the multiple, diverse patterns of knowing can be considered sets of theories. The answer to that question depends, in part, on one's view of a pattern of knowing and a theory. A pattern of knowing can be thought of as a way of seeing a phenomenon. The English word "theory" comes from the Greek word, "theoria," which means "to see," that is, to reveal phenomena previously hidden from our awareness and attention (Watson, 1999). For the purposes of this paper, a theory is defined as a way of seeing through "a set of relatively concrete and specific concepts and the propositions that describe or link those concepts" (Fawcett, 1999, p. 4). Theories constitute much of the knowledge of a discipline. Moreover, theory and inquiry are inextricably linked. That is, theories of various phenomena are the lenses through which inquiry is conducted. The results of inquiry constitute the evidence that determines whether the theory is adequate or must be refined.

Collectively, the diverse patterns of knowing constitute the ontological and epistemological foundations of the discipline of nursing. Inasmuch as both patterns of knowing and theories represent knowledge, and are generated and tested by means of congruent, yet diverse processes of inquiry (Table 4-1), we maintain that each pattern of knowing may be regarded as a type of theory. These four types of theories are subject to different types of inquiry. Henceforth, then, we will refer to the patterns of knowing as empirical theories, ethical theories, personal theories, and aesthetic theories. Our decision to regard the patterns of knowing as types of theories is supported by Chinn and Kramer's (1999) reference to ethical theories and Chinn's (2001) articulation of a theory of the art of nursing. Other global perspectives indicate the direction of diverse patterns of knowing as types of theories. For example, Scandinavian nurses view nursing within a caring science model, and they acknowledge personal knowing, personal characteristics, and moral and aesthetic knowing of caring practices as theoretical ways of knowing that elicit diverse forms of evidence (Dahlberg, 1995, Fagerstrom & Bergdom Engberg, 1998; Kyle, 1995; Snyder, Brandt, & Tseng, 2000; von Post & Eriksson, 2000).

Furthermore, we, like some of our international colleagues, maintain that the content of ethical, personal, and aesthetic theories can be formalized as sets of concepts and propositions, just as the content of many empirical theories has been so formalized (Fawcett, 1999; von Post & Eriksson, 2000). Moreover, regarding all four patterns of knowing as types of theories reintroduces the notions of uncertainty and tentativeness that typically are associated with empirical theories (Fagerstrom & Bergdom Engberg, 1998; Morse, 1996; Polit & Hungler, 1995).

The four types of theories constitute much, if not all, of the knowledge needed for nursing practice. A potentially informative analysis, which follows from the conclusion that the patterns of knowing can be regarded as sets of theories, is the examination of extant theories to determine in which pattern of knowing each is located. That analysis is, however, beyond the scope of this paper and will not be pursued here. Rather, we are attempting to make connections between the four types of theories, representing the four patterns of knowing, and what constitutes evidence for nursing practice.

On Evidence

These four types of theories underlie all methodological decisions, and they are the basis for generating multiple forms of evidence. The question of what constitutes evidence depends, in part, on what one regards as the basis of the evidence. We maintain that theory is the reason for and the value of the evidence. In other words, evidence itself refers to evidence about theories. Similarly, theory determines what counts as evidence. Thus, theory and evidence become inextricably linked, just as theory and inquiry are inextricably linked.

Any form of evidence has to be interpreted and critiqued by each person who is considering whether the theory can be applied in a particular practice situation. This view indicates acknowledgment of diverse forms of knowing as inherent in any global or cultural

interpretation of knowledge or theory (Zoucha & Reeves, 1999). The four types of theories are diverse ontological and epistemological lenses through which evidence is both interpreted and critiqued. The current emphasis on the technical-rational model of empirical evidence denies or ignores the existence of a theory lens. In contrast, our theory-guided model of evidence requires and acknowledges interpretation and critique of diverse forms of evidence. As shown in Table 4-1, we regard the scientific data produced by empirical research as the evidence for empirical theories. We count as scientific both qualitative and quantitative data and we support the call for qualitative outcome analysis (Kyle, 1995; Morse, Penrod, & Hupcey, 2000; Snyder et al., 2000). The evidence for ethical theories is illustrated in formalized statements of nurses' values, such as standards of practice, codes of ethics, and philosophies of nursing. The evidence for personal theories is found in autobiographical stories about the genuine, authentic self. The evidence for aesthetic theories is manifested or expressed as aesthetic criticism of the art and act of nursing and through works of art, such as paintings, drawings, sculpture, poetry, fiction and nonfiction, dance, and others.

Our view of the reason for evidence differs from the prevailing discussion in the literature. In current literature, typically a procedure or intervention is presented in isolation from the theory that undergirds that procedure or intervention, and in isolation from the value of the evidence. Hence the term, "evidence-based practice." We maintain that the more appropriate term is "theory-guided, evidence-based practice" (Walker & Redmond, 1999). Given the diversity of kinds of theories needed for nursing practice (See Table 4-1), evidence must extend beyond the current emphasis on empirical research and randomized clinical trials, to the kinds of evidence also generated from ethical theories, personal theories, and aesthetic theories.

Our view of the diversity of types of theories and the type of evidence needed for each type of theory addresses, at least in part, current criticisms of the evidence-based practice movement. We agree with Mitchell (1999) that the "proponents of evidence-based practice have … grossly oversimplified and misrepresented the process of nursing" (p. 34). Mitchell was particularly concerned that "The notion of evidence-based practice is not only a barren possibility but also that evidence-based practice obstructs nursing process, human care, and professional accountability" (p. 30). We respond to Mitchell's concern by including evidence about personal theories, which include authenticity in nurse-patient interpersonal relationships. Moreover, Mitchell (1999) maintained that "Evidence-based practice does not support the shift to patient-centered care, and it is inconsistent with the values and interests of consumers" (p. 34). Here, we respond to Mitchell's concerns by including evidence about ethical theories, which include the values of nurses. Mitchell (1999) also was concerned that "Evidence-based practice, if taken seriously, may restrain some nurses from defining the values and theories that guide the nurse-person process" (p. 31) and relationship. This point relates to our view that the art of nursing is expressed through the nurse-person process and the evidence derived from interpretations of tests of aesthetic theories and ethical theories.

Furthermore, our view of the diversity of types of theories and corresponding types of evidence needed for theory-guided, evidence-based nursing practice elaborates Ingersoll's (2000) definition of evidence-based nursing practice. Her definition is as follows: "Evidence-based nursing practice is the conscientious, explicit, and judicious use of theory-derived, research-based information in making decisions about care delivery to individuals or groups of patients and in consideration of individual needs and preferences" (p. 152). Our view makes explicit the multiple kinds of theories—ethical, personal, aesthetic, and empirical—whereas Ingersoll's reference to theory could easily be construed to mean only empirical theory or, perhaps because of the reference to individual needs and preferences, to include empirical and aesthetic theories.

We maintain the appropriateness of recognizing and appreciating empirical, ethical, personal, and aesthetic theories and the corresponding critique and interpretation of the evidence about each kind of theory. Such critique and interpretation of evidence is crucial for nursing practice because it is embedded in the values and phenomena located within a broad array of nursing theories. Moreover, by recognizing the four types of theories, more nurses and other health professionals may appreciate and use theories. They may agree with us that theories and values are the starting point for the critique and interpretation of any evidence needed to support clinical practices that may enhance the quality of life of the public we serve.

Conclusions

We invite readers to expand the dialogue about theory-guided, evidence-based practice. We urge nurses everywhere to consider the implications and consequences of the current virtually exclusive emphasis on empirical theories and empirical evidence-based nursing practice. We urge our nurse colleagues throughout the world to join us and those who have accurately pointed to the limitations of viewing nursing as a strictly empirical endeavor (Bolton, 2000; Dahlberg, 1995; Fagerstrom & Bergdom Engberg, 1998; Hall, 1997; Zocha & Reeves, 1999) to consider what might be gained by recognition and development of ethical, personal, and aesthetic theories and by formalization of those kinds of theories. Accordingly, we encourage all nurses to actualize their claim of a holistic approach to practice by adopting a more comprehensive description of evidence-based nursing practice, a descriptive that allows for critique and interpretation of evidence obtained from inquiry guided by ethical, personal, aesthetic, and empirical theories, as well as by any other kinds theories that may emerge from new understandings of nursing as a human science and a professional practice discipline.

REFERENCES

Bolton, S. C. (2000). Who cares? Offering emotional work as a "gift" in the nursing labor process. *Journal of Advanced Nursing, 32*, 580–586.

Carper, B. A. (1978). Fundamental patterns of knowing in nursing. *Advances in Nursing Science, 1*(1), 13–23.

Chinn, P. L. (2001). Toward a theory of nursing art. In N. L. Chaska (Ed.), *The nursing profession: Tomorrow and beyond* (287–297). Thousand Oaks, CA: Sage.

Chinn, P. L., & Kramer, M. K. (1999). *Theory and nursing: Integrated knowledge development* (5th ed.). St. Louis, MO: Mosby.

Dahlberg, K. (1995) Qualitative methodology as Caring Science Methodology. *Scandinavian Journal of Caring Science, 9*, 187–191.

Fagerstrom, L., & Bergdom Engberg, I. (1998) Measuring the unmeasurable: A caring science perspective on patient classification. *Journal of Nursing Management, 6*, 165–172.

Fawcett, J. (1999). *The relationship of theory and research* (3rd ed.). Philadelphia: F. A. Davis.

Hall, E. O. C. (1997). Four generations of nurse theorists in the U.S.: An overview of their questions and answers. *Vardi Norden: Nursing Science and Research in the Nordic Countries, 17* (2), 15–23.

Ingersoll, G. L. (2000). Evidence-based nursing: What it is and what it isn't. *Nursing Outlook, 48*, 151–152.

Kyle, T. V. (1995). The concept of caring: A review of the literature. *Journal of Advanced Nursing, 21*, 506–514.

Mitchell, G. J. (1999). Evidence-based practice: Critique and alternative view. *Nursing Science Quarterly, 12*, 30–35.

Morse, J. M. (1996). Nursing scholarship: Sense and sensibility. *Nursing Inquiry, 3*, 74–82.

Morse, J. M., Penrod, J., & Hupcey, J. E. (2000). Qualitative outcome analysis: Evaluating nursing interventions for complex clinical phenomena. *Journal of Nursing Scholarship, 32*, 125–130.

Polit, D. F., & Hungler, B. P. (1995). *Nursing research: Principles and methods* (5th ed.). Philadelphia: Lippincott.

Snyder, M., Brandt, C. L., & Tseng, Y. (2000). Measuring intervention outcomes: Impact of nurse characteristics. *International Journal of Human Caring, 5*(3), 36–42.

Stein, K. F., Corte, C., Colling, K. B., & Whall, A. (1998). A theoretical analysis of Carper's ways of knowing using a model of social cognition. *Scholarly Inquiry for Nursing Practice, 12*, 43–60.

Upton, D. J. (1999). How can we achieve evidence-based practice if we have theory-practice gap in nursing today? *Journal of Advanced Nursing, 29*, 549–555.

von Post, I., & Eriksson, K. (2000). The ideal and practice concepts of "Professional Nursing Care." *International Journal for Human Caring, 5*(3), 14–22.

Walker, P. H., & Redmond, R. (1999). Theory-guided, evidence-based reflective practice. *Nursing Science Quarterly, 12,* 298–303.

Watson, J. (1999). *Postmodern nursing and beyond.* New York: Churchill Livingstone.

Zoucha, R., & Reeves, J. (1999). A view of professional caring as personal for Mexican Americans. *International Journal of Human Caring, 3*(3), 14–20.

THE AUTHORS COMMENT | On Nursing Theories and Evidence

This article was the result of a meeting convened by Patricia Hinton Walker, then dean of the University of Colorado School of Nursing, with Jean Watson, Betty Neuman, Joyce Fitzpatrick, and me. Our task was to identify the major issues in nursing theory development. I took the lead in writing a paper that addressed the need for a comprehensive view of evidence-based nursing practice. The result was this article, the content of which we drew from the seminal work by Carper on patterns of knowing in nursing and the expansion of that work by Chinn and Kramer. If the discipline of nursing is to advance in the 21st century, nurses must acknowledge multiple types of theories and sources of evidence for theory-guided evidence-based nursing rather than rely solely on empiric theory and evidence from only controlled clinical trials.

JACQUELINE FAWCETT
JEAN WATSON
BETTY NEUMAN
PATRICIA H. WALKER
JOYCE J. FITZPATRICK

Integration of Nursing Theory and Nursing Ethics*

MICHAEL YEO, PhD

*N*ursing theory and nursing ethics are two main areas of inquiry in nursing scholarship today. Each addresses common themes and each, in its own way, speaks not only about but for nursing. In spite of this commonality there is remarkably little dialogue between them. Both theory and ethics shall benefit from increased integration.

Nursing today is a profession in flux and a profession profoundly self-critical and self-examining. This self-examination is primarily taking place in two proliferating areas of scholarship, nursing theory and nursing ethics. A rich dialogue exists within each of these areas but remarkably little communication occurs between them.

One important shared factor behind the rapid growth of scholarship both in nursing theory and nursing ethics is the ascending importance of professionalism in nursing. Although the rhetoric of professionalism has been around for some time—as early as 1900 Nightingale[1] was proclaiming that nursing had become a profession—developments in the 1950s marked a decisive turning point.[2,3] This is evidenced by increased emphasis on fundamental questions having to do with the education, role, and responsibility unique and proper to nursing. A more radical questioning has occurred about the nurse's role and responsibility in relation to patients, other health care professionals, and society in general. Both nursing theory and nursing ethics attempt to come to terms with such issues and define a distinct professional identity for nursing.

Dispute about the necessary requirements for a profession exists, but there is some consensus on at least two demarcating criteria: a profession must possess a distinct knowledge base and it also must possess some ethical standards to which its practitioners can be held accountable.[4,5] Nursing theory addresses the first requirement, nursing ethics the second.

There is a remarkable lack of communication between nursing theory and nursing ethics. They address common questions and themes but, judging from the scant cross-referencing, each does so independently of the other. For example, Roy,[6] in her most recent account of the adaptation model, does not cite any works

in the nursing ethics literature. Conversely, Muyskens,[7] in a major investigation of the philosophical and ethical foundations of nursing, cites none of the major theorists. Although nursing theory and nursing ethics are mutually relevant, for the most part this has gone unremarked.

Relevance of Nursing Ethics to Nursing Theory

In order to disclose the relevance of nursing ethics to nursing theory, it is important to call into question what might appear to be a fundamental difference separating the two. This difference centers on the idea, or better, the ideal of science. Science is highly valued in the nursing theory literature. To be sure, the sense in which a nursing theory could be said to be scientific, and the sense in which nursing science is science, has been much debated. This debate has taken into account the discussions among philosophers of science about the nature of science and of scientific method.[8,9] Nevertheless, the requirement much in evidence is that theory, if it is to be legitimate, must meet some criteria for being scientific.

This valuation of science is largely a response to the search for a legitimate knowledge base for nursing, which in turn is part of nursing's general drive for professionalism.[10] Science commands authority and power in this society, and was bound to appeal to nursing theorists as a sure route to professional legitimacy and status. Even while attempting to define a professional identity distinct from medicine, nursing theory chose the same proven path to professional legitimacy.

Nursing ethics, on the other hand, has not conferred such value on science. It has not, and in the nature of the discipline, could not have, aspired to being scientific. Ethics is almost by definition a nonexact discipline, although a discipline nonetheless.

*This article was supported by a grant from Associated Medical Services and the Richard and Jean Ivey Fund.

ABOUT THE AUTHOR

MICHAEL YEO is a philosopher who special-izes in ethics, particularly professional ethics. He received his PhD in philosophy from McMaster University. He was a researcher at the Westminster Institute for Ethics and Human Values for 5 years, during which time he wrote this article. He subsequently worked as an ethicist for the Canadian Medical Association for 5 years, during which time his primary area of research was (and remains) health privacy. He is a Professor in the Department of Philosophy and M.A. at Laurentian University in Sudbury, Ontario, Canada.

Ethics, and nursing ethics in particular, make use of science where appropriate, but with an awareness that science only goes so far in sorting out value questions by helping us to better understand their empirical dimension, for nursing ethics is above all concerned with values and value conflicts arising out of nursing practice and research. Ultimately questions of value must necessarily escape the scientist's probing forceps.

This difference between nursing theory and nurs-ing ethics conceals more than it reveals. Nursing theo-ries, some more explicitly than others, invariably have assumptions about the kind of value issues under dis-cussion in the nursing ethics literature, although too often these are not identified or explicitly thematized as ethical issues. The rhetoric of science, and espe-cially the pretense to objectivity characteristic of the received view, has had the effect of obscuring the val-ues dimension of nursing theory.[11] An argument could be made that other views of science might not have this effect and this may be so, but the fact is that until recently it has been a more or less standard view of science that has dominated nursing theory.

Roy's[6] model is a good example of how overvalu-ing science can obscure decisive ethical issues in nurs-ing theory. The adaptation model is thick with values and value choices, but they are concealed in the shad-ows cast by Roy's overt commitment to the ideology of science. Questions of value extend even to her choice of language. The vernacular is quite self-consciously borrowed from physiology and behavioral science, a decision already subject to ethical scrutiny. Terms like stimulus, response, and adaptation are not value neutral. They come from and yield a certain view of man (there is valuation in gender too), and are in marked contrast to terms employed in more humanistic language games.

The term managing stimuli, for example, which Roy[6] has lately adopted for describing nursing inter-vention, is not without important value assump-tions and implications. The management metaphor conceptualizes the nurse as in some sense having a superior role in the nurse-patient relationship: the nurse manages, the patient adapts. This is reinforced by carving up the patient's life-world into stimuli, a conceptualization somewhat removed from the terms in which patients conceptualize their own expe-rience. The language itself creates an epistemic barrier between patient and nurse and is less than conducive to dialogue or partnership, as nurses have learned from experience with the scientific but user-unfriendly ver-nacular of medicine.

There is also a values dimension to the definition of men as adaptive systems. Roy herself has come to see problems here. She claims that she "adds human-istic values to this scientific concept [the person as an adaptive system]" and admits that "these values received little attention in the earlier writings."[6(p25)] However, this is misleading. Rather than saying that she later adds humanistic values, it would be more accurate to say that she earlier subtracted them.

Related to the above point, there is valuation in the idea or ideal of adaptation. How does one dis-tinguish adaptation from ineffective responses? By what norms? More importantly, by whose norms, the nurse's or the patient's? Who decides? To be sure, Roy does expressly endorse "the humanistic approach of valuing other person's opinions and viewpoints."[6(p36)] Indeed, in another writing, Roy and Roberts go even further, maintaining that according to their model, "the person is to be respected as an active participant in his care. … The goal arrived at is one of mutual agreement between the nurse and patient. Interven-tions are the options that the nurse provides for the patient."[12(p47)] This rhetoric is not congruent with the rest of Roy's model, however, and especially the sec-tions of *Introduction to Nursing*[6] entitled *"Criteria for Setting Priorities," "Goal Setting,"* and *"Intervention,"* in which the patient maintains virtually no voice at all. The humanistic values are appended virtually as an afterthought, and are not integrated throughout the model. If these values are to be taken seriously, it is not enough to add them to a scientific base—the model needs to be reconstructed from the ground up.

Notwithstanding certain explicit statements to the contrary, Roy's adaptation model is heavily biased toward paternalism. The nurse is in a privileged posi-tion to set goals and plan interventions mandated by his or her guiding science. Since the patient does not have such knowledge and since this knowledge is expressed in a language that is difficult for the uninitiated to comprehend, the patient is on very unequal footing concerning setting goals, planning care, and so forth. It is difficult to achieve mutual agreement between partners who speak different languages, especially when one of the languages is highly abstract and bears the authoritative ring of science.

It is telling that in *Introduction to Nursing* (no less than 500 pages), Roy[6] does not speak expressly about patient autonomy. Given the considerable advocacy movement in nursing, this is quite remarkable. It is, however, understandable, given Roy's scientific orientation. When the person is defined as an adaptive system (a definition mainly fleshed out in physiologic terms) there is not much room for autonomy (or for the person to be humanistically understood). Roy may be an extreme example, but it is generally true that questions having to do with autonomy and paternalism, questions that reach to the core of the nursing profession, are seldom tackled directly by nursing theorists.

Nursing theory is rife with value dimensions—only a few have been touched here—but too often these are not brought to the fore and made the theme of analysis. There is a tendency for nursing theory to obscure its own operative norms. Typically, theorists present their work as if it were merely descriptive (science is not supposed to be normative), as if they were merely stating what nursing is. In fact, all of them, directly or indirectly, are also taking a stand on what nursing should be, and offering recommendations for the future direction of the profession—recommendations that cannot be evaluated on scientific grounds alone.

Thus, it is conceptually muddled and highly misleading to divide nursing theories into those that are valuational (normative) and those that are descriptive (scientific) as does Walker,[13] positing different standards of evaluation for each. All nursing theories, however scientific, are in some considerable measure normative or valuational, although some more self-consciously than others. They are structurally cemented with values throughout. The key definitions of nursing theory—human beings, nurse, health, environment (society)—are thickly laden with value. Disputes about them, for the most part, are not of a sort that science alone can be expected to resolve. As Gadow writes, "the very definition of nursing is an ethical problem—moreover the most fundamental and pressing ethical problem facing nursing today."[14(p93)]

One should not have to decipher the ethical face of a nursing theory behind the mask of science. The values dimension of nursing theories should be brought more out into the open and tackled more directly. Ethical issues should be identified as such and confronted head on. Here nursing theorists would stand to benefit from increased dialogue with those working in nursing ethics, who have taken as their

focus the values dimension of nursing. This dimension has been somewhat obscured in nursing theory owing to the value it places on science, or perhaps even on a narrow view of science, it being an open question whether other views of science might not be more congruent with ethical interests.

 ## Evaluation of Nursing Theories

The potential for overenthusiasm about science to eclipse ethical considerations in nursing theory is even more evident at the level of theory evaluation. To pick a somewhat early example, King,[15] placing a great deal of value on the scientificity of nursing theories, lists ten criteria for theory evaluation, none of which explicitly addresses the ethical dimension of nursing theories. Theory evaluation has become much more sophisticated since then, but the scientific paradigm (and frequently a very narrow interpretation of it) continues to dominate at the expense of sensitivity to ethical dimensions of nursing theory.

Parse,[16] a theorist who is more explicit about values than most, nevertheless sacrifices ethical concerns at the altar of science when it comes to speaking about theory evaluation. Following Kaplan,[17] she distinguishes between structure and process criteria for evaluation. Value considerations are implicit in the detailed analysis she gives of these criteria, but nowhere are they explicitly stated. This omission is telling, but all the more so given that she deems esthetic criteria significant enough to warrant special reference.[16] Surely if esthetics is worthy of honorable mention, ethics is all the more so, especially given nursing's traditional sensitivity to ethical matters.

Even Chinn and Jacobs,[18] who are otherwise refreshingly open-eyed about the limitations of the scientific ideal, do not escape its allure when it comes to theory evaluation. They are certainly to be lauded for acknowledging that there are other patterns of knowing besides the scientific one, and for assigning a legitimate place to moral knowledge or ethics in nursing as distinct from empirics. They call for the "integration of all patterns."[18(p17)] of knowing, and this *holistic* ideal approximates what this article advocates. Furthermore, they point out that "the assumptions and purposes of scientific theory form the template against which nursing theories have been judged, although many traits of theories in general and nursing theories in particular both draw on and reflect other patterns of knowing besides empirics."[18(p7)] Nevertheless, when it comes to presenting their criteria for evaluation, the guidelines they offer, although broader than many, remain dominated by the scientific ideal and concentrated on empirics. They list clarity, simplicity, generality, empirical applicability, and consequences (more or less a rehash of the familiar scientific standards), and neglect to include an evaluative category addressing the values dimension of theory in a direct manner.[18] Presumably, the value assumptions of nursing theory with respect to such matters as patient autonomy, nursing autonomy, advocacy, and so on, do not count. If, as the authors state, the integration of the various patterns of knowledge is desirable, what better place to start than in the evaluation of nursing theory?

Nursing theorists and those writing about nursing theory evaluation need to become more reflective about the fact that evaluation is valuation. More scrutiny needs to be given to the various elements that are valued and why this is so. Why are ethical (value) considerations typically overlooked or even excluded in theory evaluation? Why should simplicity be valued or evaluated while something like the moral basis of the theory is not valued at all? Could it be that, dazzled by the allure of science and obsessed with being scientific, evaluators have been somewhat blinded to questions of ethics and values?

Relevance of Nursing Theory to Nursing Ethics

If nursing theory stands to benefit from the kind of questioning that takes place in nursing ethics, so too nursing ethics stands to benefit from the not inconsiderable achievements of nursing theory. Just as nursing theorists have sought to carve an identity for nursing distinct from the medical model, there is also growing concern to develop nursing ethics as a unique field of enquiry, and something "more than a footnote to medical ethics,"[19(p72)] as Yarling and McElmurry have put it.

> *Nursing theorists and those writing about nursing theory evaluation need to become more reflective about the fact that evaluation is valuation.*

Nursing ethics today is reaching to find its own voice, an endeavor in which nursing theory, even if overly concerned about sounding scientific, is qualified to furnish some guidance. Gadow comments that in framing ethical problems, "nursing regrettably has retained medicine as its referent in an area of concern where nurses most need to engage in independent, critically reflective self-examination."[14(p92)] Gadow's remark should be qualified, since it would not apply to everyone working in nursing ethics, but overall her characterization of the state of affairs is insightful. The general tendency has been to adopt a ready-made ethics and bring it to bear on the nursing profession.

Scholarship in nursing ethics can be divided roughly into two streams, each borrowing its conceptual paradigm from a different source. On the one side, the ethical theory approach borrows heavily from moral philosophy. On the other the moral development approach borrows heavily from developmental psychology.

The Ethical Theory Approach

What James and Dickoff[20] have claimed about Beckstrand[21] could be applied to the ethical theory approach. They charge that "Beckstrand takes some selected version of what is ethics,"[20(p58)] as being authoritative, seemingly unaware that ethics is itself a contentious discipline, embracing a broad diversity of often conflicting opinions. To be sure, nursing ethicists do acknowledge some diversity. Almost everyone makes the standard distinction between deontologic and teleologic theories. However, the scope of this diversity is narrowly circumscribed.

Nursing ethics primarily borrows its framework for ordering ethical theories from medical ethics. By itself, this would not be so significant were it not that medical ethics has been very selective in circumscribing the discipline of ethics. The focus is placed almost exclusively on Kant and Mill, while other legitimate contenders are buried in the background. A list of neglected or even excluded voices would include names like Aristotle, Plato, Spinoza, Kierkegaard, and Nietzsche, all of whom wrote substantial works in ethics. Why has nursing ethics uncritically subscribed to the same canon as medical ethics? How different might the ethical landscape of nursing appear if existentialism, for example, enjoyed the same privilege accorded to utilitarianism in the nursing ethics literature?

Nursing ethics has borrowed from medical ethics not only its list of canonical authors, but also certain ways of relating to ethical issues. What White[22] calls formula ethics is a case in point. Formula ethics "involves applying ethical theories to specific situations and suggesting, for instance, what the contractarian versus the utilitarian position might be."[22(p42)] Carroll and Humphrey's[23] *Moral Problems in Nursing* is typical: "I feel I used Kant's theory when I refused to call the police and have Ms B committed for I was respecting her autonomy."[23(p82)] It is a mistake to think that Kant's theory can be used like a cookie cutter to shape the moral situation of nursing into tidy resolutions. Moreover, if one has to derive one's respect for autonomy from an ethical theory, one is in deep trouble. Nurses have practiced respect for autonomy long before Kant was brought into the hospital setting.

Formula ethics is misguided for several reasons, and not least of all because it simplifies ethical positions almost to the point of caricature. More importantly, however, it reduces ethical practice to correct technique, and promotes an overly mechanical (and therefore insensitive) comportment to ethical problems. The moral situation of nursing is squeezed into imported categories that are applied in a top-down fashion. The danger is that the experience of nursing will be distorted or otherwise denied.

While it would be folly to ignore the rich untapped resources of ethical theory, it is important to be critical in bringing them to bear on the moral situation of nursing. Those working in nursing ethics are becoming increasingly critical of the ethical theory approach. There is a growing desire for an ethic that issues from nursing itself, rather than one borrowed from elsewhere and applied from the top down. Bishop and Scudder exemplify this in urging that nursing ethics should begin "with the moral sense of nursing rather than with ethical theory."[24(p42)] This sentiment is echoed by Packard and Ferrara, who maintain that "the moral foundation of nursing will have to derive from bold excursions into the meaning of nursing."[25(p63)] What does it mean to speak of the "meaning of nursing," however? Where would one look to find such a thing?

Nursing theory would be a good place to start. If nursing ethics must borrow, why not borrow from the rich tradition of nursing theory, which at least has the advantage over ethical theory of being derived from nursing experience? Nursing theory could play an important role in a bottom-up approach to nursing ethics. It offers an alternative made-in-nursing framework (or rather several) in which to think about humans, health, environment, society, and the meaning of nursing. Nursing theory tackles these fundamentals at the very outset, whereas nursing ethics has tended to be somewhat more narrow in its focus. The tendency has been to focus on cases, which are analyzed along the traditional lines of autonomy, paternalism, and beneficence. Nursing theory can teach nursing ethics to think more profoundly about the meaning of nursing and help to broaden the frame of reference in which ethical questions are being examined. It may be illuminating in ways hardly imaginable to rethink the stock ethical terms—autonomy, justice, beneficence—in light of nursing theory.

The Moral Development Approach

The moral development approach in nursing ethics differs from the ethical theory approach by being more empirical. It looks at the moral situation of nursing

with an eye to how nurses actually respond to ethical issues, and analyzes the moral behavior of nurses in light of models of moral development. At one level, one could contrast the ethical theory approach to the moral development approach as the normative to the descriptive, but this would be misleading. Models of moral development are not value neutral, and norms come into play in describing moral behavior in the framework of a given model.

> *The moral development approach in nursing ethics shares with the ethical theory approach the habit of borrowing uncritically.*

The moral development approach in nursing ethics shares with the ethical theory approach the habit of borrowing uncritically. In particular, the work of Kohlberg[26] has exerted a profound influence on research on the moral development of nurses. Ketefian[27-31] has been a major catalyst in this area. Without negating the value of her work, it is fair to say that she has not been very critical in her acceptance of the paradigm for moral development laid out by Kohlberg. For the most part, she has accepted it as being authoritative without interrogating its fundamental norms. This is ironic, since the model's overarching norm is autonomy, which calls for such interrogation. Kohlberg has always had his detractors, but recent work by Gilligan[32] has cast his model in a critical light that is particularly illuminating for nursing. Gilligan found that, as a group, women score differently than men on Kohlberg's moral development scale. If one accepted Kohlberg's value premises, one would have to say that women score lower than men. Gilligan's innovation was to interpret this difference in a positive way. Rather than accepting the norms supporting Kohlberg's scale and interpreting this difference as deficiency, she made a virtue of it, and used it to call into question the fundamental values of Kohlberg's theory. Women do indeed define moral issues differently, but this difference is not a minus. Gilligan calls this difference the ethic of care, which is different from, but not subordinate to, the ethic of justice presupposed as norm in Kohlberg's theory. She celebrates the ethic of care as being the different voice of women.[32] Interestingly, Gilligan's work converges with that of James and Dickoff,[20] who, inspired by the French feminist Helene Cixous,[33] advanced a new ethic for nursing based on reciprocal nurturance.

The moral lesson to be drawn from Gilligan's critique of Kohlberg is a profound one: rather than trying to speak the language that happens to be authoritative, one should learn to speak unashamedly in one's own voice and to celebrate one's difference rather than apologize for it. This lesson has special relevance for nursing. Applying Gilligan's work to nursing, Huggins and Scalzi write, "If an ethical base for nursing practice is built on the ethics of justice, and the nurse's orientation is the ethic of care of another model, there will continue to be a denial of the nurse's own voice."[34(p46)] Uncritical borrowing can lead to the denial of the unique experience of nursing and to the disvaluation of the ethic of care to which Gilligan,[32] turning Kohlberg upside down, assigns a positive evaluation.

Directing their concerns specifically to Ketefian,[27-31] Huggins and Scalzi caution, "A theory of ethical practice, as is sought by Ketefian, is essential to the maturation of the nursing profession, but it must be carefully built to speak to the true voice and experience of nursing."[34(p44)] This is a very important point, but it raises a difficult question: What is the true voice and experience of nursing? Perhaps there is no one true voice, but there are several voices, the voices of nursing theorists speaking about the experience of nursing. Anyone undertaking to develop an ethic for nursing based on the experience of nursing would do well to begin by listening carefully to those voices.

Nursing theory and nursing ethics speak about and for nursing, an onerous challenge and responsibility for a profession so self-conscious and self-examining. Each, in its own way, is searching to find its own voice. To this end, would it not be desirable for each to broaden the parameters of its conversation and listen to the voice of the other? Only by joining together can the voices of nursing theory and nursing ethics hope to lay legitimate claim to be the voice of nursing.

REFERENCES

1. Nightingale, F., cited in Palmer IS.: From whence we came, in Chaska NL. (ed): The *Nursing Profession: A Time to Speak*. New York, McGraw-Hill, 1983.
2. Crowley, D. M.: Perspectives of pure science. Nurs Res 1968;17:497–499.
3. Aydelotte M. K.: Issues of professional nursing: The need for clinical excellence. *Nurs Forum* 1968;7(1):73675.
4. Conway, M. E.: Prescription for professionalization, in Chaska NL (ed): *The Nursing Profession: A Time to Speak*. New York, McGraw-Hill, 1983.
5. Greenwood, E.: Attributes of a profession, in Baumrin B., Freedman B. (eds): *Moral Responsibility and the Professions*. New York, Haven, 1983.
6. Roy, C.: Introduction to Nursing: An Adaptation Model, ed. 2. Englewood Cliffs, NJ, Prentice-Hall, 1984.
7. Muyskens, J. L. *Moral Problems in Nursing: A Philosophical Investigation*. Totowa, NJ, Rowman and Littlefield, 1982.
8. Meleis, A. I.: *Theoretical Nursing: Development and Progress*. New York, Lippincott, 1985.
9. Watson, J.: Nursing's scientific quest. *Nurs Outlook* 1981;29:413–416.
10. Johnson, D. E.: The nature of a science of nursing. *Nurs Outlook* 1959;7:291–294.
11. Tucker, R. W.: The value decisions we know as science. *Adv Nurs Sci* 1979;1(2):1–12.
12. Roy, C., Roberts, S. L.: *Theory Construction in Nursing: An Adaptation Model*. Englewood Cliffs, NJ, Prentice-Hall, 1981.
13. Walker, L. O.: Theory and research in the development of nursing as a discipline: Retrospect and prospect, in Chaska, N. L. (ed): *The Nursing Profession: A Time to Speak*. New York, McGraw-Hill, 1983.
14. Gadow, S.: ANS open forum. *Adv Nurs Sci* 1979;1(3):92–95.
15. King, I.: *Toward a Theory for Nursing: General Concepts of Human Behaviour*. New York, Wiley, 1971.
16. Parse, R. R.: Paradigms and theories, in Parse, R. R. (ed): *Nursing Science: Major Paradigms, Theories and Critiques*. Philadelphia, Saunders, 1987.
17. Kaplan, A.: *The Conduct of Scientific Inquiry*. Scranton, Penn, Chandlisher, 1964.
18. Chinn, P. L., Jacobs, M. K.: *Theory and Nursing: A systematic Approach*, St. Louis, Mosby, 1983.
19. Yarling, R. R., McElmurry, B. J.: The moral foundation of nursing. *Adv Nurs Sci* 1986;8(2):63–73.
20. James, P., Dickoff, J.: Toward a cultivated but decisive pluralism for nursing, in McGee (ed): *Theoretical Pluralism in Nursing*. Ottawa, University of Ottawa Press, 1982.
21. Beckstrand, J.: The notion of practise theory and the relationship of scientific and ethical knowledge to practise. *Res Nurs Health* 1978;1(3):131–136.
22. White, G. B.: Philosophical ethics and nursing—a word of caution, in Chinn, P. L. (ed): *Advances in Nursing Theory and Development*. Rockville, Md, Aspen, 1983.
23. Carroll, M. A., Humphrey, R. A.: *Moral Problems in Nursing: Case Studies*. Washington, University Press of America, 1979.
24. Bishop, A. H., Scudder, J. R.: Nursing ethics in an age of controversy. *Adv Nurs Sci* 1987;9(3):34–43.
25. Packard, J. S., Ferrara, M. S. N.: In search of the moral foundation of nursing. *Adv Nurs Sci* 1988;10(4):60–71.
26. Kohlberg, L.: The cognitive developmental approach to moral education, in Scharf, P. (ed): *Readings on Moral Education*. Minneapolis, Minn: Winston Press, 1978.
27. Ketefian, S.: Critical thinking, educational preparation, and development of moral judgment among selected groups of practising nurses. *Nurs Res* 1981;30:98–103.
28. Ketefian, S.: Moral reasoning and moral behavior among selected groups of practising nurses. *Nurs Res* 1981;30: 171–176.
29. Ketefian, S.: Tool development in nursing: Construction of a scale to measure moral behavior. *J NY State Nurs Assoc* 1982;13:13–18.
30. Ketefian, S.: Professional and bureaucratic role conceptions and moral behavior in nursing. *Nurs Res* 1985;34:248–253.
31. Ketefian, S.: A case study of theory development: Moral behavior in nursing. *Adv Nurs Sci* 1987;9(2):10–19.
32. Gilligan, C.: *In a Different Voice: Psychological Theory and Women's Development*. Cambridge, Harvard University Press, 1982.
33. Marks, E., de Courtivron, I. (eds): *New French Feminisms, an Anthology*. New York, Schocken Press, 1981.
34. Huggins, E. A., Scalzi, C. C.: Limitations and alternatives: Ethical practice theory in nursing. *Adv Nurs Sci* 1988;10(4):43–47.

THE AUTHOR COMMENTS — Integration of Nursing Theory and Nursing Ethics

Professor Marguerite Warner, who was then on the Faculty of Nursing at the University of Western Ontario, first introduced me to nursing theory. Her passion for the subject was infectious, and I learned much from her (and miss our conversations). As I worked through the nursing theory literature, I was struck by what I believed to be an uncritical and unwise deference to science and lack of attention to ethics, which was surprising to me, given nursing's rich tradition of ethical reflection. I believe that nursing theory should be grounded primarily not in science but in ethics. The articulation of this viewpoint in this article is my modest contribution to dialogue in and about nursing theory.

MICHAEL YEO

6

A Treatise on Nursing Knowledge Development for the 21st Century: Beyond Postmodernism

PAMELA G. REED, RN, PhD, FAAN

This article explicates a framework for nursing knowledge development that incorporates both modernist and postmodernist philosophies. The framework derives from an "open philosophy" of science, which links science, philosophy, and practice in development of nursing knowledge. A neomodernist perspective is proposed that upholds modernist values for unified conceptualizations of nursing reality while recognizing the dynamic and value-laden nature of all levels of theory and metatheory. It is proposed that scientific inquiry extend beyond the postmodern critique to identify nursing metanarratives of nursing philosophy and nursing practice that serve as external correctives in the critique process. Philosophic positions related to the science, philosophy, and practice domains are put forth for continued dialogue about future directions for knowledge development in nursing.

Among the transitions currently facing nursing is the ending of what someday will be referred to as 20th-century nursing theorizing. For the past several years, nurses have been feeling the ground shift with the reforming of philosophic ideas that launched nursing as a science. Not since the advent of modernism and the birth of modern nursing at the end of the 19th century has nursing science been faced with such a wealth of possibilities for knowledge development. These possibilities have their roots in modernism to be sure, but they also are nurtured by the current dialogue postmodern thought has precipitated.

Postmodernism has engaged nursing in a dialogue to reconcile a basic awareness about the uniqueness and differences in human beings and health, with basic beliefs in universals and values about human phenomena. It is a struggle, as a philosopher characterized that of feminism, to "modify the Enlightenment in the context of late modernity but not to capitulate to the postmodern condition."[1(p195)]

This article presents a framework that will help nursing science bridge modernist and postmodernist philosophies as nursing clarifies contemporary approaches to knowledge development. The framework builds on accomplishments of modernist nursing while exploiting opportunities of the postmodern context and, in this sense, is "neomodernist." The framework reaches beyond postmodern prescriptions for nursing science and proposes a neomodernist perspective on knowledge development that incorporates metanarratives of nursing philosophy and nursing practice into scientific inquiry.

Historical Background: Modernism and Postmodernism

From premodern to postmodern times, paths to knowledge have crossed through the Age of Faith, the Age of Reason, to the Culture of Critique. The once dominant religious and metaphysical approach to reasoning about reality was transformed into avenues to truth that separated philosophic "beliefs" from empiric "knowing." Empiricism supplanted the Aristotelian emphasis on rationality that had inspired early modernists. Although modern science enlightened the world and enhanced everyday life, its approach failed to deliver the anticipated empirical base for ultimate meaning and truth about human beings and their world. Also, as philosopher Popper[2] helped scientists realize during the decline of positivism, knowledge development could not be purged of biases, contradictions, and values. Theories, like the fisherman's net, inevitably influenced what data were caught by the scientist. Postmodern thought helped move scientists toward the realization about the embeddedness of research data and the transitory nature of theory.

Postmodernism is a social movement and philosophy that originated among French literary theorists in the 1960s, although postmodern ideas were expressed prior to this time.[3] Postmodernism is a perspective or intellectual style of creating art, of theorizing, of doing science. And it is influencing nursing's approach to knowledge development.

ABOUT THE AUTHOR

PAMELA G. REED is a Professor at the University of Arizona College of Nursing in Tucson, where she also served as an Associate Dean for Academic Affairs for 7 years. She is a three-time graduate of Wayne State University in Detroit, receiving a BSN, an MSN (with a double major in child–adolescent psychiatric mental health nursing and teaching), and a PhD with a major in nursing (focused on life span development and aging) in 1982. Dr. Reed pioneered research into spirituality and well-being with her doctoral research with terminally ill patients. She also developed a theory of self-transcendence and two widely used research instruments, the *Spiritual Perspective Scale* and the *Self-Transcendence Scale*. Her publications and funded research reflect a dual scholarly focus: spirituality and other facilitators of well-being in life-limiting illness, and nursing metatheory and knowledge development. Dr. Reed also enjoys time with her family, reading, classical music, swimming, and hiking in the mountains and canyons of Arizona.

Postmodernism challenges the modernist idea of a single, transcendent meaning of reality and the importance of the search for empirical patterns that correspond to and represent ultimate meaning. Metanarratives, grand or high theories, or other overarching discourses that identify essential truths and propose to represent reality are not recognized as valid. The "postmodern condition"[4] is a "crisis of confidence in the narratives of truth, science and progress that epitomized modernity"[5(p98)]—a time of paradigms lost. Instead, there is focus on understanding multiple meanings, with the belief that every representation conceals and reveals meanings and that an inextricable link exists between meaning and power.[6] Whereas modernists fragmented the whole to study parts in the attempt to ultimately unify knowledge about the world, postmodernists fragment and dissolve unities, universals, and metanarratives believed to be entangled with values and beliefs that oppress people and fabricate reality. In postmodern thought, problems are not "solved," they are "deconstructed."

Postmodernists generally deny the existence of an essence of human beings, and they have incited ardent debate on the relevance of philosophy for science, given that a central purpose of philosophy is to examine questions about the intrinsic nature of human beings and the world, truth, and knowledge.[7] In postmodern thought, then, there is no autonomous subject to study; the subject is myth. What is studied is what the culture has inscribed on the object of study; in this sense, the focus of study is text. Meaning derives from the relationship between the text and the reader, and the content is not related to an external narrative. There is no transcendent referent for the knowledge builder and no source of meaning about human beings to be discovered and re-presented to others. So, in a phrase, the gods have fled. Any truths that appear to exist have come about not through historical teleologic progress, but as a product of time and chance, contingent on someone redescribing nature in a way that is temporarily useful to the current culture and context.[8,9] Thus, there is an epistemologic shift from concern over the truth of one's findings to concern over the practical significance of the findings.

Framework for Knowledge Development

Postmodernism's iconoclastic and pluralistic attitudes are dislodging nursing from cherished norms about knowledge development that tended to dichotomize essential units of inquiry: research and practice, inductive and deductive reasoning, qualitative and quantitative data. Twenty-first century approaches to developing knowledge will transcend these dichotomies.

Nursing's knowledge development activities have not been daunted by the shifts in philosophic thought, but instead are evolving out of both modernist and postmodernist influences. Nursing is embracing a broadened definition of scholarship that employs various key sources for development of nursing knowledge. These sources derive from the empirical, conceptual, and practice activities of nurses.[10-12] However, consistent with modern science, these domains have been regarded as independent throughout most of 20th-century nursing.

Science, philosophy, and practice have typically represented "orthogonal subspaces" of a discipline; each domain exists in its own dimension and has no image or projection in the plane of the other.[13] The schisms between these subspaces are a problem inherent in knowledge development. Yet despite the orthogonality and despite even the dominance of the scientific over the spiritual or philosophic modes of thought, none has been eliminated. It is as though each subspace represents some irreducible or essential basis of knowledge development. However, the independence between the domains, as enforced by modernists, proved to be an unsatisfactory approach to inquiry.

What instead may be needed for 21st-century nursing theory development is what Polis[13] labeled an "open philosophy," which deliberately links phenomenon with noumenon and links empirical concepts that can be known through the senses with theoretical concepts of meaning and value that can be known through thought. The postmodern critique of modernism compels nursing to revisit the potential "openness" or linkages between scientific inquiry and the metanarratives of nursing philosophy and nursing practice as a means of both reforming and reaffirming nursing's approaches to knowledge development.

 ## Nursing Science: Modern and Postmodern Influences

A nursing scientist uses valid and reliable systems of inquiry to gain understanding of phenomena of human health and healing processes. The scientist links empirical findings to a conceptual level to create a theoretical story that satisfies certain epistemic criteria, such as predictive accuracy and internal coherence.[14] Nursing science's approach to linking the empirical and theoretical has changed over the history of its science.

Traditional empiricists, of which Nightingale was one, restricted their theorizing to observable processes. Nineteenth-century nursing theorizing did not include much movement up the ladder of abstraction to link empirical and theoretical. Rather than generalizing by abstraction (vertical movement), Nightingale tended to generalize by analogy (horizontal movement). For example, Nightingale's canon about the unhealthful effects of noise on sick people derived from drawing analogies across her observations of disturbing noises, such as rustling dresses, whispered conversations, musical wind instruments, and styles of speaking and reading to patients.[15] Nightingale's theorizing generated empirical generalizations. However, knowledge development by analogy left a gap between the empirical event and theoretical explanation; although this form of knowledge had some predictive power and was used to guide the practitioners of Nightingale's era, it had limited explanatory power.

Prior to and during the half-century hiatus in nursing scientific work between Nightingale and Peplau, a shift in axiology occurred in the scientific community that altered approaches to knowledge development. The shift was precipitated by scientists' growing need to theorize about entities too slow, too small, or otherwise unobservable but inferable from the empirical world, such as gravity or electromagnetism. Hypothetico-deductive logic emerged, whereby vertical links were made between the theoretical and empirical. In this modernist period of science, theory and research were linked through idealized systems of inquiry designed to keep research untainted of values and everyday life and independent of the religious and philosophic roots that once dominated knowledge development.

Peplau's[16] seminal work helped transform nursing from a "science of doing" to a "science of knowing" by reestablishing creative links between theory and research. Her mid-20th century theorizing employed deductive and inductive reasoning, moving up and down the ladder of abstraction to construct nursing knowledge, and produced a nursing practice theory on interpersonal relations.

Today, knowledge is regarded as process and product, as an open system rather than as a fixed set of propositions with truth flowing in top-down fashion, according to Aristotle's ideal of axiomatization.[7] Nursing scientists today are beginning to embrace all three forms of Peirce's[17] system of reasoning—abduction, deduction, and induction—without fragmenting the process. In *abduction* (a term coined by Peirce and similar to retroductive reasoning), the scientist makes a conceptual leap from experience, beliefs, and a preknowledge of patterns to arrive at an educated guess or theory about a phenomenon; the nursing scholar draws from clinical, conceptual, and empirical knowledge to do this. Through *deduction*, the scientist derives empirical events that may occur, given the theory. This deduction is put forth in the form of a hypothesis, research question, grand tour question, or other statement for inquiry. *Induction*, then, refers to the process of subjecting the theoretical ideas to empirical testing. All three forms of reasoning play important roles in knowledge development. Yet postmodernism has introduced some twists to this reasoning process that are relevant to clarifying contemporary approaches to development of nursing knowledge.

First, postmodern thought has sensitized scientists to the primacy of abductive reasoning. Abduction initiates the reasoning processes[18] and, by definition, introduces values and preunderstandings into science. No data can be free of values and biases.

Second, "empirical testing" is acquiring a broadened definition, whereby the postmodern "empirical" extends beyond the meaning of modernist empiricism. Empirical testing may interface with the practice realm to an extent greater than modernists could tolerate. The "test" of a theory, for example, is not demonstrated primarily (or at all, according to postmodern purists) by correspondence of the empirical with the theoretical but more by the correspondence between the practical and theoretical. The merit of a theory is found in its practical implications and usefulness in solving problems of the discipline.[19,20] Empirical includes the practical.

Third, what qualifies as empirical data has gone beyond empiricism. According to emerging nursing epistemology, acceptable data vary in observability. They include biologic indicators and self-reports, investigator perceptions and informant projections, motor behavior, and personal stories. The modernist distinction between qualitative and quantitative data is blurred for, as is implicit in abduction, no data, whether verbal or numeric symbols, are independent of theory.

Last, scientific work is broader than empirical work. Empirical and nonempirical (or conceptual) knowledge is not hierarchically ordered. Postmodern awareness of the intersubjectivity of knowledge invalidates such ordering and opens the door for valuing contributions to knowledge that are not empirically verifiable in the modernist sense. Nonempirical activities enhance scientific understanding by exposing new and unexpected ideas about a theory or clinical situation in the form of "conceptual innovations."[21] For example, the conceptual innovation from Freudian theory of the "unconscious" revolutionized science and practice of mental health disciplines. Newman's[22] "pattern recognition" and Orem's[23] "self-care" are other conceptual innovations that have attained significance through their meaning in practice as well as their inspiration for theory development.

In the absence of metanarratives about a transcendent truth, postmodernism has further blurred the distinction between the nonempirical and empirical, theory and fact. Theory is regarded as a "forestructure of what form of truth the data will take; theory has priority over what are taken to be facts."[19(p413)] Theory, then, does not represent truth, it creates truth. What Britt[24] stated in reference to the artist and his or her art also applies to the postmodern scientist: Modernists contemplated the meaning of the world and their place in it; postmodernists remake the world as their science demands it.

The Critical Stance: A Call to Armchairs

Given postmodernist influences on the process of knowledge development, the significance of the social critical perspective for science becomes apparent. Data alone do not yield up the theory any more than brushes and paint will produce a painting. Whether qualitative or quantitative, data reside in the researcher's theoretical context. This fact is not a caveat of knowledge development. It is the nature of science,

for "when theory does not play a selective role in research, data-gathering activities belong to the realm of journalism."[21(p794)]

Given the subjective and personalized context of theorizing, a critical stance in inquiry helps the scientist develop knowledge that potentially will be more meaningful and useful. More bluntly, some believe that the postmodern critique is a way of salvaging the empiricist tradition.[19,25] The critique serves to keep check on inherent biases and constraints—introduced by the researcher and research focus, the method, theoretical interpretation, and so on—that are not in the best interest of the subject and may oppress or constrain human potential in some way. Neither intuition and empathy nor scientific expertise and statistical significance are enough to reveal the full meaning of the data. A "call to armchairs"[26] is needed, whereby time is sanctioned for reflection and critique to examine one's assumptions and interpretations through discussion, debate, argument, and compromise with colleagues and participants—all who are affected by the knowledge developed.

Whether science is done using modernist methods, empiric-analytic or historist-hermeneutic, science is incomplete without a critical approach to one's work. Thus, the framework proposed in this article endorses a view put forth by Habermas[27] and other contemporary philosophers[1] that does not advocate the overthrow of modernism, but rather the modification of modernism by integrating the critique and communicative model of reasoning into empirical inquiry. But critique alone is not enough.

Beyond the Critique: A Neomodernist View

The neomodernist framework proposed here extends beyond the critique. The postmodern critique, with its methods of reflexivity and analysis to examine the process and products of the scientist, is not sufficient for knowledge development. Because the one who critiques is part of the culture being critiqued, complicity exists, as critics of postmodernism have explained.[1,28] And the critique cannot serve as its own external corrective; it describes a process but does not provide substance. Thus, it is suggested here that the nursing scientist's critique process be linked to a substantive overarching "ideal" or metanarrative. The metanarrative provides a base for examining knowledge as related to the context of a given discipline.[1] It functions as a "narrative foil"[28] against which scientists critique their work to form and reform knowledge.

Nursing knowledge development need not abandon completely modernist views about high theory or universal ideas. Rather than capitulate entirely to postmodernism, nurses can knowingly involve in their science the realm of perspectives and values, initially put forth by modernist nurses, that distinguish nursing knowledge and the caring application of that knowledge. In adopting a neomodernist view, nursing scientists would draw from the metanarratives of nursing for their critique. Metanarratives of nursing are found in nursing philosophy and nursing practice, as these two domains interface with nursing science in the development of knowledge.

 ## Nursing Philosophy: Metanarratives for Knowledge Development

Philosophy, by definition, goes beyond analysis and critique by assigning values to human experiences.[29] In so doing, philosophy is a source for explicating the metanarratives of a discipline. Nursing philosophy is a statement of foundational and universal assumptions, beliefs, and principles about the nature of knowledge and truth (epistemology) and about the nature of the entities represented in the metaparadigm (ie, nursing practice and human healing processes [ontology]). A variety of philosophic schemes have been identified for understanding the nature of nursing phenomena.

One major scheme derives from philosopher Stephen Pepper's[30] widely recognized 1942 work in which he explicated what he conceived were the major bases of truth about the world. Three of his six worldviews, particularly as modified slightly by Lerner[31] and other developmental psychologists, predominantly have been used by scientists, including nursing scientists,[32] to frame philosophic assumptions of their discipline. Pepper's work predates philosophic schemes identified in nursing, and it likely provided a basis for conceptualizing the nursing worldviews and paradigms.[32-35] These extant nursing schemes, along with Pepper's original worldviews, are useful in organizing basic assumptions about nursing phenomena and in deriving a nursing metanarrative from philosophy for knowledge development. The three predominant worldviews are the mechanistic, organismic, and developmental–contextual, the latter previously labeled the "contextual–dialectic" worldview.[36]

Within the *mechanistic* worldview, the metaphor for human beings is the machine, composed of parts that can be measured, controlled, predicted, and added together to understand the whole. The whole is equal to the sum of the parts. Human beings are viewed as inherently at rest. Stability is assumed. Any change that occurs results from external forces and is deterministic and reversible, not developmental.

The goal of change is to return to a state of equilibrium and balance. The individual's relationship with the environment is reactive. The unit of study is the part, devoid of context.

Within the *organismic* worldview, the metaphor for human beings is the biologic organism, composed of a complexity of interrelated parts. The parts are understood from the perspective of the whole, and the whole is represented in terms of the biologic organism itself. The environment assumes a more passive role, with the organism viewed as active on the environment. There is interactionism, primarily in the sense that the parts within the person interact and contribute to qualitative, developmental changes. Change is probabilistic and directed toward an end goal.

Within the *developmental–contextual* worldview, the metaphor for human beings is the historic event; that is, the individual is embedded in a context that is dynamic. Change, in both the human being and the environment, is ongoing and irreversible, innovative and developmental. Change occurs not as a result of the person's reaction to or action on the environment, but through a dialectic and interactive relationship with the environment. Change occurs in accord with Werner's[37] "orthogenetic principle" by which living systems develop through patterns of increasing complexity accompanied by increasing organization. Chaos and conflict can provide energy for progressive change. There is no one ideal goal for development that lasts a lifetime; each developmental phase (however defined) is qualitatively different and possesses its own ideals. The whole or basic unit of study is any living structure that manifests developmental patterns of change. Study of the person necessarily involves study of contextual factors.

Various philosophic systems have been put forth by nursing scholars, such as Hall's[33] change and persistence worldviews; Parse's[35] totality and simultaneity paradigms; Newman's[34] particulate–deterministic, interactive–integrative, and unitary–transformative worldviews; and Fawcett's[32] reaction, reciprocal interaction, and simultaneous action worldviews. These schemes reflect Pepper's[30] different depictions of reality and also extend his ideas by constructing worldviews that speak more directly to nursing and its phenomena of concern.

Some nursing scientists have appropriated worldviews from other disciplines, such as medicine and psychology. Medicine has advanced through three paradigms, namely the biomedical, biopsychosocial, and most recently the psychoneuroimmunologic paradigm.[38] Psychology's models of research and practice have evolved across behavioristic, psychodynamic, humanistic, and transpersonal schools of thought.[28,39]

The status quo in nursing seems to be that knowledge developers embrace the diversity of worldviews in critiquing knowledge and clarifying basic beliefs and assumptions about what are relevant and plausible issues of research and practice.[40] While this "plethora of paradigms"[41] available to nurses may be viewed in a positive way, it also may contribute to the potential for fragmentation within the discipline. This concern has been debated.[40,42] In the spirit of postmodernism, nurses must question the status quo and continue to debate the logic of diversity in worldviews underlying nursing knowledge development. From a neomodernist perspective, this kind of diversity may not be entirely desirable.

Diversity or Fragmentation?

Diversity at the level of the worldview may inhibit clarification of a nursing philosophy[43] and nursing metanarrative for research and critique. The worldviews within each philosophic scheme define and interrelate the nursing metaparadigm concepts in radically different ways. Sanctioning all available worldviews for nursing in one sense reflects the postmodernist retreat from conceptualizing the whole and identifying unifying ideals. In attempting to achieve unity by preserving disparate worldviews, as some advocate,[40] nursing may be sacrificing coherence for diversity.

Does the diversity offer important distinctions in worldviews, each of which has a rightful role in guiding inquiry and critique within a discipline? Or might the diversity in philosophic schemes represent progress in knowledge about the nature of the world, such that some provide for fuller understanding than others? The former position seems less likely. Diversity does not mean that all points of view are equally valid and acceptable for a given context or discipline.[43] Moreover, preserving differences through compromise or coexistence rather than striving to resolve differences in ontology, values, and goals—a purpose of philosophy[44]—blocks dialogue and opportunities to further develop knowledge. Opposing beliefs about the nature of human health and nursing goals can perpetuate even more differences in nursing's epistemic and ethical claims and research funding priorities, "bringing about more confusion in our discipline rather than creating a sense of coherence necessary for its development."[45(p26)]

In addition to the question of the merits of diversity in worldviews for the discipline's progress, there is the more urgent question as to whether entertaining disparate worldviews best serves patients' well-being. Diplomacy and discourse aside, when choices available are between a mechanistic and developmental worldview, or between a paradigm in which the nurse and not the patient possesses the knowledge and authority and a paradigm in which patients are knowledgeable and knowing participants in their own healing process, is not one paradigm more emancipating (for patient and nurse) and more representative of the nature of nursing than the other? The commitment for unity in diversity[42] may not be status quo but may be most appropriate in a postmodern world that tends to fragment focuses of inquiry, human beings, and their world.

To that end, then, the metanarrative of human developmental potential, transformational and self-transcendent capacity for health and healing, and recognition of the developmental histories of persons and their contexts is offered here as an external corrective of choice. It is a metanarrative originating in Lerner's[31] developmental–contextual worldview and congruent with the philosophic ideas expressed in Newman's[34] unitary–transformative paradigm and Parse's[35] simultaneity paradigm.

Given the alternatives, this metanarrative may be the best commitment to be made by the scientist and practitioner, at least at this point in the development of nursing knowledge. In proposing this metanarrative, however, one must acknowledge that inherent in this neomodernist framework is the realization that even metanarratives are temporary and "for the moment."[46] Although metanarratives by definition are more stable than lower levels of theory, their depictions of truth and reality are not fixed and must be open to developmental change themselves, subject in part to influences from the dynamic science and practice dimensions of nursing.

Nursing Practice: A Metanarrative for Knowledge Development

As if anticipating postmodernist values for the reality found in the culture and context of everyday life experiences, nurses have renewed focus on practice as connected to science. Nursing practice is regarded not only as a place of applying knowledge, but also as a place to generate and test ideas for developing knowledge. Early on, Peplau[47] identified practice as the context in which scientific knowledge was transformed into nursing knowledge. Linkages between science and practice help nursing move beyond grand theorizing and operationalize the metanarrative of "responsible participation and consideration of culture and context"[48(pviii)] and the emancipatory potential of nursing knowledge.

From a revisionist perspective of the early nursing theorists such as Peplau[47] and Paterson and Zderad,[49] it can be seen that nursing began moving beyond the reductionist and mechanistic approaches of modernism even before nursing recognition of postpositivism. As a result, nursing practice gave to nursing research a metanarrative that was patient oriented, context sensitive, pattern focused, and participatory. In her practice theory of interpersonal relations, for example, Peplau[47] incorporated practice and theory into her ideas of research. Resembling the hermeneutic circle, Peplau's research process began in practice, spiraled up, drawing in theories—or as she stated, "peeling out theories"—to explain the phenomenon, then returned to practice to examine the new knowledge in light of the experiences and reality of practice.

Paterson and Zderad[49] described a method of "nursology" as the study of nursing practice. They outlined five phases of phenomenologic nursology in which the practitioner role informed the research process: (1) preparing oneself to be an open window, (2) intuiting the rhythm of the other, (3) knowing the other scientifically, (4) synthesizing differences and similarities, and (5) arriving at a conception of the situation that has some universal meaning across many nursing practice situations.

More recently, Newman[50] described research as praxis, meaning an approach to research that takes the form of nursing practice in the researcher's relationship to the participant and in the enactment of values for human transformation through pattern recognition. Similarly, Parse[51] put forth a research methodology based on her "theory of human becoming." One essential step in the research process is "dialogical engagement," which involves establishing a therapeutic presence between researcher and participant.

These and other theorists' models of nursing depict ways in which doing science itself can be linked to the ideals and metanarratives of practice. Guidelines for evaluating the emancipatory potential of the research process and product have been detailed.[52] Nursing practice frameworks are evolving scientific methods that are tailored not only to elicit desired data while protecting research participants' rights, but also to be therapeutic.

The Esthetic Order and Nursing Practice

Postmodernism has stimulated greater awareness among nurses of the culture of practice as a source of ultimate meaning about the object of that practice, human beings' health and healing. Concomitantly, there has been increased interest in research on nursing care processes ranging from nursing care systems to nursing caring behaviors, intuition, nursing presence, and the nurse-patient relationship. Rather than characterize this focus as a return to the mid-20th century focus of research on nurses, it may be more accurately viewed as a focus of inquiry influenced in part by the postmodern emphasis on context. In postmodernism, the ultimate locus of meaning is the culture or context of the object of inquiry.[2] Professional practice is a nursing context. And nursing practice increasingly is being viewed as a legitimate source of knowledge, in part because it is regarded as an esthetic order of nursing, imbued with meaning and beauty.[53]

Amidst the postmodern emphasis on culture and context as something external to the person, nursing must not lose sight of the other context of healing—the patient. The postmodern notion of context must be broadened in nursing to include, if not to emphasize, the patient as a context of health and healing. Human beings' inner healing nature cannot be dismissed, as postmodernists might have it.[38] Patient as environment was first conceptualized by several nurse theorists (e.g., Levine,[54] Orem,[23] Paterson and Zderad,[49] and Neuman[55]) who wrote about the "internal environment" of the person as an inner reality and innate resource for health and development. The significance of an inner healing environment is supported by current worldviews about inner human potential and transformative capacity.[28,30,34,35] A basic assumption of Nightingale was that the natural source of healing resided in the patient.[15] And Rogers[56] wrote emphatically about the coexistence of person and environment, regarding the two as one "person–environment mutual process."

Thus, it is proposed that the esthetic in nursing practice refers not only to the meaningful and beautiful experienced through nursing practice by the nurse, but also, and perhaps more appropriately, to that experienced through nursing practice by the patient. As Kim stated in describing one perspective of esthetics, "Certain aspects of nursing practice may be considered 'art' insofar as they communicate aesthetic ideas to perceivers, especially *clients*."[57(p281)]

This perspective on the esthetics of nursing practice is contrary to the more commonly held view of the esthetic experience residing primarily in the nurse.[56] However, esthetic experience is not found primarily in the type of brushes the painter uses, or the way a musician holds an instrument, or the style of the conductor or poet. Rather, the esthetic is the beauty that is experienced in seeing the painting, hearing the music, and in reading or reciting the poem. Analogously, in nursing, the esthetic is not primarily that experienced by the practitioner; the esthetic is found in the beauty and meaning associated with the patient's experiences of health and healing—the phenomena of concern to nursing. The esthetic is what is desired, meaningful, beautiful—whether it is experienced through the art of a painter, a musician, or a nurse. Given the esthetic order underlying the nurse's art, then, nursing practice is recognized as possessing powerful metanarratives about health and the processes of healing.

Nursing Conceptual Models: Archetypes of Nursing Practice

The nursing conceptual models are a mechanism of translating the metanarrative of nursing practice for knowledge development. Nursing conceptual models broadly refer to extant conceptual and theoretical systems that describe the nature of nursing practice, patients as human beings, and health. Nursing conceptual models, their biases and preunderstandings notwithstanding,[58] "articulate disciplinary perspectives and underlying philosophical assumptions."[46(p56)] In the modernist era, these models were regarded as ideas to be revered, preserved, unaltered, and used in their entirety. More recently, Whall[59] noted, some are disparaging the conceptual models, reasoning that nursing has matured beyond needing the conceptual models for knowledge development and practice. This reasoning is specious. All levels of theory are needed in generating knowledge for theory-based practice.

The disregard for extant conceptual and theoretical models of nursing may be influenced in part by postmodernists' disinterest in grappling with the wholes that grand-level theories address. In their retreat from dealing with the complexity of a phenomenon, postmodernists fragment objects of inquiry by breaking them into smaller pieces and denying the need to conceptualize the whole.[1] However, from the neomodernist stance proposed in this article, unified conceptualizations of nursing and nursing practice are valued. Nursing conceptual models are more than a modernist artifact; they are archetypes of nursing practice.

Further, these archetypes are dynamic, unlike the archetypes of modernist science. Like the reality they depict, the practice and research contexts in which they are used, the theories they inspire, and the metaparadigm they represent, nursing conceptual models must be allowed to be open and alterable. As systems of knowledge, they must evolve, lest they move from being extant to becoming extinct. Other conceptual models will likely emerge out of the vestiges of earlier models and the new insights of creative nursing scientists, philosophers, and practitioners who grapple with the whole.

Nursing: A Postcritical Discipline

The neomodernist perspectives on knowledge development presented here build on modernist and postmodern ideas. Characteristic assumptions of postmodernism that all methods and sources of knowledge development are value laden and that the process of constructing and perceiving reality is a dynamic, relational endeavor undergird the framework. It is also recognized that knowledge development is more than science, science more than the empirical, and the empirical more than empiricism. Philosophic and practice dimensions in nursing generate open metanarratives for scientific inquiry that serve as external correctives to the critique of knowledge development. Postmodernism alone can never be a critical theory. As first proposed by Plato, critique of the particulars requires grounding in the universals. Metanarratives provide this grounding and are essential in intellectual pursuits.[2]

Postmodernists have challenged the metanarratives, referring to them as "totalizing discourses" that are fabrications and not representations of reality.[38] Other scholars have explained that science cannot exist in the absence of metanarratives, and they repudiate the notion that there are no legitimated metanarratives.[1,3,5] Language is not so slippery nor meanings so unstable that underlying patterns of individuals and groups cannot be identified. In failing to identify meaningful patterns in the ongoing change of person and environment, science becomes merely history. Thus, nursing, proposed here as a neomodernist science, has identified discourses of nursing philosophy and practice that converge on themes of healing environments, inner human potential, and the developmental–contextual nature of health.

The neomodernist framework proposed here also departs from postmodernism in that the object of inquiry—human processes of health and healing—is regarded as more than a "text" to be deconstructed or disentangled of the discourses that authority figures have inscribed on it.[38] Human beings are more than bodies inscribed by their context. There is text, or meaning, beyond the text that informs and stimulates scientific inquiry. The neomodernist retains a belief in an underlying esthetic order in nursing. This order is revealed through nursing practice processes that enhance healing and development.

Nursing can never return to a pre-postmodern era to regain lost and lofty assumptions about knowledge development and nursing. But nursing still possesses the innovativeness and imagination to continue progressing in the metanarrative Nightingale originally established—empowerment of human beings' natural potential for health and healing.

Nursing, by nature, is a postcritical discipline: Self-reflection, personal autonomy, innate developmental potential, connections between truth and life, emancipatory practice and research, and chaos as opportunity are all valued. These are values and conceptual orientations that distinguish the discipline from others.

Yet within this shared focus, there is a diversity in approaches to knowledge development. As a feminist philosopher recently implied, totality does not have to mean totalitarianism; unity does not mean uniformity.[1] A postcritical discipline values challenges to the status quo and critiques and exposes oppressive discourses. And a post-critical discipline is not timid in committing to an overarching discourse that enables and liberates patients and other persons.

Nursing is a metanarrative that shapes the broader scientific community's understanding of human beings. It is a metanarrative needed in health care reform. And, like all discourse, it warrants ongoing critique. A neomodernist perspective of knowledge development provides for this critique while also fostering the grounding and vision to continue scientific inquiry. An open philosophy that exercises connections between science, philosophy, and practice will help ensure that nursing's metanarratives do not become closed ideologic systems, and it will help ensure that the dialogue on knowledge development continues into the 21st century.

REFERENCES

1. Waugh P. *Postmodernism*. New York, NY: Routledge, Chapman and Hall; 1992.
2. Popper KR. *Conjectures and Refutations: The Growth of Scientific Knowledge*. New York, NY: Harper & Row; 1963.
3. Doherty J, Graham E, Malek M, eds. *Postmodernism and the Social Sciences*. New York, NY: Macmillan; 1992.
4. Lyotard J. *The Postmodern Condition: A Report on Knowledge*. Minneapolis, Minn: University of Minnesota Press; 1979.
5. Burman E. Developmental psychology and the postmodern child. In: Doherty J, Graham E, Malek M, eds. *Postmodernism and the Social Sciences*. New York, NY: Macmillan; 1992.
6. Foucault M. *The Order of Things*. London, England: Tavistock; 1974.
7. Philipse H. Towards a postmodern conception of metaphysics: on the genealogy and successor disciplines of modern philosophy. *Metaphilosophy*. 1994;25:1–44.
8. Rorty R. *Philosophy and the Mirror of Nature*. Oxford, England: Blackwell; 1980.
9. Rorty R. *Contingency, Irony and Solidarity*. Cambridge, NY: Cambridge University Press; 1989.
10. Carper BA. Fundamental patterns of knowing in nursing. *ANS*. 1978;1(1):13–24.
11. Chinn PL, Kramer MK, *Theory and Nursing: A Systematic Approach*. 3rd ed. St. Louis, Mo: Mosby; 1991.
12. Schultz PR, Meleis AI. Nursing epistemology: traditions, insights, questions. *Image J Nurs Schol*. 1989;20:217–221.
13. Polis DF. Paradigms for an open philosophy. *Metaphilosophy*. 1993;24:33–46.
14. Howard GS. Culture tales: a narrative approach to thinking. *Cross-Cultural Psychol Psychother*. 1991;46:187–197.
15. Nightingale F. *Notes on Nursing: What It Is, and What It Is Not*. New York, NY: Dover; 1969.
16. Peplau HE. The art and science of nursing: similarities, differences, and relations. *Nurs Sci Q*, 1988;1:8–15.
17. Peirce CS: Hartshorne C, Weiss P, eds. *Charles Sanders Peirce: Collected Papers*. Cambridge, Mass: Harvard University Press; 1934:5.
18. Staat W. On abduction, deduction, induction and the categories. *Transactions Charles S Peirce Soc*. 1993;29:225–237.
19. Gergen KJ. Exploring the postmodern: perils or potentials? *Am Psychol*, 1994;49:412–417.
20. Laudan L. *Progress and Its Problems: Toward a Theory of Scientific Growth*. Berkeley, Calif: University of California Press; 1977.
21. Kukla A. Nonempirical issues in psychology. *Am Psychol*. 1989;44:785–794.
22. Newman M. *Health as Expanding Consciousness*. 2nd ed. New York, NY: National League for Nursing; 1993.
23. Orem DE. *Nursing: Concepts of Practice*, 4th ed. St. Louis, Mo: Mosby; 1991.
24. Britt D, ed. *Modern Art: Impressionism to Post-Modernism*. Boston, Mass: Little, Brown: 1989.
25. Allen DG. Using philosophical and historical methodologies to understand the concept of health. In: Chinn PL, ed. *Nursing Research Methodology*. Rockville, Md: Aspen Publishers; 1986.
26. Omer H. London P. Metamorphosis in psychotherapy; end of the systems era. *Psychotherapy*. 1988;25:171–180.
27. Habermas J. Lawrence FG, trans. *The Philosophical Discourses of Modernity*. Oxford, England: Polity; 1987.
28. Wilber K. *A Sociable God*. New York, NY: McGraw-Hill; 1983.
29. Sahakian WS. *History of Philosophy*. New York, NY: Barnes & Noble; 1968.
30. Pepper SP. *World Hypotheses: A Study in Evidence*. Berkeley, Calif: University of California Press; 1942.
31. Lerner RM. *Concepts and Theories of Human Development*. 2nd ed. New York, NY: Random House; 1986.
32. Fawcett J. *Analysis and Evaluation of Nursing Theories*. Philadelphia, Pa: F. A. Davis; 1993.
33. Hall BA. The change paradigm in nursing: growth versus persistence. *ANS*. 1981;3(4):1–6.
34. Newman MA. Prevailing paradigms in nursing. *Nurs Outlook*. 1992;40:10–13.
35. Parse RR. *Nursing Science: Major Paradigms. Theories, and Critiques*. Philadelphia, Pa: W. B. Saunders; 1987.
36. Reed PG. Toward a nursing theory of self-transcendence: deductive reformulation using developmental theories. *ANS*. 1991;13:64–77.
37. Werner H. The concept of development from a comparative and organismic point of view. In: Harris DB, ed. *The Concept of Development*. Minneapolis, Minn: University of Minnesota Press; 1957.
38. Fox NJ. *Postmodernism, Sociology, and Health*. Toronto, Canada: University of Toronto Press; 1994.
39. Lundin RW. *Theories and Systems of Psychology*, 2nd ed. Lexington, Mass: Heath; 1979.
40. Barrett EAM. Response: disciplinary perspective: unified or diverse? Diversity reigns. *Nurs Sci Q*. 1992;5:155–157.
41. Fawcett J. From a plethora of paradigms to parsimony in world views. *Nurs Sci Q*. 1993;6:56–58.
42. Northrup DT. Commentary: disciplinary perspective: unified or diverse? A unified perspective within nursing. *Nurs Sci Q*. 1992;5:154–156.
43. Kikuchi JF, Simmons H, eds. *Developing a Philosophy of Nursing*. Thousand Oaks, Calif: Sage; 1994.
44. Moccia P. A critique of compromise: beyond the methods debate. *ANS*. 1988;10(4):1–9.

45. Laurin J. A philosophy of nursing: commentary. In: Kikuchi JF, Simmons H, eds. *Developing a Philosophy of Nursing.* Thousands Oaks, Calif: Sage; 1994.

46. Smith MC. Arriving at a philosophy of nursing: discovering? constructing? evolving? In: Kikuchi JF, Simmons H, eds. *Developing a Philosophy of Nursing.* Thousand Oaks, Calif: Sage; 1994.

47. Peplau HE. Interpersonal relations: a theoretical framework for application in nursing practice. *Nurs Sci Q.* 1992;5(1): 13–18.

48. Chinn PL. A window of opportunity. *ANS.* 1994;16(4):viii.

49. Paterson JG, Zderad LT. *Humanistic Nursing.* New York, NY: Wiley; 1976.

50. Newman MA. Newman's theory of health as praxis. *Nurs Sci Q.* 1990;3:37–41.

51. Parse RR. Parse's research methodology with an illustration of the lived experience of hope. *Nurs Sci Q.* 1990;3:9–17.

52. DeMarco R, Campbell J, Wuest J. Feminist critique: searching for meaning in research. *ANS.* 1993;16(2):26–38.

53. Katims I. Nursing as aesthetic experience and the notion of practice. *Schol Inq Nurs Pract.* 1993;7:269–278.

54. Levine M. *Introduction to Clinical Nursing,* 2nd ed. Los Angeles, Calif: F. A. Davis; 1973.

55. Neuman B. *The Neuman Systems Model.* 3rd ed. Norwalk, Conn: Appleton-Lange; 1994.

56. Rogers ME. Nursing: a science of unitary man. In: Riehl JP, Roy C, eds. *Conceptual Models for Nursing Practice.* 2nd ed. New York, NY: Appleton-Century-Crofts; 1980.

57. Kim HS. Response to "Nursing as Aesthetic Experience and the Notion of Practice." *Schol Inq Nurs Pract.* 1993;7:279–282.

58. Thompson JL. Practical discourse in nursing: going beyond empiricism and historicism. *ANS.* 1985;7(4):59–71.

59. Whall AL. Let's get rid of all that theory. *Nurs Sci Q.* 1993;6:164–165.

THE AUTHOR COMMENTS

A Treatise on Nursing Knowledge Development for the 21st Century: Beyond Postmodernism

I wrote this article to articulate a philosophic position for reforming nursing's approach to knowledge development. I integrated the best of modernist and postmodernist thinking, without succumbing to the narrow view of reality that each alone conveys. The approach acknowledges the wealth of knowledge found in our canon of conceptual models and, at the same time, requires a critical perspective of any nursing metanarratives. I tried to extend the traditional views about science, nursing practice, and conceptual models in proposing a "neomodernist" stance for knowledge development. I now call this stance "intermodernism." The "open philosophy" proposed in the article will hopefully encourage students to be innovative in their own thinking about how knowledge is developed in nursing.

PAMELA G. REED

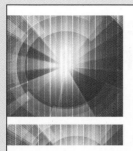

This unit was designed to increase awareness about theory as inherent in practice, and practice as a resource for theory. While it is common to hear that practice should incorporate theory, we are standing this axiom on its head to declare that *all theorizing involves practice* in some way. "Theory" refers broadly to the concepts and patterns that are drawn from observations, experiences, research, and readings to explain the everyday world of nursing. Theory entails a pragmatic thinking process that requires both action and reflection. The domains of nursing care and nursing research, particularly as practiced at the doctoral level, are not meant to be the passive recipients of others' theories and knowledge. Practitioners, like researchers, cannot shop for "ready-to-wear" theories or depend upon doctors' orders, protocols, or fancy techniques to address the unique and changing needs of their practice.

The scholarship of practice requires nurses to engage in theoretical thinking themselves—to reflect on why they do what they do in practice, to make explicit their conceptual ideas and philosophical views, to read the literature and connect the readings to their observations, and to articulate and apply this knowledge with patients and in research. Until practicing nurses fully realize this, the voice of nursing will be silent.

Scholars such as Rosemary Ellis and Hildegard Peplau promoted theoretical thinking among practicing nurses over 50 years ago—long before it was fashionable. They did this to advance nursing beyond stereotypes of the caring nurse or the automaton technical nurse that too often characterized nursing after Nightingale. Contemporary authors in this unit similarly promote theoretical thinking to foster practice that is ethical, effective, compassionate, and capable of generating knowledge through practice-informed inquiry.

QUESTIONS FOR DISCUSSION

- Is practice knowledge empirical?
- Can you use the readings in this unit to describe practice knowledge *without* using the word, intuition?
- What role do patients play in nurses' theorizing?
- How do nurses link the knowledge they use in practice to the knowledge expressed in researchers' theories?
- How might researchers use the practice knowledge of practitioners to build or evaluate their theories?

Toward Compassionate Action: Pragmatism and the Inseparability of Theory/Practice

GWENETH HARTRICK DOANE, RN, PhD
COLLEEN VARCOE, RN, PhD

Believing that the purpose of knowledge development and practice is compassionate action, in this article, we discuss how pragmatism can help us move toward that goal. Specifically, we show how pragmatic inquiry draws attention to the inseparability of practice/theory and the integral role practice experiences play in the ongoing development of theory. We demonstrate the utility of pragmatism to nursing by describing how we have explicitly approached theory development as a practical (and practice) activity of inquiry to attend to experiences of culture and diversity in family nursing.

Getting Pragmatic

Although the development of theoretical nursing practice has been a central focus within the nursing discipline over the past few decades, the practice/theory connection continues to be in need of further exploration and articulation. For example, in their research, Liaschenko and Fisher[1] noted that one rarely hears practicing nurses use the language of nursing theory unless they have been mandated to do so by accrediting bodies or institutional practices. Similarly, within nursing education, theory is often presented as an abstract body of knowledge that is learned outside of the practice arena and in isolation from everyday nursing work.[2,3] Subsequently, for many nurses, the word "theory" conjures up images of some dry, academic abstraction that has no relevance to the "real" world of practice. This tendency to objectify theory—to separate it out from everyday "real" practice and think of it as a "thing" to be applied and used—has had profound implications for theory development and nursing practice. It has not only constrained the theory-development process but also ultimately served to limit nurses' choices, clinical decision making, and their capacity for ethically responsive practice.[2]

In contrast to this objectifying approach to theory, we concur with pragmatist philosophers who believe that all so-called "theory" is always already practice.[4-6] While this idea is not necessarily a new one to nursing, we believe that its significance has not been adequately examined. Specifically, it is our intent to illustrate the integral role practice experiences play in the ongoing development of theory and the potential a

pragmatic orientation has to not only enhance theory development in nursing but also reshape the everyday moments of nursing practice. In this article, we illustrate the utility of pragmatism to nursing by describing how we have explicitly approached theory development as a practical (and practice) activity of inquiry to attend to diversity in family nursing. Although elsewhere[3] we have explicitly turned our attention to difference and diversity in terms of religion and spirituality, health and healing practices, sexual orientation, ethnicity and race, by way of illustration, we focus in this article on how a pragmatic approach to theory has enabled us to conceptualize "family" and "culture" in ways that support more responsive and socially just nursing practice.

A Pragmatic Understanding of Theory

The term *pragmatism* is derived from the Greek word meaning action, from which the words "practice" and "practical" also come.[7] Roth recounts that pragmatism was first introduced into philosophy by Charles Peirce in 1878, who pointed out that beliefs are really rules for action. Peirce contended that the sole significance of a thought or concept was the conduct it produced. Pragmatism is a process of clarifying the meaning of a thought and rests upon the principle that meaning is determined by unpacking a concept and/or theory with respect to the practical consequences in future experience.[7] So, for example, pragmatism might ask

ABOUT THE AUTHORS

GWENETH HARTRICK DOANE was born in Regina, Saskatchewan. Her educational background includes a diploma of nursing, diploma in recreational therapy, baccalaureate degree in nursing, master's degree in counseling psychology, and an interdisciplinary PhD (nursing/psychology). She is currently a Professor in the School of Nursing and Associate Dean in the Faculty of Graduate Studies at the University of Victoria in British Columbia. Her scholarly work focuses on the integration of relational ontology, knowledge and responsive action. Her key contributions have been in the areas of relational practice, family nursing, ethics, and teaching and learning in higher education.

COLLEEN VARCOE was born in rural Manitoba. She obtained her nursing diploma from the Royal Columbian Hospital School of Nursing and subsequently completed a baccalaureate in nursing, master's degrees in both nursing and education, and a doctorate in nursing. She is currently a Professor and Director Pro Tem in the school of nursing at the University of British Columbia in Vancouver. Her scholarship focuses on health inequities and social justice, with an emphasis on violence, poverty, racism, and colonialism. Her key contributions to the discipline have been in the areas of violence against women and ethical practice in nursing. She snowboards, does yoga, and runs a paragliding school with her partner in Harrison Mills, British Columbia.

what a particular concept or theory leads us to expect, to focus upon, to attend to, and to do in our nursing practice. As a process, pragmatism attempts to interpret each theory by tracing its practical consequences. Central questions pragmatism asks include the following: What difference would it practically make to anyone if this notion rather than that notion was held to be true? What concrete difference will any idea or theory make in anyone's actual life? What experiences will be different? What is the value of any theory or idea in experiential terms? If no practical difference can be traced, there is no difference and the thought (or theory) is meaningless in that particular situation.[7]

William James further developed the pragmatic perspective, highlighting that all theories are merely approximations—"They are only a man-made (sic) language, a conceptual shorthand." [6(p147)] James also contended that "truth" is something that *happens* to an idea. Ideas or theories become true, are *made* true by events, "Truth lives for the most part on a credit system. Our thoughts and beliefs 'pass,' so long as nothing challenges them, just as bank notes pass so long as nobody refuses them."[6(p163)] For example, within nursing there are many theoretical possibilities when it comes to describing and making sense of a particular situation or experience. Any number of rival formulations may be developed and any one of the theories from some point of view might be useful. As James contends, however, theories and ideas become true (are meaningful) just in so far as they help us to get into satisfactory relation with our experiences and *result in more responsive action.*

In contrast to many philosophical or theoretical perspectives, pragmatism does not stand for any special results. It is only a process. But the significance of that process is the fundamental change it offers in our approach to theory development and to nursing practice. Theory moves beyond an abstraction that is developed in isolation from everyday practice and becomes a practical activity that is central to every nursing moment. The goal of theory development is no longer to develop a truth or doctrine to follow, nor is it considered useful to compare different theories and/or argue which theory is ultimately more true. From a pragmatic perspective, one cannot look on any idea or theory as "more true" and/or as closing the quest for knowledge. Rather, the process involves setting any and all theory to work within everyday practice experiences and engaging in a continual inquiry to determine the value of the different theories to a particular situation in terms of consequences. Subsequently, theory "appears less as a solution, then, than as a program for more work, and more particularly as an indication of the ways in which existing realities may be changed. Theories thus become instruments, not answers to enigmas, in which we can rest. We don't lie back upon them, we move forward, and, on occasion, make nature over again by their aid. Pragmatism unstifles all our theories, limbers them up and sets each one at work."[6(p145)]

 ## Opening Spaces for Theory Development Through Pragmatic Inquiry

As an approach to knowledge, pragmatism does not look to any particular results but offers an attitude of orientation to take into practice. This attitude involves looking away from static abstractions and categorical ways of thinking and looking toward possibilities. As such pragmatism does not offer new knowledge "content" but rather a pragmatic "practice" process of theory construction that does not limit or confine our theorizing and/or the theoretical possibilities available to us. Berman's description[8] of the nomad who dwells in the midregion of knowing and moves into knowledge in such a way that seeks to destroy static models rather than develop them mirrors a pragmatic process of theory development. "In the nomadic mind ... the road to truth is always under construction; the going is the goal ... For nomads "truth is a verb, something you live. No sooner are you at one point than an elaboration or revision suggests itself." [8(p198)]

Engaging in a pragmatic process of theory development involves living a world presence rather than a worldview.[8] Rather than living from a unified, fixed perspective, one is grounded in immediacy, experience, and practice. As James[6] describes, "Pragmatism is willing to take anything, to follow either logic or the senses and to count the humblest and most personal experiences."[6(p157)] Subsequently, rather than being limited to an intellectual activity, theorizing is seen as an embodied, reflexive process of responsive action.[3] As such, theorizing involves tuning into and critically considering bodily sensing, intuitive and emotional responses, existing theories and research, contextual forces, and so forth. These responses and forces are seen as forms of knowing that can in-form and re-form our in-the-moment knowing actions, that is to say, theoretical practice.

Overall, pragmatism inspires an opening up to theoretical possibilities rather than the development of theoretical doctrines and truths. The pragmatic process is a process of inquiry and choice. One inquires into the different possible theories or "truths" to find a theory that works—a theory that will mediate between previous truths and new experiences. As we listen and attend to our experiences, in practice those experiences have "ways of boiling over, and making us correct our pre sent formulas."[9(p170)] Thus, in this way our practice experiences bear the fruits of theory development.

Interestingly, Dickoff and James[10] brought a similar discussion to nursing theory more than 3 decades ago. These authors described 4 levels of theory, including (a) factor-isolating theory, (b) factor-relating theory, (c) situation-related theory (including predictive and promoting/inhibiting theory), and (d) situation-producing theory. It is this idea of the fourth level of theory that we are discussing and building upon in this article. Situation-producing theory is practice-minded theory whose purpose is "to allow the production of situations of a desired kind."[10(p105)] Situation-producing theory is developed not only for the sake of producing

theory but also for producing a desired reality. These authors contend that situation-producing theory is the highest level of theory, since it exists and is produced for practice. They have argued (and we concur) that "theory for a profession of practice discipline must provide for more than mere understanding or "describing" or even predicting reality and must provide conceptualization specially intended to guide the shaping of reality to that profession's professional purpose."[10(p102)]

Theory Development: A Process of Inquiry

New truth is always a "go-between, a smoother over of transitions. It marries old opinion to new fact so as ever to show a minimum jolt, a maximum of continuity ... A new opinion counts as true just in proportion as it gratifies the individual's desire to assimilate the novel in his (sic) experience to his beliefs in stock. It must both lean on old truth and grasp new fact."[9(p150)]

Dickoff and James[10] emphasize the complexity and difficulty of developing situation-producing theory. We offer in this article a description of how pragmatism has helped us in the challenge of this complex and difficult theory development. Specifically, drawing upon pragmatist thought, we suggest a way of proceeding in practice that can support and foster the cultivation of situation-producing theory and ultimately recreate realities, both in the practice of individual nurses and the contexts of healthcare delivery.

Approaching practice with this pragmatic understanding of theory and truth compels us to take an inquiry stance—to pay attention and inquire into our own personal experiences, the experiences of others, existing knowledge such as formal theory and research, and the contextual elements and structures that shape our experiences and practice. Such an inquiry begins with the assertion of the knowledge-making capacity of people—that all people bring self-directing, self-generating, self-knowing, and self-transcending capacities.[11] A pragmatic inquiry supports us to inquire into and question the "knowing" we live in our practice, how that knowing enhances and/or constrains our in-the-moment responsiveness, and, ultimately, to remake that knowing-in-action. This knowing includes development of theory that may illuminate our action, guide and provide our action with meaning, and ultimately reshape "reality." Therefore, central to a pragmatic inquiry are questions of adequacy. Questions a pragmatist might ask as part of the theory development inquiry process include the following: Is our knowledge of things adequate to the way things are? Are our ways of describing things, of relating them to other things so as to fulfill our needs as good as possible?[4] In the context of nursing, we believe that a pragmatic inquiry includes questions such as "Are our ways of describing things, of relating them to other things so as to be responsive to patients as well as possible? Is our knowledge of things adequate to the way things are in nursing practice? Do available theories address and inform the questions and challenges that arise in our nursing work?" These questions of adequacy are essential, as according to James, any truth "has its palentology, and its "prescription," and may grow stiff with years of veteran service and petrified in men's (sic) regard by sheer antiquity."[6(p151)] We concur with Dickoff and James' admonition that "a professional is a doer who shapes reality rather than a doer who merely attends to the cogs of reality according to prescribed patterns."[10(p102)] In a similar vein, Reason and Torbert[11] contend that when we numb ourselves with knowledge (take up static doctrines), we actually become less susceptible to learning, to growth, and to people. Reason and Torbert argue that knowledge development involves learning through risk-taking in living.

As part of our work, we have intentionally engaged in a pragmatic inquiry into nursing practice in experiences of difference and diversity. This intentional inquiry was inspired through numerous experiences where we each (independently) found ourselves deeply disturbed by the inadequacy of our practice, of existing theory, and of healthcare structures and processes to attend to difference and diversity in people/families. Although we each came from different areas of nursing, we felt strongly that many of the truths and theories that dominated understandings of people/families did not do justice to their diverse living experiences and/or did not adequately support nurses to promote the health and well-being of families in their diverse everyday lives. Sharing an ethic of social justice and believing that nursing decisions and actions should be more than merely health promoting and/or economically viable, we found ourselves asking "so what?" If I do or do not do this, "so what" may the impact be? As nurses, we strive toward the ideals of compassion, respect, equitable relations, and the honoring of all life forms. The intent of our ongoing pragmatic inquiry process is to bring knowledge, compassion, and action together to produce practical knowing—to develop knowledge in service of worthwhile human purposes.[11] We concur with Reason and Torbert[11] who contend that ultimately the purpose of knowledge development is to culminate in compassion. Compassion in this sense is not just emotion but is about action—action that interferes with unnecessary pain, sorrow, and/or injustice. It is compassionate action that is both the purpose and the text of such theory development.

 ## A Pragmatic Inquiry Into Family Diversity

Overall, bringing a pragmatic orientation to our practice has directed us to (*a*) focus on the consequences of ideas and theories; (*b*) draw upon multiple theories, ideas, and perspectives examining their contradictions and complementary contributions in terms of consequences; (*c*) focus on the integrity of theory/practice rather than on the divide between them; and (*d*) remake theory and reality. The process of pragmatic inquiry has supported the development of our thinking regarding family and family nursing, and inspired further thinking about diversity in family nursing. By "diversity" we are referring both to the diversity of experiences and meanings of "family" and to other forms of diversity that relate to those experiences and meanings.

Focusing on the Consequences of Ideas and Theories

Our pragmatic inquiry was initially inspired by our experiences of discomfort in our practice. As we worked with people/families from diverse backgrounds and locations and listened to the inner rumblings of inadequacy we felt in our practice responses, it became increasingly clear that existing theoretical understandings of family that governed family nursing did not do justice to the diverse people/families with whom we worked and did not set us up well to respond in meaningful ways to their health and healing experiences. As we traced our practice experiences and responses back to explore what ideas were informing them, we began to explicitly name the consequences of holding those ideas and practicing from particular theoretical locations.[2,12] For example, as described elsewhere,[3,12] we identified how in seeing family as a literal entity—that is, as a configuration of people—we were missing the essence of family for many of those to whom we provided care and entirely discounting the experiences of many others. Furthermore, by doing so, we were drawn away from making important theoretical connections. For example, given that family is the dominant social organizing structure in society, through our practice experiences it became increasingly clear that all people live and experience family in some way regardless of whether they are part of a literal family at any given moment. Ultimately, our situation-producing theoretical work led us to retheorize family as a socially situated relational experience.[3] At the same time, we began to see ways in which our prior theoretical understanding of family (as a configuration of people)[13] served to constrain our understanding of people's health and healing experiences and our responsiveness to them. This became evident, for example, when working with women who experience violence. Statements we frequently heard nurses make such as "why doesn't she just leave" reflect an understanding of family as some 'thing' that can be left and decontextualize the complex, relational experience of both family and of violence. Such understanding led nurses to offer very limited choices to women, culminating primarily in advice to leave their partners.[13] Not only does such a limited theoretical perspective shape nursing practice in such a way that significantly hinders nurses' understanding of, and responsiveness to, women/families experiencing violence but it also leaves in place and perpetuates the larger societal discourses and theories that limit the knowing and "reality" of family and of violence.

Seeking to expand our understanding of diversity in relation to family, we have also employed our pragmatic stance as we have turned our attention to culture. We had experienced discomfort in relation to the ideas of culture and cultural diversity in our practice, and, once again, these experiences of discomfort served as points of entry into a deeper inquiry. We traced back the consequences of our ideas to the ideas themselves. That is, the impossibility of learning about the multiple "other cultures" in our multicultural, multiethnic practice settings as well as the variations we saw in people/families who were supposedly from the same culture led us to question the adequacy of how culture and nursing practice in relation to culture have been theorized. For example, drawing on others,[14, 15] we began to see the practical impact of the overriding acceptance of culture as shared values and beliefs, as something closely associated with or even equated with ethnicity or nation, and as a "thing" that belongs to groups of people. It became evident that such theoretical understandings direct nurses away from the actual experiences and meanings of families and individuals, and make their thinking vulnerable to stereotypes and assumptions. Conceptualizing culture as a thing that belongs to groups leads to a rather static understanding of culture and fosters a process of "othering"—that is, those who belong to groups in which we as nurses do not claim membership are seen as "other." Although the need to retheorize culture has certainly been addressed in the nursing literature, our pragmatic approach to theory helped us see a way of *interrupting and reshaping cultural theory at the practice level*. With the help of writers such as Swendson and Windsor,[16] we began to see how theorizing culture as shared values and beliefs of groups promoted a sensitivity to customs, habits, food preferences, health beliefs, and so on, but did not draw attention to the way in which social, economic, and political forces shaped these aspects of culture. Because "cultural sensitivity" is fundamentally concerned with learning

about "others," often distinguished from self on the basis of race, ethnicity, or nation, and is particularly concerned with learning about the values, beliefs, and practices of certain (usually nondominant) groups, in practice it leaves nurses open to assumptions, stereotypes, and inappropriate generalizations. As we inquired into the adequacy of a cultural sensitivity approach to nursing practice, it became evident that cultural sensitivity served to emphasize difference at the expense of similarities and focus upon the values, beliefs, and behaviors of particular individuals, families, and groups without drawing attention to the larger circumstances of their lives. Furthermore, this way of theorizing culture and nursing practice left Eurocentric thinking[17] unchallenged and promoted nurses to normalize Eurocentric practices and designate anything outside of those normative practices as "other."

Overall, by examining the consequences of our theories and ideas, we were able to evaluate the adequacy of those theories and ideas in everyday nursing practice, and in particular, how they optimized and/or limited responsiveness to diverse families. For example, thinking of a Canadian family as "Vietnamese" drew attention to certain dietary practices, religious practices, and so on, but did not draw attention to the ways in which immigration from Vietnam effected differently various generations of immigrants, the ways in which global politics, war, and economics shape various families' practices and experiences, or how racism might shape the family's healthcare encounters. Indeed, it became evident that the theory of culturally sensitive nursing practice offers superficial understandings of the experiences of the families and is inadequate when it comes to knowing and responding to experiences of diverse families.

A living example of this was provided by a local hospital publication entitled *The Multicultural Corner*. This periodical publication variously featured particular groups of people. One issue focused upon "Indo Canadians, "listing the "Countries of Origin" as "Pakistan, India, Sri Lanka, Bangladesh, Nepal, Fiji, East Africa, United Kingdom, and Hong Kong"; "Religion and Religious practices" as "Sikhism, Hinduism, and Islam"; and the languages spoken as "English, Hindi, Punjabi, Guharate, and Urdu. Most speak English." By theorizing culture as something belonging to groups and defining the group of concern in this manner, the authors of this publication grouped together hundreds of thousands of diverse people. The consequences included ideas that might apply to any person, family, or group (e.g., "lots of support from family and friends"), ideas that might or might not apply to people within the defined category (e.g., "role of women—caregivers, nurturers, generally submissive but respected)," and a tone of objectification (e.g., "cleanliness important," "Family spokesperson is usually the most established male"). Rather than offering guidance to greater sensitivity as was apparently intended, the publication yielded generalizations and invited stereotyping.

Drawing Upon Multiple Theories, Ideas, and Perspectives to Examine Their Contradictions and Complementary Contributions

As we came to see the consequences of the theoretical understandings that were shaping our practices, we simultaneously began looking at other theories and perspectives that could expand our view and more adequately reflect the diversity of people/family and their health and healing experiences. For example, we turned to hermeneutic phenomenology to expand our understanding of living experience and to various critical theories to enhance our "knowing" of sociopolitical family experience.[3,18] Seeking a deeper and more complex understanding of culture, we drew on the wide range of theorists who see culture as deeply imbedded within the webs of power, economics, and politics.[19-23] We began to pursue the *practical consequences* of seeing culture in this way, and of seeing culture as dynamic rather than static.

Ultimately, through this pragmatic process of theoretical inquiry, we gradually began to "retheorize our practice." This retheorizing was a highly practical process. For example, as we played with alternative views of "family" and paid attention to the way those views shaped our responsiveness, we found ourselves developing a view of "family" as a relational living experience.[3] That is, looking beyond "family" in its literal sense (as a configuration of people) as we worked with families in practice, we intentionally focused our attention on what it was that was significant to people in *relation* to family. For example, as it became clear that all people live and experience family in some way regardless of whether they are part of a literal family, we found ourselves immediately tuning into the *experience* of family rather than the configuration of people. This opened up our thinking so that we recognized family for *all* people with whom we worked, regardless of whether or not they had a visible, literal family. We began to appreciate, seek out, and understand the experience of family for people even when they were utterly alone in a literal sense. A man who had been estranged from his literal family and lived on the street for years, a woman who had been in prison and moved from town to town since, with no literal family, a youth who after living in numerous foster homes was on his own with no discernable literal family, all had important experiences of family. They characterized

some of their experiences of family as experiences of rejection, of loneliness, of "unlove," and these experiences of family were fundamental to understanding how to more responsively promote their health and healing. Furthermore, they each had other important and significant relationships (sometimes fleeting) that would not necessarily have been captured by our previous understandings of family, but were critical to understand in order to be responsive. Thus, our pragmatic inquiry expanded our "knowing" of family theoretically as well as practically. That is, we found that this ongoing inquiry process fostered a deeper knowing of the people/families with whom we worked, cultivated greater responsiveness in our practice, and simultaneously expanded our theoretical understandings.

Congruent with our view of family as a relational, situated experience, we also began to see culture as a relational experience, as something "that happens between people."[15,24] And we saw that understanding "culture" required understanding the social, economic, political, and historical webs of power within which people are embedded. At a very practical level, this led us to "look over the shoulder" of people/families with whom we worked to see the particular webs within which they had and were currently living. The consequences of this view of culture included widening our understanding of diversity within families and among families, for example, among families within particular ethnic groups. Such a view led to a more complex view than is implied through the use of ethnic or nationalist categories—rather than seeing a family as "Vietnamese," questions were immediately raised regarding the experiences of any given family. We sought to understand immigration and colonizing experiences, experiences of racism, current economic, social, and political life circumstances, and evolving variations between and among individuals, generations, and groups. We sought to understand the values, beliefs, and practices of people/families as dynamic and changing and as embedded within wider social contexts.

Seeing culture as a relational experience shifted our view of nurses in relation to culture. Rather than seeing nurses as outside some of their patients' cultures, we began to see that when nurses enter into relation, they shape and participate in culture, that is, culture is happening as patients and nurses relate. So, when a third-generation Euro-Canadian nurse enters into relation with a family who has recently immigrated from Vietnam, their histories and experiences mingle within the webs of power. They meet within multiple and shifting cultures (eg, the culture of healthcare, colonialist Canadian culture) and have the opportunity to reinforce and reproduce certain aspects of culture rather than others.

In examining multiple theories, ideas, and perspectives in relation to one another, we were led to understand both family and culture in ways that complemented and were congruent with one another. Critically examining the adequacy of our theories within the context of our everyday practice not only enhanced our capacity for responsiveness to people/families but also helped us develop appreciation for the integral relation of theory/practice.

Focusing on the Integrity of Theory/Practice

As our practice experiences fostered our retheorizing (of family as a relational experience) and we began to experience the profound difference this retheorizing made to our understanding of, and responsiveness to, the particular families with whom we worked, we came to more fully comprehend the pragmatist assertion that all so-called "theory" is always already practice.[4-6] Specifically, we came to appreciate how every nursing moment is imbued with theory/practice and is thus an opportunity for theory development—for rethinking the ideas, assumptions, beliefs, and theories that govern our practice by examining the consequences of them. Overall, our "theory" of theory and theory development shifted from a theory of objectification (where theory and practice are separate and there is a "theory-practice gap") to a relational one (where thinking is not separate from action but rather where action is understood to be integral to theory). In such situation-producing theory, action and remaking reality are inherent.

Remaking Theory and Reality

At the center of this "theory/practice" relation is a praxis process—that is, situation-producing theory means that reality is remade in every moment in nursing. It is important to distinguish this pragmatic "praxis" process from the notion of praxis that has tended to dominate nursing—that is, where praxis has been defined as theory informing practice and practice informing theory. While this view of praxis has drawn attention to the reciprocity between theory and practice, we also believe that in some ways it has reinforced the division between them. Therefore, we want to clarify that we are referring to an understanding of praxis inspired by Friere.[25] Similar to Dickoff and James' notion of situation-producing theory,[10] in Friere's definition of praxis as "reflection and action upon the world in order to transform it,"[25(p33)] action is integral to theory—it is simultaneously with, and the reason for, thinking. Thus, enacting praxis in this sense, means that *every moment in nursing is purposefully about both thinking and action that focus toward the service of worthwhile human purposes.* From this praxis perspective, it is understood that in each moment we are trying out,

evaluating, and revising our ways of thinking/acting/responding in term of ourselves, the people/families with whom we work, and importantly, as we focus "upon the world," the contexts within which we all live. And, at the heart of this praxis process is the purposeful move toward compassionate action that interrupts and addresses unnecessary pain, sorrow, and/or injustice. For example, in moving toward compassionate action to honor diversity in families, we are compelled to expose and address the underlying sociopolitical structures that are advantaging some people/families and disadvantaging others, and the theories and/or ways of knowing that keep inequities intact.[17] As we try out and evaluate the consequences of particular theoretical understandings of family, of culture, of health, and other theories that dominate healthcare practice and organizations, we gain the opportunity to identify how existing structures (for example, healthcare policies) may need revision in order to be equitable and responsive to families, particularly to those families who do not (or cannot) conform to dominant values and/or expectations.

 Implications and Conclusions

Overall, a pragmatic perspective of knowledge suggests that everyday nursing practice is a critical site for theory development. The inseparability of practice/theory and the integral role practice experiences play in the ongoing development of theory has implications for how we practice, teach, and develop knowledge. In the particular example of family diversity, pragmatism has helped us explicitly approach theory development as a practical activity of inquiry, to cultivate situation-producing theory, and ultimately to enhance our theoretical practice.

Seeing theory development as a practical activity, and practice as a theoretical activity serves to direct attention to the way in which nurses enter into practice as "knowing" practitioners. It highlights that theory development is not something that is divorced from everyday practice but is integral to it. Seeing theory/practice as inseparable draws attention to every moment of practice as a site of learning (in this example, a site of learning about families and culture). By attending to each nursing moment in this manner, we move beyond looking to see how theory informs practice or how practice informs theory to looking for the consequences of theorizing/practicing in particular ways.

Perhaps one of the most significant implications of a pragmatic approach to theory/practice is that it places "theory development" firmly in the domain of practicing nurses and recognizes the capacity all nurses have to use their inventiveness for knowledge development to address situations and challenges of everyday practice and to create and recreate their knowing in each moment of practice. In addition, such an approach opens space for people/families to inform our knowing and for us as nurses to more consciously and intentionally choose and effect our actions to be more compassionately responsive in each moment of nursing practice.

REFERENCES

1. Liaschenko J, Fisher A. Theorizing the knowledge that nurses use in the conduct of their work. *Scb Inq Nurs Pract*. 1999;13(1):29–41.

2. Hartrick Doane GA. Am I still ethical? The socially-mediated process of nurses' moral identity. *Nurs Ethics*. 2002;9(6):623–635.

3. Hartrick-Doane G, Varcoe C. *Family Nursing as Relational Inquiry: Developing Health Promoting Practice*. Philadelphia: Lippincott Williams & Wilkins; 2005.

4. Rorty R. *Philosophy and Social Hope*. London: Penguin; 1999.

5. Thayer-Bacon B. *Relational (E)pistemologies*. New York: Peter Lang; 2003.

6. James W. *Pragmatism. A New Name for Some Old Ways of Thinking*. New York: Longmans, Green & Co; 1907.

7. Roth JK. Introduction. In: Roth JK, ed. *The Moral Philosophy of William James*. New York: Thomas Y. Crowell Co; 1969:1–18.

8. Berman M, *Wandering God. A Study in Nomadic Spirituality*. Albany, NY: State of New York Press; 2000.

9. James W. *Essays in Pragmatism*. New York; Hafner Publishing; 1948.

10. Dickoff J, James PJ. A theory of theories: a position paper. In: Nicholl LH, ed. *Perspectives on Nursing Theory*, Glenview, Il. Scott, Foresman & Co; 1968/1986:99–111.

11. Reason P, Torbert WR. Toward a transformational social science: a further look at the scientific merits of action research. *Concepts Transformations*. 2001;6(1):1–37.

12. Hartrick Doane GA. Through pragmatic eyes: philosophy and the resourcing of family nursing. *Nurs Philos*. 2003;4: 25–32.

13. Varcoe C. Abuse obscured: an ethnographic account of emergency nursing in relation to violence against women. *Can J Nurs Res*. 2001;32(4):95–115.

14. Allen DG. Knowledge, politics, culture, and gender: a discourse perspective. *Can J Nurs Res*. 1999;30(4):227–234.

15. Stephenson P. Expanding notions of culture for cross-cultural ethics in health and medicine. In: Coward H, Ratanakul P, eds. *A Cross-Cultural Dialogue on Health Care Ethics*. Waterloo, Ontario, Canada: Wilfried Laurier University Press; 1999:68–91.

16 Swendson C, Windsor C. Rethinking cultural sensitivity. *Nurs Inq*. 1996;3:3–12.

17. Ladson-Billings G. Racialized discourses and ethnic epistemologies. In: Denzin NK, Lincoln YS, eds. *Handbook of Qualitative Research*. Thousand Oaks, Calif: Sage; 2000:398–425.

18. Hartrick G. A critical pedagogy for family nursing. *J Nurs Educ*. 1998;37(2):80–84.

19. Ng R. Multiculturalism as ideology: a textual analysis. In: Campbell M, Manicom A, eds. *Knowledge, Experience, and Ruling Relations: Studies in the Social Organization of Knowledge*. Toronto, Ontario, Canada: University of Toronto Press; 1995.

20. Anderson J, Perry J, Blue C, et al. "Rewriting" cultural safety within the postcolonial and postnational feminist project: toward new epistemologies of healing. *Adv Nurs Sci*. 2003;26(3):196–214.

21. Bhabha H. *The Location of Culture*. London: Routledge; 1994.

22. Giroux HA. Public pedagogy as cultural politics: Stuart Hall and the "crisis" of culture. *Cultural Stud*, 2000;14(2): 341–360.

23. Gilroy P. *Against Race: Imagining Political Culture Beyond the Color Line*. Cambridge, Mass: Belknap; 2000.

24. Clifford J. *The Predicament of Culture: Twentieth Century Ethnography, Literature and Art*. Cambridge, Mass: Harvard University Press; 1988.

25. Friere P. *Pedagogy of the Oppressed*. New York: Continuum; 1970.

THE AUTHORS COMMENT

Toward Compassionate Action: Pragmatism and the Inseparability of Theory/Practice

This article was inspired by our desire to extend the conceptualization of nursing theory and theory development beyond a "realist" perspective and to illustrate theory as inherently philosophically and practically based. The article grew out of the work we did in developing our textbook *Family Nursing as Relational Inquiry*, published by Lippincott Williams & Wilkins in 2005. In the text, we used pragmatist philosophy and relational epistemology to develop ideas for guiding nursing practice in ways that did not presume a theory/practice gap. This article allowed us to specifically demonstrate the usefulness of a pragmatic approach to nursing theory development. Our intent is to show how pragmatism has helped us to conceptualize "family" and "culture" in ways that we believe foster ethical and socially just nursing practice.

GWENETH HARTRICK DOANE
COLLEEN VARCOE

The Practitioner as Theorist

ROSEMARY ELLIS, RN, PhD

*W*hen Gulliver traveled to Laputa, land in the clouds, he found rapt theorists wandering about constructing useless ideas. And, generally, that is what we think of theorists. This author, though, says that theorists in nursing are not the ivory-tower thinkers; they are the nurses who work directly with patients. With every patient, she explains, we select an approach, then use, modify, and expand it—whether or not we are conscious of doing so. Because theories in a field have a powerful, long-term influence on the direction that field will take, the author pleads that we struggle to make already-existing, implicit nursing theories—such as TLC, for example—clear and explicit, so that nursing will develop in the direction of more skilled bedside care.

Nursing has been called an applied science. It is, in the sense that it is the application of knowledge from the basic sciences. But nursing care, or nursing practice, is something more. It is not the simple transfer of basic science knowledge. The nurse does not practice chemistry, anthropology, or sociology. She must sort out, select, adapt, and infer from her basic science knowledge. She uses some of the knowledge, orientations, processes of study, or models from these sciences as a guide to understanding patients, their pathology, and therapeutic practices.

This selection, adaptation, and sometimes interpolation from the basic sciences must be done by the practitioner. The physiologist or anthropologist cannot predict what specific knowledge or what concepts the nurse will need. The nurse must identify these, because what is needed depends on the specific purpose intended. The nurse, for nursing, uses some framework for her selection and adaptation. In this action she is a theorist. That is, some theory—often not made explicit—directs her selection of the knowledge or concepts to apply.

By "theory," I mean a coherent hypothesis, or set of hypotheses, or a concept, forming a general framework for undertaking something. Theory means a conceptual structure built for a purpose. For nursing, that purpose is practice.

But the practitioner cannot just select from a rack of ready-to-wear theories, because the knowledges and theories as we find them in the basic sciences are insufficient for practice. Instead, nursing practice requires that she structure converging, and sometimes conflicting, facts from the many fields which produce knowledge about human beings.

The nurse works within the framework of the inseparability and interdependence of one person's human life, so she attempts to relate aspects not yet clearly related in the separate sciences.

That is, we strive to act holistically, though our knowledge does not come for use from any holistic science of humans.

In this, the practitioner differs from the scientist. The scientist, due to reasons of control, feasibility, and measurement in study (due, as well, to the sheer impossibility of mastering all sciences, or even specialties within one science) isolates aspects for study. While the scientist may recognize the interrelationships of, for instance, physiologic and psychologic factors in man, he far less commonly studies these as a whole.

The practitioner of nursing, in contrast, may not have a complete science to nurse the whole man, but nurse the whole man is what she is striving to do. And, she sees the problems that result when one aspect or another is left out.

The practitioner of nursing thus finds herself working from a framework somewhat different from that within which knowledge is typically generated in the sciences. In this translation, the practitioner, of necessity, begins to *restructure* theory. She—often, at least—must apply the theory or concept in a way its originator may not have foreseen. She cannot simply take concepts from the sciences and directly apply them and hope to have the key to the biologic and psychosocial factors bound together in a patient, because this very interdependence is often a factor in response to and recovery from illness.

From R. Ellis, The practioner as theorist, American Journal of Nursing, July 1969, 69(7), 1434–1438. Copyright © 1969. Reprinted with permission from Lippincott Williams & Wilkins

ABOUT THE AUTHOR

ROSEMARY ELLIS was born in Berkeley, CA. She received an AB degree in economics and a BSN from the University of California, Berkeley-San Francisco, followed by an MA in nursing education and a PhD in human development from the University of Chicago. At the time of her death in the fall of 1986, she was a Professor of Nursing, a position she held at Case Western Reserve University since 1964. Dr. Ellis authored more than 30 articles, book chapters, and other scholarly works, including four in the *Japanese Journal* *of Nursing Research*. She emphasized the importance of pursuing questions about the substantive structure and description of nursing. Her metatheoretical writings have had a significant influence on nursing. The 1993 article "Rosemary Ellis' views on the substantive structure of nursing" by Donna Algase and Ann Whall, published in *Image: Journal of Nursing Scholarship, 25*(1), 69–72, addresses this significant contribution to nursing, drawing from both her published and unpublished works.

 ## Generalities Don't Suffice

Further, because we attempt to nurse the individual, general theories cannot suffice. General theories of human behavior describe the typical or the norm, not the exception or the individual. Or, sometimes, they describe the extremes and not the middle range.

For example, it is a useful notion that self-preservation, both in a physical and psychologic sense, is a major element in human behavior that accounts for or explains much observed behavior. Yet it is not uncommon to see patients who do not act rationally for self-preservation. They appear to have some stronger motive for action. We also see heroic acts of self-sacrifice which are not easily explained by general theories of self-preservation.

As one moves from general theories about human behavior to those relevant to all of the helping professions, and then to those relevant to patient behavior, there is need for an increasing number of conditional statements. What applies is shaped by the context, roles, and, for patients, the physical status that presents. This is yet another reason why the professional is a theorist: she is the person who must identify the conditional factors; she has to make the conditional statements.

Related to this is the fact that the professional can encounter conflicting theories, with each supported by some evidence. If she is to take some action she must choose a theory, either consciously or not, for her action is not independent of history; it stems from some framework.

For example, the concept or theory that guides the common practice of encouraging patients to talk about their problems often is not made explicit. Verbalization is generally conceived to be a good thing. But does this concept support the practice in all circumstances for all patients, or explain clearly the exceptions? Theoretically, indiscriminate practice would seem to involve some risk. Do the reasons behind this concept identify the risks and the benefits? The practitioner who follows a practice based on theory must appraise and criticize the theory if she follows it in nursing patients. She must weight the risks and benefits in a manner not required of the scholar who theorizes about a phenomenon in the specific or in general, but who does not treat the individual.

The scholar is often concerned with describing and predicting phenomena. He seeks objectivity, so he reduces, to the extent possible, the influence he may have on the variance due to the experimenter. He seeks to eliminate the human, personal element of the investigator.

This is the converse of a practice discipline. As Conant (1967) has highlighted, a practice discipline seeks not only to describe or predict phenomena, but to introduce change. Practice is goal-directed, not to the accumulation of knowledge, but to the prescription and implementation of activity to change natural outcomes to desired outcomes.

Therefore, the clinical testing of a theory is essential if it is used as a guide to practice. It is the professional practitioner who is able to criticize the theory in use, and determine its value for directing actions to achieve defined outcomes. In this she is not only a *user* of theory, but she may be a *modifier* as well. She is also a *chooser* of theory.

Consider a practice of encouraging a patient to verbalize about his operation. Talking about one's operation occurs frequently enough to have become a folk expectation and to have provoked joking. The frequency and persistence of the behavior suggests that there is some potency behind it. One could speculate, too, that there is possibly a folk norm for the time at which such talking is acceptable, excusable, and tolerated by friends and family. There may also be social norms for what content is acceptable. If such norms exist, and the patient exceeds these norms, he runs the risk of being cut off verbally or avoided by others. One hears complaints to suggest this happens.

Can this be avoided through nursing? From one theory it can be argued that if the nurse encourages a patient to talk about his operation, some of the need to continue talking about it can be extinguished, and the risk for the patient of annoying family and friends can be reduced.

But, from another theory, one could argue that if the nurse, an important figure for the patient postoperatively, encourages the patient to talk, conveys the expectation that he will talk—and thus, in effect, rewards, the behavior—she may prolong or reinforce it, causing the patient to risk violating folk norms.

It is not the originators of alternative theories who can solve a possible dilemma for the nurse. It is the nurse as practitioner and user of theory who must resolve the dilemma—in action, in critique of action, and in further theorizing.

A universal practice of encouraging patients to talk about their feelings may be questioned from another orientation. A medical patient recently talked with one of my faculty colleagues about the graduate student who was caring for him. He could not understand what the student wanted of him. This student, in her clinical course work, had time to talk with patients, and had visited with the patient after she had completed the typical morning care activities of bathing and bed making. Her conversations were patient-focused but were not probing. She did not have any specific goal in mind except to interact with the patient and to get to know him.

This patient, however, told the instructor that he was an orphan, who had learned early that people do not do things for nothing. He interpreted the student's talking with him as evidence that she wanted something from him. This man viewed even conversation as something you get or give only in exchange for something or because you want something. For him, the nurse's attempt to learn more about him by talking with him was seen as a sexual advance. He could not imagine any interaction that did not have an exploitative motive. He was, therefore, made acutely uncomfortable by a very casual attempt by a nurse to encourage him to verbalize. Her motives were significantly misperceived, to the detriment of the patient (though one could argue that perhaps we learned more about the patient because of his discomfort).

There may also be instances where attempting to get a patient to talk about his feelings is contraindicated because it may dissipate the feeling. There

may be instances where it is important for someone to experience and to recognize feelings *as feelings*. Talking about them may diminish them, objectify them, and so lose them as feelings. Joy is certainly one emotion that can be diminished by talking about it or attempting to explain it. I can recall an obstetrician father who was so profoundly moved by the birth of his own child that he burst into tears. The intensity of his own feeling totally surprised him, as well as his obstetrician colleagues. It seemed important for him to fully experience the intensity of his feeling and not diminish it until he had really felt it and absorbed it as his own feeling.

Lest I mislead, let me hasten to say that, in general, benefits seem to result from the practice of encouraging verbalization, but what are the exceptions? If benefits accrue, how are they explained? Practice could be more selective, and perhaps more effective, if we knew exactly what patient benefits to expect, and what dynamics would achieve them.

For example, benefits might be due to the patient's recognition, through talking, of the specific content of his feelings.

Benefits could also be due to the sense of companionship which can be achieved by talking with another, without regard for particular content. That is, would talking be effective without a listener? If not, what is supplied by a listener, even a nondirective listener, that is essential?

Is benefit derived from the recapitulation of an event which serves in some sense to produce mastery over, or integration of, the event, as in talking about one's operation? Or are benefits due to some reciprocal system where talking serves in place of some other potentially more detrimental form of discharge, such as acting out or somatization? Choose your theory. It is not likely to hold for all circumstances or cases, nor to support an invariate nursing practice of encouraging verbalization. Thus, the professional practitioner must become not simply a user of given theory, but a developer, tester, and expander of theory. This is not for the purpose of scholarship; it is an essential for intelligent practice.

The Need for Theory

It is essential because of the inadequacies in existing theories for the circumstances of nursing.

It is essential because of the need to synthesize, for practice, knowledge from diverse disciplines not yet fully related in theory.

It also is essential because the basic disciplines often are not pursuing the problems of importance to nurse and patient. For example, there is no extensive study, knowledge, or theory about appetite. As nurses we study nutrition, yet many of our observations and concerns with nutritional problems of patients are not solved by knowledge of nutrition. We need to know more about how to enable a patient to partake of the nutrients he needs, and about patterns of appetite in illness. For nursing, we need theories toward a science of appetite or of taste, and what happens to it in illness.

Conant (1967) gives an example of the complexities of a practice theory for back care: it must encompass maintenance of skin and underlying tissues, nutritional and fluid balance, and physical manipulation of the body. It is unlikely that the theory for back care will be developed from any other discipline than nursing. Existing theories guide the development of a field, because they guide what are seen as the interesting problems for study, the purposes for such study, and the ways in which problems are studied. Ways of defining problems, and of studying them, and what is considered worth pursuing are likely to differ from field to field. What may be significant problems for nursing may not fit with the theories, methods of study, or current focus of any other single field.

It is also unlikely that scientists in other disciplines will rush to collaborate with one another for study of a phenomenon because a nurse finds it important in nursing care. This is perhaps too pessimistic a view of collaboration in view of increasing evidence of interdisciplinary research. There remain, however, significant obstacles in orientation and method which impede cross-disciplinary research.

How Theory is Built

Of course, we theorize without knowing we do it. A nursing student last fall was relating an experience she had while walking with a young child. The child had to smell every flower in a bush. The student told the child they would all smell alike, but he had to check out every blossom, just the same.

I commented that perhaps the child had made no generalization about flowers. He hadn't yet developed a notion that flowers that are shaped and colored alike, and grown on one bush, have a high probability of smelling alike. One could say the child was operating without any general concept of flower smell, and exploring each bloom was still an adventure.

Over time, the adventure may be lost and the child will conclude—or accept someone else's conclusion—that flowers that look alike, smell alike. And he'll spend time on other adventures.

Now it occurs to me that, not being a flower specialist, I have never really thought about similarities and differences in flower smells in any scientific way. As I think about it, I very much doubt that the visual cues I use to class flowers as the same—such as shape, color, type of petal, and so on—have very much to do with smell. I associate visual similarities with olfactory similarities—probably erroneously as to cause, but not erroneously from an empiric view. But it doesn't matter. I'm not the expert. I don't practice or teach others the practice of flower smelling. Only *I* suffer from my misconceptions. But if we all acted so confused about nursing matters, we'd be in trouble.

No skillful nurse could efficiently practice like the adventurous little child—testing every detail of every nursing action each time it appeared. Instead, she arrives at some generalizations and begins to accumulate some wisdom over time that allows her to group, to classify, to identify, to focus, and to select what she will spend time pursuing. She will reach at least my level of thinking about flowers and their perfumes—it may be erroneous, but it is at least a concept.

The professional practitioner quickly recognizes differences between patients, or their responses, and accounts for them. She may not do this deliberately or make her theory explicit but, nevertheless, she adjusts her approach, her expectations, and sometimes her activities, accordingly.

She also is theorizing when she *labels* patient behavior. Many nurses have learned to recognize and label behavior as rejection even when the cues the patient gives do not exactly duplicate any specific definition of rejection. We have in some sense extended this concept or the ideas about it.

Unfortunately, we often stop when we have categorized or labeled the behavior or speculated about its genesis, just as I stopped with color, shape, and odor because I had satisfied one level of understanding. But the skillful practitioner, contrary to me and my flowers, must test out her generalization, her framework. Further, she may have an obligation to change the behavior she has observed and labeled. But too often, when she does attempt to change it, she fails to make explicit the theory which guides her action, though she implicitly is operating from some framework toward some direction. Such framework is at least incipient theory. Recognition of patterns in patient behaviors is also incipient theory.

Everyday Theorizing

We are not sufficiently conscious of the extent to which we use theory in practice, nor of the extent to which we adapt theory in practice. We also rarely recognize when we create or develop theory in practice, yet it does happen.

It is not uncommon for a nurse to sense correctly that a certain patient is not going to be able to follow some prescribed regimen, or for the nurse to predict, correctly, a patient's negative reaction to some element of therapy. Sometimes these perceptions run counter to those of the physician or others. What has happened is that the nurse has related some element of behavior to acceptance of therapy or response to it, that the other persons have not included in their framework, for some reason. And, of course, the converse can be found. Such examples illustrate the differences in the theories that are used pervasively. When the nurse's perception and prediction differ from others, she has developed a different theoretical stance.

The failure to make theory explicit is sometimes from lack of awareness of how one structures something. We do not stop to think, or possibly are not really conscious of our framework. Much of our structuring may be preconscious. Certainly, some failure to make theory explicit is because the practitioner (of necessity, and rightly so) is interested in the goal of nursing care, and not the analysis of the perceptions and processes used to achieve it. Our focus is on action, not on the analysis of it. But if we really have a commitment to the future beyond the personal accumulation of wisdom from patient to patient, and if we wish to communicate this wisdom we must try to analyze our actions and formulate theories from them. We must have practitioners in nursing who are willing to be scholars as well and who have the interest, skill, and time to pursue the analyses and formulations and test them in practice.

 ## A New Look at the Familiar

But there is another reason why theory may not be made explicit. It is because we may overlook the familiar, or perhaps we devalue it.

There is some danger of neglecting, or even rejecting, some of the traditional, familiar components in nursing as we grow in our emphasis on science and research. One such component might be what is termed TLC—"tender loving care." This something or this concept, which someone (it would be fascinating to know who) has tried to capture by a phrase, is nonscientific. We are not likely to do research on it. We do not have tools to measure it. Yet many nurses, as well as nonnurses, recognize it as an essential component in nursing for many patients.

Recently in teaching I used this vague concept, TLC, as a possible example of something that occurs in nursing for which we do not yet have a theory or perhaps, more precisely, that we have not theorized about, yet which we can sense. I felt the idea embarrassed several students. I think this regrettable, but I was not totally surprised. One of my friends has been collecting data from entering, middle, and graduating students from nine schools of nursing, baccalaureate and diploma, religious-affiliated and secular. These data included many, many examples of student dilemmas about expressing their feelings for patients. It would appear that a significant number of students enter with compassion for patients but quickly get the idea they must never convey feelings to patients. Rightly or wrongly, such an attitude will affect one's view of "tender loving care."

My own view is that tenderness and love are essential ingredients in nursing care. We need to theorize about these elements in nursing. Others have valued them as effective components in care, and occasionally TLC is actually prescribed—though I doubt the effectiveness of ordering it.

Whether or not you agree with this view about TLC, it is an example of a concept that exists, that is associated with nursing, that has been felt to be rather specific to nursing, but that we have not yet made explicit, nor yet fully conceptualized. We probably know, at least at a preconscious level, more about it than anybody else, for we can see it in so many diverse actions and situations. It does not seem unreasonable to suggest that theorizing about something as vague and yet as familiar as TLC might be valuable for understanding nursing.

At this stage in theory development I could entertain, even, the use of jargon—in the sense of a special professional language—to express some of the ideas in nursing. For instance, I would endorse the use of this term TLC for the purposes of talking about it until we can more precisely or more elegantly describe what we are talking about.

At this time in theory development it will be profitable to borrow or adapt concepts and theories from whatever source we can, if they will help us to understand and produce nursing. They must, however, be tested for their usefulness in guiding nursing practice in the arena of practice.

Intuitive exploration, speculation, trial and error, introspection, subjective impression—all can be used toward development of theory.

What is needed are attempts to make theory explicit, with tests of theories for nursing *in the practice* of nursing, and with further development or theories emerging *from the practice* of nursing.

REFERENCE

Conant, L. H. (1967). Closing the practice-theory gap. *Nursing Outlook, 15,* 37–39.

THE AUTHOR COMMENTS | The Practitioner as Theorist

I wrote this article to demystify the then-prevalent ideas that theory should be "grand theory" or that what was needed was some "theory" to justify nursing. As was evident from the literature and conferences at national meetings, there was great confusion concerning uses of theory and why nurses as practitioners needed theory. With their emphasis on theory and research, nurse scientists often rejected or at least ignored the importance of phenomena of nursing practice.

ROSEMARY ELLIS
1969

"Lest We Forget": An Issue Concerning the Doctorate in Nursing Practice (DNP)

ANN L. WHALL, RN, PhD, FGSA, FAAN

The academic community within nursing is currently discussing an interesting option to the PhD, or Doctorate of Philosophy degree. Termed the Doctorate in Nursing Practice (DNP), it is currently described as a practice-focused rather than a research-focused doctorate (such as the PhD). Several issues are being explored, including descriptions of the differences between programs of study for the DNP versus the PhD; one of these differences is sometimes described as less of a metatheoretical focus within the DNP. While this distinction is a clear and worthy one, it brought back remembrances of past nursing practices that are perhaps best seen as unexamined or at least ill informed. Before describing such practices, it is helpful to remind ourselves that one's view of science (arguably a metatheoretical issue) dictates how one practices (e.g., what is focused upon, how one approaches assessment, interventions, etc). These views of science thus determine the possibilities of and for practice, including (in part) the domains (or proper subject matter) of such practice, the truth criteria (or practice standards) accepted, as well as the persistent questions used to guide the research supporting the evidence base for such practice.

Less of a focus within the DNP upon metatheory might be interpreted as viewing nursing practice as a stand-alone phenomenon, affected remotely, if at all, by philosophic beliefs and views of science held within the discipline. Such a view would not only greatly affect nursing practice, but will concomitantly increase the influence of other disciplines upon nursing practice. When nursing in the past was not clear concerning its metatheoretical stance, practicing nurses at times assumed the practice values of other disciplines. The result might be described as analogous to a "rudderless ship," greatly influenced by the winds of the day and not by specific values of nursing.

Some cases in point include that from the time of Nightingale to roughly the mid-twentieth century, nurs-

ing education and practice was focused primarily on rote-learned nursing care procedures. Focus on carrying out technology in an expert fashion, without questioning philosophic issues involved, might have allowed nurses to expertly assist with prefrontal lobotomies, patient restraint (chemical/physical), and such events as the "syphilis experiment" with disadvantaged subjects and/or other practices ultimately seen as abhorrent. The positivistic view of science undergirding such practice included that "observables" were the only "proper" focus of science and that culture and other values were unimportant to science. This view of science was ultimately rejected within nursing, but unquestioning acceptance and "rote compliance" with existing practice norms and procedures remains a part of nursing's past. Since the mid-twentieth century, the postmodern (and including post-structural) philosophic view of science has predominated within nursing, and this view includes assessment of cultural preferences, patient input, etc.[1] However, the half-century preceding this era is a reminder that nurse leaders (especially those supporting the DNP) must understand the philosophic foundations of practice that define the nature and possibilities of advanced practice.

As nursing discusses ways to develop the DNP, it is important to keep in mind the philosophic views of science that have negatively affected nursing practice and research in the past. *Practice is not a "stand alone" phenomenon*; rather, it is a direct outcome of philosophic beliefs. DNP graduates will lead nursing practice forward, and they need a clear grounding in philosophy of science (or metatheoretical) issues that define the nature of nursing practice and research. A cursory familiarity will not do. As Nelson and Gordon[2] have argued, nursing has the tendency to approach current issues as not having a "past" and of repudiating our disciplinary past experience. Hopefully, this will not be forgotten in current discussions of the DNP.

ABOUT THE AUTHOR

ANN L. WHALL is currently holding the Allesse Endowed Chair in Gerontological Nursing at Oakland University School of Nursing, in Rochester, Michigan. She is also a Visiting Professor at the University of Cork, Republic of Ireland, and Professor Emerita at the University of Michigan, Ann Arbor. Ann is active in her program of research in the targeting of behavioral treatments for the nursing care of older adults with dementia. She also teaches doctoral level philosophic foundations of nursing theory classes in several invited venues.

REFERENCES

1. Whall A, Hicks F. The unrecognized paradigm shift within nursing: Implications, problems, and possibilities. *Nurs Outlook* 2004;50:72–6.

2. Nelson S, Gordon S. The rhetoric of rupture: Nursing as a practice with a history? *Nurs Outlook* 2004;52:255–61.

THE AUTHOR COMMENTS

"Lest We Forget": An Issue Concerning the Doctorate in Nursing Practice (DNP)

I was concerned with what I considered to be disregard for the other ways of knowing within nursing as the technical and empirical base continued to grow exponentially. I saw the suggestion that nursing metatheory was less important in the preparation for the clinical doctorate in nursing as a dangerous and "ahistoric" approach to nursing science.

I believe that the discussions of metatheoretical issues related to nursing clinical practice is a major way to ensure that nurses do not become technically driven automatons, similar to caregivers one might encounter in Orwell's "Brave New World."

ANN L. WHALL

The Link Between Nursing Discourses and Nurses' Silence

Implications for a Knowledge-Based Discourse for Nursing Practice

CONNIE J. CANAM, RN, PhD

Much emphasis has been placed on the importance of nurses' articulating what they do to counteract the invisibility of nursing practice. Yet there has been minimal focus on why nurses are silent. This article explores the link between technical and caring discourses and nurses' silence and suggests an alternative discourse that conceptualizes nursing as a knowledge-driven enterprise that shifts the focus from what nurses do to what nurses know by promoting nurses' practice knowledge as a language for articulating their practice. **Key words** *nursing knowledge, nurses' silence, practice discourses, practice language relational practice, social context*

The call for nurses to articulate the nature of their practice to address the invisibility of nursing work[1] and to illuminate the significance of their contributions to healthcare and society[2] continues to be emphasized within the nursing literature. Nurses are being urged to speak up about the work they do because it is "largely invisible to other providers, to administrators, and policy-makers"[1(p37)] and to the public.[3,4] Yet, it has been noted that nurses continue to have difficulty clearly articulating the essential contributions they make to healthcare.[2] Thus, although a case can be made for the importance of nurses' articulating their practice, the reasons why they have difficulty doing so require further exploration.

In this article, I draw on findings from a study of clinical nurse specialists' (CNSs') practice and locate these findings within the literature on the social context of nurses' practice, to make a link between technical and caring discourses that the nurses described as operating within the practice environment and their difficulty articulating their practice. I then propose an alternate discourse for nurses to use in articulating their practice and their contributions to healthcare that is based on the knowledge that informs their practice.

The aim of the study was to gain an understanding, from the perspective of CNSs, of their contributions to the healthcare of children with chronic health conditions and their families. An interpretive, descriptive methodology provided direction for accessing CNSs' understandings of their practice, the knowledge that informs it and the factors influencing it, and for explicating the ways in which their understandings are

shaped by the social context in which their practice is situated. Sixteen nurses, who worked in pediatric CNS roles in specialty programs that provided health services for children with complex health needs and their families, participated in individual, in-depth interviews that were audiotaped and transcribed.

Data consisted of several hundred pages of interview transcripts as well as participants' written comments on a copy of their interview transcript, which was sent to each participant with a request to clarify, change, or add any comments that would further capture their practice. Fourteen participants responded with written comments in the margins of their transcripts and/or in an attached note. A third source of data was field notes on my observations and reflections of all interactions with participants. For example, several participants expressed concern that they would not have anything meaningful to contribute to the study. Initially, I thought their concerns were related to my lack of clarity in describing the purpose of the study, but it became clear that this concern is reflective of their lack of confidence in their knowledge and is demonstrated in the findings related to the difficulty they have articulating their practice.

The aims of the data analysis were 2-fold: to describe CNSs' understandings of the nature of their practice, the knowledge that informs it, and the factors that influence it and to analyze the ways in which their understandings are shaped by the social context in which their practice is situated. In the descriptive analysis, participants' transcripts were examined for recurring themes and their relation to one

From C. J. Canam, The link between nursing discourses and nurses' silence implications for a knowledge-based discourse for nursing practice. Advances in Nursing Science, 2008, 31(4), 296–307.

ABOUT THE AUTHOR

CONNIE J. CANAM was born and raised in Stickney, New Brunswick, on the eastern coast of Canada. She received her BSN degree from Dalhousie University in 1973, her MSN degree from the University of BC in 1980, and her PhD in nursing from the University of Victoria in 2004. She has held various nursing positions in the field of pediatric nursing including staff nurse, nurse clinician, staff educator, and lecturer and is currently an Assistant Professor at University of British Columbia School of Nursing located in Vancouver, British Columbia, Canada. Her scholarship has focused on determining the knowledge and skills required by nurses and families to promote the health of children with chronic health conditions. Her key contributions are the development of an education program for parents of children with chronic health conditions, a framework for assessing family coping with a child's chronic health condition, and furthering the dialogue on nurses' articulation of their practice and contributions to clients' healthcare. When not working, she takes advantage of the great outdoors in British Columbia by walking near the ocean, hiking, and playing tennis.

another. Extensive use was made of participants' own words to exemplify the themes and to represent their understandings as accurately as possible.

For the interpretive analysis, I drew on the work of researchers in narrative analysis who operate from the premise that the language individuals use to articulate their understandings provides access to the social and cultural forces influencing their thinking and actions.[5-7] I was particularly informed by the approach of Lieblich et al.[8] to interpretive analysis, in which the researcher listens to 3 voices in analyzing participants' accounts; the voice of the narrator as represented by the tape or text, the voice of the researcher as monitored through self-reflection, and the voice of theory as accessed through the researcher's theoretical and empirical knowledge of the context/culture that is being studied. In examining the voice of the narrator, I focused on the language participants used to describe their understandings of their practice world and asked questions of the data such as the following: Are there particular discourses that participants draw upon to describe their practice? What contextual knowledge guides their actions? What language strategies are apparent in their accounts such as core metaphors or frequent use of a word or phrase?

The overall findings of the study illuminate the nature of CNSs' practice as predominately relational, involving education, support, advocacy, and coordination of care for individual children and families and initiatives such as program development and educational outreach for the population of children and families. Participants described approaching the care of children and families from a holistic perspective and drawing on an extensive knowledge base that includes empirical, theoretical, contextual, and sociopolitical knowledge. Factors identified as influencing their practice include an individualistic orientation of the healthcare system underpinned by a biomedical model and physician dominance, and a corporate model of healthcare focused on minimizing costs and protecting corporate interests. These findings are reported in more detail elsewhere.[9,10]

The study findings of relevance to the ideas discussed in this article relate to the ways in which CNSs' understandings were shaped by the social context in which their practice is situated. More specifically, the findings related to the difficulty CNSs had articulating their practice are linked to their understandings of the power dynamics operating within their practice environment.

Although the CNSs emphasized that their knowledge of children and families is key to the provision of quality healthcare, they described a number of situations within the healthcare setting, where they could have contributed relevant knowledge to a discussion but they remained silent. These situations often related to formal or informal discussions with other members of the healthcare team.

In exploring the reasons for their silence, it became clear that their understandings of the power dynamics operating within the practice environment influenced articulation of their perspective. They described a practice environment dominated by a biomedical model of healthcare and a technical discourse in which objective/technical knowledge is privileged and subjective/experiential knowledge is discounted. In observing the pervasiveness of a technical discourse among members of the multidisciplinary team, the CNSs felt pressured to "speak the language" if they wanted to participate in healthcare conversations. However, they claimed that the language of a technical discourse does not adequately represent the realities of their practice, which they described as primarily relational rather than technical. They viewed the subjective/experiential language of a caring discourse as more aligned with the nature of their practice and knowledge. Yet, in drawing on this language to articulate their practice, they experienced their perspectives being discounted or ignored by other members of the healthcare team.

They noted that their perspectives were rarely sought at the individual or population levels of healthcare, which sent them a message that their knowledge is not considered relevant to healthcare decisions. These experiences had the effect of undermining their confidence in their practice and knowledge, as reflected in one participant's comment, "all I do is talk to people," suggesting that her work is not significant while discounting the contributions she makes to educating, supporting, advocating for, and coordinating care for children and their families. Moreover, there was an underlying sense within their narratives of the legitimacy of nursing as a technical endeavor, whereas the nontechnical aspects of their practice were considered less legitimate, or what some participants referred to as "soft." This understanding reflects their view that much of what they do is not seen as legitimate by the dominant system.

The findings suggest that nurses' silence is related to their understandings of the power dynamics operating within their practice environment that privilege a technical discourse and objective/technical knowledge and discount a caring discourse and subjective/experiential language. Given that the language of the dominant discourse does not represent CNSs' practice or the knowledge that informs it, and the language of a caring discourse is discounted by the dominant system, they did not have a language for articulating their practice.

These findings are located within the theoretical and research literature on the social context of nurses' practice to further explore the relationship between power dynamics operating within the practice environment and nurses' articulation of their practice and knowledge.

The Social Context of Nurses' Knowledge and Practice

Liaschenko and Fisher are among the few theorists who emphasize the importance of connecting the knowledge that directs nurses' work to "the social reality in which nursing is situated."[11(p30)] They maintain the current literature on practice knowledge, while moving nursing practice beyond a dependence on biomedical knowledge, has taken only a limited account of the influence of context on knowledge and action.

Traditionally, the knowledge-practice relationship was viewed as a simple application of knowledge to practice with little consideration for the context in which it was enacted. A second view, proposed by Benner,[12] is that knowledge and practice interact and in the process knowledge is transformed. Benner's contention that expert nurses base their expertise on pattern recognition that influences future actions has been criticized as ignoring the context of interaction from which the pattern emerges.[13]

A third view is that nurses draw on knowledge of the social and in particular on "readings of the social context in which nursing is practiced"[13(p116)] to engage in the production and reproduction of institutionalized practices.

Although there are several factors within the practice environment that can influence nurses' understandings of their practice and knowledge, a factor particularly relevant to the CNS study is participants' perceptions of the power dynamics operating within the healthcare environment, evident in the dominance of a technical discourse and the discounting of a caring discourse that nurses took up to make sense of their practice.

The Language of Power in Healthcare

Smith's work[14–16] explores how male-dominated institutions maintain power by ideological practices that discount subjective forms of knowledge and reify objectified forms of knowledge. These practices are maintained through language, and Smith suggests that women end up with a split relationship to language. On one side of the split are the subjective forms of knowledge that come out of their lived experiences and on the other side are the objectified forms of knowledge, which is the language of the relations of ruling. Smith contends that the language of those in positions of power is maintained by the ideological practices of converting people's perspectives of their own experience into objectified forms of knowledge. Thus, power is maintained and reproduced through knowledge, and because language is central to the production of knowledge,[17] it is also central to the maintenance and reproduction of power relations. Which discourse becomes the dominant one depends on the power of the various political interests that the discourses represent.[18]

Understanding power as inherent in our ways of thinking and speaking is associated with a postmodern perspective of power relations as embedded in various discursive positions.[19] Thus, the discourses that one takes up have within them a predetermined script for enacting power relations. This idea is reflected in Fisher's argument that doctors and nurses are professionals "whose identities are produced by their location in a gendered profession,"[20(p179)] which prompts them to represent how the system works "in ways that reinscribe or resist hegemonic discourse."[20(p180)]

If power is seen to reside in the various discourses that one takes up, deconstructing the power scripts inherent within these discourses provides a way of disengaging from the dynamics by changing these scripts or creating new discourses with different power scripts.

A Technical/Rationalist Discourse

It has long been noted within the nursing field that nurses practice in a healthcare environment dominated by physicians and a technical rationalist discourse, in which the central values are objectivity and efficiency.[21] Nursing practice within this model of care is viewed as instrumental and task oriented.[22] A central assumption underlying a technical/rationalist discourse is that empirical forms of knowledge are of the highest order and provide the only valid evidence for healthcare decisions.[23] Following from this is the assumption that that experiential forms of knowledge are subjective and therefore not evidence. Associated with these assumptions is the view of nursing knowledge as subjective and physician knowledge as objective.[2]

The privileging of objective/empirical knowledge and the discounting of subjective/ experiential knowledge maintain the dominance of physicians in healthcare.[15] Moreover, it has the effect of undermining nurses' confidence in their knowledge that, in the current study, they viewed as less legitimate than that of the technical discourse. As Ceci and McIntyre[24] note, when one's way of understanding the world is unacknowledged, there is a sense of somehow being incorrect in one's understandings. Brown sees this sense of being incorrect as a gender issue, commenting that "ironically, as women and as nurses our first response is often to consider our own inadequacies."[25(p170)] It has also been noted that when nurses discuss evidence-based practice, they ignore the multiple patterns of knowing in nursing and draw on a medical perspective of evidence,[26] which reflects a view of objective/empirical knowledge being more legitimate.

Thus, one explanation for CNSs' difficulty articulating their practice is their perception that the objective/empirical language of the dominant discourse is more legitimate than the subjective/experiential language of the caring discourse but because it does not fit with the nature of their practice they could not draw on it to articulate their practice. Consequently, a technical rationalist discourse and the privileging of empirical knowledge had the effect of silencing them.

Psychosocial/Caring Discourse

Smith[15] suggests that in addition to exploring and disclosing the conceptual practices of the ruling relations, as women we also need to become aware of how our own ideological practices contribute to and maintain the power relations within dominant systems and then work toward different social practices and different ways of thinking and knowing the society in which we live.

Nursing's ideological practices can be examined through the discourses that have developed around various conceptualizations of nursing. Several authors have initiated exploration of the discourses that shape nursing practice. For example, in exploring nursing from a poststructural perspective, Cheek and Rudge[27] examined language with regard to the role it plays in both constructing and conveying understandings about nursing. They raised key questions about how nursing knowledge is produced and used and point to the potential of developing different discourses for nursing knowledge.

Over the years, various conceptualizations of nursing have been put forward in the form of nursing models and theories in an attempt to define nursing and distinguish it from medicine. Although it has been pointed out that nurses in practice rarely use the language that composes these conceptual models,[11] I would argue that their practice is influenced by the discourses that develop around these various conceptualizations, particularly as they take up certain discourses to make sense of their practice.

A discourse that has been most associated with nursing is holism. Boschma[28] contends that a holistic ideology has been used to legitimize an independent and unique role for nurses since the beginning of the 20th century. Initially, notions of holism encompassed the physical, psychological, and social needs of individuals as well as their environment. However, during the 1960s and 1970s the language of holism began to shift from the concept of "total" patient care to "psychosocial" care and "the nurse-patient relationship," which was considered central to resolving the patient's psychosocial problems.[28] In this reconfiguration of holism, the physical aspects of patient care and the context in which care occurs faded into the background. The concept of holistic care was replaced by the concept of psychosocial care and nursing distanced itself from the physical aspects of care, at least in the language of its discourse.

Boschma[28] claims that the exclusive focus on psychosocial needs and the nurse-patient relationship as a way to meet those needs, served an ideological function by defining nursing's unique and independent role in the hospital setting. However, focusing on the psychosocial aspects of care as the exclusive domain of nursing was misguided in 2 critical ways. First, constructing a psychosocial/caring discourse that excluded the patient's physical needs did not reflect the realities of nurses' practice, which clearly involved physical care as well as psychosocial care. Ironically, in trying to establish a unique role for itself, nurses became guilty of fragmenting the patient in their exclusive focus on the psychosocial, as it accused medicine of doing in their exclusive focus on the physical aspects of care. Second, the creation of a psychosocial/caring discourse to represent nursing set up an arbitrary dichotomy between nursing knowledge as subjective/relational and physician knowledge as objective/technical, which is still in evidence today.[2] This dichotomy led to a binary thinking in which knowledge and practice were viewed as either technical or relational[29] and became linked with particular practice settings. This understanding of nursing as either technical or relational is illustrated in the comment of a participant in the current study: "It's sort of like the ICU nurse versus the psychiatric nurse and I've always been the more technical kind of nurse."

Although many nurses embrace a biomedical/technical discourse to guide their practice, particularly those who work in high-acuity areas, others educated in the height of the caring movement enter the practice arena with a caring discourse firmly embedded in their understanding of nursing practice. Either discourse can create dissonance for nurses if it does not fit with the realities of the practice setting. An example of this dissonance is illustrated in a study of nursing practice on 2 surgical units in an acute care hospital. The practice environment is described as specialized, fast paced, complex, and uncertain as patients' conditions could quickly change. The nurses required advanced clinical skills to work on the units and their work was task oriented, with wound care taking up much of their time. The researcher notes "for many of the nurses, being able to develop a trusting relationship with patients was what made nursing work meaningful."[30(p355)] She comments that while the relational aspects of nurses' work were seen as "important to their personal understanding of themselves as nurses, it did not seem to be part of the nursing services as officially defined on the unit,"[30(p356)] which suggests that the caring discourse that directed nurses' understandings of themselves as nurses and their practice did not fit with the mandate of the clinical setting in which their practice was carried out. It was noted that the official discourse on the units seemed to be objective and impersonal (technical) whereas the "private" discourse (caring) of the nurses was driven underground.

A disconnect between the discourse that nurses take up to guide their practice and the reality of the practice setting places them in a "no-win" situation. If their identity as nurses and the meaningfulness of their work is tied to developing a trusting relationship with patients, and they are in a setting where this is not a priority or not possible, this sets them up to be frustrated and dissatisfied with their work. It could also be argued that it decreases nurses' credibility by not having a language that reflects the patient's reality and the reality of the practice setting. Moreover, it has been noted in a recent study that nurses' allegiance to a caring discourse that is not valued by the hospital's administration undermined the credibility of the nursing department's assertion that its services were highly effective.[31]

The discrepancy in the above study between what nurses see as important to their self-definition as nurses and what the healthcare institution sees as nurses' work suggests that theorists have not taken account of "the social reality in which nursing is situated"[11(p30)] in their development of nursing practice models. When claims are made that caring is the essence of nursing, or the nurse-patient relationship is central to nursing practice, or that nursing is a technical or task-oriented practice, there is an underlying assumption that these theories or discourses are universal and do not require consideration of the context in which nurses practice. Yet, clearly, a high-tech acute care setting in which many of the patients may not be able to communicate requires different practice models than an ambulatory setting in which patients and families are, for the most part, managing their own care.

A further problem with technical and caring discourses is the arbitrary dichotomy that has been set up between technical practices as underpinned by objective/ empirical knowledge and associated with medicine and relational practices as underpinned by subjective/experiential knowledge and associated with nursing.[29,32] Consequently, the psychosocial/caring discourses that provide the basis for a relational language of nursing practice are often discounted by the dominant system of healthcare, so nurses who do not "speak the language" of the dominant system find themselves excluded from healthcare conversations.

Cheek and Rudge posed the question, "is the difficulty that nursing has in defining itself because it attempts to do so in terms set by others?"[27(p18)] Initially, I considered the "terms set by others" as the technical rationalist discourse of the dominant system of care, and the CNSs indeed had difficulty defining their practice within that discourse. However, the "terms set by others" could also be the psychosocial and caring discourses that have provided the basis for a relational language of nursing practice. Although the CNSs maintained that their attempts to communicate their practice in relational language were ignored or discounted, it could be that this language also does not accurately reflect the nature of relational practice. This premise is supported by participants' narratives, in which there are many examples of them struggling to find the words to articulate their practice within the language of a caring discourse as the following quote illustrates:

> You can teach anybody those task things. What's harder is the interpersonal stuff, the family stuff, the "how do I know that you're not coping?" I don't even know how to say it; maybe that's the thing they call the art, you know, the caring piece. It's the stuff that's harder to get at.

Given the premise that neither the language of a technical discourse nor the language of a caring discourse captures the reality of nurses' practice, a second explanation for their difficulty articulating their practice is that they do not have a language that accurately represents it. The premise that nurses are silenced because they do not have a language for articulating their practice offers another perspective on the power dynamics within the healthcare system and a different approach to addressing these dynamics. Rather than trying to change the system, which is perceived as discounting nurses' knowledge, the focus is on helping nurses develop a language that accurately represents the nature of their practice, placing the power for change in their hands. Moreover, having a language that accurately represents their practice and their knowledge can enhance their confidence in contributing their perspective to the healthcare conversations as equal members of the healthcare team.

A Knowledge-Based Discourse for Nursing Practice

Chinn and Kramer's[33] suggestion that the knowledge nurses draw on to inform their understandings and their actions can provide a language for articulating their practice points to a discourse for nursing practice that is knowledge based rather than task or caring based. If, instead of a technical or caring discourse, nurses take up the discourse of nursing as a knowledge-driven enterprise in which nurses contribute important knowledge to client healthcare, the power script within this discourse is that nurses are equal members of the healthcare team who make valuable contributions to the healthcare of the public.

The key to developing a language of nursing practice is connecting it to the social context in which nursing is situated. In other words, the language should come from the knowledge nurses draw on in their actual practice rather than from theorists who are removed from the practice situation. Findings from the current study support the premise that nurses' practice knowledge can provide a knowledge-based rationale for their actions and thus a language for their practice. Participants' narratives reflected their practice knowledge as intricately tied to the nature of their practice and their practice goals, which they described as assisting families to understand and manage the ongoing care of the child at the individual level, and contributing to the design and delivery of effective healthcare services at the population level.

Although the CNSs described their practice as predominantly relational rather than technical, they demonstrated extensive knowledge of the chronic conditions of children served by the specialty program in which they worked and of the latest technology used to monitor and treat a particular health condition. Biomedical and technological knowledge were drawn upon to educate parents about their child's condition and to assist them in developing the technical skills they require to care for the child. Empirical knowledge was also drawn on in consultations with other healthcare professionals and agency personnel from across the region. Participants said they spent a great deal of time in phone consultations with a variety of people in regards to biomedical or technical aspects of a health condition. They maintained that because the programs in which they worked are specialized and associated with a tertiary care institution, they are a visible place to contact for information related to specific chronic conditions. The CNSs also drew on their extensive empirical knowledge base to develop services and programs that addressed the health needs of the population of children and families within their specialty.

To assist families in managing their child's ongoing care, the CNSs described drawing on theoretical knowledge of family coping, child development, social determinants of health and so forth, which provided direction for gathering and interpreting knowledge of the particular context in which the child and the family are situated. For example, in discussing a child and family she had recently assessed, one CNS identified "new marriage, new child, major health problems from birth, infant in hospital for 2 months, ESL family, working parents, supportive grandparents" as an important contextual knowledge to consider in determining a plan of care.

Another example in which theoretical and contextual knowledge provided a knowledge-based rationale for a plan of care relates to a mother whose infant was born with a cleft lip. In discussing the situation, the CNS's statement, "If you are only measuring mom's coping by the fact that she can change the [infant's] dressing, then you've missed all of it, I think," reflects knowledge of coping theory, which is brought to bear on the particular situation of the birth of a child with a disability. Theoretical knowledge alerted the nurse to determine the stressors this family is facing, the resources they have available to assist them, and the mother's perception of the situation. By drawing on both theoretical knowledge and knowledge of the particular context, the nurse determines, in conjunction with the family, what they need in the way of assistance to cope with the situation and manage their child's ongoing care.

Participants made a distinction between the knowledge they draw on to determine the best approach to care and the knowledge physicians draw on. One participant related a situation in which parents had refused consent for their child to have surgery to prevent further spread of a brain tumor. The physicians, drawing on biomedical knowledge, strongly recommended surgery to prolong the child's life, "basically insisting that we had to make them get treatment for the child." The CNS had talked with the family and knew that it was a decision that had been difficult for them but one that was informed by their concern for their daughter's quality of life. She talked with the physicians about respecting the family's decision and justified her reasoning by drawing on both contextual and ethical knowledge in considering the family's values and the family's right to make the decision. When she articulated the knowledge behind her position, the physicians agreed that the family's decision should be respected.

In the broader context of the CNSs' practice at the population level, there were several examples of situations in which a knowledge-based rationale for actions and decisions was articulated. For example, in lobbying for change in a policy that impacted families of children who require palliative care, one participant provided a knowledge-based rationale for suggested changes that included theoretical and contextual knowledge. The current policy was if the child does not require tasks related to symptom management, they do not qualify for a nurse in the home. The CNS emphasized that "palliative care nursing is holistic, it's complex" and often having a nurse in the home means that families have a choice about where their child dies. If there is not a nurse within the home, families are often reluctant to take their child home or to remain at home. And while having their child die in hospital may be difficult for many families, it can be particularly so for those living in other areas of the province.

> You take, not only the child, but the family out of their community and fly them down to another community and you take them out of their support system, and it medicalizes dying in a way that being at home doesn't.

She believes that providing options for families is an important criterion of quality healthcare and consequently is lobbying the committee to expand their definition of nursing care.

There are a number of advantages to a knowledge-based discourse of nursing practice. One advantage is that it has the potential to improve working relations between doctors and nurses by decreasing the tension created by the conceptualization of nursing knowledge as subjective/relational and physician knowledge as objective/technical. In providing a knowledge-based rationale for relational care, nurses can move beyond the binary thinking of technical knowledge as medicine's domain and relational knowledge as nursing's domain. The following story told by Street [34] provides an example to illustrate how nurses can provide a knowledge-based rationale for relational care and the potential impact this could have on dissolving the conceptual boundaries that currently pervade nurse-doctor communication.

A nurse was working in a neonatal ICU and calming a newborn who was crying and thrashing about, while 2 doctors were trying to get an IV started on the infant. The nurse placed one hand under the infant and stroked his brow with the other, while speaking in soothing tones. The infant calmed quickly and his heart and respiratory rate dropped dramatically, and he remained still while the doctor inserted the IV. When the doctor asked the nurse what she was doing, she said, "I'm looking after the baby's emotional needs"

to which the doctor replied, "we need strapping." The nurse called out for someone else to get the strapping and continued to hold the infant. Later, she said that the doctor was irritated with her because she would not get the strapping and run the IV through. She interpreted this as him thinking she was there to assist him and seeing the technical tasks as more of a priority than caring for the baby's emotional needs. There is, however, another way of interpreting this story. Perhaps "looking after the baby's emotional needs" did not have a lot of meaning for the doctor who was trying to get the IV stabilized. What if the nurse had responded to his question by saying, "I am calming the baby, to make it easier to insert the IV. Research shows that talking in soothing tones and stroking the infant calms them"? It is possible that it might not have made any difference to the doctor's response, but it is a much more descriptive rationale for her actions than "looking after the baby's emotional needs" and it demonstrates knowledge-based practice. Furthermore, it demonstrates a collaborative approach in which the nurse is working with the doctor to provide care for the infant, which suggests a different tone than "assisting him."

Another advantage of developing a knowledge-based discourse of nursing practice is that it can provide a basis for examining the evidence nurses draw on to address the health needs of individuals and populations Nurses' practice knowledge is derived from multiple sources including empirical research, practice theories, clients' experiences, and their own experiences/observations of being at the intersection of healthcare delivery and people's lives. All these sources of knowledge can be drawn on to provide evidence for nurses' practice decisions.[26] Thus, a knowledge-based discourse of nursing practice has the potential for broadening our understandings of the kinds of evidence required to improve patient and system outcomes.[35]

 ## Implications of a Knowledge Discourse for Nursing Practice

The premise that nurses are silenced because they do not have a language for articulating their practice suggests that we need to revisit the interpretation of nurses' silence as reluctance on their part to talk about what they do. For instance, Buresh and Gordon's [36] book *From Silence to Voice* is based on the premise that nurses do not have a public voice because they are reluctant to "tell the world what they do" and their solution is to teach them the skills they need to communicate with the public and to help them overcome their ambivalence to being more vocal. I would argue that conceptualizing the issue as nurses' reluctance to talk about what they do rather than their inability to communicate what they know has sent us in the wrong direction for addressing the issue. By focusing on competencies and skills rather than on nurses' knowledge, we continue to perpetuate the idea that nursing is a task-oriented, rather than a knowledge-driven enterprise. Creating a knowledge discourse for nursing practice provides an alternate approach to assisting nurses to articulate their practice, which focuses on recognizing, valuing, and articulating the in-depth knowledge that informs their practice.

The findings from this study suggest that a knowledge discourse is foreign to nurses practicing in the current healthcare environment, in which technical/rationalist and caring discourses continue to dominate healthcare communications. Introducing the idea that nurses can articulate their practice by drawing on the knowledge that informs it presupposes that nurses can articulate their knowledge. This may not be the case, so a beginning step is to encourage nurses to reflect on the knowledge underpinning particular practice decisions and actions.

As educators we can engage graduate students in learning activities that draw out their knowledge. For example, have them walk through their day and examine the knowledge required for the activities with which they are involved and the decisions they make. Class presentations could also provide students with opportunities to articulate their practice with one another. In addition, learning activities that connect students' knowledge to client outcomes can assist them in developing confidence in what they know and the difference this knowledge can make to healthcare. As Falk-Rafael[37] notes, nurses' contributions to healthcare must first be made visible by nurses acknowledging their own expertise before expecting others to recognize it.

Educators can also convey the expectation that nurses have a responsibility to clients, themselves, and the profession to articulate the knowledge that underpins their practice. This responsibility involves contributing to the provision of quality healthcare by making their knowledge available to inform healthcare decisions. It also involves educating other members of the healthcare team, regarding the nurse's role on the team and the knowledge they can contribute to healthcare decisions. Moreover, nurses need to be aware that by not articulating their practice and the knowledge that informs it, they are participating in maintaining the status quo and the power dynamics they see as constraining their practice. By remaining silent, they also contribute to the invisibility of their practice.

Research is needed that explores the potential usefulness of a knowledge-based discourse for facilitating nurses' articulation of their practice. Qualitative methods that access nurses' voices can serve the purpose of assisting nurses to reflect on their practice and the knowledge that informs it. Studies that employ action research methods could involve small groups of practicing nurses who reflect on and describe the knowledge that informs particular practice decisions

and actions, using this knowledge to articulate their practice with others in the research group and then in their practice setting. Research could be conducted to develop, implement, and evaluate educational approaches to teaching students to identify, value, and articulate the knowledge that informs their practice.

Further research is needed to continue developing the kinds of knowledge that inform nurses' practice. In particular, studies are needed that build on our understandings of the knowledge that informs the relational dimensions of healthcare.

 ## Conclusion

The premise is put forward that nurses are silenced because the technical and caring discourses operating within the healthcare environment do not provide an appropriate language for articulating their practice. An alternate nursing discourse is proposed that conceptualizes nursing as a knowledge-based enterprise in which nurses draw on the knowledge that informs their practice as a language for articulating it. It is proposed that having a language that accurately represents their practice and their knowledge can enhance their confidence in contributing their perspective to healthcare conversations as equal members of the healthcare team to promote coordinated and relevant healthcare. Promoting a practice environment in which nurses' practice knowledge is recognized, valued, and articulated will increase the visibility of nurses' work and recognition of the significant contributions they make to the healthcare of individuals and society.

REFERENCES

1. Rodney P, Varcoe C. Toward ethical inquiry in the economic evaluation of nursing practice. *Can J Nurs Res.* 2001;33(1):35–57.
2. Litchfield M, Jonsdottir H. A practice discipline that's here and now. *Adv Nurs Sci.* 2008;31(3):79–91.
3. Baer E. Philosophical and historical bases of advanced practice nursing roles. In: Mezey M, Mc-Givern D., eds. *Nurses, Nurse Practitioners: Evolution to Advanced Practice.* New York: Springer Publishing Company; 1999:72–91.
4. Gordon S. Necessary nursing care. *Nurs Inq.* 2000;7:217–219.
5. Chase S. Taking narrative seriously: consequences for method and theory in interview studies. In Josselson R, Lieblich A, eds. *Interpreting Experience: The Narrative Study Lives.* Vol. 3. London: Sage Publications; 1995:1–26.
6. Anderson K, Jack D. Learning to listen: interview techniques and analyses. In: Gluck S, Patai D, eds. *Women's Words: The Feminist Practice of Oral History.* London: Routledge; 1991:11–26.
7. Mishler E. *Research Interviewing: Context and Narrative.* Cambridge: Harvard University Press; 1986.
8. Lieblich A, Tuval-Mashiach R, Zilber T. *Narrative Research: Reading, Analysis, and Interpretation.* Thousand Oaks: Sage Publications; 1998.

9. Canam C. *The Place of Advanced Practice Nurses in the Community-Based Health Care of Children With Complex Health Needs and Their Families* [Doctoral dissertation]. Victoria, British Columbia, Canada: University of Victoria; 2004.

10. Canam C. Illuminating the clinical nurse specialist role of advanced practice nursing. *Can J Nurs Leadership*. 2005;18(4):70–89.

11. Liaschenko J, Fisher A. Theorizing the knowledge that nurses use in the conduct of their work. *Sch Inq NursPract*. 1999;13(1):29–41.

12. Benner P. *Interpretive Phenomenology: Embodiment, Caring, and Ethics in Health and Illness*. Thousand Oaks, CA: Sage Publications; 1994.

13. Purkis M. Entering the field: intrusions of the social and its exclusion from studies of nursing practice. *Int J Nurs Stud*. 1994;31(4):315–336.

14. Smith D. *The Everyday World as Problematic: A Feminist Sociology*. Toronto, Ontario, Canada: University of Toronto Press; 1987.

15. Smith D. *The Conceptual Practices of Power: A Feminist Sociology of Knowledge*. Toronto, Ontario, Canada: University of Toronto Press; 1990.

16. Smith D. *Writing the Social: Critique, Theory, and Investigations*. Toronto, Ontario, Canada: University of Toronto Press; 1999.

17. Morrow R, Brown D. *Critical Theory and Methodology*. Thousand Oaks, CA: Sage; 1994.

18. Fraser N. *Justice Interrupts*. New York: Routledge; 1997.

19. Street A. *Nursing Replay. Researching Nursing Culture Together*. Tokyo: Churchill Livingstone; 1995.

20. Fisher S. A discourse of the social: medical talk/ powertalk/ oppositional talk? *Discourse Soc*. 1991;2(2):157–182.

21. Browne A. The influence of liberal political ideology on nursing science. *Nurs Inq*. 2001;8(2):118–129.

22. Bjornsdottir K. Language, ideology, and nursing practice. *Sch Inq Nurs Pract*. 1998;12(4):347–362.

23. Higgs J, Burn A, Jones M. Integrating clinical reasoning and evidence-based practice. *AACN Clin Issues*. 2001;12(4):482–490.

24. Ceci C, McIntyre M. A "quiet" crisis in health care: developing our capacity to hear. *Nurs Philos*. 2001;2:122–130.

25. Brown Response to "An interpretive study describing the clinical judgment of nurse practitioners practice." *Sch Inq Nurs Prac. Int J*. 1999;13(2):167–173.

26. Fawcett J, Watson J, Neuman B, Walker P, Fitzpatrick J. On nursing theories and evidence. *J Nurs Sch*. 2001;33(2): 115–119.

27. Cheek J, Rudge T. The panopticon re-visited?: An exploration of the social and political dimensions of contemporary health care nursing. *Int J Nurs Stud*. 1994;31(6): 583–591.

28. Boschma G. Ambivalence about nursing's expertise: the role of a gendered holistic ideology in nursing, 1890–1990. In: Rafferty A, Robinson J, Elkan R, eds. *Nursing History and the Politics of Welfare*.New York: Routledge; 1997:164–176.

29. Reed J, Ground I, Dunlop M. *Philosophy for Nursing*. London: Arnold; 1997.

30. Bjornsdottir K. Language, ideology, and nursing practice. *Sch Inq Nurs Pract*. 1998;12(4):347–362.

31. Weinberg DB. When little things are big things. In: Nelson S, Gordon S, eds. *The Complexities of Care: Nursing Reconsidered*. Ithaca, NY: ILR/Cornell UniversityPress; 2006:30–43.

32. Carnevale F. Book review: the complexities of care: nursing reconsidered. *Can J Nurs Res*. 2007;39(3):213–215.

33. Chinn P, Kramer M. *Theory and Nursing: Integrated Knowledge Development*, 6th ed. Toronto, Ontario, Canada: Mosby; 2004.

34. Street A. *Nursing Replay. Researching Nursing Culture Together*. Tokyo: Churchill Livingstone; 1995.

35. Reimer Kirkham S, Baumbusch J, Schultz A, Anderson J. Knowledge development and evidence-based practice. *Adv Nurs Sci*. 2007;30(1):26–40.

36. Buresh B, Gordon S. *From Silence to Voice. What Nurses Know and Must Communicate to the Public*. Ottawa: Canadian Nurses Association; 2000.

37. Falk-Rafael A. Speaking truth to power. *Adv Nurs Sci*. 2005;28(3):212–223.

THE AUTHOR COMMENTS

The Link Between Nursing Discourses and Nurses' Silence: Implications for a Knowledge-Based Discourse for Nursing Practice

I was inspired to write this article, based on my dissertation research, to offer an alternative perspective on nurses' silence, one that draws attention to a critical aspect of nursing practice that has been overlooked: the language that nurses use to articulate their practice. Findings from the study demonstrate that although nurses have a rich body of practice knowledge they draw on to inform their practice, they have difficulty articulating their perspective within the health care setting because they draw on the language of caring or technical discourses that do not accurately represent their practice. Conceptualizing nursing as a knowledge-based practice provides the basis for an alternative language for nurses to draw on to articulate their perspective.

I see this article as contributing to nursing theory in the 21st century by focusing attention on the critical importance of nurses having access to a language that accurately represents the nature of their practice. Drawing on the knowledge that informs their practice can provide nurses with a language to articulate their unique perspective and has the potential to empower nurses to own their contributions to healthcare. It is my hope that this article will stimulate an ongoing dialogue and further research toward the development of a common language for nursing practice.

CONNIE J. CANAM

11

Transcending the Limits of Method: Cultivating Creativity in Nursing

GWENETH A. HARTRICK, RN, PhD

*I*n this article the author suggests that by nurturing the development of creativity in individual nurses and cultivating a culture of creativity in the profession, our knowledge and practice as a discipline could be strongly enhanced. This cultivation process, however, requires that we move beyond "using" theory to develop methods of practice. Such an approach to theory serves to solidify and constrain practice and inhibits the full contribution of nursing theory and knowledge. Drawing on the work of philosophers in the pragmatist tradition, the author considers how we might redescribe form to better support the creative process and ultimately enhance the development and contribution of nursing knowledge and theory. **Key words:** *creativity, nursing creativity, family nursing*

As a discipline, nursing continues to develop an ever-growing body of knowledge and theory. However, as an educator who also consults with nurses in many areas of clinical practice, I have experienced a continuum of attitude toward this knowledge and theory. At one end of the continuum are nurses who are clamoring for theory to "follow." At the other end of the continuum are nurses who are adamantly critical of the very idea of theory—some have described it as useless "gobbly gook" that has no relevance to their everyday work. And, of course there are nurses at many other places along that continuum.

Although we typically think of these responses as a problem of theory (e.g., we need to make theory more relevant, we need to bridge the gap between theory and practice) it has seemed to me that the problem is more one of language, conception and attitude. The problem lies not in theory, but in how we think about and employ theory. Similar to Wittgenstein's (1953) description of false problems, the language we use that separates theory from practice (e.g., theory-based practice) and conceptualizes theory as something apart from practice creates "the problem of theory." And, particularly problematic is our tendency to think of theory as something that can be "used" to develop methods of practice. That is, based on the conception of theory as something that exists apart from practice, *theoretically based methods* are developed to provide a systematic and scientific foundation for practice.

Paradoxically, this attitude of "using" theory to develop method serves to thwart our very intent. Rather than serving to open up and expand our practices, theory and knowledge is used to solidify them. That is, theories and frameworks are often employed and/or turned into proscriptive and definitive methods of practice. Not only does this attitude inhibit the full contribution of nursing theory and knowledge to our practice, it serves to create "the problem of theory," and contravenes the development of an essential element of nursing—that of creativity.

Through my work as a nurse educator and consultant, I have come to believe that creativity is central to nursing work and to knowledge development. It has become increasingly evident that by nurturing the development of creativity in individual nurses and cultivating a culture of creativity in the profession, our knowledge and practice as a discipline could be strongly enhanced. I begin my discussion of creativity in nursing by exploring our inherent desire for method and form. Drawing on the work of philosophers in the pragmatist tradition, I consider how we might redescribe form to better support the creative process. Finally, I discuss how nurturing creativity in practice can enhance the development and contribution of nursing knowledge and theory.

 ## Method: An Answer to Our Problems

As nursing has sought to increase knowledge and create standards in the profession, there has been a strong emphasis on developing methods of practice.

ABOUT THE AUTHOR

GWENETH A. HARTRICK was born in Regina, Saskatchewan. Her educational background includes a diploma of nursing, diploma in recreational therapy, baccalaureate degree in nursing, master's degree in counseling psychology, and an interdisciplinary PhD (nursing/psychology). She is currently a Professor in the School of Nursing and Associate Dean in the Faculty of Graduate Studies at the University of Victoria in British Columbia. Her scholarly work focuses on the integration of relational ontology, knowledge, and responsive action. Her key contributions have been in the areas of relational practice, family nursing, ethics, and teaching and learning in higher education.

The assumption has been that by delineating *methods* our ability to practice scientifically and knowledgeably is enhanced. For example, in the area of family nursing, family and nursing theories have been used to develop structured assessment methods and tools that nurses can use to determine a family's health status and to direct nurses' attention to aspects of family functioning that "theoretically" might be problematic. The assumption underlying these methods and tools is that, since they are theoretically based and have been developed by experts in family nursing, they provide a systematic and solid foundation for family nursing practice. Subsequently, it is assumed that by following these methods and tools nurses can feel fairly certain that their practice is competent and knowledgeable.

Caputo (1987) contends that our desire for method is a result of our metaphysical belief that there is a "master key" that can still the flux of life and control its course. According to Caputo (1987) this belief evolves out of the deductive model of rational thought we have come to equate with science. Berman (1981, 2000), one of many writers who have explored the historical roots of modern science, has highlighted that, although this view of science has become the hegemonic "truth," it was actually the social and economic milieu of modern Europe that served to sustain this deductive-rational model of science. Berman argues that this mechanistic view of science has equated science with a structure of discipline, with a particular method rather than with a process of freedom and creativity. And, the social constraints this deductive-rational model produces has resulted in an alienated, nonparticipatory consciousness.

Within this nonparticipatory consciousness, people are no longer at the center of their experience or action. Epistemology (how we know) is separated from ontology (how we are), action is separated from being, and people are no longer participants in the drama of life. The dominant discourse of this nonparticipatory consciousness has ultimately served to arrest the free movement of science and form.

Our nursing lives have been played out against this historical and scientific background. Understanding our nursing work through this nonparticipatory consciousness we have justifiably felt the need for scientific and theory-based methods. Believing that the difficulties and angst that arise in practice can be "scientifically" eradicated through form, we have looked for methods that can provide structure and certainty for our practice. However, as we have tried "to nail things down" (Caputo, 1987, p. 213) we have become further bound by the rule of fixed technique. Our focus on employing methods further alienates us from ourselves and our own creative and scientific potential. Structure and method overrule responsive nursing practice. As Caputo describes, "... method rules instead of serving, constrains instead of liberating, and fails conspicuously to let science be" (1987, p. 213). As we have developed and given precedence to method, we have simultaneously lost and/or not developed the confidence and courage to open up to our own creative and scientific potential.

Our "non-participatory consciousness" can be seen in the way we have approached relational nursing practice. Separating epistemology from ontology and being from action, we have sought to control the human flux of relationships by employing behavioral and communication research and theories to develop methods and techniques such as behavioral communication skills. Most communication courses in nursing education today continue to take this method-based attitude that assumes relational practice is "done" through a structured method such as behavioral skills. Subsequently, the central content of interpersonal/relational practice courses usually includes a variety of "methods" of communication such as open-ended questions, clarification, nonverbal communication, and so forth. This emphasis on method not only serves to alienate nurses from their own human capacity to be in relation (Hartrick, 1997) it paradoxically limits the contribution of nursing theories (e.g., Newman, 1986; Paterson & Zderad, 1976) that could potentiate creativity and ultimately enhance the development of nurses' relational capacity.

The Authority of Method

The somewhat daunting challenge that lies before us is that of releasing ourselves from the authority of method in order to become participants in the drama of nursing work. That is, the challenge is that of willingly opening up to the flux of human experience rather than enclosing ourselves in the protective form of method and technique. The challenge involves seeing methods and techniques as merely artifacts at our disposal rather than as structures for guiding practice. As Kohak (1984) describes while there is nothing wrong with artifacts, there is something wrong with us, "we have lost sight of the sense, the purpose of our production and our products. Artifacts, finally, are good only extrinsically as tools. They have no intrinsic sense of their own" (p. xii).

Nursing is not a line of action (a method). Rather, as Paterson and Zderad (1976) describe, nursing is an experience lived between people. Nursing as a science makes its way by a "free and creative movement whose dynamic baffles the various discourses on method" (Caputo, 1987, p. 211). Science (and nursing) is a creative venture that involves doubt, risk, uncertainty and experimentation (May, 1975). As such the "form" of nursing must be fluid, arising in the creative moment.

It is time, therefore, to reverse the relationship between nursing and method. Rather than having nursing subservient to the artifact of method, we need to make method subservient to the art and science of nursing. As Caputo (1987) contends, method needs to be replaced with a deeper appreciation of *methodos*—the creative way in which we pursue a matter.

 ## Beyond Mental Theme Parks to Experience

Philosopher Ludwig Wittgenstein contended that it was possible to make people drunk with ideas. However, the problem was whether they knew how to use those ideas soberly (cited in Berman, 2000). Two years before his death, Wittgenstein had decided that his ideas and teachings had perhaps done more harm than good. The reason for his despair was that people had begun to use his ideas as a formula (Bouwsma, cited in Berman, 2000). Students had turned his philosophical teachings into a method. They imitated his gestures, adopted his expressions, and began "doing" Wittgenstein philosophy. Paradoxically Wittgenstein's philosophy emphasized the destroying of formulas and idols and the importance of *not* creating new ones to follow.

This tendency to create and follow idols—to turn to new theories and ideas and shape them into yet another formula or method continues to dominate nursing. This quest for new theories and methods is resonant of John Ralston Saul's contention that we hold the "unshakeable belief that we are on the trail to truth—and therefore to the solution to our problems" (1995, p. 19). This belief is so integral to our thinking that it prevents us from seeing the fallacy of our actions. As Ralston Saul describes, it has created a paradigm-shift addiction that perpetuates an unending search for new and better mental theme parks. These mental theme parks come not only in the form of ideas, but also in the form of people who either hold themselves up or who are held up by others, as possessing a new truth. That is, of possessing a new way of thinking, a new method or technique that can soften or alleviate the struggles that are part of nursing work.

The problem with these mental theme parks is that they take us away from ourselves and our experience. They most often trade in generalities and simplifications which make it easy to forget that human experience (and nursing) is particular and complicated. Life is a moving affair in which any truth quickly ceases to apply (Berman, 2000). For that reason we need the courage and willingness to live in our experiences. Helpful as mental theme parks and discrete methods might be, something more lies beyond. No method can guide us as we navigate through the unknown terrain of human experience and relationships. Methods do not offer certainty and autonomy. Rather, they merely serve to subordinate our creative and scientific potential.

According to Dewey (1929) the quest for truth and solutions should be replaced with the demand for imagination. Imagination is a form of playful analogical thinking where previous experiences are drawn on and combined in unusual ways, generating new patterns of meaning (Policastro & Gardner, 1999). Imagination is the outreaching of mind (May, 1975) and involves the meeting of doubt and opposition head on (Whitehead, 1933). Progress in knowledge development is not a matter of getting closer to the truth or closer to the right action but rather it involves increasing our imaginative power (Rorty, 1999) to responsively "form" our nursing care in the moment of experience.

 ## Shifting the Authority

It is important to clarify that I am not advocating for throwing away nursing frameworks or methods. Rather, I am calling for a shift in authority. Specifically, I am suggesting that we shift the authority that governs our practice from that of method to that of experience and creativity. In considering how we might move toward an "authority of experience" I have found philosophers in the pragmatist tradition helpful. For pragmatists, there is no deep split between theory, practice and experience. Pragmatists believe that all so-called "theory" is always already practice (Rorty, 1999). Rorty (1999) explains that pragmatists do not aim at truth and/or at doing the right thing since they contend it is impossible to know if you have hit the mark. Long after you are dead, better informed people may judge your knowledge or action to have been a terrible mistake (Rorty, 1999). The changing truths of health and disease care throughout the past few decades certainly bear witness to this argument.

Instead of aiming for truth or right action, pragmatists aim for ever more sensitivity to people, striving to take people's needs and experiences into account more than she or he did previously. In contrast to knowledge development in nursing, which most often involves a process of critique where the pros and cons of existing knowledge or methods are contested by new evolving ones that offer more promise, pragmatists focus on redescribing themselves and their practice. Since there are no possible criteria to determine which theory or method is more true, or more representational, criticism is neither helpful nor pragmatic (Rorty, 1999). Rather, for pragmatists, the most useful way to develop knowledge is through redescription and re-redescription. This redescription involves a creative process of reimagining one's self and one's practice and is inspired by the hope "to make the best selves for ourselves that we can" (Rorty, 1989, p. 80).

Being a Creative Ironist

Rorty (1989) explains that ironism is an essential feature of a pragmatist. Ironism is an attitude adopted by people who are convinced of their contingency. That is, they are convinced that they and their actions are dependent upon everything else in a particular situation and must be fluid enough to respond to the unforeseen circumstances and elements of particular people and situations. What helps ironists live this contingent attitude is their understanding that their way of thinking, their theories and their methodologies are merely "contrivance—possibly wise, useful, and well-motivated contrivance, but contrivance nonetheless, and something that may well be found laughable from another time and place" (Flanagan, 1996, p. 207). According to Flanagan (1996) the ironist relishes and is amused by contingency, including the contingency of her or his aspirations, projects, theories, ways of practice, and so forth. She is not confident that she has things right—she is confident she doesn't. "She is a confident unconfident" (Flanagan, 1996, p. 207). As such, the ironist is a realist and this realism provides an avenue into authenticity and experience (Flanagan, 1996).

The ironist is similar to Berman's (2000) description of the nomad who dwells in the midregion and seeks to destroy images and static models rather than develop them. "In the nomadic mind ... the road to truth is always under construction; the going is the goal ... For nomads 'truth' is a verb, something you live. No sooner are you at one point than an elaboration or revision suggests itself" (Berman, 2000, p. 198). In this way, the creative ironist lives a world presence rather than a worldview (Berman, 2000). Rather than living from a unified, fixed perspective, she or he is grounded in immediacy and experience.

With experience as the integrating form, the creative ironist uses her or his imaginative power to revise, adapt, expand, and alter knowledge and practice. The focus of knowledge development and skillful competent practice is one of continuous, vital redescription. Rather than willfully following a method that requires setting oneself apart from the flux of human experience, the creative ironist courageously holds oneself open and alive to hear what "being" may speak (May, 1975).

Fostering the Creative Process of Nursing

Although creativity and imagination are often taken as the frosting to life rather than as the solid food (May, 1975), my experiences as a nurse educator have led me to wonder: What if imagination and creativity were not frosting at all, but the core of nursing practice? What if knowledge and form in nursing evolved from creativity and were fundamentally dependent upon it? Exploring these questions in my work as an educator and consultant the following is a glimpse of what I have experienced.

Creativity and Family Nursing

Having practiced, taught, and written in the area of family nursing, I am often invited to consult and/or speak with nurses who are attempting to enhance their family nursing knowledge and skill. I have found this work to be both inspiring and disconcerting. I have been profoundly inspired by the passion, commitment, and deep caring I have witnessed in the nurses I have worked with. At the same time, I have felt great concern at the lack of self-confidence and self-trust many of these nurses experience. Governed by the authority of method many seem to have either not developed, or to have lost touch with their creative capacity to shape and determine their practice. Their belief that there is a "right method" to use when promoting health in families often hinders their spontaneous, responseability to families.

Similar to Ralston Saul's (1995) mental theme park, many nurses often assume that I am going teach them how to "do" family nursing based on the approach I use and have published in nursing journals. When I invite them instead to open up to their own creative and imaginative power and suggest that they use the knowledge and ideas to inspire their own process of redescription, I am usually met with a combination of excitement (at the possibility of there being no truth they "have to" follow) and angst or frustration (that there is no ready made method they can apply).

Similar to Doll's (1993) suggestion that human openness contains a paradox, as the nurses take up my invitation and begin to open up to wider possibilities for their practice, they simultaneously have a desire to make sense of that which they are opening up to. They want to bring form and a sense of cohesive closure to the ideas and possibilities they are exploring. May (1975) contends that this passion for form is a way of trying to find and constitute meaning in life. And, according to May this passion for form is the essence of creativity. As we try to make meaning of our self-world relationship, we create and give life to our creation through form. Form provides the essential boundaries and structure for the creative act. In creative endeavors the imagination operates in juxtaposition with form—imagination infuses form with its own vitality (May, 1975). However, in contrast to developing defined and static methods, this creative form is fluid and everchanging.

I have found that creativity arises out of the tension between spontaneity and limitations. Limits are not only unavoidable in human life; they are also valuable. Creativity itself requires limits. That is, the creative act arises out of the struggle of human beings with and against that which limits them (May, 1975). As the nurses I have worked with have faced limitations in their practice and have been invited to spontaneously open up to, and inquire into those limitations, the creative process has been sparked.

A sine qua non of creativity is the freedom to give all the elements within oneself free play (May, 1975). "Considerable evidence demonstrates that a playful approach to the task at hand increases the likelihood of producing creative results" (Policastro & Gardner, 1999, p. 217). This free play requires the courage to risk one's self. So for example, as the nurses and I have "played" with our knowing—with past experiences, with nursing theory, with family theory, with the ideals and principles of health promotion, and with possible strategies and techniques, I have encouraged them to "risk" trying them on for size. Rather than having to mold themselves to fit the theory or method, I ask them to explore how a particular knowledge fits with them and how it might enhance their sensitivity and response-ability to the families they work with.

Following May's suggestion that creative courage involves the paradox of commitment to knowledge and the simultaneous awareness that one might possibly be wrong, I have encouraged nurses to play with both their convictions and their doubts. Often this takes the form of exploring the "what ifs." For example, through simulations we might explore the doubts nurses have about the usefulness of a particular theory or idea in their particular practice environment or doubts they have about their own potential to creatively and scientifically respond in-the-moment. As Kneller (1965) describes, creative thought is innovative, exploratory, and venturesome, and is attracted to the unknown and the undetermined. Risk and uncertainty stimulate it. Through this imaginative, playful process each nurse has the opportunity to continually redescribe—to recreate—her or his own family nursing practice.

As nurses begin to describe and redescribe their practice with families, they are not so much breaking with existing knowledge and approaches as they are contributing to them. Kneller (1965) argues that creative novelty springs largely from the rearrangement of existing knowledge. Such a rearrangement might reveal unsuspected connections between nursing theories or ideas long known but not previously coupled. "Just as the writer transforms her or his experience of the human scene into a novel or play, so the scientist tests and probes the data he has acquired in order to produce a new theory. Both rearrange existing knowledge and experience, their own and others, into a new form or pattern … moreover both the writer and the scientist work through intuition as well as intellect" (Kneller, 1965, p. 12). It is this bringing together, and honoring of both intuition and intellect that seems to spark the sense of freedom and the courage needed to "risk" redescription.

However, Kneller reminds us that novelty alone does not make an act or an idea creative. Relevance is also a factor. Since the creative act is a response to a particular situation, it must respond to, or in some way clarify the situation that has caused it to arise. "In sum, an act or an idea is creative not only because it is novel but also because it achieves something that is appropriate to a given situation" (Kneller, 1965, p. 7). For practicing nurses, this relevance to the situation is a vital and pragmatic thread underpinning the creative process.

 ## Transcending the "Problem" of Theory

Existing research and writing on creativity (Hart, 1998; May, 1975; Montuori, Alfonso, & Purser, 1995; Runco & Albert, 1990) has an amazing synchronicity with the art and science of nursing work. For example, May's (1975) description of the creative process echoes Paterson and Zderad's (1976) description of humanistic nursing. According to May, the creative act involves an intimate encounter with the world. World in this sense is the pattern of meaningful relations in which a person exists and in the design of which he or she participates. Scientists encounter their experiments, an artist may encounter a landscape, nurses encounter the people they care for. An important aspect of this encounter is the degree of absorption. Similar to Paterson and Zderad's (1976) description of nursing, May contends that the creative process requires a special quality of engagement in which one is absorbed and wholly involved. In essence, "creativity is the encounter of the intensively conscious human being with his or her world" (May, 1975, p. 54).

This "wholly involved" engagement extends to how it is we engage with theory and knowledge. It has seemed to me that paradoxically our quest for methods and certainty has hindered our ability to fully engage with theory and knowledge. My experience working with nurses who creatively engage in a process of redescription has highlighted the potential of such a process for knowledge development. For example, each time I consult with a group of nurses I find that my own knowledge and practice is deepened. Through these experiences I am compelled to redescribe what it is I know about family nursing. For that reason, as an "unconfident confident" I suggest that if imagination and creativity served as the core of nursing practice and if knowledge and form in nursing evolved from creativity and were fundamentally dependent upon it, the "problem" of theory and the limitations of method might cease to exist.

Concluding Thoughts

Our conception of creativity and the domains to which its applications are rewarded and valued has tended to distract our attention from putting creativity to work in professional disciplines such as nursing. Yet, May (1975) contends that every profession requires creativity and the courage to develop its creative potential. According to May, the need for creative courage is in direct proportion to the degree of change the profession is undergoing since creativity is the process of making and bringing change into being. In this sense, creativity is a special case of cultural evolution.

In thinking about how we might cultivate a culture of creativity in nursing we must look beyond the level of the individual nurse. Csikzentmihalyi (1990) contends that to foster creativity by focusing on the individual alone is like trying to understand how an apple tree produces fruit by looking only at the tree and ignoring the sun and the soil that supports life. According to Csikzenetmihalyi, the social environment (e.g., cultural environment of nursing)

not only facilitates the expression of individual creativity, it is always an essential component of the creative process. How creativity develops or even if it develops is greatly affected by the field of knowledge within which it arises. The field can serve as a source of acceptance or rejection of potentially creative contributions (Feldman, 1999).

Creativity requires the ability to change our approach to nursing and to knowledge development. When one moves beyond method, to a more "wholly-involved engagement" with theory—as in creative engagement—there is no longer the possibility of following theory or rejecting it. We become theoretical through our redescriptive process.

Cultivating the creative potential of nursing involves moving beyond a quest for methods and answers to embrace the uncertainty and questions we experience. Creativity involves the generation of ideas that are both relevant and unusual, to see beyond the immediate situation, to redefine understandings regardless of the activity. And, finally, creativity involves opening up to our intuitive, embodied experience of right-relatedness, of—"this is the way things are meant to be" in this moment. The paradox is that at that moment of right-relatedness we are simultaneously opened up to the limitations and potential that lie beyond it.

REFERENCES

Berman, M. (1981). *The reenchantment of the world*. London: Cornell University Press.

Berman, M. (2000). *The wandering god*. Albany, NY: State University of New York Press.

Caputo, J. (1987). *Radical hermeneutics: Repetition, deconstruction, and the hermeneutic project*. Bloomington, IN: Indiana University Press.

Csikzentmihalyi, M. (1990). The domain of creativity. In M. A. Runco & R. S. Albert (Eds.), *Theories of creativity* (pp. 190–212). Newbury Park, CA: Sage.

Dewey, J. (1929). *The quest for certainty: A study of the relation of knowledge and action*. New York: Minton, Balch & Company.

Doll, W. E. (1993). *The postmodern perspective on curriculum*. New York: Teachers College Press.

Feldman, D. H. (1999). The development of creativity. In R.J. Sternberg (Ed.), *Handbook of creativity* (pp. 169–186). Cambridge: Cambridge University Press.

Flanagan, O. (1996). *Self expressions. Mind, morals and the meaning of life*. New York: Oxford University Press.

Hart, T. (1998). Inspiration: Exploring the experience and its meaning. *Journal of Humanistic Psychology*, 38(3), 7–29.

Hartrick, G. A. (1997). Relational capacity: The foundation for interpersonal nursing practice. *Journal of Advanced Nursing*, 26, 523–528.

Kneller, G. F. (1965). *The art and science of creativity*. New York: Holt, Rinehart and Winston, Inc.

Kohak, E. (1984). *The embers and the stars. A philosophical inquiry into the moral sense of nature*. Chicago: University of Chicago Press.

May, R. (1975). *The courage to create*. New York: W. W. Norton & Co.

Montuori, A., & Purser, R. E. (1995). Deconstructing the lone genius myth: Toward a contextual view of creativity. *Jorunal of Humanistic Psychology*, 35(3), 69–86.

Newman, M. (1986). *Health as expanding consciousness*. St. Louis, MO: Mosby.

Paterson, J. G., & Zderad, L. T. (1976). *Humanistic nursing*. New York: John Wiley & Sons.

Policastro, E., & Gardner, H. (1999). From case studies to robust generalizations: An approach to the study of creativity. In R. J. Sternberg (Ed.), *Handbook of creativity* (pp. 213–225). Cambridge: Cambridge University Press.

Ralston Saul J. (1995). *The unconscious civilization*. Concord, Ontario: Anansi Press.

Rorty, R. (1989). *Contingency, irony, and solidarity*. Cambridge: Cambridge University Press.

Rorty, R. (1999). *Philosophy and social hope*. London: Penguin Books.

Runco, M. A., & Albert, R. S. (Eds.). (1990). *Theories of creativity*. Newbury Park, CA: Sage.

Whitehead, A. (1933). *Adventure of ideas*. New York: Macmillan.

Wittgenstein, L. (1953). *Philosophical investigations*. New York: Macmillan.

THE AUTHOR COMMENTS | **Transcending the Limits of Method: Cultivating Creativity in Nursing**

This paper was inspired by the concern I felt about the way in which existing theories and methods were being taken up or not taken up in nursing practice. It seemed to me that many nurses, as governed by the authority of extant theories and methods, had either lost touch with or lacked the opportunity to develop their own creative capacity as knowers—to be "wholly involved" creators of knowledge in nursing moments. Subsequently, their trust in themselves as knowledgeable practitioners and their response-ability to people in complex nursing situations was diminished. My intent was to highlight the significance of creativity as an ontology of knowing that opens up possibilities for theorizing, knowledge development, and more responsive nursing practice.

GWENETH A. HARTRICK

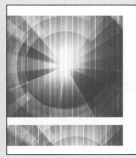

3

Theory and Knowledge Translation

The chapters in this unit present a variety of methods by which theory is involved in knowledge translation. Theory informs a range of nursing activities in research and practice, from systems-level implementation research to the intimate nurse-patient interactions to alleviate pain. Translating conceptual ideas, empirical evidence, and other data into meaningful knowledge is not an atheoretical endeavor. Nursing contexts are imbued with the "theoretical", that is, the philosophies, values, frameworks, concepts, and perceptions of human beings. *Theory-informed* means reflecting on and explicating these theoretical elements that reside within nursing practices of research and caregiving.

Theory is translated through practice into knowledge for practice. For some, theory is a guide; for others, theory arises out of the practice situation. Whether we speak of nursing theory–guided practice or practice-guided theory, a key to developing nursing knowledge derives from recognizing the nonlinearity of the theory-practice process.

QUESTIONS FOR DISCUSSION

- What does knowledge translation mean to you?

- In your opinion, what value, if any, is there in clarifying whether theory guides practice, or practice guides theory?

- What conceptual underpinnings influence your practice or research?

- How might the context of practice influence the way practitioners translate research findings to generate knowledge in practice, for practice?

- The authors of some of these chapters present theory-based strategies or methods to generate knowledge. What approaches discussed in these chapters best suit you in your own knowledge translation work?

Knowledge Translation in Everyday Nursing
From Evidence-Based to Inquiry-Based Practice

GWENETH HARTRICK DOANE, RN, PhD
COLLEEN VARCOE, RN, PhD

The interconnection of theory, evidence, and practice is most often conceptualized as an epistemological enterprise. In this article, we shift the discussion from one that is solely concerned with epistemology to one that considers the significance of ontology and the way in which epistemology and ontology are intricately intertwined in every nursing action. Drawing on deconstructive hermeneutics, we contend that to understand and affect the interconnection of theory, evidence, and practice, an ontological inquiry at the action level is required. Using a nursing practice example, we illustrate the complexities of knowledge translation and how effective integration of knowledge into practice involves an embodied process of ontological inquiry and action. This inquiry process draws on theory and evidence to enlarge and imagine possibilities for action in particular moments, situations, and contexts and rests in a way-of-being in which the interconnection of theory, evidence, and practice is embodied. **Key words:** embodiment, epistemology, hermeneutics, inquiry, knowledge translation, ontology

This article was inspired by our deeply felt concern with the profound disparity that often exists between what nurses *know* and what nurses *do*. Although many of the questions and ideas we raise here have been discussed in the nursing literature under various epistemological and/or theoretic topics, we enter the discussion of the interconnection among theory, evidence, and practice from a somewhat different vantage point—that of nursing action. We take this "action turn" because we believe that ultimately safe, competent, theoretically informed, evidence-based nursing practice is about action. As nurses, we are at the service and behest of society; thus, the significance of the interconnection lies in the difference it makes in the everyday actions in which nurses engage as they seek to promote people's health and healing. We also take this action turn because although as a profession we have engaged in critical work to explicate the interconnections among theory, evidence, and practice at the discursive level (e.g., within the scholarly literature), where we seem to have run into problems is translating the interconnection into action. That is, at times we have had difficulty "walking the talk."

In this article, we contend that the difficulty in translating theoretic discourse into nursing action may lie in how we are conceptualizing the interconnection of nursing knowledge and nursing action.

Specifically, the emphasis on epistemology may be inadvertently contributing to the problem. For example, despite nursing literature emphasizing the importance of ontology, discussions within the academic literature have framed the "theory practice gap" as an epistemological problem of a theoretic practice and emphasized the importance of integrating sound theory and evidence into practice. At the same, time practitioners have bemoaned the irrelevance of theories espoused in research, academic literature, codes, practice guidelines, and so forth. In both cases, the interconnection of theory, evidence, and practice is framed as an epistemological concern and the "gap" is framed as an epistemological problem. That is, the problem is discussed as though it is about knowledge—what is known and how knowledge is used or applied.

In this article, it is our intent to shift the discussion of knowledge translation from one that is primarily concerned with epistemology to one that considers the ontological dimension. That is, we contend that the relationship among theory, evidence, and practice is also a question of how we *are*—our ways of being and relating to ourselves, to knowledge, to one another, and to our environments. As others have done previously, we assert that ontology and ontological motivation are central to how we live/translate/enact knowledge in complex moments of practice.

From G. H. Doane, & C. Varcoe, Knowledge translation in everyday nursing from evidence-based to inquiry-based practice. Advances in Nursing Science *Vol. 31, No. 4, pp. 283–295. Copyright © 2008 Wolters Kluwer Health | Lippincott Williams & Wilkins.*
Reprinted with permission from Lippincott Williams & Wilkins.

ABOUT THE AUTHORS

GWENETH HARTRICK DOANE was born in Regina, Saskatchewan. Her educational background includes a diploma of nursing, diploma in recreational therapy, baccalaureate degree in nursing, master's degree in counseling psychology, and an interdisciplinary PhD (nursing/psychology). She is currently a Professor in the School of Nursing and Associate Dean in the Faculty of Graduate Studies at the University of Victoria in British Columbia. Her scholarly work focuses on the integration of relational ontology, knowledge, and responsive action. Her key contributions have been in the areas of relational practice, family nursing, ethics, and teaching and learning in higher education.

COLLEEN VARCOE was born in rural Manitoba. She obtained her nursing diploma from the Royal Columbian Hospital School of Nursing and subsequently completed a baccalaureate in nursing, master's degrees in both nursing and education, and a doctorate in nursing. She is currently a Professor and Director Pro Tem in the school of nursing at the University of British Columbia in Vancouver. Her scholarship focuses on health inequities and social justice, with an emphasis on violence, poverty, racism, and colonialism. Her key contributions to the discipline have been in the areas of violence against women and ethical practice in nursing. She snowboards, does yoga, and runs a paragliding school with her partner in Harrison Mills, British Columbia.

However, we take this assertion further by considering how an ontological understanding of the interconnection of theory, evidence, and practice offers new possibilities for nursing practice, education, and research. This ontological exploration is an attempt to respond to Gadow's assertion that within nursing we need to restore "the physical substance that has fallen away from the philosophical discourse"[1(p208)] to turn our attention to the tangible, embodied actions of giving and receiving nursing care.

Lost in Translation? Critiques of Knowledge Translation

The interconnection among theory, evidence, and practice has been conceptualized and explored under various topics within the nursing literature including the theory-practice gap, nursing praxis, evidence-based practice (EBP), research utilization, knowledge transfer, research dissemination, research uptake, innovation diffusion, and so forth. Although it could be argued that while related, these terms and/or topics are somewhat distinct, Graham et al[2] explain that many of the terms are used interchangeably. As a whole, they encompass the subject of knowledge use—that of "how to get knowledge used" and "translated" into practice.[2–4]

An Epistemological Frame

There have been wide-ranging critiques of the way knowledge translation has been conceptualized within the various topic areas above. In undertaking these critiques, authors in nursing have often grappled with

knowledge translation through an epistemological frame. That is, they have articulated the epistemological limitations inherent within both the conceptualizations of knowledge translation and the strategies meant to enhance the interconnection of theory, evidence, and practice. Examples include the long tradition of concern with and inquiry into research dissemination and utilization.[5–9] Similarly, nurses have explored extensively the idea of a theory-practice gap.[10,11] For example, it has been argued that the "theory-practice gap" is not "real" but rather the result of a particular epistemological stance—that any gap is due to the realist perspective that shapes the understanding of theory.[12–14] In other words, for a theory practice gap to be "real," theory must be conceptualized as a "real thing" that exists independent of practice. In contrast to the realist perspective of theory, discussions of nursing praxis have highlighted the integral connection of theory and practice and the way in which all practice is inherently theoretic, with every moment of practice already imbued with theory.[15]

A Question of Epistemology?

Given the epistemological frame that has been used within the topic of EBP, a central epistemological critique has been that the perception of a knowledge "gap" has been fostered by the *kinds* of knowledge that are assumed to constitute valid theory or evidence and on which practice is subsequently based. For example, Kirkham Reimer et al describe that although EBP focuses on the integration of research evidence, clinical expertise, and patient values in clinical decision making, the overriding assumption has been that "epidemiological and statistical research findings could be useful for influencing the effectiveness of clinical practice."[4(p27)] These authors argue that the privileging of empirical knowledge has limited the consideration of evidence from a variety of other research methodologies and related knowledges emphasizing that "nurses clearly rely on knowledge beyond that which can be empirically verifiable."[4(p28)] According to these authors, the result is "incomplete epistemologies" that segregate empirical knowledge from other forms of knowledge and ultimately limit knowledge generation and application in everyday nursing practice. By privileging empirical knowledge and emphasizing the application of that knowledge in nursing practice, EBP strategies such as best practice guidelines favor evidence from randomized clinical trials and offer linear approaches that fail to address the complex realities of nursing practice situations.[4] Overall, epistemological critiques in EBP discussions highlight the way in which the *kinds* of knowledge privileged ultimately shape what "counts" as evidence, what knowledge is translated, where "translation" occurs, who is active in the translation process, and what constitutes "successful" EBP.

A Question of Ontology?

Ricoeur describes that both Heidegger and Gadamer challenged the assumption of interpretation and translation as being solely about epistemology. Both philosophers attempted "to dig beneath the epistemological enterprise itself to uncover its properly ontological conditions."[16(p64)] This was not to create a duality between the 2 and/or to subordinate epistemology to ontology. Rather the intent was to articulate the way in which epistemologies reflect the conscious and unconscious ontologies of their creators and vice versa. Ricoeur highlights the interrelationship of meaning, interpretation, subjectivity, and context. He contends that understanding, including interpretation and translation, is not simply mode of knowing but way of being and way of relating.

Cecci[14] has pointed to the significance of this ontological dimension within nursing knowledge. She contends that rather than focusing concern on the *kinds* of knowledge conceptualizations, there is a more fundamental question that might "change the tenor of the conversation ... (that of) how we understand ourselves as knowers to be related to what we think we know."[14(p58)] Cecci describes the way in which our ontological assumptions (e.g., seeing people as disembodied and detached beings) shape our knowing processes. Drawing on Harding's[17] work (1991), Cecci explains that there is no possibility of disinterested knowledge that is separate from ourselves—from the values, beliefs, and assumptions we hold. Similarly, in highlighting this ontological dimension, writers in deconstructive hermeneutics (e.g., Ricoeur, Derrida, and Caputo)

have emphasized that epistemology is fundamentally a values matter—it arises through people and is inherently about what is of value, what is privileged, what is marginalized, and so forth. For example, Caputo explains that evidence (including that which arises empirically) is not a "given... for what is important evidence in one view is not important in another."[18(p218)]

It is this value-laden, ontological dimension on which we wish to focus in considering the interconnection of theory, evidence, and practice. We assert that the interconnection is not only an epistemological matter. Rather, ontology and ontological motivation are central to how we live/translate/enact knowledge in complex moments of practice. Therefore, understanding and enacting the interconnection of theory, evidence, and practice require an examination of how epistemology and ontology are intricately intertwined in every nursing action.

Mind the (Ontological) Gap

Our work as researchers and educators over the past several years has focused on addressing the chasm that often exists between nursing knowledge and nursing actions. Yet in some ways, rather than lessening, the chasm seems to be deepening. At the level of everyday bedside nursing, our research on ethical practice in nursing[19-21] and the work of others on moral distress[22-24] has illustrated the gulf between nurses' knowledge of "good" practice and their actions. Similarly, in response to epistemological discussions in the nursing literature, Cecci[14] and Thorne et al[25] have described the epistemological positioning and "othering" practices that are at times undertaken in the name of advancing nursing knowledge. For example, Thorne et al describe how during disputes over knowledge claims nurse scholars are inclined to rely on binaries (such as conceptualizing nursing theory into 2 competing paradigms—the simultaneity versus totality paradigms) and "in some cases, this adoption of a binary position has led to a passionately held form of 'othering' that prohibits a healthy and critical engagement with ideas."[25(p208)] Suggesting that fear is at the root of this binary positioning, Thorne et al emphasize the need to "begin to understand its dynamics as they play out in our intellectual engagements, and to learn what options there might be to reconsider its impact on our intellectual processes and products."[25(p210)]

These othering practices are enacted within nursing scholarship despite relational, caring values and goals, theories, and philosophic positions being espoused within that same scholarship. Thus, it seems that even those of us focused on knowledge development and "bridging the gap" between knowledge and action are not being all that successful in "translating" the theoretic and/or research knowledge we value into our everyday actions. Moreover, these considerations highlight that the gap is not only an epistemological problem. It is not merely that we privilege some epistemological camps over others or that there is a gap between what we know (theory and evidence) and what we do (practice). There seems to be a much more fundamental disconnect at the ontological level. To understand that disconnect, we turn to the site of everyday nursing practice. The following is a real experience of one of the authors, with minor details changed to protect the identity of the nurse involved.

An Illustration: Beginning in Everyday Nursing Action

I sit up and reach for the nasal prongs, I turn the oxygen on and take some slow, deep breaths. Funny, my breathing has been so stable over the past couple of days—why am I suddenly feeling so short of breath? Sitting upright I take my pulse and go over the possibilities in my mind. The cardiograms have been normal; my pulse is strong and steady. Maybe its just tightness from the fractured ribs. But why now? It could be an embolus—maybe the blow from the steering wheel injured more than my ribs— maybe I have more than contused lungs. I reach for the call bell and wait for the nurse. My nurse walks in smiling—"What can I do for you?" she asks cheerfully. "I am feeling quite short of breath—it's different than it has been. I'm due to go home this afternoon so I am wondering if maybe I could get it checked before I leave just in case something has developed." The nurse frowns—"it's probably nothing—just your ribs." She takes my vital signs, shrugs and says "don't worry about it—it's nothing." "Well yes," I reply, "it may be just my ribs but I wonder if I could get checked out before I leave just to be on the safe side." The tone of her voice changes—gone is the friendly demeanour. In an authoritative tone she states "I'll think about it." With that she turns and walks out of the room.

I wait.

An hour later she has not returned, my breathing has eased somewhat and lying in my bed I contemplate my next step—do I let it go or do I persist? An x-ray porter calls out my name as she wheels a stretcher into the room. I raise my head to identify myself. "I'm having an x-ray?" I ask. The porter looks surprised. "That's what the requisition says." "Great," I reply as I attempt to move to the stretcher before she can question further—I want that x-ray! ½ an hour later as I settle in my bed after returning from x-ray the nurse walks in. "Oh there you are. I just wanted to check that you were back and everything is ok." She smiles at me, "you know I didn't make the connection earlier." "The connection?" I ask, confused. "Yes, I read your articles when I was a nursing student—about relational practice. I so believe everything you write about." With great conviction in her eyes she declares, "and I practice exactly as you describe."

In considering this situation, it is important to emphasize that what is not known is what else was happening for the nurse that day, what the unit was like to work on, the demands she faced, and the contextual forces that were pressing in on her. However, we have chosen this experience because of what we *do know*. We know the baccalaureate nursing program that the nurse went through and thus that she was exposed to what we consider to be exemplary nursing knowledge and education. The curriculum was built on theoretic constructs such as health promotion, culture/context, personal meaning, social justice, and collaborative, relational practice. Within the curriculum, there is a concerted focus on praxis and "practice-based learning." As part of her nursing education, she would have been introduced to theories from human science and critical, feminist, interpretive, and biomedical paradigms and the way in which nursing practice requires the integration of those different knowledges. So how was it that this passionate, committed young nurse acted as she did? Obviously her actions were grounded in evidence and theory—she carried out an assessment and made a clinical decision to request an order for an x-ray. Yet, given the knowledge to which she had been exposed in her educational program, the theory and evidence she drew on was quite limited. For example, her actions did not reflect the collaborative, relational theories she had studied and with which she had obviously deeply resonated as a student. She "knew" them well enough to actually identify the theories with a particular author, yet did not enact them in her practice. What is perhaps more perplexing is that she believed that she *was* acting in a way that was congruent with the theories she had read in her nursing program and later described those "ways-of-knowing" and "ways-of-being" as being central to *who she was* as a nurse. However, as existing critiques have outlined and the above nursing experience illustrates, theoretic, evidence-based knowledge is not necessarily "translated" into nursing action.

An Ontology of Knowing-in-Action

We are interested in understanding the disconnect between the knowledge that the nurse in the above story valued and saw as integral to her identity and way-of-being as a nurse, the knowledge, and evidence that she used and/or did not use to inform her response and how that all translated into action. As we have grappled with trying to make sense of this situation, we have found current understandings of knowledge translation inadequate. Moreover, it seemed to us that some of the normative understandings that currently govern knowledge translation discourse are serving to limit understanding. Subsequently, we found ourselves turning toward Caputo's[26] description of an ontological approach to knowledge development.

Drawing on the work of Heidegger, Caputo[26] describes progress in science as possible on 2 levels. Knowledge can be developed to fill in the existing horizon—to build the known body of knowledge to confirm and refine predictions and hypotheses. However, consistent with Kuhn's[27] well-known description of scientific progress, Caputo argues that "it is possible, and sometimes necessary that the horizon undergo revision, and that can occur by a discontinuous revision or a shift of horizons … (by) a reorganization of the whole field of disciplinary activity."[26(p164)] According to Caputo, this latter approach is carried out at the level of regional ontology—at the ontological horizon within which the work in the field is conducted.

This latter approach, that of developing knowledge at the level of regional ontology, seemed potentially fruitful for advancing understandings of knowledge translation and the interconnection of theory, evidence, and practice toward the particular goals of nursing. Toward that end, we have drawn on deconstructive hermeneutics and in particular, the work of Ricoeur, Derrida, and Caputo. Caputo[26] describes deconstructive hermeneutics as the ontology of understanding. Although a thorough consideration of deconstructive hermeneutics is well beyond the scope of this article, there are 2 particular ideas that we wish to draw forth for the purposes of this discussion. First, meaning, interpretation, and translation "begin where we are" and, therefore, are shaped by not only who we are but *where* we are—by the communities and contexts within which we know and act. Second, "the world of action is the basis for all meaning"[28] and action is fundamentally ontological.[16]

Knowing Begins Where We Are

Ricoeur[16] argues that context is critical to interpretation and translation. Knowledge is translated through contextual features with both subjectivity and context shaping the capacity for knowing and knowledge translation. Drawing on the idea that epistemologies reflect the ontologies of their creators and vice versa, and taking into account the reciprocity between contexts and knowers, it has seemed to us that the ontology underlying the epistemological "cultural code" in nursing may be contributing to the experiential disconnect among theory, evidence, and practice. As Ricoeur contends, "epistemological difficulties, although perhaps diverse and irreducible to one another, often have the same origin. They stem from the very structure of a being that is never capable of distancing itself from the totality of its conditioning."[(p266)] That is, what is often interpreted as inadequate knowledge or inadequate application of knowledge may from an ontological view be more related to how, as situated beings, we have come to be. The nurse in the situation we described did not necessarily lack knowledge—rather the problem seemed to be in translating knowledge (e.g., knowledge of relational practice) ontologically.

In discussing the ontological foundation of knowing—of interpretation and translation—Ricoeur[16] describes the autonomization of action in which *action is detached from its agent and develops consequences of its own.* It has seemed to us that the nurse in the above story illustrated this autonomization of action. Although she had studied and resonated with other more collaborative models of practice, ontologically she responded by *being* the "knowing nurse" to the "unknowing patient" and *automatically* assumed the power and privilege of that knowing position. Her action became routine and automatic in the context within which she worked. Although her espoused theoretic claims were inconsistent with her actions in the situation, she was seemingly unaware of that inconsistency and thereby of the consequences of her action, including the effect of those actions on her patient.

According to Ricoeur, this autonomization is a social phenomenon in which individuals are conscripted into the actions of the social group. For example, the nurse's enactment of power evident in her statement "I'll think about it" does not merely reflect her actions. It also reflects her social conditioning into understandings that dominate healthcare settings—understandings regarding what knowledge is relevant, who is knowledgeable, how knowledge should be used, and so forth. The nurse's actions reflect how this particular nurse has taken up these ideologic features and how ontology and epistemology are mutually shaped within particular contexts.

Ricoeur is but one of many authors (e.g., Derrida, Caputo, Dewey, Foucault, and so forth) who in differing ways have articulated the ideologic shaping of ontology, epistemology, and practice. "The interpretive code of ideology is something *in which* men (sic) live and think, rather than a conception *that* they pose. In other words, an ideology is operative and not thematic. It operates behind our backs, rather than appearing as a theme before our eyes. We think from it rather than about it."[16(p251)] In this way, epistemology is intertwined with social relations. Ideology becomes the glue that shapes how theory, evidence, and practice are connected. "Ideology falls within what could be called a theory of social motivation … something that justifies and something that carries along…. Hence ideology is both interpretation of the real and obturation of the possible."[16] In the above situation, the nurse acts from the ideology of the expert professional, justified by her position within the healthcare hierarchy. A consequence of this automization of action was the inability to see the impact of her actions and/or to consider other possibilities such as a collaborative relationship with the patient, despite her valuing of such theories and exposure to the evidence supporting his or her health-promoting outcomes.

Action is Fundamentally Ontological

Elias[29,30] offers a description of the way in which ideology including attitudes, beliefs, and social practices shapes people's experiences—even the way they experience themselves bodily. He describes, for example, how people in the Enlightenment era experienced a division between emotions and intellect because they were enmeshed in social controls and norms that perpetuated that way of being and thinking. Although those controls were externally perpetuated by Descartes and other thinkers of that time, people took this division up bodily. They experienced and knew themselves in that disembodied way. The division between intellect and emotion was not "the source of experience; rather, one of its products."[31(p18)] As people took up this division bodily, it became an ingrained and unconscious way-of-being in the world.

The above example of the nurse illustrates both the disembodied way-of-being Elias describes and also the way in which action is fundamentally ontological. For example, the nurse's actions arose out of her way-of-being as a knower into which she had been socialized. Moreover, her way-of-being shaped her actions and the way she drew on knowledge and evidence. The nurse's response that she would *"think* about it" is 1 illustration of the disembodied ideology that continues to dominate knowledge translation in healthcare. The patient's felt bodily sense that something was "different" was not only *not* explored, it was dismissed as the nurse took up a rationalist ontology telling the patient "it's probably nothing." This response implies that what mat-

tered (what constituted valid evidence) was what could be measured by observable, physical evidence. Thus, as the "knowing nurse," she assumed the authority to determine, translate, and make the ultimate decisions for intervention based on that particular evidence.

There have been many discussions in the nursing literature about ideology and also about how the discipline has inadvertently adopted epistemologies that are contrary to nursing values and goals. However, such discussions tend to emphasize the *epistemological* aspect of ideology, without fully considering the *ontological* dimension. Similarly there have been discussions about embodiment and disembodied approaches to care. *However, there has been little exploration into embodiment/disembodiment and the living relation of epistemology and ontology.* Moreover, little consideration has been given to the way in which existing ideologies and in particular the ontological foundations and ways of relating to and around knowledge may be contrary to embodying our nursing goals and furthering the interconnection of theory, evidence, and practice.

Ricoeur describes that it is in moments of action—at the "level of the meaningful, mutually oriented, and socially integrated character of action that the ideological phenomenon appears in all its originality."[16(p249)] It is in particular moments of nursing action that one sees ideology and the ideologic shaping of people and ontology. For this reason, Ricoeur contends that "the critique of ideology can be and must be assumed in a work of self-understanding, a work that organically implies a critique of the illusions of the subject."[16(p268)] That is, to understand and affect the interconnection of theory, evidence, and practice, an ontological inquiry at the action level is required because it is at the action level where the connections and disconnections of theory, evidence, and practice are experienced and embodied by people.

Ontological Inquiry: Examining Knowing-in-Action

Flaming[32] describes that when researching students' experiences of becoming a nurse, all of the participants in the study related "being a certain type of person" with good nursing practice. Moreover, asking students to translate their nursing actions through who they wished to be at an ontological level, through their ontological motivation, resulted in more responsive nursing actions. Flaming's research points to the significance and potential of ontological inquiry within everyday nursing practice.

From a deconstructive hermeneutics perspective, it is understood that any action and/or practice of knowledge translation proceeds from somewhere—from an already existing network of presuppositions. For example, who we are as people including how we identify ourselves to ourselves and how we identify ourselves to others is translated through a network of relations. The "kind of person I wish to be" is already relationally shaped by the discourses and practices of the larger world. Ontological motivation arises through this network of relations among oneself, others, and the contexts within which we are situated.

Ontological inquiry, like scientific inquiry, involves a conscious, intentional, and responsive process of reflexive inquiry into how particular ontologies and the knowledge and knowledge practices stemming from those ontologies are supporting the goals and values of nursing within particular practice situations. It involves recognizing the relational nature of one's own ontology and responding by questioning the meaning and consequences of that way-of-being. From this perspective, the central focus of knowledge translation is not how to get theory and research evidence used in practice. It is understood that practice is always, already evidence-based and theoretically informed. Therefore, the focus of knowledge translation becomes inquiring into one's way-of-being and how the prescribed intelligibility (and the automatization of being, knowing, and acting) is shaping the interconnection of theory, evidence, and practice—and in particular how it is limiting and/or enhancing action toward particular goals. The intent is to acknowledge and enlist existing knowledge and sensibility while simultaneously examining one's way-of-being (including the knowledge and sensibility informing that way-of-being).

A fundamental distinction within this knowing/translating process is in the ontological motivation. While existing theoretic knowledge and research evidence certainly inform one's actions ontologically, the nurse as subject does not so much follow and/or apply knowledge as *respond* to the possibilities any knowledge implies. The nurse does not act from "*behind* the text… but in *front of* it, at that which the work unfolds, discovers, reveals. Henceforth, to understand is *to understand oneself in front of the text* … (it is a matter of) exposing ourselves to the text and receiving from it an enlarged self … corresponding in the most suitable way to the world proposed."[16(p88)]

The nurse in the earlier example can be seen to have been acting from behind the text as reflected in her statement "I practice exactly like you describe." She did not appear to reflect on her actions within the particular situation and what those actions revealed about her way-of-being and knowing as a nurse and/or about the context within which she was practicing. Consequently, although she "knew" and valued relational theories, the opportunity to stand in front of these theories, be enlarged by the possibilities they offered, and ultimately translate herself and her actions into effective, responsive nursing practice was hindered.

 ## Shifting the Horizon: From Evidence-Based to Inquiry-Based Practice

As the ontological horizon of knowledge translation is reenvisioned to focus on what transpires in specific nursing situations, *knowledge translation becomes a process of apprehending a possibility of being.*[33] It involves active inquiry in which questions and answers arise through and in the everyday pragmatics of nursing situations.[12,15] As such, the form and emphasis of practice shift from *evidence-based* to *inquiry-based* practice.

Embodied knowing is central to inquiry-based practice. Within nursing, embodiment has been used to describe the use of the body as a vehicle for knowing the world, as an ethical stance of conscious action, as a material form of subjectivity and experience, and in reference to meaning-centered conceptualizations of culture rather than, for example, ethnicity-centered ones.[1,34] Interestingly, Gadow contends that nursing understandings of embodiment "remain discouragingly disembodied."[1(p90)] In this article, our use of the term *embodiment* is in line with Wilde's[34] explanation that embodiment "is not a theory, or a group of theories, but a different way of thinking about and knowing human beings." Somewhat in contrast with the goals of rationalist understandings, embodiment highlights the physical substance of knowing.[1] As Polanyi contends, whether we are aware of it or not "Every time we make sense of the world, we rely on our tacit knowledge of impacts made by the world on our body and the complex responses of our body to these impacts."[35(p147)] Our bodies are the site where knowledge converges in a far more intricate manner than any intellectual conceptualization.[36] "Our body is the ultimate instrument of all our external knowledge, whether intellectual or practical. In all our waking moments, we are *relying* on our awareness of contacts of our body with things outside for *attending* to those things."[37(p16)]

Inquiry-based nursing involves a conscious tuning into this implicit, intricate knowing process as a way-of-being in nursing situations.[38] Within inquiry-based practice, the first function of understanding is to orientate within a particular situation.[16] "To understand is to contextualize, to situate a thing within the contextual arrangement in which it belongs … to 'cast' it in the appropriate terms."[26] The epistemological ground—the ground of knowing—is each person's tacit experiential presence in the world in relation with everyone and everything in the world.[15,39] The knowing process entails looking toward the primary constituents—people, context, research and theoretic knowledge, meaningful purposes, excellence of practices, and effectiveness of outcomes.[39] Evidence of successful knowledge translation lies in the pragmatic outcomes of any action, for example, how nursing actions respond to and correspond with people's health and healing experiences and ultimately effect health outcomes.

As an inquirer, the goal is to enter each situation experiencing theoretic and research knowledge anew. We attend to the possibilities seen in the light of a particular theory and are aware of the theory/evidence/knowledge in an active way. That is, theory/evidence is considered in relation to that which it opens up in terms of understanding, interpretation, selection, and action. Like a scientific inquiry, inquiry-based practice involves picking out clues that seem relevant to the present moment, examining what it is they appear to indicate while simultaneously responding with possibilities for action.[39] As Gendlin[36] describes, it involves "thinking with experiential intricacy. "Through such experiential intricacy, practice is permitted to surprise theory and theory/evidence is translated into more intricate ways of acting.[36] For example, taking an inquiry-based approach the nurse in the example we provided might have engaged herself differently by *inquiring into* the patient's sensation that "something was different." Purposefully attending to the interconnection of ontology ("who I want to be") and epistemology ("how/what knowledge might I enlist as a knower") she might have gone beyond the automized ontology/action of "knowing nurse to unknowing patient." Rather than limiting her evidence-gathering actions to vital signs she might have *been* with the patient in a more relationally responsive manner and as such expanded her actions to intentionally open the possibilities for other forms of knowledge and evidence to inform her clinical decision making. In this way, the interconnection among her espoused nursing values and goals, the theory and evidence she enlisted to inform her practice, and her actions might have been enhanced.

Remaking Knowledge and Ideology

In addition to promoting informed, responsive, competent actions in nursing situations, ontologically informed inquiry-based practice also serves to "make knowledge and ideology over." Purposefully theorizing and enacting epistemological and ontological possibilities that might better support the values and goals of nursing involve a meaning-making process in which knowledge and ideology are reinterpreted. As one examines the interconnection of ideology, theory, evidence and practice in a particular situation, that interconnection is understood and reshaped.[15] Moreover, the "doing" of nursing is melded with qualities of being and knowing through that translation process.

Reason and Torbet[40] describe that through such an inquiry process, "all movements of the attention,

all knowing, all acting, and all gathering of evidence is based on at least implicit fragments of *normative theory of what act is timely now*."[40] This idea of normative theory is an important one given the ideologic shaping of knowledge and the experiential "gap" outlined earlier. For example, ideologically if one examines the nursing literature it is possible to see that "the gap between theory and practice" has become a common sensibility. Similar to Elias' example of people in the Enlightenment who experienced their own bodies in disembodied ways, the discourse of the theory-practice gap of EBP and so forth has served to normalize this sensibility to the point that the gap is a "real" "normal" experience. However, entering nursing situations as an inquirer automatically sets one up to remake the normative values and discursive practices within that dominant ideology. Translation becomes a process of reshaping our ways of being, knowing, relating, and acting.

This remaking of knowledge and ideology is in many ways akin to Dickoff and James'[41] description of "situation-producing theory." These authors contend that situation-producing theory is the highest level of theory because it exists and is produced for practice. Moreover, it has the potential to translate and reshape nursing knowledge and action to be more responsive in particular moments of practice. They have argued (and we concur) that "theory for a profession of practice discipline must provide for more than mere understanding or 'describing' or even predicting reality and must provide conceptualization especially intended to guide the shaping of reality to that profession's professional purpose."[41(p102)]

Derrida emphasizes the importance of this remaking process describing the "tension between memory, fidelity, the preservation of something which has been given to us, and at the same time heterogeneity, something absolutely new."[42(p6)] The goal of inquiry is to know and understand the intelligibility well enough that one can see through its gaps and inconsistencies to select, filter, interpret, and transform it. "Consequently and paradoxically, one can be faithful to one's heritage only in as much as one accepts to be unfaithful to it, to analyze it, to critique it, to interpret it, relentlessly."[43(p19)] In this way, reinterpreting the relationship among theory, evidence, and action in nursing practice and the dominant conceptions of knowledge translation serves nursing goals.

 ## Toward the Embodiment of Theory/Evidence/Practice

Recently there has been a call for theory to shape the design and implementation of knowledge translation.[3,44] Estabrooks et al[3] contend that theories are needed to develop testable and useful interventions. We concur that greater understanding of knowledge translation and better support of the interconnection of theory, evidence, and practice are needed. At the same time, we are cognizant of Caputo's[26] contention that we ought not to presuppose "a hard and fast distinction between practice and theory—as if theory did not have a praxis of its own, and practice did not have a 'sighting' of its own."[(p159)] That is, from a hermeneutic perspective any theory originates from our involvement in the world and any practice is already imbued with theory. Thus, it is important to think carefully about the theories one enlists to shape knowledge translation processes. If interpretation, translation, and action are relationally and ontologically mediated through subjectivity, context, and ideology, there is, as Cecci[14] has previously contended, no neutral, disinterested theory. Given the epistemological concerns that have already been raised about the limited conceptualizations of knowledge translation and the forms of nursing practice to which they give rise, a careful *ontological* consideration of the theories and ideologies shaping understandings of knowledge translation seems vital.

Within his theory of translation, Ricoeur[33] describes that a central characteristic of a spoken language is that it is in a sense "untranslatable" from one language to another. The question with which we are currently grappling in our own inquiry process is: Can any theory and/or group of theories "translate" across the complexity of nursing situations and result in competent, safe, ethical practice? Ricoeur[33] suggests that "it is through a 'doing' in the pursuit of theory that the translator gets over the (translation) obstacle."[(p32)] Might it be more fruitful to "stand in front" of Ricoeur's suggestion and focus on *acting* in the pursuit of theory?

Along this line, Caputo[26] contends that perhaps our best epistemological bet is to take up an antiessentialist open-ended nonknowing approach. This nonknowing keeps the door open to evidence that has not yet come in and will multiply the opportunities for seeing something we did not see coming—to potentialities we cannot presently conceive. Rather than focusing our attention on using and/or developing theory, Ricoeur[33] suggests that "we need to get beyond ... theoretical alternatives ... and replace them with practical alternatives, stemming from the very exercise of translation, the faithfulness versus betrayal alternatives, even if it means admitting that the practice of translation remains a risky operation which is always in search of theory."[(p14)]

Nursing education informed by an understanding of nursing as an embodied process of critical inquiry and translation might emphasize the development of ways of being. For example, while attending to questions such as "what do you need to know in this situation?," we ask our students continuously to consider "what kind of nurse do you want to be in this situation?" Such questions evoke commitment, engagement, and "response-ability," and help students bring together more effectively multiple forms of knowledge (e.g., empirical, ethical, esthetic, contextual) and work within the potential contradictions between those differing knowledges. Similarly, nursing research informed by an ontological understanding might seek to derive implications and recommendations for nurse's ways-of-being with patients. For example, in the area of violence against women, ways-of-being that validate the woman's worth as a human being and abuse as undeserved are the most important aspects of an effective response and the foundation for a trusting relationship.[45,46]

Seeing competent nursing practice as involving more than the application of theory and evidence, as an embodied process of critical inquiry and translation, one that draws on theory and evidence to enlarge and imagine possibilities for action in particular moments, situations, and contexts offers a *way-of-being* in which the interconnection of theory, evidence, and practice is lived. Moreover, it sets us up to question the role and purpose of any knowledge and inquire into the ontological motivations that shape our knowing-in-action. Finally, an ontological understanding of the interconnections among theory, evidence, and practice highlights that any knowledge translation process should be guided by the question "how might (this) theory and evidence inform and enlarge the possibilities for being with and responding to this particular patient in this specific situation?" In this way an ongoing ontological inquiry not only enhances the interconnection of theory, evidence, and practice but also has the potential to transform the ideologies currently shaping nursing education, nursing scholarship, and nursing practice.

REFERENCES

1. Gadow S. Philosophy as falling: aiming for grace. *Nurs Philos.* 2000;1:89–97.
2. Graham ID, Logan J, Harrison MB, et al. Lost in translation: time for a map? *J Contin Educ Health Prof* 2006;26(1):13–24.
3. Estabrooks C, Thompson D, Lovely J, Hof meyer A. A guide to knowledge translation theory. *J Contin Educ Health Prof.* 2006;26(1):25–36.
4. Reimer Kirkham S, Baumbush JI, Schultz A, Anderson JM. Knowledge development and evidence-based practice. Insights and opportunities from a postcolonial feminist perspective for transformative nursing practice. *Adv Nurs Sci.* 2007;30(1):26–40.
5. Tarlier D. Mediating the meaning of evidence through epistemological diversity. In: Reed P, Shearer N, eds. *Perspectives on Nursing Theory.* 5th ed. Philadelphia, PA: Lippincott Williams & Wilkins; 2008:365–376.
6. Schultz P, Meleis AI. Nursing epistemology: traditions, insights, questions. In: Reed P, Shearer N, eds. *Perspectives*

on *Nursing Theory*. 5th ed. Philadelphia, PA: Lippincott Williams & Wilkins; 2008:385–394.

7. Funk SG, Tornquist EM, Champagne MT. Barriers and facilitators of research utilization: an integrative review. *Nurs Clin North Am*. 1995;30:395–406.

8. Estabrooks CA. Mapping the research utilization field in nursing. *Can J Nurs Res*. 1999;31(1):53–72.

9. Dobbins M, Ciliska D, DiCenso A. *Dissemination and use of Research Evidence for Policy and Practice: A Framework for Developing, Implementing and Evaluating Strategies*. Ottawa: Canadian Nurses Association; 1998.

10. Reed P. The practice turn in nursing epistemology. In: Reed P, Shearer N, eds. *Perspectives on Nursing Theory*. 5th ed. Philadelphia, PA: Lippincott Williams & Wilkins; 2008: 693–697.

11. Marrs J, Lowry LW. Nursing theory and practice: connecting the dots. In: Reed P, Shearer N, eds. *Perspectives on Nursing Theory*. 5th ed. Philadelphia, PA: Lippincott Williams & Wilkins; 2008:3–12.

12. Hartrick Doane G, Varcoe C. Toward compassionate action: pragmatism and the inseparability of theory/practice. *Adv Nurs Sci*. 2005;28(1):81–90.

13. Flaming D. Nursing theories as nursing ontologies. *Nurs Philos*. 2004;5:224–229.

14. Cecci C. Not innocent: relationships between knowers and knowledge. *Can J Nurs Res*. 2000;32(2):57–73.

15. Hartrick Doane G, Varcoe C. *Family Nursing as Relational Inquiry: Developing Health-Promoting Practice*. Philadelphia, PA: Lippincott Williams & Wilkins; 2005.

16. Ricoeur P. From *Text to Action. Essays in Hermeneutics, II*. Evanston, IL: Northwestern University Press; 1991.

17. Harding S. *Whose Science? Whose Knowledge? Thinking from Women's Lives*. New York: Cornell University Press; 1991.

18. Caputo J. *Radical Hermeneutics: Repetition, Deconstruction and the Hermeneutic Project*. Bloomington, IN: Indiana University Press; 1987.

19. Varcoe C, Doane G, Pauly B, et al. Ethical practice in nursing—working the in-betweens. *J Adv Nurs*. 2004;45(3): 316–325.

20. Rodney P, Varcoe C, Storch J, et al. Navigating towards a moral horizon: a multisite qualitative study of ethical practice in nursing. *Can J Nurs Res*. 2002;34(3):75–102.

21. Doane GH, Pauly B, Brown H, McPherson G. Exploring the heart of ethical nursing practice: implications for ethics education. *Nurs Ethics*. 2004;11(3):240–253.

22. Hamric AB. Moral distress in everyday ethics. *Nurs Outlook*. 2000;48:199–201.

23. Peter E, Liaschenko J. Perils of proximity: a spatiotemporal analysis of moral distress and moral ambiguity. *Nurs Inq*. 2004;11(4):218–225.

24. Corley MC, Minick P, Elswick RK, Jacobs M. Nurse moral distress and ethical work environment. *Nurs Ethics*. 2005;12(4):381–390.

25. Thorne S, Henderson AD, McPherson G, Pesut BK. The problematic allure of the binary in nursing theoretical discourse. *Nurs Philos*. 2004;5:208–215.

26. Caputo J. *More Radical Hermeneutics*. Blooming-ton, IN: Indiana University Press; 2000.

27. Kuhn TS. *The Structure of Scientific Revolutions*. Chicago: University of Chicago Press; 1962.

28. Valdes MJ. Introduction: Paul Ricoeur's poststructuralist hermeneutics. *Ricoeur Reader: Reflection and Imagination*. Toronto: University of Toronto Press; 1991:3–40.

29. Elias NJ. *The History of Manners: The Civilizing Process*. Vol 1. Oxford: Blackwell; 1978.

30. Elias NJ. *State Formation and Civilization: The Civilizing Process*. Vol 2. Oxford: Blackwell; 1982.

31. Burkitt I. The shifting concept of the self. *Hist Human Sci*. 1994;7(2):7–28.

32. Flaming D. Becoming a nurse: "it's just who I am." *Med Humanitarian Rev*. 2005;31:95–100.

33. Ricoeur P. *On Translation*. Madison, NY: Routledge; 2006.

34. Wilde MH. Why embodiment now? *Adv Nurs Sci*. 1999;22(2):25–38.

35. Polanyi M. *Knowing and Being*. Chicago, IL: University of Chicago Press; 1969.

36. Gendlin ET. Thinking beyond patterns: body, language and situations. In: den Ouden B, Moen M, eds. *The Presence in Feeling and Thought*. New York: Peter Lang; 1992:21–51.

37. Polanyi M. *The Tacit Dimension*. Glouchester, MA: Peter Smith; 1983.

38. Doane G. Being an ethical practitioner: the embodiment of mind, emotion and action. In: Storch J, Rodney P, Starzomski R, eds. *Toward a Moral Horizon: Nursing Ethics for Leadership and Practice*. Toronto, Canada: Pearson Publishing; 2004:433–446.

39. Reason P, Bradbury H. Inquiry and participation in search of a world of worthy human aspiration. In: Reason P, Bradury H, eds. *Handbook of Action Research: Participative Inquiry and Practice*. London: Sage; 2001:1–14.

40. Reason P, Torbert WR. Toward a transformational social science: a further look at the scientific merits of action research. *Concepts Transform*. 2001;6(1):1–37.

41. Dickoff J, James PJ. A theory of theories: a position paper. In: Nicholl LH, ed. *Perspectives on Nursing The*ory. Glenview, IL: Scott, Foresman & Co; 1968/1986.

42. Derrida J. The Villanova roundtable: a conversation with Jacques Derrida. In: Caputo J, ed. *Deconstruction in a Nutshell. A Conversation With Jacques Derrida*. New York: Fordham University Press; 1997:3–30.

43. Egea-Kuehne D. The teaching of philosophy: renewed rights and responsibilities. In: Trifonas P, Peters M, eds. *Derrida, Deconstruction and Education. Ethics of Pedagogy and Research*. Victoria, Australia: Philosophy of Education Society of Australasia; 2004:17–30.

44. Eccles M, Grimshaw J, Walker A, Johnston M, Pitts N. Changing the behavior of healthcare professionals: the use of theory in promoting the uptake of research findings. *J Clin Epidemiol*. 2005;58:107–112.

45. Gerbert B, Caspers N, Bronstone A, Moe J, Abercrombie P. A qualitative analysis of how physicians with expertise in domestic violence approach the identification of victims. *Ann Intern Med*. 1999;131(8):578–584.

46. Gerbert B, Caspers N, Milliken N, Berlia M, Bronstone A, Mof J. Interventions that help victims of domestic violence. *J Fam Pract*. 2000;49(10):889.

THE AUTHORS COMMENT

Knowledge Translation in Everyday Nursing: From Evidence-Based to Inquiry-Based Practice

This article was inspired by a somewhat bewildering experience that I (Gweneth) had as a patient. Together, Colleen and I grappled with the complexities of knowledge translation and sought to examine the complacent underpinnings of knowledge-based nursing practice. We wrote the article to raise what we consider to be vital questions of knowledge translation, hoping to invite a reconsideration of the epistemological emphasis and the inscribed epistemological and ontological dichotomies that seem to dominate nursing discourse. We have long decried the existence of a 'theory-practice gap', arguing that every moment of nursing practice is theoretical, even if the theoretical underpinnings are not made explicit. We hoped that this article might inspire nurses to consider their own ontology and ontological motivation—to question 'to what end' they integrate knowledge in their practice and how they might embody nursing knowledge in a way that is responsive to particular people and situations.

GWENETH HARTRICK DOANE
COLLEEN VARCOE

13

Nursing Theory as a Guide to Practice

WILLIAM K. CODY, RN, PhD, FAAN

After much deliberation, I find myself more convinced than ever that in the discipline of nursing today, given a forced choice between these two general propositions represented in Dr. Fawcett's questions about theory and practice, it is far more accurate and meaningful to assert that *theory guides practice*. To assert the alternative, that theory arises from practice to an equal or greater extent than theory guides practice, would be a misrepresentation of the contemporary art and science of nursing theory development. In actuality, this assertion has been made widely and, I would venture to say, that is to the detriment of theory development in nursing.

Reflections on Practice: Yes, Guided by Theory

As I reflect on my own experience, I think about the first 10 years of my work in nursing. During those years—the 1970s and the 1980s—nursing was nearly devoid of nursing theory *per se*. In contrast, the next 15 years were inundated with nursing theory. I realize that there always was some identifiable body of knowledge that provided an underpinning to my work. In the early days of my career—and I suspect that this experience is shared with many nurses now around my age, in their 40s and 50s—the knowledge that guided my work could be overwhelmingly categorized as rudimentary knowledge of anatomy and physiology, medicine, pharmacology, physics, chemistry, microbiology, hygiene, psychology, and communication. There was some vague introduction to core ideas (I now know to be) from Virginia Henderson and Dorothea Orem, but their names and the name of any *theory* had been removed from the content. I was simply taught to care for people who were ill in such a way that they could, it was hoped, return to doing as much as possible to care for themselves, as soon as possible.

In the 1980s, I worked in a major urban medical center with a reputation for fine nursing practice. There, my nurse colleagues and I were constantly

challenged by the nursing leadership to think critically and to consider the scientific rationale behind every element of patient care. Thus, I found myself obliged to take the rudimentary knowledge that had been the bedrock of my then-biomedical practice and make it broader and deeper, although keeping it almost completely categorizable as anatomy and physiology, medicine, pharmacology, and so on. When I consider these memories from 10 years of intensive bedside nursing, I cannot think of any other domain of life—other than the subsequent 15 years in which my work has been nursing theory intensive—in which my activities (homemaking, my own healthcare, relationships, recreation, participating in the arts, car maintenance, or anything else) have been so *thoroughly* guided by a specified body of knowledge. It was not nursing theory, but it was theory.

Problem-Solving and Common Sense: Guided by, Not Producing, Theories

To be sure, there were many creative ideas that emerged in my shared nursing worklife, ideas that surfaced in direct problem-solving efforts, brainstorming, being asked by my supervisors for input to resolve various situations, and other instances of making-do, jury-rigging, and flying by the seat of one's pants. We came up with different ways of taping intravenous lines to withstand restlessness and confusion, ingenious methods of affixing complicated dressings to large wounds, and clever ways of explaining complex concepts of medicine to lay people so that they might understand what was happening to them. We experimented with different ways of preventing and minimizing pressure sores; we learned when to test serum electrolytes and how to restore fluid, electrolyte, and hemodynamic stability with a minimum of direction from the physician; we organized the work of caring for groups of patients to be more efficient; shared ways of minimizing discomfort while passing various tubes

From W.K. Cody, Nursing Science Quarterly 2003, 16(3): 225–231.
Copyright © 2003, SAGE Publications. Reprinted by permission of SAGE Publications, Inc.

ABOUT THE AUTHOR

WILLIAM K. CODY was born in Hampton, VA, and grew up in North Carolina. He began his career in nursing as a Licensed Practical Nurse and later received ASN and BSN degrees from Regents College; a BS in communication from New York University; an MSN from Hunter College, where he met his mentor, Rosemarie Parse; and a PhD in nursing from the University of South Carolina.

He is currently Dean and Professor, Presbyterian School of Nursing at Queens University of Charlotte in Charlotte, North Carolina. He is perhaps best known for his articles on theoretical concerns written for *Nursing Science Quarterly*. As a Robert Wood Johnson Executive Nurse Fellow, 2003–2006, his leadership foci included nurse-managed health centers and community–campus partnerships.

into persons' orifices; and we mentored each other in talking with patients and families about death and dying. I witnessed my associates and myself gradually becoming more and more expert in various aspects of the job.

I admired many of my colleagues for the vast expanse of their knowledge and for their creativity in problem solving. However, upon much reflection, I would have to say that I do not find it accurate or useful in any way to think of the activities just described as developing, generating, or inventing theory. Indeed, I find that reflecting on my own experiences in light of a robust notion of what constitutes theory development strongly contradicts the notion that *theory arises from practice*. To my knowledge, although I worked with a number of brilliant people and, along with them, solved many hundreds of practical problems with creative solutions, none of those activities rose to the level of generating theory, few were deeply rooted in any philosophy of nursing or anything else except practicality, none were published or widely disseminated, and some were later shown to be misguided by theory development and research.

Applying known principles of science and common sense to activities that are performed repetitively for months or years and coming up with incrementally better ways of doing things, to me, is not theorizing, and it is not useful to think of it as such. It is problem-solving; it is the benefit of practical experience; it is common sense at work. Even if one were to grant that this kind of creative thinking is *theorizing*, if it is neither grounded in a philosophy of nursing nor intended specifically to guide the work that is the specialized mission of nursing, then I see no reason to think of such creative ideas as *nursing* theories. It cannot substitute in any way for the fullness and richness of practice that is guided by nursing theory, and it pales in comparison in meaningfulness and effectiveness in enhancing quality of life.

My view is, to put it simply, that one learns to practice nursing by studying nursing theories, and one learns to practice nursing *very well* by studying nursing

theories very intensely over a long period of time. One does not learn to practice in the discipline and profession of nursing by merely practicing what is commonly called nursing but is not specific to nursing, and one does not learn to practice nursing very well by practicing nursing that is bereft of nursing theory, even if it is practiced very intensely over a long period of time.

Contexts of Repression: Likelihood and Limitations

I essentially agree with Dr. Parker when she says that "practice must first be guided by theory, and then the theory can be studied and further developed as a result of expert practice" (Fawcett, 2003, p. 131). The difficulty that resides in connecting higher levels of nursing theory development in general with something called *expert practice* in nursing today is plain to see. By what are today's frontline, bedside nurses guided? I believe that for the most part, now as in the early years of my own career, they are guided by rudimentary principles and empirical generalizations from medicine and pharmacology, with a little social science and an eclectic mélange from a variety of other disciplines as needed for working in their settings and with their populations. Elements of the nursing theories that are taught in schools of nursing are, as often as not, taught sketchily and half-heartedly, and the majority of practice settings do not reinforce, value, or encourage the use of nursing theories. Innate good will, and a modicum of professionalism and ethical reflection upon one's practice can go far toward keeping basic care decent, but these clearly are not substitutes for a coherent vision of one's profession and its unique mission with an articulated practice methodology.

In the United States, nursing practice is carried out in a context of for-profit healthcare that demands skeleton staffing and production-line care, while about a third of the population is uninsured, underinsured, or a paycheck away from being uninsured.

It is carried out in a context in which many persons must do without needed medicine because they cannot pay for it. It is carried out in a context in which a sizable proportion of the diagnostic tests performed are ordered as defensive measures against the possibility of malpractice lawsuits. It is carried out in a context in which the majority of the leaders and decision-makers in healthcare and health policy remain straight, White, males from middle- or upper-class backgrounds. And, much of medicine remains prone to the glorification of machismo and dominance in both physician-patient and physician-nurse relationships. The mammoth barrier to nursing theorizing arising in everyday nursing practice is not merely that the dominant ideas that permeate contemporary healthcare are *non-nursing*, although that is certainly the case; the greater barrier is that many of the ideas actually guiding practice (explicitly or implicitly) are alien to nursing's tradition of *caring for whole people where they are and as they are*, and even anathema to such an ideal. Ironically, perhaps, I do see nursing theory-based practice as the primary source of hope for altering these contexts.

The graduate students to whom I teach nursing theory have several common, salient reactions to the proposition that nursing practice should be guided by nursing theory. One reaction is that they (nurses) are far too busy in the chaotic, high-pressure environments of contemporary hospitals to take time to do "all that touchy-feely stuff," as some say. Another is to question why, if this knowledge is important, did the nursing establishment—so famously intent on control of many aspects of nursing education and practice—let them progress through their careers to see themselves and be seen as expert nurses without ever having seriously studied nursing theories? And still another reaction is that it is already hard enough to learn and remember all the medicine and pharmacology, and all the regulations, policies, and procedures required in everyday nursing practice, without trying to remember even more ideas and to practice differently from the habits of thought and action with which they have been indoctrinated over many years. Without a thorough education in nursing theory and the opportunity to engage over time in nursing theory-based practice, these *expert* nurses cannot be expected to develop nursing theory or contribute to nursing theory. This would be analogous to saying that the next great school of thought in psychology is likely to spring up spontaneously from the discipline of engineering.

 ## Contexts of Understanding

I agree with Dr. Parker when she says that "our concepts guide what we 'look for,' and take in … and the experience then may be reflected on and described

to enhance concepts" (Fawcett, 2003, pp. 131–132), a process she describes as a spiral. It seems that Dr. Parker is picturing something akin to the Heideggerian circle of understanding, which moves circularly or, as Dr. Parker prefers, spirally, from one's current understanding and that which is familiar to that which is new and unfamiliar and back again, continuously integrating the unfamiliar into one's unfolding experience in accord with one's worldview, values, and beliefs. That which is utterly new to one's experience, completely unfamiliar, incommensurate with one's worldview, or contradictory to one's values and beliefs, is likely to be passed over, rejected, or avoided. I believe this is particularly so when the new idea hovers close to cherished values and beliefs or deeply ingrained patterns of daily life, challenging or contradicting them. We weave the fabric of our day-to-day personal and professional experience using by-and-large the threads and patterns that we know, recognize, and are comfortable with. Yet I deeply wish we (nurse leaders) would better provide young nurses with a deeper familiarity with and appreciation for the richness of the fabrics, yarns, and patterns that constitute *bona fide* nursing philosophy and science, that is, the extant theories and theoretical literature delineating nursing ontologies, epistemologies, and methodologies.

 ## Contexts of Possibilities

When we have a critical mass of bachelor's, master's, and doctorally prepared nurses working in everyday healthcare guided predominantly by theories of nursing—an image that you, Dr. Fawcett, elicited in your exchange with Dr. Parker—perhaps the whole question of whether theory arises from practice will appear different. This would be a nursing workforce that could participate more fully in the work of developing and testing (in the broad sense) nursing theories. I don't believe that this attitude is elitist. I have provided leadership to an ongoing project of teaching the fundamentals of Parse's (1998) theory in a hospice facility staffed with nursing assistants, and I fully believe that the pattern of practice there is grounded in and consistent with nursing theory.

The majority of the contemporary workforce of registered nurses, however, offer a very different challenge to nurse educators, theorists, theoreticians, administrators, and other nurse leaders. They have learned, absorbed, and identified with a body of knowledge and skills that they believe to be nursing—which coincides for the most part with the stark requirements for licensure and the expectations of corporate employers of frontline nurses, and *not* with the body of knowledge that has emanated from 150 years of nursing scholarship rooted explicitly in philosophies of nursing. Naturally, these nurses are prone to respond to their first exposure to nursing theory with the reaction that it has little or nothing to do with *nursing* as they know it. I was one of those nurses for a long time, and in 25 years of working more than full-time in nursing I have met, worked with, or taught thousands of such nurses. The transformation of the educational preparation of nurses and the culture of nursing could yet bring about an environment in which the everyday practice of nursing is grounded in and intersects with *bona fide* nursing scholarship. But what is required to get to that future phase of our development in which "all nurse educators, nurse administrators, nurse researchers, and practicing nurses … view nursing from the lens of nursing models and theories" (Fawcett, 2003, p. 133), is nothing short of revolution. This is the revolution that should have occurred in the discipline of nursing, *circa* 1970, with the publication of Rogers' seminal work, *Introduction to the Theoretical Basis of Nursing*, but did not.

The Revolution That Didn't Come and the Potential That Yet Remains

As I refer to something I have called *bona fide* nursing scholarship, I find myself reflecting on exactly what I mean by that. In pondering the meaning, I am reminded of Orem's (1985) early work examining the question of who is a legitimate recipient of nursing services. She eventually came to say:

> *Persons with a legitimate need for nursing are characterized (a) by a demand for discernible kinds of and amounts of self-care or dependent-care and (b) by health-derived or health-related limitations for the continuing production of the amount and kind of care required. (p. 31)*

Orem's declaration, along with Henderson's (Harmer & Henderson, 1955) famous definition of nursing, clearly has directly or indirectly influenced the nurse educators who taught me and legions of other students in the 1970s. The beliefs and values reflected in those definitions that were generated in the first decades of self-conscious nursing theory development include the image of the nurse as a kind of surrogate mother. Peplau even stated as much directly in her 1952 book, which was, I believe, the first instance of a nurse deliberately naming her ideas a theory of nursing. Delineated there as one of the roles of the nurse was indeed "mother surrogate" (Peplau, 1952, p. 54). Surely the works of Henderson, Orem,

Peplau, and those who carry on their work are *bona fide* nursing scholarship. But I cannot help wondering what may be the lingering effects of the 1950s conceptualization, in that first decade of deliberate and self-conscious nursing theory development, of *the nurse as someone whose central vocational duty is to perform a wide range of personal care for the other in an essentially maternal manner*. To be sure, it is miraculous that a field of human endeavor occupied 95% and led by women was able to assert at all that it was *a science with a unique body of knowledge* in the repressive and sexist era of the 1950s.

The works the early nurse theorists produced were commensurate with the actualities of the everyday work of nurses in their time. Similarly, Orlando (1962) produced a framework that offered as its central contribution a guide to actually thinking through nursing care situations rather than responding automatically. Such conceptualizations, it seems to me, likely merely adduced and formalized dimensions of nursing care embedded in the everyday worklives of nurses and offered a formal structure for implementing the best of then-current nursing practices.

It seems to me that the *next* major wave in nursing theory development, historically, which brought about the radical ideas of Martha Rogers (1970), Paterson and Zderad (1976), Parse (1981), and Watson (1985), got far *ahead* of the vast majority of nurses, leading to a rift between ordinary practice and the leading edge of nursing theory that has continued for 30 years. We will probably never fully understand how or why this happened. My impression is that many nurse leaders in the 1970s, 1980s, and 1990s, without advanced education in nursing theories, deliberately resisted and undermined efforts to advance nursing theory-based practice and research. The federally funded Nurse Scientist programs of the 1960s apparently did much to advance the status of academic nurses in universities, while ironically doing little or nothing to advance nursing science, since the doctorates it supported were all in other fields.

I believe that probably the key dynamic in the nonadoption of nursing theories by nurses has been the overwhelming societal need for professional/vocational care givers trained for biomedical/technical care in huge numbers, juxtaposed with the immense intellectual challenge, on the other hand, of mastering the creatively synthesized new knowledge generated by a newly emergent discipline. To rise to both of these challenges while also struggling to rise above enforced second-class-citizenship as nurses and as women represents a monumental challenge. And yet a large and growing body of literature continues to emanate from the works of such visionary nurse scholars as Rogers, Paterson and Zderad, Parse, Watson, and their followers. This seems to me a testament to the value of the ideas that have arisen within nursing theory development over the past 50 years. The notions that were born of and are central to nursing—humans as unitary beings, human-environment mutual process, health as much more than wellness alone, life as rhythmic patterning, the centrality of meaning and of interpersonal caring in human experience, the nonlinearity and paradoxicality of human experience, the profundity of the nurse-person relationship, and that relationship as the locus of nursing practice—are all too important to be lost to humanity by a lack of attention to the further development of bona fide nursing science.

 ## The Hijacking of Nursing Science

A glance at the emerging mainstream meaning of *nursing science* is instructive. One might almost think the emergent meaning is being propelled by a reaction against nursing theory. I have before me as I write a list of all the grants funded by the National Institute for Nursing Research (NINR) in fiscal year 2001, retrieved from the World Wide Web (NINR, n.d.). It is easy to see from the titles of the studies that the foci deemed legitimate by the NINR are overwhelmingly those that relate to the kinds of interests that biomedically-trained nurses have held for the past several decades. Some topics of recurring interest to the NINR include arterial disease, hormone therapy, symptoms of angina, thromboembolism, hypertension, hyperlipidemia, nutrition, pulmonary aspiration, mechanical ventilation, genetic testing, smoking cessation, and medication adherence. Upon investigation, one can also ascertain that a small but significant portion of the studies that the NINR funds (perhaps about 10%) are not only conceptually unrelated to nursing but also conducted by nonnurses without any apparent connection to nursing. I also have noted that the American Academy of Nursing now has two disparate and nonoverlapping councils, one focused on nursing theory and one focused on something called *nursing science*, which appears to be code for *funded research*. I believe that these two situations, and the thousands of smaller echoes of these situations among groups of nurses all around the world, are the complex multilayered consequences of the rift between theory and practice that occurred many years ago.

As a nurse theoretician, I see this historic rift and its sequelae as first, the emergence of the best that nursing as a discipline has to offer humankind, truly the most original and most important leap forward in the discipline of nursing since Nightingale, and then, the near or complete rejection of that great gift by much of the discipline, after strangely little investigation or effort. The parallel developments over the past 15 years of the nurse practitioner movement, rooted largely in a biomedical perspective, and the nonnursing emphases of the much-coveted NINR funded research would seem to have brought us to the verge of the eclipse of the nursing theory movement.

Can nursing survive as a discipline without a specified body of knowledge of its own? Can a discipline that is fragmented and discontinuous, a discipline with many major stakeholders *within* it who have no real commitment to higher education in nursing and no commitment to the philosophies, theories, or methods specific to nursing survive? I think not. More and more these days one hears academics in healthcare disciplines assert that interdisciplinary research on so-called middle-range theories is where the action is now and that this approach constitutes the wave of the future. Such research is what is most commonly funded by the NINR today. This kind of research is generally focused at a relatively concrete level of scientific understanding, cause-effect in its ontology, and problem-solving in its real purpose.

But the great contributions of any and all disciplines do not reside in the thousands of particular transient projects focused on middle-range or concrete phenomena that its scholars conduct from year to year. Rather, the greatest contribution of a discipline resides in the articulation of its central reason for being, its central mission, and the major conceptualizations of its phenomena of concern. Consider the centrality of the concept of evolution in biology, the concept of the unconscious mind in psychology, or the concept of society itself in sociology. The great contributions of these disciplines to civilizations over centuries do not reside in the experiments in problem-solving on a concrete level that pepper the journals like so many refrigerator drawings, but in the great and lasting ideas central to the discipline. That is what is missing in the so-called nursing science that is not rooted in philosophies and theories of nursing. This is why I am moved to say that the dominant thrust of so-called nursing science today, toward interdisciplinary cause-effect research on concrete phenomena, is in fact detrimental to the future of the discipline. In the unique context of nursing as it exists today, this is tantamount to selling our soul to buy the respect of members of other disciplines—who may never come to know the unique scholarship that resides in the specific literature of nursing philosophy and theory.

Recently, I had experiences with two unrelated, well-respected academics from psychology and audiology. Each, separately, in the midst of conversations, blithely and unabashedly stated something to the effect that "I have read some of that *nursing theory* and I have found it to be nonsense." Actually, one said he found it to be "neither broad nor deep" and the other said it was garbage. Both of these men, by the way, have actually worked closely over time with nurses, but those nurses had no ties to nursing theories. Yet these experiences do not sadden me so much as the fact that a very great many of my colleagues in nursing academia are not only *unwilling* to defend nursing science against such attacks, but are also *unable* to do so, due to their own lack of knowledge.

As a scholar with broad interests, I have read and studied hundreds of books and journal articles from several disciplines outside of nursing. Certainly it would never occur to me (nor, I am sure, to most of our readers) to label and declare a large, heterogeneous, and multidimensional body of knowledge from another discipline to be essentially worthless. I think that the willingness of persons both inside and outside the discipline of nursing to subject the body of knowledge specific to nursing to this kind of ridicule is likely related to the *lack of respect for women and nurses* that is so prominent in our history. It has sometimes surprised me that feminists in nursing have not more assertively defended the body of knowledge that is specific to nursing. (There are, after all, as yet no widely recognized men nurse theorists.) The early 20th century leaders of nursing strongly identified with and interacted with the leading feminists of their day in creating and building the very discipline of nursing. Lillian Wald (1934), a self-described feminist at the turn of the century, later wrote, "The nurse question had become the woman question" (p. 76).

With perhaps one third of nurse academics unable to defend against this kind of disparagement, and possibly another third joining in, it is sometimes hard to be optimistic about the future of nursing theory. I must remind myself that the nursing theory movement is *stronger than ever*, although perhaps *relatively* weaker in relation to other national and international developments, such as the NINR priorities or the nurse practitioner movement. There is more literature on nursing theory-guided practice today than ever before, more nurse scholars are educated in nursing theories today than ever before, and there is a growing number of projects and practice settings (funded by other sources) guided explicitly by nursing theories.

Continuing the Unfinished Revolution

What I find truly most encouraging—and I always come back to this in my musings—is the fact that nursing theory-guided practice can be shown to enhance health and quality of life when it is implemented seriously with strong, well-qualified guidance. Demonstration projects rooted in philosophies

and theories of nursing are probably the most valuable means of generating acceptance and buy-in and, in my experience, these *work* brilliantly. Examples include Dr. Parker's (2001) many projects in South Florida, Dr. Gail Mitchell's (see for example, Cody, Bunkers, & Mitchell, 2001) implementation of patient-centered care principles drawn from Parse's theory at Sunnybrook and Women's College Health Science Centre in Toronto, Dr. Sandra Bunkers' many projects in South Dakota (see for example, Cody, Bunkers, & Mitchell, 2001), and our implementation of the Charlotte Rainbow PRISM Model based largely on Parse's theory at the Nursing Center operated by the School of Nursing of the University of North Carolina at Charlotte (Cody, 2003).

What the mid-range problem-solving scholars don't buy into is that *to bring about transformation of healthcare, one needs the whole gestalt of philosophy, theory, and method, aligned with administration and education.* It is much easier to work with unwieldy and stagnant (but powerful) institutions when you merely lay claim to having a circumscribed study or a project that will solve a particular concrete problem for them. What is vastly more challenging but *essential* for the transformation of healthcare is the adoption of a whole different revolutionary way of approaching healthcare. This is what true nursing theory-based practice, after Rogers or Parse or other revolutionary nurse theorists, can do. And it is, however poorly funded or disparaged it may be, still extremely threatening to the powers that be. It may be that *people*—consumers, in today's business-of-healthcare parlance—may be our strongest allies as they become more and more aware of the transformational power of innovative nursing models.

From a global, multigenerational perspective—a very long view—if nursing as we know it does not survive long into the future as an autonomous discipline called nursing, its *loss* does not have to be a catastrophe for humankind. Great ideas, when challenged and repressed, can often seem tenuous, even teetering on the brink of nonexistence, but they are hard to kill. The ideas that are embedded in the great nursing theories of our time may reemerge in some future synthesis that doesn't get called nursing, but they could still be implemented and be of great benefit to humankind. My thinking about this eventuality is simply that it may well happen, given current conditions, and that would be a great pity because these ideas are here, now, ready and available to be put into practice—and when they are, human betterment happens.

Leaders in nursing, especially academics and community-oriented nurses, have long viewed nursing as very much an autonomous profession. Indeed, it has been shown many times in a variety of settings that increased autonomy of nurses is associated with improved quality of care and outcomes (Alfano, 1969;

Havens, 2001; Wald, 1934). The truly original, radically visionary nursing frameworks that were put forward by nurse scholars in the 1970s and 1980s offered (and still offer) nurses the best opportunity we have ever had to move into a demonstrably unique and autonomous practice to the greater benefit of humankind. This is a transformational shift, a bold movement toward a new vision of nursing, rooted in concepts and theories that could only have emerged in the unique context of nursing and can only be learned through the extensive study of nursing. Indeed, despite the previously mentioned movement of powerful stakeholders in nursing in the opposite direction, this transformation may still be happening, albeit slowly and quietly, one-by-one, among nurse scholars like those who may be reading this journal. I have not yet known any nurse scholar who, having thoroughly learned how to interpret experience and practice from the perspective of a nursing theory, and having had the opportunity to put the theory into practice in an organization supporting implementation of the theory, to subsequently turn his or her back on nursing theory completely. The value of the turn toward nursing theory is obvious to those who take this path. The power of autonomous nursing practice guided by nursing discipline-specific theories to enhance quality of life in a meaningful way, when experienced directly by practicing nurses, is very persuasive. It is a whole different order of experience from merely implementing various interdisciplinary concrete problem-solving measures based on mid-range research devoid of a philosophical basis in nursing or a coherent vision of nursing and health. Many among us may yet be persuaded to reclaim the uniqueness of nursing.

 Full Circle

To come full circle in the discussion, allow me to share my own evolution. I encountered Parse's theory in the 10th year of my nursing career, having by then earned two bachelor's degrees, graduated with honors, climbed a clinical ladder to management, and mentored many new nurses. Yet it still took me 3 to 4 years to learn how to practice well in accord with Parse's theory and method. I am convinced that the vision of nursing theory-based practice that many of us embrace, that of a world in which nursing theory-based practice is universal, is achievable only through a renewed attention to depth in nursing education, greater appreciation of the human condition and our lived experiences, and thorough study of the history and philosophy of nursing, nursing theories, and nursing's unique research and practice methodologies.

Nursing theories guide nursing practice. Nursing theories are more than middle-range problem-solving algorithms. Some nursing theories are revolutionary and transformational. All nursing theories require in-depth study over time to master. Nursing practice will be transformed to the betterment of humankind when all nursing practice is fully autonomous and guided predominantly by nursing theory. A salubrious future for nursing includes a rapid shift toward the vast majority of nurses being educated at the bachelor's level and above, with far greater engagement among nurse scholars in theory development, research, and practice, in a context in which the intellectual domain of nursing is universally recognized as nursing theory. When that time comes, we should perhaps revisit the question of whether theory arises from practice.

REFERENCES

Alfano, G. (1969). The Loeb Center for Nursing and Rehabilitation. *Nursing Clinics of North America, 4,* 487–493.

Cody, W. K. (2003). Human becoming community change concepts in an academic nursing practice setting. In R. R. Parse, *Community: A human becoming perspective* (pp. 49–71). Sudbury, MA: Jones and Bartlett.

Cody, W. K., Bunkers, S. S., & Mitchell, G. J. (2001). The human be-coming theory in practice, research, administration, regulation, and education. In M. E. Parker (Ed.), *Nursing theories and nursing practice* (pp. 239–262). Philadelphia: F. A. Davis.

Fawcett, J. (2003). Theory and practice: A conversation with Marilyn E. Parker. *Nursing Science Quarterly, 16,* 131–136.

Harmer, B., & Henderson, V. A. (1955). *Textbook of the principles and practice of nursing.* New York: Macmillan.

Havens, D. S. (2001). Comparing infrastructure and outcomes: ANCC magnet and nonmagnet CNEs report. *Nursing Economics, 19,* 258–266.

National Institute for Nursing Research, (n. d.). *NIN R funded grants.* Retrieved March 7, 2003, from http://www.nih.gov/ninr/ research/grants_index.html

Orem, D. E. (1985). *Nursing: Concepts of practice* (3rd ed.). New York: McGraw-Hill.

Orlando, I. J. (1962). *The dynamic nurse-patient relationship: Function, process, and principles.* New York: G. P. Putnam's Sons.

Parker, M. E. (Ed.). (2001). *Nursing theories and nursing practice.* Philadelphia: F. A. Davis.

Parse, R. R. (1981). *Man-living-health: A theory of nursing.* New York: Wiley.

Parse, R. R. (1998). *The human becoming school of thought: A perspective for nurses and other health professionals.* Thousand Oaks, CA: Sage.

Paterson, J. G., & Zderad, L. T. (1976). *Humanistic nursing.* New York: Wiley.

Peplau, H. E. (1952). *Interpersonal relations in nursing.* New York: G. P. Putnam's Sons.

Rogers, M. E. (1970). *An introduction to the theoretical basis of nursing.* Philadelphia: F. A. Davis.

Wald, L. D. (1934). *Windows on Henry Street.* Boston: Little Brown.

Watson, J. (1985). *Nursing: Human science and human care.* Norwalk, CT: Appleton-Century-Crofts.

THE AUTHOR COMMENTS | **Nursing Theory as a Guide to Practice**

I wrote this article as a part of a dialogue with Marilyn Parker and Jacqueline Fawcett. I was, in-the-main, simply responding to the questions posed by Dr. Fawcett, "Do you think that theory arises from practice? Or, do you think that theory guides practice?" Certainly, I was aware that many before me had provided very scholarly answers to these questions. I aspired to stake out new territory in this piece, by taking a strong stand that *theory guides practice* and providing what I hoped was a cogent and original analysis of some of the contexts in which this occurs. My favorite parts of the article are the most controversial, "The Revolution that Didn't Come" and "The Hijacking of Nursing Science." I believe the comments therein really needed to be said—and still need to be said today.

WILLIAM K. CODY

The Situation-Specific Theory of Pain Experience for Asian American Cancer Patients

EUN-OK IM, RN, PhD, MPH, CNS, FAAN

Studies have indicated the need for theories that explain and target ethnic-specific cancer pain experiences, including those of Asian Americans. In this article, I present a situation-specific theory that explains the unique cancer pain experience of Asian Americans. Unlike other existing theories, this situation-specific theory was developed on the basis of evidence, including a systematic literature review and research findings, making it comprehensive and highly applicable to research and practice with Asian American patients with cancer. Thus, this theory would strengthen the interconnections among theory, evidence, and practice in pain management for Asian American cancer patients.
Key words: *Asian American, cancer, pain, situation-specific theory*

Theories on cancer pain experience tend to aim at cancer patients generally and have usually been developed on the basis of findings from white cancer patients.[1,2] Consequently, the underlying assumption of the existing theories has been that cancer pain experience is the same across both gender and ethnicity.[3] However, recent studies have reported specific racial and ethnic differences in cancer pain experience[4,5] and suggested the need for theories that could explain ethnic-specific cancer pain experiences and strengthen the interconnections among theory, evidence, and practice.[2]

Of the various ethnic groups in the United States, Asian Americans are the least observed in cancer pain studies primarily because it has been reported in the literature that they are less likely to experience severe pain in comparison with other ethnic groups.[6-8] Moreover, it is well-established in the literature that Asians, including Asian Americans, rarely seek help until their pain becomes severe.[6-9] In other words, Asians suffer through pain that could potentially be managed with existing pain management methods. Several reasons for this have been postulated: (1) stoicism is highly valued by Confucianism[8] and Taoism, philosophies embedded in many Asian cultures[10]; (2) Asian cultural beliefs hold that pain helps build strong character[8]; (3) Asians may desire to be considered "good" patients by their healthcare providers[8]; and (4) Asians may have misconceptions about the use of opioids to relieve pain (eg, that they shorten life or are addictive).[9] These findings strongly support the need for a theory to specifically explain and target the pain experience

of Asian American cancer patients so that it could be translated into nursing practice for these patients.

In this article, I present a situation-specific theory that aims to explain the pain experience of Asian American cancer patients while outlining the theory's development process. This situation-specific theory is not simply a theory developed for whites adapted to Asian American cancer patients. Rather, my aim was to develop a theory specific to Asian American cancer patients on the basis of contextual understanding of their cancer pain experiences. In nursing, as in other healthcare fields, there have been increasingly loud calls for theory-based investigations and clinical studies, especially in the field of knowledge translation.[11] Situation-specific theories may be the answer to these calls because they focus on specific nursing phenomena that reflect clinical practice and are limited to one population or field of practice.[12,13] Because of their level of specificity, nursing scholars have asserted that situation-specific theories are undoubtedly applicable to nursing practice and research because they can explain a population's unique health/illness experience with a limited scope of generalizability but with a specificity that can provide a comprehensive view and explanation of the nursing phenomenon.[12]

In this article, I first outline the methods used to develop this situation-specific theory. Next, I present the situation-specific theory that was developed, the assumptions made during theory development, the sources for theory development, and the major concepts of the theory. In this article, *culture* is defined as the totality of socially transmitted behavioral patterns,

From E. Im, The situation-specific theory of pain experience for Asian American cancer patients.
Advances in Nursing Science, 31(4), 319–331. Copyright © 2008 Wolters Kluwer Health / Lippincott Williams & Wilkins.
Reprinted with permission from Lippincott Williams & Wilkins.

ABOUT THE AUTHOR

EUN-OK IM was born in South Korea and moved to the United States in her 20s. She received a PhD in nursing from the University of California, San Francisco, where she also held a postdoctoral position. She is currently a Professor at The University of Pennsylvania School of Nursing. Professor Im has gained national and international recognition as a methodologist and theorist in international cross-cultural Internet research through more than 90 peer-reviewed publications and over 150 professional presentations. Her published articles on situation-specific theories, feminist critique, and Internet research methodologies are cited by many researchers around the world. Her hobbies include reading novels, knitting, and watching movies.

arts, beliefs, values, customs, lifeways, and all other products of human work and thought characteristic of a population of people that guides their worldview and decision making.[14] This definition of culture assumes the inclusion of health and healthcare beliefs and values and the dynamic nature of culture.[14] *Ethnicity* refers to a cultural group's sense of identification associated with that group's common social and cultural heritage,[14] and *ethnic identity* refers to a subjective sense of social boundary and self-definition.[15] Ethnic identity was used in this study as a concept representing one's cultural background. Here, *Asian American* refers to people having origins in any of the native populations of the Far East, Southeast Asia, or the Indian subcontinent.[16]

The Method

To develop the situation-specific theory of pain experience for Asian American cancer patients (SPEAC), I used the integrative approach.[17] This approach is based on the assumption that the processes of conceptualizing and formulating a theory can occur simultaneously;

otherwise, it might take years to complete the process and the theory might never evolve into a useful integrated view of reality.[13,17] In addition, the approach is based on the assumption that the theory development process may not occur sequentially or continuously; rather, some steps of the process might be skipped and others might occur repeatedly.[13,17] The integrative approach suggests that developing a theory needs to include the following steps: (1) checking the assumptions made in theory development; (2) exploring multiple sources; (3) formulating the theory; and (4) reporting, sharing, and validating the theory developed.[13,17] Using these steps, I developed the SPEAC, which I present in this article along with details of the theory development process. The SPEAC is illustrated in Figure 14-1.

Assumptions

In this section, I describe the assumptions made in developing the SPEAC, the sources used, and the SPEAC's major concepts. In developing the SPEAC, I made several assumptions suggested by the integrative

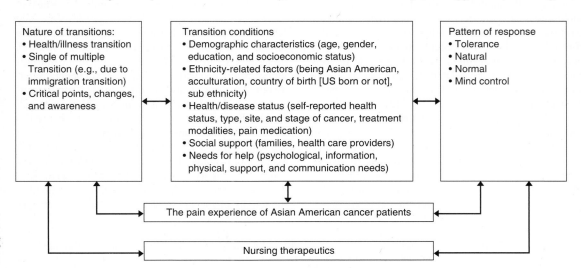

Figure 14-1 *The situation-specific theory of pain experience for Asian American cancer patients.*

approach.[17] First, in the theory development process, I took into consideration the diversity and complexity of the cancer pain experience. In other words, I considered the ethnic differences in the cancer pain experience, as well as the ethnic variations among Asian American ethnic groups (despite a small sample size for some of these groups). Second, I assumed that the theory development process was cyclic and evolutionary. In other words, the pain experience of Asian American cancer patients explored in the development of this theory is current but may not be valid in the future. Consequently, the primary assumption made in developing this situation-specific theory was that it might not be applicable to the same population at a different time or in a different sociopolitical context. Third, in developing this theory, I assumed that the sociopolitical context of nursing phenomena— that is, the pain experiences of Asian American cancer patients—occurs in specific sociopolitical contexts. Thus, again, the theory presented in this article may not be applicable to any other historical time, social structure, or political situation because of its limited generalizability and specific focus. Finally, the process of formulating the theory was based on a feminist nursing perspective. Consequently, the process of conceptualizing and formulating the SPEAC may be different from how a medical doctor, who may only be interested in the physiological or pathological aspects of the cancer pain experience, might do it. In the development of the SPEAC, I focused on cancer patients' whole being in the context of their daily lives. Using this feminist nursing perspective, I also viewed ethnicity and gender as significant factors influencing the pain experience of Asian American cancer patients.

Sources

An integrative approach[17] suggests that the sources for developing a situation-specific theory could be diverse. In developing the SPEAC, I used multiple sources: (1) the midrange transition theory, (2) an integrative literature review, and (3) research findings. I describe the details about these sources below.

The Midrange Transition Theory

I used the transition theory of Meleis et al[18] as a source for developing the SPEAC. The transition theory is a midrange theory based on the theories of transition proposed by Chick and Meleis[19] and Schumacher and Meleis,[20] an integrative literature review, and 5 research studies. These research studies aimed to uncover emerging themes that were not originally in the framework suggested by Schumacher and Meleis.[20] I used both inductive and deductive reasoning to develop the SPEAC from this midrange transition theory.

I based the SPEAC on the midrange transition theory because the pain experience of Asian American cancer patients is linked to the health/illness transition that they experience because of their disease. Generally, pain experience of cancer patients has a specific beginning, even before the diagnosis of cancer, and progresses or improves throughout diagnosis and treatment.[17] On the other hand, their pain experience may not influence their life, depending on the type, site, and stage of cancer.[17] In addition, their pain experience may have a specific ending point.[17] When cancer patients die or remit, their pain ends.[17] However, if their cancer becomes chronic, their pain will continue intermittently or constantly, with or without adequate management.[17]

Other major concepts of the midrange transition theory may also be relevant to developing a theory about the pain experience of Asian American cancer patients. The midrange transition theory included 6 major concepts[18]: (1) types and patterns of transitions, (2) properties of transition experiences, (3) transition conditions (facilitators and inhibitors), (4) process indicators, (5) outcome indicators, and (6) nursing therapeutics. First, the midrange transition theory includes the following types of transitions: developmental, health and illness, situational, and organizational.[18] The pain experience of Asian American cancer patients can be linked to their health/illness transition as described above. Just as the midrange transition theory conceptualized transitions as having multiple and complex patterns,[18] the pain experience of Asian American cancer patients' can be explained by their multiple and complex health/illness experiences. Depending on their individual financial situations, some patients might seek help in the US healthcare system, whereas others might suffer through the pain that they can adequately manage it with currently available cancer pain management regimens. In addition, depending on their immigration status, some patients might return to their countries of origin for more affordable treatment of their disease and/or management of their pain. In addition, in the midrange transition theory, essential properties of the transition experience included awareness, engagement, change and difference, time span, and critical points and events,[18] all of which are also prominent in the pain experience of Asian American cancer patients. For instance, Asian American cancer patients are aware of their health/illness transition; they are engaged in the transition by participating in their own diagnosis and treatment; they experience physical, psychological, and social changes because of the disease itself, the diagnosis process, and the treatment modalities; and they experience specific critical transition points, such as their diagnosis, which is a beginning point, and death or ultimate survival, which are critical ending points.[21] The midrange transition theory also addresses transition conditions at the personal (including meanings, cultural beliefs and attitudes, socioeconomic status, preparation, and knowledge), community, and societal levels.[18] These transition conditions also describe the pain experiences of Asian American cancer patients. At a personal level, their cultural attitudes toward complementary and alternative medicines are related to their choice of pain management; as members of unique cultural groups, their community conditions influence the resources available to them; and they are subjected to societal conditions that tend to marginalize them because they are immigrants or because they are members of ethnically oppressed groups.[21] In addition, the midrange transition theory includes indicators or patterns of responses that characterize healthy transitions.[18] Process indicators included feeling connected, interacting, location and being situated, and developing confidence and coping skills.[18] Outcome indicators included (1) mastery of the skills and behaviors needed to manage new situations or environments and (2) fluid rather than static integrative identities that are reformulated during the transition.[18] These indicators of the health/illness transition can also describe the pain experience of Asian American cancer patients. Those who may have adequate information and support through resources already available to them may feel connected and interact with others in a positive way, thus developing confidence that they can cope with their disease.[21] However, more recent immigrants who do not have health insurance may feel marginalized, isolated, and frustrated by the US healthcare system.[21]

The Literature Review

As suggested by the integrative approach,[17] I conducted an extensive systematic review of the literature as a source for developing the SPEAC, extensively searching databases such as PubMed. In a PubMed search of the literature from 1998 to 2008 using the key words "Asian American, cancer, pain, and experience," I retrieved only 3 articles. Therefore, I modified the literature search to include the key words, "Asian American, cancer, and pain," and retrieved 9 articles. I again modified the search to include the key words "Asian American and cancer," and retrieved 496 articles. However, only 24 of these were studies relevant to the literature review. I identified additional articles from the reference lists of the articles retrieved in these searches, adding 15 additional articles to the literature review. I then sorted the articles according to the major factors that were the focus of formulating the SPEAC: (1) cancer pain, generally; (2) the pain experience of Asian American cancer patients; and (3) transition conditions/predictors of the cancer pain experience (eg, demographic factors, ethnicity-related factors, health/disease status, social support, and needs for

help). I then analyzed the major findings of the articles and incorporated the literature review into the theory development process as described previously.

The Decision-Support Computer Program Study

In the integrative approach,[17] sources for formulating theories are the findings and experiences from research studies, educational programs, and/or clinical practice in hospital and/or community settings. In the process of developing the SPEAC, I used the findings from a multiethnic Internet study on cancer pain aimed at the development of a decision-support computer program for cancer pain management (the DSCP study).[21-25] In short, the purpose of the DSCP study was to explore gender and ethnic differences in the cancer pain experience of 480 cancer patients in 4 major ethnic groups in the united States (participants included 105 Hispanics, 148 non-Hispanic whites, 109 non-Hispanic African Americans, and 118 non-Hispanic Asian Americans). The Asian American participants included 90 Chinese, 10 nonspecified Asians, 2 Koreans, 3 Vietnamese, 6 Taiwanese, and 2 others, which limits the generalizability of the theory that I present in this article. Because 67% of the Asian American participants in this study were Chinese, the SPEAC is probably most appropriate for Chinese American cancer patients, as opposed to other ethnic groups of Asian Americans. The DSCP study was a cross-sectional multimethod study with a feminist approach that sought to gather information from the views, perspectives, opinions, and experiences of the research participants themselves. The instruments included questions on sociodemographic characteristics and health/illness status, 3 unidimensional cancer pain scales (the verbal Descriptor Scale [VDS], the Visual Analog Scale [VAS], and the Wong-Baker Faces Pain Scale [FS]), 2 multidimensional cancer pain scales (the McGill Pain Questionnaire-Short Form [MPQ-SF] and the Brief Pain Inventory [BPI]), the Memorial Symptom Assessment Scale (MSAS), the Functional Assessment of Cancer Therapy Scale-General (FACT-G), and 9 online forum topics. Detailed information about the methods and findings of the DSCP study are published elsewhere.[21-25] A situation-specific theory that explains white cancer patients' unique cancer pain experience on the basis of the DSCP study is also published elsewhere.[2]

 Major Concepts

As stated previously, the SPEAC includes 5 major concepts, including (1) the nature of transition, (2) transition conditions, (3) patterns of response, (4) the pain experience of Asian American cancer patients, and (5) nursing therapeutics. Four of the major concepts are almost identical to components of the midrange transition theory,[18] except 1 major concept related to the pain experience of Asian American cancer patients that was added because it is the focus of the theory being developed. These major concepts influenced the pain experience of Asian American cancer patients by interacting with each other. For example, the terminal or chronic nature of the health/illness transition influences the pain experience, and cancer patients' ethnicity (eg, Korean, Chinese) influences the pain experience. At the same time, cancer patients' ethnicity influences their cultural attitudes toward the terminal or chronic nature of cancer (eg, they stigmatize the experience or view it as a normal experience); ethnicity also influences their patterns of response to the transition. I discuss each of these major concepts in detail in the following sections except the concepts of the pain experience of Asian American cancer patients and nursing therapeutics because these 2 concepts are just to explain the relationships among the major concepts. Because of the lack of literature on the cancer pain experience of Asian American patients, the literature review included in the conceptualization process, described in the subsequent text, incorporates the literature on other ethnic groups, as well as that for Asian Americans.

The Nature of Transition: The Health/Illness Transition

The type of transition that Asian American cancer patients experience is obviously a health/illness transition. This health/illness transition is terminal or chronic, depending on the type, stage, and site of cancer for each individual.[22] Most of the Asian participants in the DSCP study viewed their pain experience as normal and part of the natural process of transitioning to being a cancer patient.[21] One participant wrote:

> The pain of cancer, just like birth, aging, illness, and death as the must-be process in human being, is just one among those. Do not be scared. The medicine is progressing and the environment is changing.

The Nature of Transition: Single or Multiple Transitions

The transition that Asian American cancer patients experience might consist of only 1 transition, or possibly multiple transitions at the same time, depending on each individual's situation. For example, most participants in the DSCP study were first-generation immigrants from Asian countries,[24] meaning that they were in the health/illness transition and at the same time were experiencing the situational transition of

immigrating to a new country. Interestingly, several participants went back to their country of origin to receive treatments, although they were residing in the United States at that time. These participants were managing the health/disease transition caused by their cancer, as well as a reverse cultural transition back to their country of origin while receiving cancer treatments. One Asian participant in the DSCP study wrote:

> I had treatment alone in Taipei. When in pain, I could only tolerate and cry. Also, cheer up self! I took care of myself alone. There was no way to express the pain and suffering of chemotherapy … The suffering from chemotherapy had led me to stop having treatment in the end. I once told to my family about giving up the treatment and going back to the United States. They all said the same thing and asked me to cheer up and to be hanging there until the completion of the 12 cycles of treatment.

The Nature of Transition: Critical Points, Changes, and Awareness

In the DSCP study, the starting point of the transition was quite clear to all of the Asian participants, who vividly remembered their health/illness transitions and pain experiences in detail. One Asian participant mentioned:

> I was diagnosed with breast cancer about 3 years ago. Mammogram exams were negative at that time. Luckily, I got an extra step—the ultrasound and it was confirmed that I had cancer… I also went through mastectomy, lymph nodes dissection, and hysterectomy. I have been taking aromasin since last July after 2 years of tamoxifen to control/reduce the recurrence risks.

Many participants mentioned the changes in their lives because of their cancer, which at first inhibited them from functioning normally. Later, with a new awareness of and subsequent adjustment to these life changes, participants changed their attitudes toward their cancer and pain; they tried to be strong and live through it. To many of them, the diagnosis of cancer was a shock, and at first, they considered it a death sentence. Later, however, during the health/illness transition, they came to recognize that they could live with the pain and/or were strong enough to overcome the pain. One participant wrote:

> When I first faced cancer and chemo, the fear and pain was too horrible to tolerate. At

that time, pain, body damage, not eating, not sleeping, not walking, vomit, bleeding, etc... I felt that life was no meaning at all... I ate 96 pills of amien at once. Fortunately, I survived after that. Since then, I read many books and articles. Mainly, they are related to how to view life, fate, life and death ... I did meditation, yoga, and deep breathing ... Many strong cancer patients moved my heart and gave me some teaching so that I become strong and have new perspective on the meaning of life. In this way, the pain also becomes less...

The Transition Conditions: Demographic Factors

In general, demographic factors such as age, gender, education, and socioeconomic status are associated with the cancer pain experience[26-31]; thus, these factors would also influence the pain experience of Asian American cancer patients. Pfefferbaum et al[26] reported a significant inverse relationship between age and pain distress. Deimling et al[27] indicated that age-related factors accounted for 14% of the variance in pain, whereas cancer-related factors explained only 2% of the variance. Gender is also associated with the cancer pain experience[28]; healthcare providers tended to underestimate the pain severity of female patients. Barragan-Berlanga et al[29] reported that pain was more frequent in women than in men (48.3% vs 33.6%) and increased with age. Van den Beuken-van Everdingen et al[30] reported that a positive predictor of the prevalence of pain was a lower education level. Cancer patients with high incomes had fewer symptoms, including pain,[2] and those with low incomes were more likely to have pain because of their lack of access to healthcare.[31] In contrast, comparing patients from all socioeconomic classes, Larson and Marcer[32] found no significant differences in their cancer pain experiences. However, we know little about the reasons for the inconsistent findings about the influences of socioeconomic status on the cancer pain experience or the specific pain management strategies that cancer patients from different socioeconomic classes might use.

In the DSCP study,[24] a multiple-regression analysis showed that some of these demographic factors influenced the pain experience of Asian American cancer patients. Age, income satisfaction, and gender explained 4.9% of the total variance of the VDS scores ($P < .01$), 5.4% of the total variance of the VAS scores ($P < .01$), 4.8% of the total variance of the FS scores ($P < .01$), 6.2% of the total variance of the MPQ SF scores ($P < .01$), 9.6% of the total variance of the BPI scores ($P < .01$), 9.4% of the total variance of the MSAS scores ($P < .01$), and 6.3% of the total variance of the FACT-G scores ($P < .01$).

The Transition Conditions: Ethnicity-Related Factors

Ethnicity-related factors also influence the cancer pain experience, generally.[33-35] For example, some cultural norms may encourage stoicism in the face of pain resulting in the underreporting of pain,[28,35] a phenomenon confirmed by the DSCP study. Asian Americans, African Americans, and Hispanics all had stoic attitudes toward their cancer pain.[21,23-25]

In the literature, it is often assumed that acculturation, or taking on the cultural values and practices of the host population, is a desired health-related outcome of immigration; in addition, acculturation is reportedly associated with the health/illness conditions of immigrants[36] Although I located almost no studies about the association between acculturation and cancer pain in a search of PubMed, I located a few studies about the association between acculturation and the experience of general pain.[37-39] These studies reported the following: (1) a strong negative association between acculturation scores and widespread pain; (2) less acculturated Hispanic women reported more bodily pain and impaired social functioning than non-Hispanic white women; (3) less acculturated Japanese women were less likely to report problems on the role-emotional scale; and (4) patients with rheumatoid arthritis who were partially acculturated tended to report higher symptom scores compared with those who were fully acculturated. On the basis of these findings, I could conclude that more acculturated Asian American cancer patients (having been longer in the United States and having higher acculturation scores) are less likely to report pain and symptoms accompanying pain.

Most of these studies, however, clumped Asian Americans into a single group and did not consider the differences among Asian American ethnic groups. Consequently, very little is known about the cancer pain experience of Asian American ethnic groups; in fact, most of our knowledge comes from studies of Chinese Americans. However, each ethnic group of Asian Americans has its own unique cultural values, beliefs, and attitudes toward cancer pain.[6] Indeed, in the DSCP study,[21] findings from an online forum for Asian American cancer patients also showed differences in the cancer pain experience among Asian American ethnic groups. In these forums, about 67% of the Asian American participants were Chinese from Mainland China; about 7% were Chinese from Taiwan; about 4% were Chinese from Hong Kong; about 4% were Eastern Indians; and about 19% were from other ethnic groups (eg, Koreans, Japanese, Vietnamese, Filipinos). Despite commonalities in their cancer pain experience, there were specific differences among these ethnic groups. Chinese from Mainland China and Taiwan tended to return to their countries of origin to obtain affordable cancer treatment and pain management. Koreans and Japanese, however, tended to depend on the Western healthcare system in the United States, but they preferred healthcare providers from their own ethnic groups.

In the DSCP study,[24] a multiple regression analyses showed an association of ethnicity related factors to cancer pain experience. Being non-Hispanic Asian or not explained about 3% of the total variance of the VDS scores ($P < .01$), about 3% of the total variance of the FS scores ($P < .01$), about 5% of the total variance of the MPQ-SF scores ($P < .01$), and about 3% of the total variance of the BPI scores ($P < .01$). In addition, there were significant differences in the cancer pain scores ($P < .05$) by country of birth; those born outside the United States consistently reported lower VDS, VAS, FS, MPQ-SF, and BPI scores than those born in the United States.

The Transition Conditions: Health/Disease Status

Health/disease status is another transition condition that may influence the pain experience of Asian American cancer patients. Factors related to health/disease status that are known to influence the cancer pain experience include the type, site, stage of cancer, and treatment modalities.[40] Zabora et al[41] reported an overall prevalence rate of pain (35.1%), with lung cancer patients reporting the highest degree of pain (43.4%), and those with gynecological cancers reporting the lowest (29.5%). The mechanism(s) by which the cancer site influences the cancer pain experience is believed to involve hormonal changes, neurotransmitters, digestive enzymes, or bicarbonate.[42] Van den Beuken-van Everdingen et al[30] also reported that the positive predictors of the prevalence of pain included disease that is more advanced.

In the DSCP study,[24] there were significant associations between cancer pain and health/disease status. Self-reported health status and pain medication accounted for 28% of the total variance of the VDS scores ($P < .01$), 33% of the total variance of the VAS scores ($P < .01$), 34% of the total variance of the FS scores ($P < .01$), 28% of the total variance of the MPQ-SF scores ($P < .01$), 30% of the total variance of the BPI scores ($P < .01$), and 11% of the total variance of the MSAS scores ($P < .01$).

The Transition Conditions: Social Support

My literature review showed that social support is associated with the cancer pain experience generally, which implies that social support would be another transition condition that may influence the pain experience of Asian American cancer patients. Social support also influences the quality of life in cancer patients, including both their physical and psychosocial needs, including pain and symptom management.[43,44] A lack

of social support can be a significant stressor for some patients because they depend on social interaction to sustain their mood and morale as they endure cancer pain.[40] Functional status related to cancer pain is also reportedly influenced by social support.[45]

The DSCP study[21] showed a significant association between social support and the cancer pain experience of Asian American patients. Most patients mentioned how helpful their families and healthcare providers had been during their health/illness transition, which positively influenced their cancer pain experience. One participant said:

> *During my treatment period, my families go online to search information to encourage me. The volunteers and nurses in American Chinese Cancer Institution often call me to inquiring my situation and come to visit me at home. They answer my questions very thoroughly and instruct me the disease condition and the strategies of management.*

For some of the participants, however, their families also inhibited the adequate management of their cancer pain. Because participants were concerned about their families and did not want them to worry about them, they often did not report pain and simply endured it. One participant wrote:

> *To my family, I seldom mention my pain to prevent them from worries. I remember that once I had a side effect from chemotherapy and was very uncomfortable. I called the nurse who did chemotherapy for me and asked how to handle ... (rather than asking help to my family).*

The Transition Conditions: The Need for Help

The *need for help* is another transition condition that may influence the pain experience of Asian American cancer patients. In this article, the *need for help* refers to the physiological, psychological, and social requirements for well-being that cancer patients perceive.[46,47] *Psychological needs* are defined as patients' perceived needs with regard to psychological and emotional issues; *information needs* are those related to diagnosis, investigative tests, family issues, and financial issues; *physical needs* pertain to coping with physical symptoms and the side effects of treatment, performing the usual physical tasks and activities of daily living, and self-management of medical treatment routines and healthcare at home; *support needs* are defined as those related to connections with family, friends, and healthcare professionals; and *communication needs* are those related to interpersonal relationships and the interaction skills and communication styles of healthcare providers.[46,47] In the literature, multiple reports indicate that these needs influence the daily experiences of cancer patients,[46,47] which subsequently influences their cancer pain.

The online forums in the DSCP study[21] indicated significant associations between the *need for help* and the cancer pain experience of Asian Americans. Asian American cancer patients tended to ignore and minimize their pain because of the stigmatization of cancer in their cultures. Thus, even when they had strong support needs (when they needed support from their family members or friends), they tended not to report these needs or seek help. Consequently, even when they suffered pain, they did not ask for help with pain control. Rather, they regarded being stoic and dealing with pain alone as the best strategy to manage their cancer pain. Thus, the perception that they did not need support might have negatively influenced their cancer pain experience. One participant mentioned the stigma attached to cancer:

> *Usually when talking about cancer, Chinese will change the color of their faces. Not only have few people had the fearful heart toward cancer. Therefore, when a family member gets cancer, all people will hide the diagnosis for patient, from doctors to families. This is a big difference from Western culture…*

Patterns of Response

The patterns of response identified in Asian American cancer patients can be conceptualized into 4 subconcepts: (1) tolerance, (2) natural, (3) normal, and (4) mind control.

Tolerance

The literature on the pain experience of Asian American cancer patients is limited. However, it is repeatedly reported in the literature that Asians rarely complain about pain, tolerate pain well, and delay seeking help until their pain becomes severe.[6-8] As mentioned above, stoicism is regarded as the primary reason Asian Americans may avoid seeking relief from pain.[8] Many Asian cultures are based on Confucianism, which emphasizes harmony in social relations and subsequently discourages the expression of potentially disruptive and distressing emotions like pain.[6] Asians' stoic attitudes toward pain and minimum treatment of pain are perhaps also explained by the prevalent influence of Taoism in many Asian cultures.[10] The philosophy of Taoism prescribes that people understand "change" and accept it harmoniously.[48] Consequently, Asian American cancer patients tend to tolerate pain

instead of treating it aggressively. As mentioned above, there are also reports in the literature that Asian American cultural beliefs hold that pain helps build strong character.[8] In other words, most Asian cultures view someone who can overcome pain as a strong person.[6] Consequently, being stoic about pain is viewed as a symbol of bravery, which is considered a virtue.[6] Finally, reports in the literature note that Asian American cancer patients often desire to be considered a "good" patient by their healthcare providers[8] and that they have misconceptions about the use of opioids to relieve pain (eg, opioids shorten life or are addictive).[9]

Natural

As mentioned above, in the DSCP study,[21] participants considered their pain experience a natural consequence of having cancer. One participant explained:

> *… disease tortures human body… the body will react to it spontaneously and the reaction is pain… People experience different pain in life, not just cancer. Some other diseases can cause more pain than cancer… it is natural that cancer patients have pain.*

Normal

In the DSCP study,[21] having the attitude that their pain was a natural part of having cancer, participants attempted to normalize their cancer pain experience by trying to live normal lives despite their disease and its consequences. It was obvious in the DSCP study[21] that Asian cultures stigmatize cancer; in fact, many patients hid their disease because they did not want their children's future marriages affected by it. The participants sought to overcome the stigma attached to cancer by "normalizing" it or "shrinking" cancer into just one small problem in the totality of their lives. One participant said:

> *… In my culture (Chinese), we consider cancer as a result of "bad karma" from the previous life … as a punishment on a sin of the person … because of this view, I did not disclose my disease to others … some people even keep a distance from cancer patients … (I) just see it as a headache or stomachache. …*

Mind Control

In the DSCP study,[21] one unique aspect of Asian Americans' responses to cancer and cancer pain was that they tried to control their disease mentally. The participants valued positive thinking as a treatment modality throughout the disease process. They thought that a strong mind and positive thinking would help reduce pain and increase a sense of hope in their daily lives. One participant explained:

> ... *Before I get up, I always tell myself that I am going to be a happy person today... your body cells will follow.... This "mind over body" attitude is essential to cope with pain. I have to focus on the positive side to cope with pain and mental fear .... Only strong mind can make patients tolerate and endure pain... I mainly use "mental therapies," such as reading Sutra and talk with family members and close friends.*

Conclusions

As mentioned in the introduction, there have been increasingly loud calls for theory-based investigations and clinical studies in the field of knowledge translation.[11] Situation-specific theories might be one answer to the call because they are easily translated into nursing research and practice due to their specificity. As mentioned above, situation-specific theories can provide a more specific and comprehensive view of a nursing phenomenon,[12,13] which makes them more applicable to nursing research and practice compared with other types of theories.[12] In other words, by developing and using situation-specific theories, nursing phenomena could be more closely and comprehensively described and understood, and thus, more closely linked to nursing research and practice.

In this article, I proposed a situation-specific theory of the pain experience of Asian American cancer patients, with descriptions of the assumptions, sources for theory development, and the major concepts of the theory. Because this situation-specific theory was evidence-based (evolving from a systematic review of the literature and research findings), as well as grounded in an existing theory, it is more comprehensive and more easily translated into research questions and nursing practice with Asian American cancer patients than the existing theories.

This article completes the first 2 parts (reporting and sharing) of the last step of the integrative approach (ie, reporting, sharing, and validating the theory).[17] Starting with the situation-specific theory proposed in this article, I expect that in future studies and nursing practice, the SPEAC will be further validated and developed, and the interconnections between theory, evidence, and practice in the field of pain management for Asian American cancer patients, as well as of other ethnic minorities, will be further strengthened in the process.

REFERENCES

1. Cleeland CS. Cancer-related fatigue: new directions for research. Introduction. *Cancer* 2001;92(6):1657–1661.
2. Im EO. A situation-specific theory of Caucasian cancer patients' pain experience. *ANS Adv Nurs Sci.* 2006;29(3): 232–244.
3. Vallerand AH. Measurement issues in the comprehensive assessment of cancer pain. *Semin Oncol Nurs.* 1997;13(1): 16–24.
4. Green C, Anderson K, Baker T, et al. The unequal burden of pain: confronting racial and ethnic disparities inpain. *Pain Med.* 2003;4:277–294.
5. Rabow M, Dibble S. Ethnic differences in pain among outpatients with terminal and end-stage chronic illness. *Pain Med.* 2005;6:235–241.
6. Lipson J, Dibble S. *Culture and Critical Care.* San Francisco, CA: UCSF Nursing Press; 2005.
7. Streltzer J, Wade T. The influence of cultural group on the undertreatment of postoperative pain. *PsychosomMed.* 1981;43:397–403.
8. Wills B, Wootton Y Concerns and misconceptions about pain among Hong Kong Chinese patients with cancer. *Cancer Nurs.* 1999;22:408–413.
9. Morita T, Miyashita M, Shibagaki M, et al. Knowledge and beliefs about end-of-life care and the effects of specialized palliative care: a population-based survey in Japan. *J Pain Symptom Manage.* 2006;31:306–316.
10. Chung JWY Wong TKS, Yang JC. The lens model. *Cancer Nurs.* 2000;23:454–461.
11. Rycroft-Malone J. Theory and knowledge translation: setting some coordinates. *Nurs Res.* 2007;56(suppl 4):S78–S85.
12. Im EO, Meleis AI. Situation-specific theories: philosophical roots, properties, and approach. *ANS Adv Nurs Sci.* 1999;22(2):11–24.
13. Meleis AI. *Theoretical Nursing: Development and Progress.* 3rd ed. Philadelphia, PA: Lippincott; 1997.
14. Purnell LD, Paulanka, BJ. *Transcultural Health Care: A Culturally Competent Approach.* 3rd ed. Philadelphia, PA: FA Davis; 2008.
15. Meleis AI, Lipson JG, Paul SM. Ethnicity and health among five Middle Eastern immigrant groups. *Nurs* Res. 1992;41:98–103.
16. US Census Bureau. *Resident Population Estimates of the United States by Sex, Race, and Hispanic Origin.* Washington, DC: US Census Bureau; 2000.
17. Im EO. Development of situation-specific theories: an integrative approach. *ANS Adv Nurs Sci.* 2005;28(2):137–151.
18. Meleis AI, Sawyer LM, Im EO, Messias DK, Schumacher K. Experiencing transitions: an emerging middle-range theory. *ANS Adv Nurs Sci.* 2000;23(1):12–28.
19. Chick N, Meleis AI. Transitions: a nursing concern. In: Chinn PL, ed. *Nursing Research Methodology: Issues and Implantation.* Gaithersburg, MD: Aspen Publisher; 1986.
20. Schumacher KL, Meleis AI. Transitions: a central concept in nursing. *Image J Nurs Sch.* 1994;26:119–127.
21. Im EO, Liu Y, Kim YH, Chee W. Asian American cancer patients' pain experience. *Cancer Nurs.* 2008;31(3): E17–E23.
22. Im EO. White cancer patients' perception of gender and ethic differences in pain experience. *Cancer Nurs.* 2006;29(6):441–450.
23. Im EO, Guevara E, Chee W. The pain experience of Hispanic patients with cancer in the United States. *Oncol Nurs Forum.* 2007;34(4):861–868.

24. Im EO, Chee W, Guevara E, et al. Gender and ethnic differences in cancer pain experience: a multiethnic survey in the United States. *Nurs Res.* 2007;56(5):296–306.

25. Im EO, Lim HJ, Clark M, Chee W. African American cancer patients' pain experience. *Cancer Nurs.* 2008;31(1):38–46.

26. Pfefferbaum B, Adams J, Aceves J. The influence of culture on pain in Anglo and Hispanic children with cancer. *J Am Acad Child Adolesc Psychiatry.* 1990;29(4):642–647.

27. Deimling GT, Bowman KF Wagner LJ. The effects of cancer-related pain and fatigue on functioning of older adult, long-term cancer survivors. *Cancer Nurs.* 2007;30(6):421–433.

28. Anderson KO, Mendoza TR, Valero V et al. Minority cancer patients and their providers: pain management attitudes and practice. *Cancer.* 2000;88(8): 1929–1938.

29. Barragan-Berlanga AJ, Mejia-Arango S, Gutierrez-Robledo LM. [Pain in the elderly: prevalence and as- sociated factors]. *Salud Publica Mex.* 2007;49(suppl4):S488–S494.

30. van den Beuken-van Everdingen MH, de Rijke JM, Kessels AG, Schouten HC, van KleefM, Patijn J. High prevalence of pain in patients with cancer in a large population-based study in The Netherlands. *Pain.* 2007;132(3):312–320.

31. Rannestad T, Skjeldestad FE. Pain and quality of life among long-term gynecological cancer survivors: a population-based case-control study. *Acta Obstet Gynecol Scand.* 2007;86(12):1510–1516.

32. Larson AG, Marcer D. The who and why of pain: analysis by social class. *Br Med J.* 1984;288(6421):883–886.

33. Beck SL. An ethnographic study of factors influencing cancer pain management in South Africa. *Cancer Nurs.* 2000;23(2):99–100.

34. Lubeck DP, Kim H, Grossfeld G, et al. Health related quality of life differences between black and white men with prostate cancer: data from the cancer of the prostate strategic urologic research endeavor. *J Urol.* 2001;166(6): 2281–2285.

35. Alberque C, Eytan A. Chronic pain presenting as major depression in a cross-cultural setting. *Int J Psychiatry Med.* 2001;31(1):73–76.

36. Im EO, Yang KR. Theories on immigrant women's health. *Health Care Women Int.* 2006;27:666–681.

37. Palmer B, Macfarlane G, Afzal C, Esmail A, Silman A, Lunt M. Acculturation and the prevalence of pain amongst South Asian minority ethnic groups in the UK. *Rheumatology (Oxford).* 2007;4(6):1009–1014.

38. Avis NE, Colvin A. Disentangling cultural issues in quality of life data. *Menopause.* 2007;14(4):708–716.

39. Escalante A, del Rincon I, Mulrow CD. Symptoms of depression and psychological distress among Hispanics with rheumatoid arthritis. *Arthritis Care Res.* 2000;13(3):156–167.

40. WoolMS, MorV. Amultidimensionalmodelforunderstanding cancer pain. *Cancer Invest.* 2005;23:727–734.

41. Zabora J, BrintzenhofeSzoc K, Curbow B, Hooker C, Piantadosi S. The prevalence of psychological distress by cancer site. *Psychooncology.* 2001;10(1):19–28.

42. Almeida OP, Waterreus A, Spry N, Flicker L, Martins RN. One year follow-up study of the association between chemical castration, sex hormones, beta-amyloid, memory and depression in men. *Psychoneuroendocrinology.* 2004;29(8):1071–1081.

43. Henoch I, Bergman B, Gustafsson M, Gaston-Johansson F, Danielson E. The impact of symptoms, coping capacity, and social support on quality of life experience over time in patients with lung cancer. *J Pain Symptom Manage.* 2007;34(4):370–379.

44. Yan H, Sellick K. Symptoms, psychological distress, s o c i a l support, and quality of life of Chinese patients newly diagnosed with gastrointestinal cancer. *Cancer Nurs.* 2004;27: 389–399.

45. Wan GJ, Counte MA, Cella DF, et al. The impact of sociocultural and clinical factors on health-related quality of life reports among Hispanic and African-American cancer patients. *J Outcome Meas.* 1999;3:200–215.

46. Foot G. *Needs Assessment in Tertiary and Secondary Oncology Practice: A Conceptual and Methodological Exposition* [dissertation]. Newcastle: University of Newcastle; 1996.

47. Foot G, Sanson-Fisher R. Measuring the unmet needs of people living with cancer. *Cancer Forum.* 1995;19:131–135.

48. Stanford Encyclopedia of Philosophy. Taoism. http://plato.stanford.edu/entries/taoism/ Accessed July 31, 2006.

THE AUTHOR COMMENTS

The Situation-Specific Theory of Pain Experience for Asian American Cancer Patients

Because many students in my doctoral class wanted clear directions for theory development, especially for development of situation-specific theories, I wrote an article on the integrative approach to development of situation-specific theories. However, the article tends to be too abstract for students to follow in actual theory development, and I thought that I should give a practical example of theory development for my students. At the same time, I conducted an NIH-funded R01 study on cancer pain management of four major ethnic groups in the United States and thought about developing a theoretical basis for my next study on Asian cancer patients' pain experience. That was why I developed this situation-specific theory and wrote this article. I believe that this article can contribute to nursing theory in the 21st century by giving a practical example of theory development that can provide a direct and substantive theoretical basis for nursing research and practice.

EUN-OK IM

Theory and Knowledge Translation
Setting Some Coordinates

JO RYCROFT-MALONE, RN, PhD, MSc, BSc (Hons)

In a healthcare context in which research evidence is not used routinely in practice, there have been increasingly loud calls for the use of theory from investigators working in the field of knowledge translation. Implementation researchers argue that theory should be used to guide the design of testable and practical intervention strategies, and thus, contribute to generalizable knowledge about implementation interventions. The purpose of this commentary is to critique model papers writing by a team of scholars who aimed to disentangle some of the relationships determining research utilization, by scrutinizing an existing conceptual framework that acknowledges, along with other factors, the importance of contextual factors in knowledge translation. These papers are used as a vehicle to explore theory application in knowledge translation research. As theory use and development is in its infancy, some key issues, including different ideological perspectives, factors for and against theory use, ensuring conceptual clarity, selecting coherent overarching frameworks, and choosing appropriately among theories, are considered. Finally, an agenda for theory-informed research is outlined, which highlights the need for scholarly, pluralistic, and collaborative activity if the state of knowledge translation science is to advance.

Key words: *knowledge translation, theory*

A science does not truly become mature until it develops a predictive capability. (Peter Medawar, 1984)

There have been increasingly loud calls for the use of theory from investigators working in the field of knowledge translation. Although loud, the calls are not unanimous, with those in favor of theory use in one camp (e.g., Estabrooks, Thompson, Lovely, & Hofmeyer, 2006; ICEBeRG Group, 2006), and those against theory use in the other (e.g., Bhattacharyya et al., 2006; Oxman, Fretheim, & Flottrop, 2005). Theory use and development is presented by supporters as a promising approach to better understanding the *black box* of implementation, and the reasons this is often not translated into healthcare practice and improved outcomes for patients.

Estabrooks et al. (in this supplement) aim to unpick some of relationships determining research utilization by nurses. While building on research utilization theory by scrutinizing an existing conceptual framework, the authors also aim to make a methodological contribution to the field. In this commentary, these papers are examined critically from the perspective of theory use and development. As theory development and use in knowledge translation activity within the healthcare setting is in its infancy, there are

a number of key issues that require consideration if the knowledge base is to advance, which are explored here from the perspective of a knowledge translation researcher. Where appropriate, a critical reflection on the work of Estabrooks et al. is presented, and the implications are considered. Finally, an agenda for theory-informed implementation research is outlined.

Theory-Informed Knowledge Translation

Appeals for theory use in knowledge translation have occurred over the last four decades (Estabrooks et al., 2006). Notably, however, it has been relatively recently that these calls have come from those working in knowledge translation in the context of healthcare, particularly in relation to implementation research (e.g., Eccles, Grimshaw, Walker, Johnston, & Pitts, 2005; Estabrooks, in this supplement; ICEBeRG Group, 2006; Michie, Hendy, Smith, & Adshead, 2006). This turn to theory can be understood in a context where, politically, there has been a focus on pushing out research evidence, and on developing the skills

ABOUT THE AUTHOR

JO RYCROFT-MALONE qualified as a nurse in London in 1987 and then completed an undergraduate degree in psychology, a master's in occupational psychology, and a PhD in health sciences. Over the last decade, my research has focused on evidence synthesis and the implementation of evidence in practice, supported by national and international research funding. I am part of the team that has developed the Promoting Action on Research Implementation in Health Services (PARIHS) framework, which is now widely known and used by those engaged in implementation activities. I am a Professor of Implementation Research and Director of Research, Centre for Health-Related Research School of Healthcare Sciences in the University of Wales College of Health and Behavioural Sciences located in Bangor, United Kingdom. I am also Editor in Chief for the journal, *Worldviews on Evidence-Based Nursing*.

and knowledge of individual practitioners to appraise research and make rational decisions, with variable results (e.g., Grol, 2001; McGlynn et al., 2003).

It has been suggested that theory should be used to guide the design of testable and useable intervention strategies, and thus, contribute to generating generalizable knowledge about implementation interventions. Specifically, Eccles et al. (2005) make a case for theory use, based on their view that previous implementation research has been "an expensive version of trial and error" (p. 108), a trial that has provided limited knowledge about what factors influence implementation efforts. Furthermore, reviews of implementation research have highlighted that researchers do not pay attention to the theoretical underpinnings of their work, nor provide sufficient contextual details for an assessment of transferability (e.g., Grimshaw et al., 2004). Currently, there are no clear directions to help healthcare researchers, practitioners, or managers make decisions about what implementation strategies to use, in which contexts, and with what groups of stakeholders. If using and developing theory can help to design studies that increase the chances of knowledge translation and enable a coherent interpretation of findings while contributing to generalizable knowledge, most would agree to sign up.

Naturally, there are some skeptics (e.g., Bhattacharyya et al., 2006; Oxman et al., 2005). Broadly, these authors argue that: (a) there is a lack of evidence to support the idea of theory use; (b) theory selection can only at best be arbitrary because there are limited criteria to help us choose among them, and some theories are unsubstantiated; and (c) common sense, sound logic, and rigorous evaluation should prevail when designing implementation interventions. In addition, it is suggested here that a challenge for theory users is in accounting for the complexities of knowledge translation processes. Being confined to theory-driven interventions may mean key processes, interactions, and relationships are neglected because attention is focused too specifically on the theory, or theories, being tested. Rather than an either-or approach to theory use, perhaps a more sophisticated view would be for researchers to consider the application of theory along a continuum. The continuum might extend from implicit to explicit theory use, where different questions, settings, and circumstances dictate the type and extent of theory use.

Although the literature on theory use in knowledge translation is extremely limited, the literature concerning theory *development* is even more scarce. Here, theory use refers to the use and testing of existing explicit theory, implicit theory, or both, and theory development refers to the construction or formalization of theory from theory use research or inductively from, for example, practice-level activity (e.g., Kitson, Ahmed, Harvey, Seers, & Thompson, 1996). To date, authors who discuss theory use tend not to explicitly consider explicitly how the findings from their studies of use may be linked to theory construction; there has been an emphasis on testing the transferability of existing theory (e.g., Eccles et al., 2005).

Theory has been and can be applied in knowledge translation research in three main ways:

1. *Developing knowledge translation interventions based on theory or theories*. It is argued that using theory in this way enables the designing of testable theories, which may predict changes in behavior and other outcomes (e.g., Eccles et al., 2005). This view assumes that changing behavior and outcomes takes a linear path; that is, identify theory -> develop intervention -> put into practice = change (or not). On the other hand, developing interventions using theory is likely to provide clarity of focus, aid explanation of findings, and enable the generation of transferable knowledge, which is important for theory development.

2. *Using theory to assist in the identification of appropriate outcomes, measures, and variables*. Choosing theoretically sensitive outcomes should facilitate more robust theory development. Clearly, outcomes also need to be measurable and include both intermediate and summative consequences.

3. *Using theory to guide the evaluation of knowledge translation processes*. Until recently, there has been a relative lack of attention to the processes of implementation, particularly in relation to

the impact of context on knowledge translation. Developing evaluation strategies that are guided by existing theoretical frameworks and theory or conducting studies that are designed to develop theory inductively may facilitate knowledge translation theory testing and building.

It is likely that as the field advances, the ways in which theory could be applied will evolve and develop, providing more creative examples.

Theory and Knowledge Translation: World Views

The most prevalent definition of theory derives from positivism (Charmaz, 2006). Through this lens, a theory is made up of specific concepts that are organized systematically in a statement of relationships to represent or characterize particular phenomena (Fawcett, 2000), which may provide a partial view or perspective on reality (Kramer, 1997). Therefore, the root of theory development is conceptual meaning and clarity; concepts are the building blocks of theory (e.g., Walker & Avant, 2005). From this view, the objectives of theory are explanations and prediction, with positivist theory favoring deterministic explanations (Charmaz, 2006). Charmaz (2006) argues that although often parsimonious, these theories can result in narrow and reductionist explanations. In contrast, interpretive theory emphasizes understanding rather than explanation. This type of theory "assumes emergent, multiple realities; indeterminacy; facts and values as linked; truth as provisional; and social life as processual" (Charmaz, 2006, p. 126). Rather than seeking causality and linearity, interpretive theories are used to prioritize connections and patterns.

Theory use and development, like any other form of knowledge generation, are open to study through adopting different ontological and epistemological perspectives. Like anything, it depends on one's own world view. Knowledge translation research and activity has been dominated by those rooted in logical positivism, a philosophical system that recognizes only scientifically verifiable facts and propositions as meaningful. Examples of theory use by, for example, Eccles et al. (2005) and Estabrooks et al. (Cummings, Estabrooks, Midodzi, Wallin, Hayduk, in this supplement; Estabrooks, Midodzi, Cummings, Wallin, Adewale, in this supplement; Midodzi, Hayduk, Cummings, Estabrooks, Wallin, in this supplement; Estabrooks, in this supplement; Wallin, Estabrooks, Midodzi, & Cummings, 2006) are illustrations of a deductive, positivistic approach to theory use. In these cases, theory has been isolated from context and used to generate hypothesis to predict causal relationships, which are then tested using reductionist approaches.

To date, there has been no debate in the knowledge translation literature about these complex issues. Given that knowledge translation is a multidimensional and multilayered process, the questions that need to be debated include determining the most appropriate approaches to applying and developing knowledge translation theory, understanding how different epistemological approaches contribute to understanding the black box of implementation, and how to design studies to incorporate plural perspectives.

Conceptual Clarity: The Building Blocks of Theory Development

The issue of conceptual clarity is a problematic issue in knowledge translation generally (see Graham et al., 2006 for a fuller description). Although the terms are often used interchangeably, they are not necessarily synonymous, and many concepts are contested (e.g., Rycroft-Malone, 2006; Scott-Findlay & Pollock, 2004). Terms and associated concepts rarely are made explicit or used consistently, which is problematic for theory use and development.

Cummings et al. (in this supplement) clearly state they use the term *research utilization* to mean the processes involved in using research knowledge to inform clinical decisions. Knowledge translation has been defined as "the exchange, synthesis and ethically sound application of knowledge—within a complex system of interactions among researchers and users…" (About Knowledge Translation, 2006), where knowledge is broader than scientific research. Arguably, therefore, research utilization is a more specific type of knowledge translation activity. Consequently, it could be suggested that a theory about the concept of research utilization may be different from a theory about the concept of knowledge translation. Clearly, there is likely to be some overlap in the concepts articulated in theories about research utilization and those about knowledge translation; however, the ways in which concepts interrelate and are organized (ie, the theory) may differ. If advances in the science of knowledge translation are to be made, and in particular, in relation to theory development, it is essential that investigators are clear about the concepts they use.

Selecting a Coherent Overarching Framework

Although there is no single knowledge translation theory, there are numerous models and frameworks available to guide knowledge translation activity, each at varying levels of development and maturity. Estabrooks et al. (Cummings et al., in this supplement; Estabrooks, in this supplement; Estabrooks et al., in this supplement; Wallin et al., 2006) state their preference for using and developing knowledge translation theory, and have chosen the Promoting Action on Research Implementation in Health Services (PARIHS) conceptual framework to guide their assumptions and analysis (Kitson, Harvey, & McCormack, 1998; Rycroft-Malone et al., 2002; Rycroft-Malone, Harvey et al., 2004). Modeling techniques, such as those used by Estabrooks et al., require that models are built from theory that is well-grounded and include variables that reflect the phenomenon under investigation (Hickey, 1993). Specifically, there is a danger in forcing researchers to make strong assumptions in order to make stronger conclusions.

The PARIHS framework represents the complexity of the factors involved in implementing evidence into practice. Specifically within the framework, successful implementation (SI) is explained by a function of the dynamic, simultaneous relationship among *evidence* (E),[1] *context* (C),[2] and *facilitation*[3] (F) (containing subelements): SI = f(E,C,F). Despite an ongoing development process, questions about the PARIHS framework remain, including:

1. How do the elements and subelements interrelate and interact?
2. Do the elements and subelements have equal weighting in getting evidence into practice?
3. Is the content of the framework comprehensive?
4. How does individual behavior fit into the framework?

Specifically, the concept analyses undertaken on each of the elements concluded that the concepts (ie, elements) were developed partially but in need of delineation and comparison (Harvey et al., 2002; McCormack et al., 2002; Rycroft-Malone, Seers, et al., 2004). These are critical issues for theory development because they provide direction for further work. From a traditional theory development perspective, only when there is a unified set of relationships can the goals of predication and explanation be met (Walker & Avant, 2005). It has been acknowledged that the suggestions and propositions generated through the PARIHS conceptual framework require further testing through research and practice (e.g., McCormack et al.,

---

[1] Includes evidence types from propositional and nonpropositional sources of knowledge.
[2] The setting in which evidence is implemented.
[3] Refers to the process of enabling (making easier) the implementation of evidence into practice. Facilitation is achieved by an individual carrying out a specific role (a facilitator), who aims to help individuals, teams, and organizations apply evidence into practice.

2002; Rycroft-Malone, Harvey, et al., 2004). Therefore, whether the PARIHS framework could be considered to be a well-grounded theory, and therefore, one that should be used in modeling, is open for debate.

Providing a Focus

Although further testing is required, the PARIHS framework provides a useful heuristic for examining relationships and variables of interest in knowledge translation activity, and therefore, for theory development. The idea that context is a potentially important mediator of knowledge translation has empirical support from multiple evaluation studies (e.g., Dopson & Fitzgerald, 2005; Dopson, Fitzgerald, Ferlie, Gabbay, & Locock, 2002). However, context is often neglected by investigators in the design and conduct of implementation research.

Wallin et al. (2006), Estabrooks et al. (in this supplement), and Cummings et al. (in this supplement) aimed to explore context, as conceptualized in the PARIHS framework; to test the hypothesis that the use of research is more likely in contexts that are receptive; and to understand the relative contributions of different predictors of research use at three levels: individual, unit, and hospital. As the authors indicate, they have tested this relationship somewhat independently of evidence and facilitation, which for the theoretical advancement of the PARIHS framework as a whole may be limiting. Additionally, because of the nature of their inquiry (ie, the use of statistical modeling), the interactions integral to knowledge translation are neglected. Their work is founded on a set of theoretical assumptions about causality and predictive capability which, arguably, may not be appropriate for understanding fully the complexities of knowledge translation. However, in exploring context, and its relationship to nurses' use of research, a number of other findings emerged (discussed further below) that may contribute to informing the design of future intervention studies.

Wallin et al. (2006) and Midodzi et al. (in this supplement) describe a complex statistical process for deriving and validating variables of interest from existing data sets because direct measures of research utilization and PARIHS related variables were missing. Rightly, the authors suggest that possible existing databases should be mined thoroughly, and their work demonstrates a novel approach to doing so. However, this approach also presents some challenges. It is important that modeling includes variables that reflect the phenomenon under investigation (Hickey, 1993). In this case, the research team selected the variables of interest based on their knowledge of the literature and framework of choice (Estabrooks et al., in this supplement). It is possible that other research teams and other stakeholders may have made different choices, which may serve to limit the reliability and validity of these findings. Additionally, the operationalization of context may be problematic, based on the following items:

Culture: freedom to make important patient care and work decisions

Leadership: a nurse manager or immediate supervisor who is a good leader or manager

Evaluation: praise and recognition for a job well-done

and an assumption that context is static. The team made pragmatic decisions based on available information (Wallin et al., 2006), and at face value these items reflect a notion of culture, leadership, and evaluation. Equally, however, it could be argued that they are not particularly sensitive, and do not fully operationalize the conceptualization of context (McCormack et al., 2002; Rycroft-Malone, Harvey et al., 2004; Wallin et al., 2006).

Similarly, the finding that facilitation had no effect on nurses' research utilization may be a consequence of the inadequate operationalization of the concept of facilitation (Cummings et al., in this supplement). The item chosen for the statistical model "opportunity for staff to consult with clinical nurse specialists or expert nurse clinicians/educators" does not equate to the conceptualization of facilitation in the PARIHS framework (Harvey et al., 2002). Ideally, items that more specifically operationalizes concepts would have been available to the team. Therefore, a challenge for the future theoretical development of the PARIHS framework is to develop, utilize, and test *true* indicators. The same could be said of other frameworks and theories.

Theory Selection

Whether for or against theory use, the menu of potentially useable existing theories is vast, originating from a variety of sources including, for example, health promotion, social science, organizational development, and marketing (see Table 15-1 for an overview, and Grol, Wensing, Hulscher, & Eccles, 2005 for a detailed summary). In healthcare, knowledge translation scholars have only recently begun to use theory to guide implementation research (e.g., Eccles et al., 2005; Grol & Grimshaw, 2003; Walker, Grimshaw, Armstrong, 2001). These early attempts have tended to be focused on relatively straightforward clinical issues (e.g., sore throat) and on an individual practitioner's (usually physicians) change in behavior

TABLE 15-1	Overview of Relevant Theories for Knowledge Translation
Level	**Theory Examples**
Individual (relevant to practitioners and patients)	• Decision-making and cognitive theories • Educational theories • Attitudinal theories • Motivational theories • Marketing theories • Professional development theories • Changes theories
Group	• Social network theories • Communities of practice theories • Social capital theories • Communication theories • Leadership theories
Organization	• Institutional theory • Organizational culture theories • Agency theory • Change theories • Complexity theory • Economic theories • Organizational learning theory • Configuration theory • Actor-network theory • Structuration theory

(e.g., prescribing practice) applying single theories (e.g., theory of planned behavior). Studies guided by theory that examine complex, multifaceted issues; acknowledge the dynamics of the context of action; consider behavior within and across professional groups; and consider the interactions of all these elements have yet to be conceptualized, designed, conducted, and evaluated.

Criteria that might assist decision making about which theory to apply include, for example, whether it is robust, logical, generalizable, testable, and useful (Eccles et al., 2005; ICEBeRG, 2006). These provide a starting point; however, there are two problems. First, applying these criteria will narrow down the potential number of theories but not identify which particular theory to use in what circumstance or context.

Second, it is likely that in the implementation of complex interventions, more than one theory will be required. In such cases, there is no guidance to help researchers choose an appropriate theory or suite of coherent theories. One practical suggestion would be to link the choice of theories to the overarching theoretical framework of the study. For example, in applying the PARIHS framework, it may be appropriate to consider using the following theories in a study that aimed to improve outcomes while evaluating how and why interventions worked or not:

- Dual processing models of reasoning (e.g., Sladeck, Phillips, & Bond, 2006), which would help identify and explain individual differences in the way practitioners moderated their decisions to incorporate new *evidence.*

- Structuration theory (e.g., Giddens, 1984), which would be helpful in discovering the links between *context* (structure) and action (in this case, behavior of practitioners in incorporating evidence into practice) and in understanding the dynamic processes between context and action.

- Adult learning theory (Knowles, 1984), which facilitators use as part of a *facilitation* intervention could be tested along side the application of, for example, social influence theory (Mittman, Tonesk, & Jacobson, 1992).

Although not intended to be exhaustive, these examples illustrate how an overarching conceptual framework can guide the choice of multiple theories in an organized way. Crucially, it would be important to design studies to ensure the interaction between the various elements, and thus, theories are captured and made sense of. However, this approach is an illustration of a deductive approach to theory application whereby theories are borrowed and applied to different settings, people, and topics; an alternative approach would be to develop theory inductively from, for example, practice and practitioners using methodologies such as grounded theory, action research, and realistic evaluation. The advantages of inductive theory development are contextual relevance, and rather than focusing attention on the applicability of borrowed theory, there is the potential to develop a more inclusive understanding of knowledge translation action.

Cummings et al. (in this supplement) and Estabrooks et al. (in this supplement) describe a number of findings that also may be helpful in providing further direction about the types of theories useful in guiding the development of implementation interventions. Overall, findings demonstrate that the better the contextual conditions (as operationalized by the team

in relation to the PARIHS framework), the higher nurses' research utilization scores. This relationship supports the theoretical proposition that in receptive contexts there will be greater use of evidence. Broadly, this indicates that implementation projects should (a) pay attention to context and (b) use organization-level theory. However, the authors also report that individual factors accounted for most of the variance in the multilevel model. Perhaps this is unsurprising given that individuals interact with all levels of an organization, but serves to further highlight the absence of individual factors in the PARIHS framework. Furthermore, although individual factors accounted for most of the variance, the factors that impact at the contextual level are multiple.

Findings at the levels of individual, group, and organization are summarized in Table 15-2. To better understand the direct and indirect influences of the factors on nurses' research utilization, some have been labeled here as *antecedent* findings. This approach has been taken because a number findings described by Cummings et al. (in this supplement) may be precursors for the results reported by Estabrooks et al. (in this supplement) and for nurses' use of research more generally. For example, hospital size has a positive relationship with opportunities for staff development, staffing, and support services (antecedent), which in turn contributes to higher research utilization in larger hospitals.

Findings indicate that it might be appropriate to target interventions at micro-, meso-, and macrolevels of context (McNulty & Ferlie, 2002). However, there is a danger in considering context as a layered set of relationships because it may lead to a lack of attention to the interactions across boundaries. That is, the boundaries are artificial and do not represent the complexity of the practice context in which knowledge translation occurs. It would therefore be critical to evaluate relevant theories at different levels (including the individual), but also capture the myriad of processes and interactions among them.

The findings provide an indication of the sort of theories that could be evaluated in future intervention studies. For example, if greater nurse-to-nurse collaboration is related to an increase in research utilization, an intervention based on social network theory (e.g., West, Barron, Dowsett, & Newton, 1999) or communities of practice theory (Wenger, 1998) would be appropriate to evaluate. Both these theories are concerned with how networks and groups produce, communicate, and transfer knowledge and so relate closely to the idea of nurse-to-nurse collaboration, although in future studies this could apply equally to multiprofessional groups. Additionally, a *unit's ability to control its own practice* could be considered to be a feature of a learning organization (Senge 1990). In applying learning organization theory

TABLE 15-2	Summary of Findings at Individual, Group, and Organization Levels		
	Findings		
Source	**Individual**	**Group**	**Organization**
Estabrooks et al. (in this supplement) and Cummings et al. (in this supplement)	Emotional exhaustion—higher reported levels of were associated with lower levels of research use.	Greater nurse–nurse collaboration—greater reported use of research.	Hospital size—the larger the hospital, the higher levels of research utilization.
	Internet use—increased time on Internet associated with higher levels of research use.	Unit's ability to control own practice—associated with higher levels of research use.	Responsive administration (antecedent)—led to reports of greater unit-level autonomy, increased staffing, support services, and support for innovation.
		Increased relational capital (antecedent)—led to greater nurse-to-nurse collaboration and lower emotional exhaustion.	Hospital size (antecedent)—larger positive relationship with opportunities for staff development, staffing, and support services.
			Higher staffing and support services (antecedent)—more staff development, nurse-to-nurse collaboration, time to nurse, and lower emotional exhaustion.
			Greater use of research—fewer patient adverse events.
			In specialized units—increase in research utilization scores.

to implementation intervention design, one therefore might pay attention to learning, self-regulation, clinical leadership, and decentralization. The signposts that Estabrooks et al. provide are preliminary, and require substantiation and replication particularly as the databases they used are now relatively old and relate to nurses in Alberta, Canada. Furthermore, the research agenda with respect to theory use and development in knowledge translation is significant.

 ## Theory-Informed Knowledge Translation: A Research Agenda

Eccles et al. (2005) suggest that we should not underestimate the time and investment required to raise implementation research to the level of other clinical sciences. Some would challenge whether this should indeed be the goal. It may not be possible, or even appropriate, to think about implementation research as a field of inquiry akin to biology or pharmacy. In contrast to many clinical science interventions, implementation strategies are acknowledged to be complex, involving multiple actors and factors, which are not always amenable to randomized controlled trials. Building on the issues introduced above, the following outlines some initial ideas for advancing the field through research.

Theory-driven implementation research has been criticized because it potentially stifles creativity and innovation (e.g., Oxman et al., 2005). This is a fair critique given the type of theory application research conducted to date. The challenge then is to design studies that not only pay attention to theory (implicit and explicit) but also allow for an exploration beyond the parameters that a theory might be used to determine. Necessarily, ideological clashes will need to be avoided, and the use of positivist and interpretative approaches should be embraced in order to capture both outcomes and processes. Walach, Falkenberg, Fonnebo, Lewith, and Jonas (2006) suggest that rather than relying on randomized controlled trials when evaluating complex interventions, circular models using different designs and multiple methods would result in rigorous and pragmatic findings. For example, a knowledge translation research question focused on evaluating the effectiveness of a particular approach to audit, and feedback is amenable to action research embedded within a randomized trial. Making sense of the relationship between outcomes and processes should be facilitated by the adoption of an overarching theoretical or conceptual framework that offers propositions and hypothesis, or through methods that do this as part of the research process.

Little is known about the operationalization and transferability of theory-driven interventions across professional groups or settings and patient groups. For example, it could be predicted that nurses and physicians are likely to respond differently to the same theory-based intervention because their respective socialization and education are likely to impact on individual behavior. Similarly, interventions may result in different outcomes in different clinical settings with different patient groups. An approach would be to develop micro- or practice theory that could be used to understand and explain knowledge translation in specific disciplines and stakeholders, in specific contexts. Addressing and evaluating these assertions in a way that others can judge transferability will aid the development of context-appropriate theory.

It has been argued that multiple theories within intervention studies are likely to be more powerful and explanatory than single theory use (e.g., Estabrooks et al., 2006). Designing studies that coherently link multiple theories to interventions and outcomes will be challenging. Research designs that incrementally and sequentially test theoretically based interventions within the same study may enable the development of clearer links and make it easier to disentangle relationships. In reality, pragmatic yet informed decisions will need to be made.

One rationale for theory use is in helping us gain a better understanding of the black box of implementation. Arguably to date, particular assumptions about what is in this black box have been made by those applying theory, which include linearity, prediction, and generalizability. Scholars who have looked into the box through empirical inquiry report multiple modifiers and context-specific outcomes. This makes isolating strong effects difficult (e.g., Dopson & Fitzgerald, 2005). There is a strong platform from which to argue that any advances made in the field of knowledge translation theory use and development will result from an acceptance and incorporation of the multiple interactions, processes, and outcomes that coexist. In acknowledging this complexity, it may be appropriate to apply existing

theories but, in doing so, also notice unexpected consequences and events that occur over time. The multiple (and often unpredictable) interactions that arise in particular contexts are likely what determine the success or failure of the implementation efforts; it will therefore be important to conduct studies so these are not stripped away. For example, Pawson and Tilley's (1997) approach to realistic evaluation acknowledges that "outcomes are explained by the action of particular mechanisms in particular contexts and this explanatory structure is put in place over time by a combination of theory and experimental observation" (p. 59). The emphasis on *what, why*, and *how* questions not only requires the development of explanatory theoretical frameworks, but also stresses empirical observation. Studies that include both evaluative and intervention streams of work, which are integrated theoretically, are likely to produce more informative findings than those focused purely on implementing interventions. Furthermore, in acknowledging that context is not a static entity, longitudinal research studies that enable the changing nature of context to be captured will provide a richer picture and will enhance transferability.

Estabrooks et al. have demonstrated through statistical modeling that both individual and contextual factors are important mediators of nurses' use of research. This has implications for the PARIHS framework, which does not explicitly acknowledge the role of individuals, and for research. Researchers exploring the individual factors impacting on research use tend to focus on barriers, are many, and provide consistent messages (e.g., Rycroft-Malone, Harvey, et al., 2004). Perhaps in the next generation of research the individual practitioner should be acknowledged as an actor in the context of practice. In doing so, theories appropriate to individual clinical decision making and those relevant to modifying and understanding better contextual factors should be evaluated. Importantly, the findings of this statistical modeling exercise need to be verified in the reality of the clinical setting.

As Estabrooks (in this supplement) notes, such an agenda does not lend itself to unidisciplinary work. It could be argued that advances in the field have not been made because there is a tendency for scholars to work within professional and methodological silos. Therefore, it is essential that in attending to the research agenda, meaningful collaborations are developed and sustained.

 ## Conclusion

If, as Medawar (1984) suggests, a science does not truly become mature until it develops a predictive capability, then what is the status of knowledge translation research? If a positivistic view of science is taken, knowledge translation research is immature. If an interpretive lens is used, some progress has been made. Scholars have begun to develop understanding about the factors that are important to the success of knowledge translation and therefore develop theory inductively from their observations.

If the knowledge translation field is to advance, scholars need to attend to a large research agenda, which includes theory use and development, among other issues. Estabrooks et al. have taken the opportunity to develop and test new statistical modeling techniques, resulting in a novel analysis of some of the factors that influence nurses' use of research evidence. This is one approach; there are many others to explore. Additionally, their ideas now need further testing. Although some coordinates may have been set, the journey remains long. Although this will present challenges, it also offers exciting opportunities. This agenda should be carried forward by conducting scholarly research, guarding against reductionism, embracing pluralism, encouraging collaboration, and entering into open and critical dialogue. In this way, not only may the art and science of knowledge translation be advanced, but positive and enduring changes to patient outcomes may be reported.

REFERENCES

About Knowledge Translation. (2006). Retrieved May 18, 2006, from www.cihr-irsc.gc.ca/e/29418.html.

Bhattacharyya, O., Reeves, S., Garfinkel, S., & Zwarenstein, M. (2006). Designing theoretically-informed implementation interventions: Fine in theory, but evidence of effectiveness in practice is needed. *Implementation Science, 1,* 5.

Charmaz, K. (2006). *Constructing grounded theory: A practical guide through qualitative analysis.* London: Sage.

Dopson, S., Fitzgerald, L., Ferlie, E., Gabbay, J., & Locock, L. (2002). No magic targets! Changing clinical practice to become more evidence based. *Health Care Management Review, 27,* 35–47.

Dopson, S. & Fitzgerald, L. (Eds.). (2005). *Knowledge to action? Evidence-based health care in context.* Oxford: Oxford University Press.

Eccles, M., Grimshaw, J., Walker, A., Johnston, M., & Pitts, N. (2005). Changing the behaviour of healthcare professionals: the use of theory in promoting the uptake of research findings. *Journal of Clinical Epidemiology, 58,* 107–112.

Estabrooks, C. A., Thompson, D. S., Lovely, J. E., & Hof meyer, A. (2006). A guide to knowledge translation theory. *Journal of Continuing Education in the Health Prof essions, 26,*25–36.

Fawcett, J. (2000). *Analysis and evaluation of contemporary nursing knowledge: Nursing models and theories.* Philadelphia: FA Davies.

Giddens, A. (1984). *The constitution of society: Outline of the theory of structuration.* Cambridge: Polity.

Graham, I. D., Logan, J., Harrison, M. B., Straus, S. E., Tetroe, J., Caswell, W. et al. (2006). Lost in knowledge translation: Time for a map? *Journal of Continuing Education in the Health Prof essions, 26,*13–24.

Grimshaw, J. M., Thomas, R. E., MacLennan, G., Fraser, C., Ramsay, C. R., Vale, L., et al. (2004). Effectiveness and efficiency of guideline dissemination and implementation strategies. *Health Technology Assessment, 8,*1–72.

Grol, R. (2001). Success and failures in the implementation of evidence-based guidelines for clinical practice. *Medical Care,* 39(Suppl. 2), 1146–1154.

Grol, R., & Grimshaw, J. M. (2003). From best evidence to best practice: Effective implementation of change to patients' care. *Lancet, 362,* 1225–1230.

Grol, R., Wensing, M., Hulscher, M., & Eccles, M. (2005). Theories in implementation of change in healthcare. In R., Grol, M., Wensing, & M., Eccles (Eds.), *Improving patient care. The implementation of change in clinical practice* (pp. 15–40). London: Elsevier.

Harvey, G., Lof tus-Hills, A., Rycrof t-Malone, J., Titchen, A., Kitson, A., McCormack, B. et al. (2002). Getting evidence into practice: The role and function of facilitation. *Journal of Advanced Nursing, 37,* 577–588.

Hickey, M. (1993). Structural equation models: Latent variables. In B. H., Munro & E. B., Page (Eds.), *Statistical methods for health care research* (2nd ed., pp. 295–320). Philadelphia: Lippincott Company.

ICEBeRG Group. (2006). Designing theoretically-informed implementation interventions. *Implementation Science, 1,* 4. Retrieved April 10, 2006, from www.implementationscience/com/content/1/1/4.

Kitson, A., Ahmed, L. B., Harvey, G., Seers, K., & Thompson, D. (1996). From research to practice: One organisational model for promoting research-based practice. *Journal of Advanced Nursing, 23,* 430–440.

Kitson A., Harvey G., & McCormack B. (1998). Enabling the implementation of evidence based practice: a conceptual framework. *Quality in Health Care, 7,* 149–158.

Knowles, M. S. (1984). *Andragogy in action.* San Francisco: Jossey Bass.

Kramer, M. K. (1997). Terminology in theory: Definitions and comments. In I. M., King & J., Fawcett (Eds.), *The language of nursing theory and metatheory* (pp. 51–61). Indianapolis: Sigma Theta Tau International, Centre Nursing Publishing.

McCormack, B., Kitson, A., Harvey, G., Rycroft-Malone, J., Titchen, A., & Seers, K. (2002). Getting evidence into practice: the meaning of context. *Journal of Advanced Nursing, 38,*94–104.

McGlynn, E. A., Asch, S. M., Adams, J., Keesey, J., Hicks, J., DeCristof aro, A., et al. (2003). The quality of care delivered to adults in the United States. *New England Journal of Medicine,* 348, 2635–2645.

McNulty, T., & Ferlie, E. (2002). *Reengineering health care: The complexities of organizational transformation.* Oxford: Oxford University Press.

Medawar, P. (1984). *The limits of science.* Oxford: Oxford University Press.

Michie, S., Hendy, J., Smith, J., & Adshead, F. (2006). Evidence into practice: A theory based study of achieving national health targets in primary care. *Journal of Evaluation in Clinical Practice, 10,* 447–456.

Mittman, B. S., Tonesk, X., & Jacobson, P. D. (1992). Implementing clinical practice guidelines: Social influence strategies and practitioner behaviour change. *Qualitative Review Bulletin,* 18, 413–422.

Oxman, A. D., Fretheim A., & Flottrop, S. (2005). The OFF theory of research utilization. *Journal of Clinical Epidemiology*, *58*, 113–116.

Pawson, R., & Tilley, N. (1997). *Realist evaluation*. London: Sage Publications.

Rycroft-Malone, J. (2006). The politics of the evidence-based practice movements. Legacies and current challenges. *Journal of Research in Nursing*, *11*, 95–108.

Rycroft-Malone, J., Harvey, G., Seers, K., Kitson, A., McCormack, B., & Titchen, A. (2004). An exploration of the factors that influence the implementation of evidence into practice. *Journal of Clinical Nursing*, 13,913–924.

Rycroft-Malone, J., Kitson, A., Harvey, G., McCormack, B., Seers, K., Titchen, A. et al. (2002). Ingredients for change: Revisiting a conceptual framework. *Quality in Healthcare*, *11*, 174–180.

Rycroft-Malone, J., Seers, K., Titchen, A., Harvey, G., Kitson, A., & McCormack, B. (2004). What counts as evidence in evidence-basedpractice?*Journal of Advanced Nursing*, *47*,81–90.

Scott-Findlay, S., & Pollock, C. (2004). Evidence, research, knowledge: A call for conceptual clarity. *Worldviews on Evidence-Based Nursing*, *1*, 92–97.

Senge, P. M. (1990). *The fifth discipline: The art and practice of the learning organisation*. New York: Doubleday/Currency.

Sladek, R. M., Phillips, A., & Bond, M. J. (2006). Implementation science: A role for parallel dual processing models of reasoning? *Implementation Science*, *1*, 12. Retrieved May 1, 2006 from www.implementationscience/com/content/1/12.

Walach, H., Falkenberg, T., Fonnebo, V., Lewith, G., & Jonas, W.B. (2006). Circular instead of hierarchical: Methodological principles for the evaluation of complex interventions. *BMC Research Methodology* 6(29). Retrieved March 28, 2007 from www.biomedcentral.com/1471–2288/6/29.

Walker, A. E., Grimshaw, J. M., & Armstrong, E. M. (2001). Salient beliefs and intentions to prescribe antibiotics for patients with a sore throat. *British Journal of Health Psychology*, *6*, 347–360.

Walker, L. O., & Avant, K. C. (2005). *Strategies for theory construction in nursing* (4th ed.). New Jersey: Pearson Education, Inc.

Wallin, L., Estabrooks, C. A., Midodzi, W. K., & Cummings, G. G. (2006). Development and validation of a derived measure of research utilization by nurses. *Nursing Research*, *55*, 149–160.

West, E., Barron, D. N., Dowsett, J., & Newton, J. N. (1999). Hierarchies and cliques in the social networks of health care prof essionals: Implications for the design of dissemination strategies. *Social Science & Medicine*, *48*, 633–646.

Wenger, E. (1998). *Communities of practice: Learning, meaning, and identity*. Cambridge: Cambridge University Press.

THE AUTHOR COMMENTS Theory and Knowledge Translation: Setting Some Coordinates

At the time of writing the article, there had been little discussion about the theoretical underpinnings of implementing evidence in practice; therefore, this was a timely opportunity to stimulate some discussion. More specifically, a traditional view of theory use was dominant within the implementation science literature. This manuscript provided an opportunity to open up the debate to begin consideration of different, more creative ways that theory could be both used and developed.

JO RYCROFT-MALONE

Unitary Appreciative Inquiry
Evolution and Refinement

W. RICHARD COWLING III, RN, PhD, AHN-BC, APRN-BC, FAAN
ELIZABETH REPEDE, PhD, CMH, FNP-BC

Unitary appreciative inquiry (UAI), developed over the past 20 years, provides an orientation and process for uncovering human wholeness and discovering life patterning in individuals and groups. Refinements and a description of studies using UAI are presented. Assumptions and conceptual underpinnings of the method distinguishing its contributions from other methods are reported. Data generation strategies that capture human wholeness and elucidate life patterning are proposed. Data synopsis as an alternative to analysis is clarified and explicated. Standards that suggest enhancing the legitimacy of knowledge and credibility of research are specified. Potential expansions of UAI offer possibilities for extending epistemologies, aesthetic integration, and theory development. **Key words:** *life patterning, methodology, nursing science, nursing theory, science of unitary human beings, unitary appreciative inquiry, unitary science, wholeness*

The purpose of this article is to present the evolution and refinement of the unitary appreciative inquiry (UAI) method as previously described and explicated in 15 articles and book chapters since 1990.[1-15] The refinements have arisen from the use of UAI by a number of researchers who have sought to address challenges and concerns that have occurred in planning and implementing research.[16-23] There has also been a need to clarify assumptions and conceptual underpinnings of the method distinguishing its contributions to an evolving nursing science of wholeness. In addition, certain aspects of UAI have been wanting in explicitness in such areas as data generation procedures, data synopsis, and credibility and legitimacy of findings. The further elaboration of UAI and clarification of its refinements are essential for researchers who are seeking methods that purport to offer a window into human wholeness.

Overview and History

In studying the science of unitary human beings, it became evident that the conceptual framework had potential for offering a wholeness-focused path to nursing care. However, there seemed to be a huge disconnection between the conceptual system with its assumptions of wholeness and its theoretical tenets of unique human patterning, and the available practice approaches and research methods for those seeking

to apply these ideas and concepts. In addition, if there were attention to be given to the development of theories derived from the conceptual system, there would need to be methods consistent for generating and testing such theories.

Unitary appreciative inquiry grew from conceptual development aimed at creating a practice approach centered on human field pattern as explicated by Rogers[24] rather than on disease or diagnosis.[13,15] One of the critical questions addressed in this conceptual development work was differentiating unitary knowing from other forms of knowing in practice.[14] This work evolved toward a conceptualization of pattern-focused practice called first unitary pattern appraisal[15] and later unitary pattern appreciation, wherein the goal of practice was to appreciate fully the wholeness of human life as a reference point for care consistent with the science of unitary human beings. Unitary knowing was differentiated from systems knowing offering guidance in how to interpret data through a synoptic rather than analytic lens. This was derived from the notion of synopsis as considering various aspects of human experience that might not be generally linked together to try to get at an underlying integration. There was a gradual evolution toward bridging science and practice using unitary pattern appreciation.[11]

The intent and focus of unitary pattern appreciation were described as "perceiving, being aware of, sensitive to, and expressing the full force and delicate distinctions of [energy field pattern]

From W. R. Cowling & E. Repede, Unitary appreciative inquiry evolution and refinement.
Advances in Nursing Science 2010, 33(2), 64–77. Copyright © 2010 Wolters Kluwer Health | Lippincott Williams & Wilkins.
Reprinted with permission Lippincott Williams & Wilkins.

ABOUT THE AUTHORS

W. RICHARD COWLING III is currently a Professor and Director of the PhD Program in Nursing at the University of North Carolina Greensboro and Editor of the *Journal of Holistic Nursing*. The accomplishments that he is most proud of in relation to nursing are in the areas of research and practice relevant to women's survivorship of childhood abuse and depression. He has sought to integrate theory, research, and practice from a unique holistic and unitary perspective. Outcomes of the work include the creation of innovative practice and research methods, implementation and support of research, conception of a theory of healing, and formulation and implementation of a practice model for intervention with women who have experienced abuse in childhood. He is certified as an Advanced Practice Nurse in both mental health and holistic nursing. In 2008, he was awarded a Department of Health and Human Services' grant to support a PhD program focused on health disparities and health promotion. He was named the 2008 Holistic Nurse of the Year by the American Holistic Nurses Association. Dr. Cowling was inducted as a Fellow in the American Academy of Nursing in 2010. His hobbies and personal interests revolve around the activities with his partner, daughter, and granddaughters who add immeasurable joy to his life.

ELIZABETH REPEDE is an Assistant Professor of Nursing at Western Carolina University in Enka, North Carolina. She was born in Highland Park, IL, and received her Diploma in Nursing from Evanston Hospital School of Nursing in 1976. Moving steadily south, she received a BSN from the University of Kentucky, a master's degree in Nursing as a Family Nurse Practitioner from the University of South Carolina, and a PhD in Nursing at the University of North Carolina, Greensboro. It was under the tutelage of Dr. Richard Cowling III that she developed her passion for scholarship into nursing theories and methods for the deep transformation of nursing knowledge and science through a contextual framework of wholeness. Her hobbies and interests include reading, the study of healing arts, spending time with family and friends, and travel. In addition to teaching in the Family Nurse Practitioner Program at Western Carolina University and research with women who have experienced abuse, she maintains a private practice in holistic healing using hypnosis, imagery, and various energy modalities.

while sympathetically recognizing its excellence as experienced in gratefulness, enjoyment, and understanding."[11(p130)] Unitary pattern appreciation was specified to have a particular process, orientation, and approach. The process was described as reaching for the essence of pattern through its manifestations of experience, perceptions, and expressions including all realms of information or data. The orientation outlined guiding assumptions and characteristics as well as elements related to the implementation for science and practice. In addition, the synoptic, participatory, and transformative features of unitary pattern appreciation were explicated.

A transition in the use of unitary pattern appreciation occurred in the development of a case study method called unitary case inquiry[1,5,10] and eventually into a research approach that could be integrated into practice as a praxis approach. Praxis was used to denote the synthesis of research, theory, and practice similar to participatory action research. It was also intended to convey the potential use by both researchers and practitioners. Unitary appreciative inquiry is essentially a praxis approach that can enable knowledge to be generated in both practice and research enterprises.[3,6] However, this is an area that warrants further clarification because of the potential confusion about how UAI can be used and broader conceptual disagreements about what praxis really means.

Unitary appreciative inquiry evolved into its current form through application of the approach in a variety of studies described in the literature review section of this article. Knowledge gained from research aided in the refinement of UAI specifying:

- clarification of aim of inquiry as life patterning of individuals, groups, families, and communities;
- conceptualization of life patterning as an indicator of unitary energy field patterning that integrates human-environment mutual process;
- elaboration of 3 major strands of inquiry as appreciative, participatory, and emancipatory;
- suggestions for data generation and data management procedures that create the most

complete picture possible of the wholeness of life patterning;

- consideration of data in synthesizing and synoptic ways as an alternative to analysis that might enhance possibility of fragmentation of information;

- delineation of credibility and legitimacy standards and procedures; and

- representation of findings that express the wholeness of life patterning that include experiential, presentational, propositional, and practical adopted from cooperative inquiry.[25]

Unitary appreciative inquiry draws upon a history of development that included a general description and conceptualization of unitary pattern appreciation, an explanation and differentiation of unitary knowing and systems knowing, and specification and delineation of unitary pattern appreciation as an orientation, process, and approach. Unitary appreciative inquiry in its current version grew out of unitary pattern appreciation as a case study approach that provided a means of systematically implementing pattern-focused care and reporting the results of these endeavors. In its present state of development, UAI provides an opportunity for researchers to generate knowledge relevant to answering research questions, generating or testing theories, or exploring approaches that have as their major concern of capturing the wholeness of life patterning in individuals, groups, families, or communities.

 ## Unitary Appreciative Inquiry Research

Research using UAI is presented through a review of published studies available in the literature. The original 3 studies on despair in the lives of women using UAI[5,6,8] are discussed, as well as 5 other studies found through a search of PubMed, CINAHL, and EBSCO completed in August of 2009 and a recently completed dissertation. Consistent with a unitary-participatory paradigm, evaluation of research is not based on predetermined outcomes. These studies occurred while legitimacy and credibility standards were under development.

Initially developed as a case method for research and practice,[12,13] UAI was further expanded in a series of 3 projects exploring the life patterning of women experiencing despair.[2-5,8] These 3 projects resulted in the development of a "... unitary healing praxis model for women in despair."[3(p128)] The initial project was a case study method involving 6 women who explored despair in their lives. Data were collated synoptically from participant drawings, dreams, and narratives; from researcher experiences with the participant;

and from the unfolding dialogue that reflected the expression and experience of despair in the lives of each of these women. The researcher developed narratives called pattern profiles that synthesized major patterns within each woman's life story. The profiles integrated metaphor, images, and music and became a focal point for helping these women better understand their lives within the context of a larger life story reflecting their unique patterning. It also created an opportunity to explore alternative ways of approaching life.[3]

Given critical assumptions of a unitary participatory paradigm, expectations of particular changes or outcomes were suspended.[8] The *desire* for positive changes existed without a need to *expect* specific outcomes. The researcher sought to capture the wholeness of the life patterning as a reference point for both the researcher and the participant to consider what was and what could be. This process was aimed at capitalizing on the phenomenon that Rogers described as "knowing participation in change,"[24] which was further conceptualized as a theory of power by Barrett.[26]

The appreciative orientation of the researcher allowed for an unconditional regard for the uniqueness of each participant's life patterning suggesting a case study perspective. The unitary appreciative case study approach created time and space in the research process for reflection without judgments about how the participants wanted to change their life situations. The process allowed for the participant to be self-determining. The unitary appreciative case study approach resulted in a natural unfolding of a participatory-appreciative-reflective process without the researcher or practitioner projecting outcomes that might limit the exploration.

The second UAI project[5] was a qualitative, participatory study of despair in 14 women within the context of 10 life situations: major depression, addiction, sexual abuse, child abuse, homelessness, loss of a loved one, terminal illness, spinal cord injury, infertility, and chronic illness.[3,5] The design did not limit the gender of participants; however, all respondents were female. Ten described some history of abuse (verbal, physical, sexual). Interviews were conducted focusing on descriptions, features, and contexts of despair, transformational processes, if any, associated with despair, and what was helpful personally and with healthcare experiences. The researcher created 4 documents from the data collection process: (1) the original transcript of the interview; (2) a researcher-developed synopsis of despair using the participants' words written in the first person for the participant; (3) a pattern profile using metaphor, images, and music from the themes and content of the transcriptions in a story format; and (4) a summary document including general information about despair from the individual participant's perspective. These were shared with participants to determine whether the documents represented the participant's life patterning as they experienced and understood it.

By shifting the focus of the study of despair to study of the life patterning of women in despair, the richness of despair was found to be a transformational opportunity for appreciating wholeness in all of its complexity in the lives of these women. Pattern profiles helped the participants move toward a journey of self-discovery and knowledge. While some common features of despair were described, the contextual features of despair remained unique to each woman and distinct from any generalizability. Shifting from a symptom-based model of praxis in nursing research to a pattern-based model added to the richness of individual experience and guided the clients toward self-knowing.[3,5]

The third UAI project by Cowling,[2,3,5] used to develop the unitary healing praxis model for women in despair, evolved from the prior 2 studies and was a cooperative inquiry group that focused on the connection between despair and abuse. Six women in a community domestic violence program, a staff member, a graduate nursing student, and the researcher comprised the study group.[2,3] Meeting for six 3-hour sessions over a 10-week period, the group discussed the relationship of abuse and despair. In contrast to a phenomenological approach that would have looked at the lived experience of despair, the researcher used a patterning focus to generate "unitary knowledge concerning despair as experienced by abused women and their perceptions of ways to improve their chances for self-determination and life enhancement."[3(p128)] The exploration included general discussions both about the context of despair in relation to abuse in life patterning and on the specific focus of living in despair.

The study findings were synthesized into an appreciative pattern profile that was developed by participants and used as the foundation for a study report shared with the funding agency.[3] There was a clear benefit from working cooperatively with other women who had experienced both abuse and despair. Positive effects occurred through the use of artistic expressions such as poetry, music, stories, and movies to represent the nature of despair. Words, images, and stories were successfully used to convey feelings of vulnerability, fragility, and anger experienced by the women. Practical knowledge was generated by developing strategies that ameliorated feelings of despair.

Extending Cowling's ongoing research with women abused as children, 11 women participated in a UAI study exploring a facilitated waking dream process called participatory dreaming[21] as a method of unitary healing.[20] The focus of this study was on the appreciation of healing in the lives of the women subsequent to their abuse as children. Over 2 full days in a retreat-like setting, the women participated in repeated cycles of imagery, journaling, group discussion, and art that focused on healing from the abuse. Using both synoptic and analytic processes, a group patterning profile was created using music videos developed by the researcher that described healing in the lives of women abused as children. The study findings, validated by the participants, suggested that healing from abuse is a lifelong process described as a journey taking them more deeply into themselves and potentiating their process of self-discovery and empowerment. Participatory dreaming was a unitary process that was ideal for informing, illuminating, and transforming the appreciation of wholeness in the women's lives and suggesting practical skill development.

Rushing[22] explored the unitary life pattern of serenity with 9 participants from 12-step addiction recovery programs. Following individual interviews, a data synthesis method was used to develop a matrix of manifestations of serenity shared among the group of participants. Common experiences, perceptions, and expressions of participants led to the identification of 4 pattern facets. These included addiction, turning points, early sobriety, and serenity. The researcher prepared a unique appreciative profile using storytelling in a creative format for each individual participant. Serenity was "… a way of living and being, an orientation to life, and a transformation of personality … a healing quality that seemed to emerge as each experienced a spiritual awakening or a transcendence of experiences."[22(p204)]

In a UAI study of the life patterns of 8 persons who had experienced a spinal cord injury at least 2 years prior to the study, 3 shared pattern manifestations were identified.[16] Despite what were considered "good" physical outcomes, each participant with spinal cord injury shared the 3 pattern manifestations of profound depersonalization, loss, and hopelessness.

Cox[17] conducted a study grounded in UAI emphasizing the participatory strand of the research. His innovative research engaged 8 bedside nurses in the development of appreciative profiles of their experiences of professional caregiver despair related to healthcare financing.[17] The impact of insurance risk transfers (managed care, cost shifting, diagnosis-related groups, and healthcare financing) on RNs and the care they provide to clients was explored using UAI. An a priori theory of professional caregiver despair related to insurance risk transfers (cost shifting) was supported by the data synopsis and analysis. Strategies were identified to reduce professional caregiver despair and improve working situations.

Kemp[19] explored the life patterns of women who returned from deployment during the first war in the Persian Gulf, using a UAI methodology emphasizing pattern appreciation. The researcher and the participants cocreated metaphorical stories of the women's lived experiences of being deployed. Data synopsis and analysis highlighted postdeployment life patterning associated with social limitations, military sexual trauma, and a loss of trust in persons and institutions. Prospective pattern profiles for future hopes and dreams were codeveloped by the participants and the researcher.

Nursing presence was studied from both the patient and the nursing perspectives, using the UAI methodology.[18] A combination of data synopsis and analysis were used to identify patterns and to extract themes from interviews. Nurse participants were included in the synopsis/analysis process. Nurse themes included knowing the patient, responding to needs, nurse/patient attitudes and beliefs, bonding between nurse and patient, influencing others, and relationships. Patient themes included knowing me, bonding, supporting me, encouraging me/others, accessibility, and healing. The study findings suggested that nursing presence was felt to be more important than technical care by patients and that healing as a theme evolved spontaneously without researcher suggestion.

Unitary appreciative inquiry was used for a community assessment project in a small southern town by RN-BSN students and their faculty.[23] Because of a lack of unitary framework for community assessment in the nursing literature, the authors/faculty engaged the UAI process to appreciate the wholeness, uniqueness, and essence of the community field pattern under study. A pattern profile of the community was developed using a creative distillation process. Poetry, stories, and photography were used to capture the "feel" of the town and made into a music video shared with community members. The culmination of the pattern profile led to a community action project codeveloped by students and community members that aimed at smoking prevention education for middle-school children and diet and exercise classes for the community at large.

Reported research occurred over several years while the method was being developed and refined by Cowling. These studies, with the exception of the community assessment, were dissertation studies. They reflected the current thinking regarding the method and its potential use to answer a variety of research questions. These studies attempted to capture field patterning through its manifestations by creating profiles providing a picture of wholeness. Unintentionally, some of the studies leaned toward essentializing phenomena rather than giving the fullest attention to the patterning associated with these phenomena. The shift by Cowling to the level of abstraction delineated as life patterning was intended to bring greater clarity to the focus of research. These studies added incrementally to the refinement of the method and provided an opportunity for the originator to consider critical issues related to the intent and implementation of UAI.

 ## The Process of UAI: Praxis of Appreciation, Participation, and Emancipation

The process of UAI was intentionally developed to provide flexibility in uncovering life patterning through innovative approaches in a praxis context. Inquiries can be initiated by either a researcher or participants seeking a researcher to undertake a study project of mutual concern.[3] Sampling is purposive and done by linking the researcher(s) and participants who are interested in a unitary understanding of the research topic. Participants are considered coinquirers or coresearchers consistent with the tenets of participatory research.[27] The primary mode of data generation is mutually engaged dialogue, reflection, and action among individuals and the researcher(s) or as a group process.[3] Participants are invited to participate in dialogue, reflection, aesthetic expression, and action as indicated by the participant-researcher dyad or the group of participant-researcher. Cycles of reflection and action may be used similar to the processes associated with participatory action research.[25] However, the reflection-action cycle is not essential to all projects as determined by the aims and purposes of the inquiry. The reflection and action can occur in either an individual or group format and between dialogue sessions. The data include dialogue, experiential descriptions, expressive products, journals, and whatever is determined by participants to be reflective of life patterning.[3] Borrowing from cooperative inquiry designs, a study may have an informative or a transformative aim or a combination.[25] some research projects provide an opportunity for participants to explore strategies focused on desired changes in life patterning. Depending on the particular project, participants are involved to varying degrees in design and implementation of the study, including data collection, interpretation of data, evaluation of the study, and preparation of the final report. Participants may be involved in coauthoring manuscripts or other publications. This section provides an explication of the elements of the UAI praxis process.

Description of the Unitary Design as Praxis

The ability to enter into an evolving patterning process with clients over time is viewed as particularly relevant to nursing because it seeks to integrate the empirical, interpretive, and critical dimensions of a practically oriented theoretical foundation for nursing science.[28] Unitary appreciative inquiry has been described by Newman[28] as praxis because it is an active synthesis of theory, research, and practice. As praxis, UAI creates opportunities for participants to open themselves to new unitary understandings of their lives in process with an appreciative stance toward what is, rather than what should be,[3] all the while providing a context for discovering what could be. Emancipation occurs with the freedom from a preconceived set of expectations, allowing the energy of transformation to be creatively mobilized toward practical ways of doing and being in the world that support growth. Inquiry projects that encompass reflection and participation support "generative theorizing" wherein action and knowledge are simultaneously informed.[3,6] The reflection inherent in UAI requires a critical and appreciative examination of one's own practices as well as an awareness of what maintains the status quo.[3] This is participatory both within the individual and within the collective. The generative capacity of praxis[3] allows for the development of propositional knowledge (theory), experiential knowledge (group encounters and endeavors), presentational knowledge (imaginative and creative ways of comprehending life patterning and illuminating new possibilities), and practical knowledge (actions or practices that evolve from the first 3 ways of knowing and that advance change and transformation).[25] The foundation of UAI as praxis lies in the core process components of appreciation, participation, and emancipation.[1]

Appreciation

Appreciative knowing incorporates "perceiving, being aware of, sensitive to, and expressing the full force and delicate distinctions"[11(p130)] of life pattern[ing] through an attitude of gratefulness. Appreciation implies an empathy or resonance of the perceiver with the pattern perceived as it manifests in its entirety.[6,8] As a healing practice, the focus is on appreciating the wholeness within this pattern. In UAI, pattern is appreciated through the intimacy of the encounter with self and other.[5,6]

Appreciating is the antithesis of essentializing.[6] Essentializing implies stereotyping or generalizing, whereas appreciation in UAI refers to the deliberate process of seeking out of that which is unique for the individual or group. Essence, the root of essentializing, is a static phenomenon. This is in direct contrast to the appreciation of life patterns as ever-changing and fluid in their relationship between the individual and the cosmos. When essence is referred to in UAI, it implies the dynamic flux of patterning expressed through one's life versus a more static dimension of phenomena.[7]

In the work of Cowling[5,6] with despairing women, the appreciation as praxis evolved in 4 directions. Describing what worked, reflecting on adversity and power, envisioning possibilities, and contemplating life patterning as an informational resource for change were the foci of appreciation for participants because they reflected upon wholeness in their lives. These 4 dimensions have become the structural framework for the development and sustainability of a healing process that potentially exists within UAI projects.

Encouragement and support through journaling, dialogue, and creativity are provided to illuminate the ways in which participants have known or felt personal power, made positive life changes, or influenced others.[5,6] Individual and/or mutual reflection provides opportunities for understanding the relationship between personal power, life choices, and personal sustenance in the midst of adversity. Dreaming or imaging of new possibilities is accomplished through creative expression, collages, imagining, imagery, writing, and dialogue. Goals or desired outcomes may be written, expressed, drawn, or performed. Outcomes are not static representations of what is expected to occur but rather a suggestive delineation of the possibilities of what could occur. Contemplation of life patterning through these techniques can provide a source of information for both individuals and groups about what currently exists and the desire for knowing transformation and change.

Unitary appreciative knowing is distinct but informed by an understanding of appreciative knowing in organizational life described by Cooperrider and Srivastva.[29] Appreciative knowing is distinct from critical knowing. Appreciative knowing assumes a stance of mystery that can never be fully known. Critical knowing seeks to answer a question or problem. In UAI, the mystery is something to be caught up in rather than a problem to be solved. Knowledge cannot be categorized with diagnoses or language. The researcher is an inquirer who comes into relationship with the coinquirers through an act of affirmation based on mutual trust in the absolute integrity of universal wholeness. Thus, UAI as praxis is a theoretical precept of wholeness, a research method centered on the appreciation of inherent wholeness in human life as expressed in patterning. Unitary appreciative inquiry has as its primary agenda to discover and explore human wholeness through appreciation aspiring to find practical ways of transforming life patterning through knowing participation in change.

Participation

The concept of participation in UAI is as much a metaphysical stance as a method of inquiry.[7,4,27] There is the assumption of a participatory consciousness in which each person has a personal relationship with the universe in UAI.[7] As an inquirer-participant, each individual is a direct participant in the cocreation of the cosmos. In unitary nursing and research, this is reflected in mutual relationship, an openness to discovery without preconceptions, negotiation of process, and the release of predicted or proscribed outcomes.[8,7] The human capacity for knowing participation in change and patterning is a central tenet of unitary theory. The participant is considered as the expert on and the author of his or her own life in UAI. Change may be the outcome of knowing participation; however, the researcher/practitioner releases the *expectation* of change for the participant.[8,7]

The relationship of pattern, participation, power, and praxis to knowledge generation was elaborated in a matrix model by Cowling.[6] Participation is described as engagement, shared reflection, cooperation, and dialogue that contributes to sensemaking through experiential knowledge.[6] The mutuality of participation inspires and encourages imagery generation and creative expression for presentational knowledge. Propositional knowledge arises from and is grounded in the mutual reflection inherent in a participatory design. Also, practical knowledge is developed as skills through participation in the inquiry process.[6]

Participation can be between individuals and the researcher or between groups and the researcher. A number of studies focused on experiences in women's lives, including despair and abuse, have demonstrated the capacity for UAI to create a participatory context for women to share life experiences, examine the wholeness of lives, discover life patterning, and consider and, in some cases, experiment with practical strategies for change. Individual and group inquiries require the creation of time and space that offers safety and comfort to share experiences. In a group encounter, there is opportunity for dialogue and creation of social space that leads to clarification and elaboration of information, formulation of both common and individual impressions and perceptions, and the consideration of collective action based on shared understandings.[5,27]

Emancipation

Cowling[7] makes a case for UAI as both interpretive and emancipatory. Hermeneutic inquiry is the exemplar of the interpretive paradigm of nursing science. The ontological assumptions of both UAI and the interpretive paradigm include a complex, holistic, and contextual reality.[30] However, the goal of UAI is not to understand and interpret the meaning of human experiences. Rather, it seeks to illuminate the inherent wholeness and uniqueness of human life through discovering and understanding the patterning that expresses that life. The purpose of this illumination, discovery, and understanding is to provide a referent point for nursing knowledge development that is both theoretical and practical. Human life is meant to encompass the wholeness of individuals, groups, families, or communities. Emancipation arises from the praxis nature of

UAI as a potential, rather than as a specified, end point similar to what is seen in critical inquiry approaches. However, the agenda of UAI is distinctive from the critical inquiry paradigm, although sharing common interests and concerns. Emancipation is also a function of newly perceived possibilities, visionary innovations, and personal explorations that emerge from fully engaging others in the appreciative process.

Praxis through power is also a feature of emancipation.[6] Power is experienced through the experiential component of UAI as a result of being in process with other(s) in the inquiry. Power lies in the creative expressions of an appreciated life. The propositional or theory generating capacity of UAI lends power to participants through expanding knowledge and also creates a venue in which their voices are heard through research and activism within the community. And finally, through the UAI process practical skills are developed that support emancipation.

Concerns and Challenges: Refinements

Several concerns and challenges have arisen during the evolution of UAI over the past decade. These have led to significant refinements in the UAI method associated with assumptions and conceptual underpinnings, data generation approaches, data synopsis, and credibility and legitimacy standards.

Assumptions and Conceptual Underpinnings

Unitary appreciative inquiry is grounded in the science of unitary human beings[24] and was developed to offer a method for researchers interested in generating and testing theories derived from that conceptual system. The linkages to the unitary conceptual system have been made explicit through the pattern appreciation, case study, and UAI stages of evolution. The developments and refinements of UAI have consistently been shaped considering the compatibility of method choices with the assumptions and conceptualization of a unitary perspective. The assumptions and conceptual underpinnings need to be made more explicit reflecting current theoretical developments in unitary science.

The 4 general assumptions and conceptual underpinnings derived specifically from the science of unitary human beings on which UAI is based are as follows:

1. Humans are essentially and inherently whole unified beings—derived from humans as energy fields.

2. Human life coexists and emerges through its relationship and participation with the environment—derived from human-environment mutual process.

3. Human life expresses itself in patterning that can be known through its manifestations, some directly and some indirectly sensed—derived from human as energy field pattern.

4. Human life has infinite potentials for expansion, growth, health, and well-being—derived from pandimensionality and unpredictability as the nature of change.

The assumptions and conceptual underpinnings refined and specified to serve as a broader foundation for UAI are as follows:

1. Individuals, groups, families, and communities are characterized by inherent wholeness that takes the form of a unique patterning.

2. The patterning of human wholeness is reflected in a variety of phenomena that provide information about the patterning but cannot singularly represent fully the nature of patterning. These phenomena include those labeled as physical/physiological, mental/emotional, social/cultural, and spiritual/mystical.

3. The patterning of human wholeness is signified by experiences, perceptions, and expressions of human life conceptualized as life patterning.

4. The unitary appreciation of life patterning involves the elucidation, affirmation, comprehension, and representation of the factors and forces within individuals and groups that serve to nourish human living and well-being.

5. Unitary appreciation of life patterning is a form of knowing participation in change that leads toward transformation and emancipation of those involved.

6. Unitary appreciative inquiry creates a participatory context from which to launch and sustain projects that seek to answer questions, address issues and concerns, and generate and test theories regarding human wholeness and life patterning. It also creates the context for the exploration of strategies that use a unitary appreciation of life patterning as a reference point for promoting health and well-being for individuals and groups.

In addition to providing a research method that is compatible with unitary science, the method might serve researchers seeking to understand life patterning from a perspective of wholeness. These assumptions and conceptual underpinnings are meant to clarify the relevance of UAI for directing and guiding projects. These also serve to differentiate UAI from other qualitative and participatory methods such as grounded theory, phenomenology, ethnography, and participatory action research.

Data Generation

Data generation methods are chosen on the basis of the purpose and research questions of the study as with any research approach. Previous researchers using UAI have relied heavily on dialogical engagement with participants in interviews or group encounters as a source of generating data. These dialogical engagements have been focused on the primary research question and related content with varying degrees of structure. For one of the studies on despair in women, the advertisement for recruiting participants set the stage by having as the lead: "Despair: Your Story?"[5] Participants were interviewed individually and engaged in a dialogue with the interviewer. The initial interview question was, "What is it like to have despair in your life?" A series of suggested questions was used as a guide. These questions included topics related to the experience of despair, how it manifested itself in the life of the person and in their relationships, the ways in which despair may have enhanced or limited the person's life, things learned from having a life in which despair was central, remedies and treatments of and challenges of a despairing life, experiences in the healthcare system, and life changes and transformations that might have occurred in association with despair. These questions were grounded in the purpose of the study that explored the life patterning of women with despair.

In addition to the dialogical engagement, researchers have used a variety of approaches for generating data relevant to the life patterning of individuals or a group. In some cases, researchers have asked participants to create aesthetic products that reflect their life patterning, to write a chapter representing what might transpire in their lives,[19] to engage in a guided dreaming experience,[20,21] to create a collage storyboard that shows their life experience, to identify a character from a play, novel, or movie or a piece of music that reflects their life patterning, and to create a symbol, image, or photograph or share an object that represents the way life is experienced. In many cases, researchers have combined data generation strategies. Although thus far all data generation strategies have been qualitative in nature, depending on the purpose of the project, quantitative data may offer information highly relevant to life patterning.

Some guiding principles for data generation include the following:

1. Ideal sources of data are ones that have the greatest potential for capturing the fullest and richest picture possible of life patterning.

2. Given the perspective of the uniqueness of life patterning for those experiencing it, approaches that rely on the perspective of the person or group of people are most desirable.

3. Critical to the efficiency of data generation is the need to explore sources of data that are most parsimonious in providing the linkages necessary to portray life patterning, that is, building a compelling case for data as indicators of life patterning.

4. Data generation approaches that synthesize life patterning information (such as narratives and symbolic representations) will assist in the movement from data to interpretation of data in a synoptic format.

5. Involving participants in identifying data sources and approaches to securing data is advantageous, considering the strong participatory strand within UAI and the attempt to reach an appreciative understanding of life patterning.

6. Data generation to portray life patterning relies upon an inclusive stance of what counts as pattern information and often goes beyond what is observable or directly sensed.

Data Synopsis

Unitary appreciative inquiry relies on a synoptic perspective for considering information generated in projects. The synoptic perspective is derived from the idea of synoptic empiricism[31] described by Murphy[32] in his groundbreaking work synthesizing knowledge related to human transformation. According to Broad, "Synopsis is the deliberate viewing together of aspects of human experience which for one reason or another, are generally kept apart by the plain man and even by the professional scientist or scholar."[31(p8)] Recently, Purnell[33] and Schoenhofer[34] have referred to synoptic knowing as a defining feature of the discipline of nursing reflecting its unitary nature. They cite the work of Phenix, which describes the integrative function of synoptic meanings that creates a pathway to "uniting meanings from all the realms into a unified perspective, that is, providing a single vision."[35(p235)]

Unitary appreciative inquiry employs synopsis as the primary approach to considering the various data generated in a project. The goal of synopsis in UAI is to sense an emerging pattern that reflects the wholeness and uniqueness of human life.[5,6] Thus, data such as experiences, perceptions, and expressions of the participants as well as phenomena that are categorized as physical/physiological, mental/emotional, social/cultural, and spiritual/mystical are viewed together in an inclusive way. It is not necessary to collect all these types of data, but these data may provide indicators of human life patterning. In many cases, data generation

approaches themselves are synoptic, such as asking a person to write a story that reflects their lives or create a collage of images and words.

While data may be collected across the spectrum of forms of phenomena, the critical feature of synopsis is to search for the connections, themes, commonalities, and relationships among the data.[7] In 1993, Cowling[14] differentiated systems knowing and unitary knowing. This differentiation was recently updated conveying how a systems perspective and unitary perspective are contrasted in gathering and using information. In a systems perspective, the focus is on the parts (physical/physiological, emotional/mental, spiritual/mystical, social/cultural) to make sense of the whole. In a unitary perspective, the focus is on considering all observations and information as unique expressions of the life patterning of human wholeness. This requires that the researcher appreciate "each area of information and observations as an expression of wholeness—not as an expression of subsystems or parts."[1(p85)] Researchers are challenged to develop approaches that give a greater emphasis to synopsis and synthesis rather than analysis. This will require "creative ways of organizing information and observations to be able to see the patterning beyond the parts."[1(p85)]

Credibility and Legitimacy

Issues of credibility and legitimacy were addressed in the early stages of unitary pattern appreciation following general tenets of qualitative research such as member checking, auditing, and peer review.[11] Later, in describing UAI, standards of credibility of research and legitimacy of knowledge were suggested using the perspective of Ford-Gilboe and her colleagues[36] because they were described as transcending paradigm boundaries. They identified 4 issues in evaluating the quality of research: "(1) quality of data; (2) investigator bias; (3) quality of the research process; and (4) usefulness of the study findings."[36(p23)] Since UAI has interpretive and emancipatory strands, interpretive phenomenology and critical inquiry standards were considered and modified because UAI is clearly not the same as these 2 methods. The gold standards for each of the methods were presented and then approaches to achieving these standards in UAI were provided.

While the standards and approaches originally provided remain relevant, additional refinements have occurred from using UAI for a variety of projects. These refinements relate directly to enhancing the unitary, appreciative, participatory, and emancipatory strands of UAI:

1. The quality of data is considered in terms of how well the data chosen give the fullest and most comprehensive picture of wholeness as expressed

in life patterning, whether the data provide inclusive and synoptic information for researcher appreciation of the life patterning, the degree to which the data generation incorporates the perspective of the person or group that is the focus of the research, and the extent to which the data bring clarity to the potential in life patterning for greater freedom.

2. Investigator bias is considered in terms of how well the researcher prepares himself or herself to sense patterning within human wholeness, how sensitive the researcher is in appreciating all that is uncovered, how vigilant the researcher is in using and integrating perspectives of participants, and how attentive the researcher is in generating data that identify the oppressive and liberating qualities of life patterning.

3. Quality of the research process is considered in terms of the use of design and procedures developed to capture life patterning in human wholeness, use of data generation processes that create an appreciating orientation to sense life patterning in individuals and groups, use of research protocol that enhance participation of coinquirers across all stages of the inquiry process, and use of strategies aimed at creating an inquiry that is responsive to the liberating inclinations of the participants.

4. Usefulness of findings is considered in terms of the ability of the research to elucidate life patterning to provide information for desired change, the capacity of the research to generate knowledge that expands the appreciation of life patterning, and the potential of the research to explicate the ways in which participatory knowing supports development of important knowledge and skills relevant to transforming life patterning.

5. The emancipatory intent of UAI requires attention to the support and promotion of the liberation of participants. Findings are considered on the basis of the possibilities of the research to illuminate the ways in which knowledge of life patterning can lead to emancipatory changes in the lives of the participants. Standards might include the capacity of the design to release constraints on the fullest self-expression of participants and the potential of the research to support and sustain conditions of human uplifting.

Conclusions and Expanding Potentials

The development and evolution of UAI since 1990 has provided for the exploration of life patterning and human wholeness in the context of a number of nursing studies. The use of UAI in these studies, the dialogue among UAI scholars, and the ongoing examination and critique of UAI have led to further elaborations and refinements. Three areas of potential future expansion are in the realm of extended epistemologies, the integration of aesthetics into the process of inquiry and representation of human wholeness, and the development of a unitary theory of healing.[1]

One of the primary aims of UAI is to generate multiple forms of knowledge relevant to human wholeness and life patterning. Unitary appreciative inquiry employs unitary, appreciative, and participatory ways of knowing that take shape and form in synoptic knowing reflecting the patterning of the whole.[6] Recently, the examination of emancipatory knowing in nursing offers the potential for integrating more precisely this way of knowing into UAI processes. Borrowing from participatory research in general and cooperative inquiry in particular, several UAI researchers have used experiential, presentational, propositional, and practical forms of knowledge to organize findings from their studies.[25] The major challenge for future development is the construction of findings into forms of knowledge that describe and explain the dynamic nature of life patterning and wholeness without resorting to categorical representations. One potential resolution is for researchers to convey the interrelatedness of the forms of knowledge used to present the findings. Another is to rely upon aesthetic representations such as plays, digital and other forms of storytelling, dances, performances, and exhibits.

Unitary appreciative inquiry researchers have relied heavily on aesthetic forms of data generation as well as aesthetic representations of human wholeness and life patterning. There is an apparent and compelling argument for the inclusion of aesthetics into UAI, given its potential to obtain more unitary information from participants and its ability to portray the unitary nature of life patterning. There is need for further consideration and expansion of aesthetics into the design of UAI projects. A recent dialogue among students and staff at the University of Bournemouth generated expanding potential and examples of aesthetic approaches that could be used in UAI to reveal wholeness in human life patterning. Critical reflection and examination are required to explain and clarify the relationship of aesthetics and unitary knowing.

Finally, researchers and participants have alluded to transformation and healing that are often observed and experienced in the conduct of UAI projects. Early explication of healing as appreciating wholeness recognized this potential within unitary pattern appreciation.[8] More recently, a unitary healing praxis model for women in despair was formulated on the basis of completed UAI projects.[3] An evolving unitary theory of healing that goes beyond any single group or population was suggested as having potential for general nursing practice.[1] According to Cowling and Repede, "Unitary healing is viewed as appreciating human wholeness through participating knowingly in emancipatory change and transformation."[1(p87)] The descriptions of UAI experiences by researchers and participants indicate that there is a realization of potentials for change and transformation through participating in the inquiry process. Perhaps unwittingly, UAI researchers, regardless of intent, may have unleashed the potential for unitary healing by the construction and conduct of their studies. This warrants further exploration as a benefit of participation in UAI studies.

REFERENCES

1. Cowling WR, Repede E. Consciousness and knowing: the patterning of the whole. In: Locsin RC, Purnell MJ, eds. *A Contemporary Nursing Process: The (Un)Bearable Weight of Knowing in Nursing*. New York, NY: Springer; 2009:73–98.
2. Cowling WR. An essay on women despair, and healing: a personal narrative. *Adv Nurs Sci*. 2008;3(3): 249–258.
3. Cowling WR. A unitary healing praxis model for women in despair. *Nurs Sci Q*. 2006;19(4):123–132.
4. Cowling WR. Despairing women and healing outcomes: a unitary appreciative nursing perspective. *Adv Nurs Sci*. 2005;28(2):94–106.
5. Cowling WR. Despair: a unitary appreciative inquiry. *Adv Nurs Sci*. 2004;27(4):287–300.
6. Cowling WR. Pattern, participation, praxis, and power in unitary appreciative inquiry. *Adv Nurs Sci*. 2004;27(3):202–214.
7. Cowling WR. Unitary appreciative inquiry. *Adv Nurs Sci*. 2001;23(4):32–48.
8. Cowling WR. Healing as appreciating wholeness. *Adv Nurs Sci*. 2000;22(3):16–32.
9. Cowling WR. A unitary-transformative nursing science: potentials for transcending dichotomies. *Nurs Sci Q*. 1999;12(2):132–135.
10. Cowling WR. Unitary case method. *Nurs Sci Q*. 1998;11(4):139–141.
11. Cowling WR. Unitary pattern appreciation: the unitary science/practice of reaching for essence. In: Madrid M, ed. *Patterns of Rogerian Knowing*. New York, NY: National League for Nursing; 1997:129–142.
12. Barrett EAM, Cowling WR, Carboni JT, Butcher HK. Unitary perspectives on methodological practices. In: Madrid M, ed. *Patterns of Rogerian Knowing*. New York, NY: National League for Nursing; 1997:47–62.
13. Cowling WR. Unitary practice: revisionary assumptions. In: Parker MS, ed. *Patterns of Nursing Theories in Practice*. New York, NY: National League for Nursing; 1993:199–212.
14. Cowling WR. Unitary knowing in nursing practice. *Nurs Sci Q*. 1993;6:201–207.
15. Cowling WR. A template for unitary pattern-based nursing practice. In: Barrett EA, ed. *Visions of Rogers' Science-Based Nursing*. New York, NY: National League for Nursing; 1990:45–65.
16. Alligood R. *The Life Pattern of People With Spinal Cord Injury* [dissertation]. Richmond: Virginia Commonwealth University; 2007.
17. Cox T. *Risk Induced Professional Caregiver Despair: A Unitary Appreciative Inquiry* [dissertation]. Richmond: Virginia Commonwealth University; 2004.
18. Duis-Nittsche ER. *A Study of Nursing Presence* [dissertation]. Galveston: The University of Texas Graduate School of Biomedical Sciences; 2002.
19. Kemp JE. *Women Deployed: Pattern Profiles of Women Who Served During the Persian Gulf War* [dissertation]. Denver: The University of Colorado Health Sciences Center; 2004.
20. Repede E. *Participatory Dreaming and Women Abused As Children: A Study of Unitary Healing* [dissertation]. Greensboro: The University of North Carolina; 2009.
21. Repede E. Participatory dreaming: a conceptual exploration from a unitary appreciative inquiry perspective. *Nurs Sci Q*. 2009;22(4):360–368.
22. Rushing AM. The unitary life pattern of persons experiencing serenity in recovery from alcohol and drug addiction. *Adv Nurs Sci*. 2008;31(3):198–210.
23. Talley B, Rushing A, Gee RM. Community assessment using Cowling's unitary appreciative inquiry: a beginning exploration. *Visions*. 2005;1(1):27–40.
24. Rogers ME. Nursing science and the space age. *Nurs Sci Q*. 1992;5:27–33.
25. Heron J, Reason P. The practice of co-operative inquiry: research "with" rather than "on" people. In: Reason P, Bradbury H, eds. *Handbook of Action Research: Participative Inquiry and Practice*. Thousand Oaks, CA: Sage; 2001:179–188.
26. Barrett EAM. A nursing theory of power for nursing practice: derivation from Rogers' paradigm. In: Riehl-Sisca JP, ed. *Conceptual Models for Nursing Practice*. 3rd ed. Norwalk, CT: Appleton-Century-Crofts; 1989:207–217.
27. Reason P, Bradbury H. Introduction: inquiry and participation in search of a world worthy of aspiration. In: Reason P, Bradbury H, eds. *Handbook of Action Research: Participative Inquiry and Practice*. Thousand Oaks, CA: Sage; 2001:1–14.
28. Newman MA. The pattern that connects. *Adv Nur Sci*. 2002;24(3):1–7.
29. Cooperrider DL, Srivastva S. Appreciative inquiry in organizational life. *Res Org Change Dev*. 1987;1:129–169.
30. Monti EJ, Tingen MS. Multiple paradigms of nursing science. *Adv Nurs Sci*. 1999;21(4):64–80.
31. Broad CD. *Religion, Philosophy and Psychical Research*. New York, NY: Harcourt Brace & Co; 1953.
32. Murphy M. *The Future of the Body: Explorations Into the Further Evolution of Human Consciousness*. San Francisco, CA: Tarcher Press; 1992.
33. Purnell MJ. Phoenix arising: synoptic knowing for a synoptic practice of nursing. In: Purnell MJ, Locsin RC, eds. *A Contemporary Nursing Process: The (Un)Bearable Weight of Knowing in Nursing*. New York, NY: Springer; 2009:3–16.
34. Schoenhofer SO. Transcending boundaries: nursing—a synoptic discipline? In: Purnell MJ, Locsin RC, eds. *A Contemporary Nursing Process: The (Un)Bearable Weight of Knowing in Nursing*. New York, NY: Springer; 2009:17–30.
35. Phenix PH. *Realms of Meaning: A Philosophy of the Curriculum for General Education*. New York, NY: McGraw-Hill; 1964.
36. Ford-Gilboe M, Campbell JC, Berman H. Stories and numbers: coexistence without compromise. *Adv Nurs Sci*. 1995;18(1):14–26.

THE AUTHORS COMMENT | **Unitary Appreciative Inquiry: Evolution and Refinement**

I was inspired to write this article because I wanted to articulate more precisely and clearly the nature and practice of unitary appreciative inquiry in its most contemporary form. The inclusion of the perspective of Elizabeth Repede was central to this work as she did a systematic integrated review of unitary appreciative inquiry for her dissertation research. I also sought to highlight her work and the work of others that contributed to the evolution of unitary appreciative inquiry. I believe the major contribution of this article to nursing theory is that it demonstrates the potential of unitary appreciative inquiry for advancing a science of nursing grounded in a unitary transformative theoretical perspective.

W. RICHARD COWLING III
ELIZABETH REPEDE

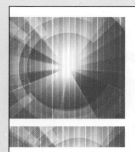

Philosophies of Nursing Science in Research

This unit presents a variety of philosophic perspectives about science embraced within nursing and found to be useful in research. The chapters present clear and stimulating writing about a complex topic of knowledge development. A wide variety of philosophic perspectives are addressed, all of which have been used in nursing research and theory development. These philosophies include critical realism, neopragmatism, postcolonialism, Eastern and Western nursing philosophies, as well as other interpretive views and post-positivism. They are lenses for transcending and then reflecting on the immediate context to evaluate one's research or clinical practice.

The chapter authors also present ideas about how to use these philosophies. They pose arguments about best philosophic approaches for research or theory development. This unit not only informs readers about the various philosophies, but it also stimulates discussion questions relevant to the knowledge-building process.

QUESTIONS FOR DISCUSSION

- What philosophical views do you embrace? What views do you have difficulty accepting or understanding?

- Should the nurse's focus or approach in inquiry be congruent with the nurse's philosophy (personal beliefs about human health, the environment, and nursing)? If it is important, why, and if it is not important, why not?

- Use the readings in this and other units to extend descriptions of research-based knowledge beyond what is solely "empirical."

- What guidelines do philosophies of nursing science offer for judging the trustworthiness of qualitative research?

- In your opinion, should multiple perspectives be entertained in one's research, or are certain philosophies more useful than others to nursing?

- Using DeGroot's guidelines and the ideas on *epistemology* from Unit 5 and on *nursing ontology* from Unit 8, can you articulate your own philosophy of nursing science?

Complex Critical Realism
Tenets and Application in Nursing Research

ALEXANDER M. CLARK, RN, PhD, BA(Hons)
SUE L. LISSEL, MA
CAROLINE DAVIS, PhD

Aim: To outline the main tenets of critical realism (CR), its use, and future application in nursing. **Background:** Little work has been done to discuss how CR can be applied to nursing research. **Findings:** The tenets of CR include recognition of reality independent of human perceptions, a generative view of causation in open systems, and a focus on explanations and methodological eclecticism using a postdisciplinary approach. Critical realism is useful for (1) understanding complex outcomes, (2) optimizing interventions, and (3) researching biopsychosocial pathways. Such questions are central to evidence-based practice, chronic disease management, and population health. **Conclusions:** Critical realism is philosophically strong and potentially useful for nursing research. **Key words:** *framework, nursing research, ontology, philosophy, realism, realist, theory*

Although method and design are important, it is vital to reflect on the assumptions about reality that can and do underpin method. Failing to do so or relying on unsupported "common sense" arguments can result in work that lacks wider credibility, is inadequately justified, or even lacks internal coherence.[1]

Over the last decade, the metatheory known as critical or complex realism (CR) has emerged in Europe as a promising basis for theorizing in the human sciences, including nursing.[2–4] However, far less work has examined the theoretical application of CR in research studies. The aim of this article is to identify the types of research questions relevant to nursing to which CR has appropriate application. To do this, the article identifies the main tenets of CR, discusses previous work in nursing guided by CR, and considers the wider uses of CR for nursing research.

The origins of CR lie with philosopher Roy Bhaskar, whose early work addressed what reality must be like for science to be possible.[5] This work criticized positivist accounts of the natural sciences that emphasized the existence of universal law-like explanations for phenomena and a view that research was based only on what could be observed.[6] A number of influential academics, such as Wittgenstein, Popper, Kuhn, and Feyerabend, also attacked this positivistic approach to science.[5] Yet, the natural conclusions of these critiques were often problematic variations of relativism, a sense that not only knowledge development was a social process but also knowledge itself was relative to the perspective of the individual. As a consequence, arguments based on reason could not resolve competing claims to knowledge.[5] It was not clear who or what could determine what was true and, indeed, whether the very notion of truth itself was legitimate.

Currently, these initial arguments appear polarized and narrow. Bhaskar presented a direct critique of positivism as an epistemology that viewed the world as being overly uniform and "reduced to the ways in which we know it."[7(p254)] He argued that human perceptions of the world (epistemology) could not be synonymous with the world's objective state (ontology).[5] Proponents of relativism argued for the centrality and unacknowledged role of language in research and critiqued the claims of Western science to truth as being unjustifiably universalistic and dogmatic.[7] Other perspectives, such as idealism, sought some middle ground through claims that the objects to which science refers are not fully objective but are consensual models that are not determined by the mind of any one individual.[5]

The challenges of engaging with these arguments are evident in the health sciences.[8,9] Debate is mired in different labels and subtle variations. Positivism has been called objectivism, empiricism, or universalism and can be discussed generically or taken to be synonymous with a specific school, such as logical positivism. Similarly, relativism has been used interchangeably with terms such as *constructivism, perspectivism, intepretivism,* or *antifoundationalism;* it also has a number of variations, including cognitive or epistemic relativism (the claim that truth is relative to an individual or groups) and moral relativism (the claim that moral principles are relative to settings).

ABOUT THE AUTHORS

ALEXANDER M. CLARK is a Professor in the Faculty of Nursing at the University of Alberta in Canada. He grew up in the United Kingdom, obtaining his PhD from the Department of Nursing and Community Health, Glasgow Caledonian University, United Kingdom. His work uses critical realism to explain and understand health outcomes and involves qualitative and quantitative methods and systematic review—mostly in the field of cardiovascular disease. This research has guided health policy and guidelines on both sides of the Atlantic. In his spare time he enjoys being with his wife and children; supporting, coaching, and sometimes playing soccer; and reading.

SUE L. LISSEL is a health services researcher and a member of the faculty of nursing at the University of Alberta in Canada. **CAROLINE DAVIS** is a Medical Anthropologist as well as a researcher in the faculty of nursing at the University of Alberta in Canada.

Both Sue Lissel and Caroline Davis were researchers who worked with Clark on a series of research projects drawing on critical realism. These studies sought to explain why some people with heart disease engage in more healthy behaviors (and some people do not); why some patients consume their medications (and some patients do not); and how to improve health in indigenous populations.

Debate in nursing has not sufficiently recognized some of these distinctions or has fallen too readily into polarized arguments framed by discredited forms of relativism[3] or stereotypical views of positivism.[9] However, although researchers are unlikely to claim positions that reflect more extreme versions of positivism and relativism,[10] these positions can be adopted implicitly. They are reflected not only in the positions researchers overtly claim to hold but also in what they do with, and the claims they make, for data. Positivist assumptions can be made when researchers overly generalize from data,[11] such as when extrapolating findings from data generated in a small region to a diverse country. Relativistic assumptions are reflected when researchers assign an objective truth value on human perspectives[8]; for example, when lay perceptions of a disease are viewed as being synonymous with the disease itself.

That said, there are merits of variations of positivism and relativism to nursing. Positivism points to the possibility of wider knowledge of the world that can be developed and built systematically through research. This resonates with nursing as a discipline that is informed by knowledge from the natural and human sciences.[3] Conversely, relativism points to the centrality of human experiences, social and cultural constructs, values, perspectives, and language. This connects with nursing as a discipline that focuses with sensitivity and respect on individual holism, patient advocacy, communities, and context.[3]

Complex realism emerged as a wider attempt to harness the strengths and address the weaknesses of positivism, idealism, and relativism. It acknowledges the possibility of science but recognizes the social dimensions of humans and science in a manner that does not fall into problematic versions of relativism or positivism. Taking the middle ground, it does not reduce the world to unknowable chaos or a positivistic universal order, nor does it place objective truth value on the perspectives of human beings or remove the influence and importance of human perspectives. These characteristics are evident in the following overview of its main tenets.

The Existence of Independent Social and Physical Reality: Reconciling the Objective and Subjective Values

Complex realism views physical and social entities as having an independent existence irrespective of human knowledge or understanding. Although social structures and phenomena exist as a product of the existence of human beings (eg, class, culture, or discrimination), these entities are seen to be as independent of individual human beings as physical entities. Structures also exist and exercise power irrespective of whether this is known or recognized by individual humans. For example, gender-based discrimination may exist in an organization whether or not it is recognized by management or workers.

This stance can still incorporate human meaning and experiences (the hermeneutical dimension) and recognize that these can influence behavior and sometimes wider social structures.[12] However, human social processes and perceptions (including science), as with physical phenomena, are fallible and perspectival, that is, discourse around or perceptions of social phenomena and science are not synonymous with objective truth. Judgments regarding the accuracy of these accounts should be made with recourse to other arguments or available data.[12]

Consider, for example, a patient with colon cancer who sincerely believes he or she does not have cancer and acts accordingly.[8] In CR terms, the individual can be judged to be wrong on the basis of recourse to wider evidence, such as the results of pathology tests, professionals' opinions, and symptoms conventionally recognized to signal the disease.[8] It remains important, especially to nursing, that the patient's representation of his or her condition has intrinsic subjective value. This is likely, for example, to influence the patient's emotions and disease management. However, in epistemological terms, other evidence indicates that the patient is highly likely to be wrong. Hence, the perspectives of the patient, professionals, and those derived from other data make claims to truth, which like those from witnesses in a courtroom trial, have to be reconciled, weighed, and ultimately judged regarding their reliability and what they say about reality. Here, then, is an acknowledgment of the value of multiple data sources relating to the same phenomena as well as a recognition of the need to reconcile these perspectives and any claims made against each other.

A Stratified Emergent Generative Ontology: Understanding Reality and Causation

Bhaskar[5] argued that for experiments to be possible, underlying structures, powers, and processes must act together under certain circumstances to influence observable events. These underlying phenomena are as real as the observable effects and outcomes they cause. Reality is divided or *stratified* into 3 domains: the actual (events and actions that are more likely to be observed), the real (underlying powers, tendencies, and structures whether exercised or not that cause events in the actual domain), and the empirical (fallible human perceptions and experiences, including science).

For example, a high school physics experiment involves the artificial creation of a vacuum around a ringing electronic bell. Upon creation of the vacuum, the "ringing" bell can be seen but no longer heard. This, the physics teacher would ensure, provides knowledge of the processes underlying the progression of sound and light through the earth's atmosphere. Hence, in the experiment described, the sound and the movement of the bell occur in the actual domain. The changes observed when the vacuum is created point to the underlying nature of the unseen structures and processes of the progression of sound and light through air in the real domain.

Finally, human perceptions and interpretations of both of these realms are in the empirical domain.

Two further concepts are relevant here. *Transfactuality* refers to the frequent misalignment of the actual, real, and empirical domains. Human perceptions in the empirical domain are fallible representations of the real and actual domains that are prone to incompleteness and inaccuracy in perception and inference. Students' experiences and inferences from the bell jar experiment can and may well differ. Similarly, scientists' ways of understanding and explaining phenomena such as the motions and forces guiding the earth's atmosphere have been and continue to be revised over centuries. Dimensions of the empirical domain should never be taken to be synonymous with those in the actual or the real domain. For example, sound and light traveled through the earth's atmosphere in the same ways before humans knew or devised experiments to explore this. Phenomena in the real domain may not be visible or exercise influence on the actual domain at any one point in time.[5] Yet, under the right circumstances, the power of these structures in the real domain can become active and influential.

Complex realism also offers an *emergent* ontology. *Emergence* is defined as "a relationship between two features or aspects such that one arises out of the other ... [but] remains causally and taxonomically irreducible to it."[13(p63)] In practice, this means entities can be classified hierarchically into strata at macro and micro levels. Although CR acknowledges that humans are composed of huge numbers of subatomic particles acting in accordance with principles of physics, humans can also be understood at higher levels, for example, at the cellular, chemical, biological, psychological, and various social levels. Phenomena occurring at these higher levels are dependent on those at lower levels for existence; humans can function only at the social level because they exist as cellular matter. However, the notion of emergence comes from the sense that the social emerges from, but is also conceptually distinct from and more than, an individual's cells, biology, or psychology. This approach indicates the social is "emergent, distinctive and non-reducible ... and thereby respects the autonomous logic of sociological theory."[14(p46)]

Phenomena within and between each of these levels can act together to create different phenomena that are irreducible to the underlying components. Water is composed of hydrogen and oxygen but is very different in nature from these 2 components in their isolated forms.[12] Yet, when these 2 elements come together in the right combination, a substance with very different properties emerges. Similarly, factors in the social realm can be causally influenced by a myriad of elements from the biological, geographical, and cultural factors but remain distinct from and irreducible to these other factors.

Finally, in CR terms, causation is not linear or successionist in the sense that event A must cause event B if A precedes B regularly[15]; that is, an approach that infers causation from regular sequences of events.[12,15] Rather, CR views events as being a product of many factors coming together in certain combinations and given the right circumstances or context to causally *generate* new events. Sayer summarizes the difference between these successionist and generative approaches as: "What causes something has nothing to do with the number of times we have observed it happening. Explanation depends instead on identifying causal mechanisms and how they work, and discovering if they have been activated and under what conditions."[12(p14)] To use another analogy, understanding of how a clock works is not based only on observation of the regular movement of its hands over time but necessitates a deeper examination to explore its underlying mechanics, the physics guiding these and possibly even the social meaning of the clock to different groups.[12] Hence, events in the actual domain are generated from complex interactions of factors in the real domain. To explain why phenomena occur, researchers therefore need to go beyond the surface of observable factors (the actual) to explore what is happening underneath (the real).

In the social realm, there is a high degree of flux within this generative model. Potentially small changes in underlying factors could have significant and large effects on the nature or the possibility of a certain event arising in the actual domain.[14] Hence, an event that appears to be straightforward and linear requires a distinct set of conducive circumstances and factors to align together in the right combination.

An Explanatory-Focused Open-Systems View: Understanding Deep Causation in a Complex World

Social phenomena occur in "open systems" rather than the artificially controlled "closed systems" of laboratory experiments. Complex realism wholeheartedly ascribes to the open nature of the social world in which numerous factors are present and interact in highly complex and variable ways over time and context.[12] Although humans can understand more about the world by trying to artificially control some of these factors in an experimental situations, this is not possible or desirable in social research owing to the difficulties of generalizing from closed to open systems.[15] Lawson,[16] writing on closed and open systems

in economics, views markets as being the epitome of complex open systems. He argues that mathematical modeling in economics is based on a closed-systems view that has had very limited success in explaining and preventing major economic events in the real world (an open system). Although economists may know some of the main components of economies and have a reasonable knowledge of how economies function, it is a step further to be able to understand at a deeper level how these interact to cause outcomes.

Healthcare researchers often examine correlates and predictors or describe patterns in data. Similar to economics,[13] efforts are devoted to evaluating interventions or developing more accurate predictions via increasingly sophisticated mathematical techniques such as structured equation modeling or multiregression.[17] However, this often occurs in preference to attaining a sufficient understanding of causes and mechanisms.[18,19] Event regularities are rare outside laboratory experiments and prone to all manner of other influences in the real world,[13] be these social, physical, or psychological in nature.[15] To understand outcomes and patterns, researchers still need to examine regularities in the world but search for explanations *beneath* these patterns to account for why they did or did not occur.

This does not reduce the world to chaos; rather, the world is complex and somewhat patterned. This notion is captured in the CR term "demi-regularity,"[13] which is

> the occasional, but less than universal, actualization of a mechanism or tendency over a definite region of time-space. The patterning observed will not be strict if countervailing factors sometimes dominate (but) ... there is evidence of relatively enduring and identifiable tendencies in play.[13(p204)]

Such tendencies are familiar to nursing—found in fields such as health inequalities, cardiovascular risk, patient infections, and health improvement programs—in which enduring and consistent patterns are evident but not always predictable or persistent.

To recap, to identify causes researchers need to understand outcome *patterns* not identify outcome *regularities*.[20] These patterns are not the product of a small number of entities but of a larger number of factors coming together to *generate* an outcome of interest. Complex realism challenges nursing research to address generative causation over or before developing other types of knowledge. For example, Clark et al[21] identified that low usage of health services is often correlated with a lack of patient transport facilities. Researchers adopting a successionist view could conclude that the low uses of health services are caused by a lack of transport. However, CR-driven research that has sought to explore this pattern in people who both followed and deviated from it identified that at a deeper level, usage patterns are caused by patient conceptions of the self, other comparable patients, and general heart diseases. These generate a lack of perceived benefit that in the absence of sufficiently accessible transport fails to outweigh the perceived costs of participation. The mechanisms linking service usage to transport are therefore complicated and involve mechanisms associated with self-identity, disease conceptions, and views of other people.

Recognition of Complex Agency and Structure Interactions

Complex realism, somewhat obviously, views the world as being complex. It draws attention to the primacy of the world in leading both conceptualization and method.[12] The logic of this is that because the world exists independently of human beings, those attempting to discover knowledge of the world need to ensure their conceptions minimize distortion of the actual domain. These conceptualizations are problematic; for example, if they: "divide what is in practice indivisible, or if they conflate what are different and separable components So much depends on the modes of abstraction we use, the way of carving up and defining our objects of study."[12(p19)] This position may seem self-evident, but arguably the social sciences are beset with poor categorization and impoverished abstraction.[12]

Complex realism advocates that both agency and structural factors and mechanisms cause events. This reflects long debate in the social sciences of the relative importance of individual ("agency") factors (such as beliefs, attitudes, and personal meanings) and contextual ("structural") factors (such as social norms, culture, geography, and environment)[22], as well as the argument that this weight of research must be taken into account. The influence of both of these types of factors is recognized in nursing. This may be due to nursing's long-standing holistic focus or the strength of evidence that both individual and contextual factors affect health.[23] However, there has been far less historical recognition of the influence and interplay of these factors in economics[13] and social science[24] in which debates have overemphasized one over the other. Yet, even in modern healthcare, a wealth of discourse around health maintenance, patient self-care, and "compliance" presupposes high levels of personal agency to the neglect of structural determinants.[17] Complex realism urges nursing research to address the nature and complex interplay of agency and structural factors.

Methodological Eclecticism and Postdisciplinary Study

All that is useful in explaining phenomena cannot be quantified.[13] The tenets of CR do not restrict researchers to adopt quantitative or qualitative approaches, or a particular method or disciplinary approach. Rather, researchers should acknowledge the complexity of the world and its open systems and let methodological choice be led by the nature of research question and the conceptualization of the phenomena under study.[12] That said, some researchers drawing on CR advocate a greater reliance on qualitative work,[12,13] whereas others argue for the contribution that mixed methods[25] or quantitative approaches can make,[26] for example, in cluster analysis[14] and regression analyses.[27]

Although this eclectic stance is now more accepted in nursing, this has not always been the case and mixed-method approaches are often argued for without resource to any underlying philosophical principles.[9]

Similarly, researchers from different disciplines seek to look beyond the conceptualizations and parameters of any one discipline[12] because approaches from a single discipline can lead to "disciplinary imperialism … reductionism, blinkered interpretations, and misattributions of causality."[12(p7)] This will ensure that conceptualizations are more responsive to the nature of the phenomena being examined rather than potentially narrow and loaded disciplinary perspectives and ideologies.[12] Although interdisciplinary research involving nursing is now well accepted politically and with funding bodies, CR offers a philosophical rationale for this approach. Moreover, via the notion of "postdisciplinary study,"[12] it challenges all researchers to focus on the phenomena being studied rather than disciplinary orientation.

Using CR to Inform Research: Research Questions

These tenets provide a basis for understanding reality and the world that has implications for research. Complex realism is congruent with the purposes and values of practice-based disciplines that must, by nature, address issues in the complex other.[28] However, this does not tell researchers when and how they can and should use CR as an underling to guide their inquiries. Although CR has methodological and theoretical implications, it does not itself constitute a method.[29]

To convey how CR can be applied throughout the research process, we now outline 3 main types of research areas of relevance to nursing that CR is particularly suited to and discuss how it can inform method in these areas.

Health Outcomes: Explaining Events in Contexts

Which policies lead countries to sustainable economic growth over the long term?[13]

Why are some crime prevention programs effective while others are not?[15]

How do health inequalities arise?[30]

Although these questions come from different disciplines and address different fields, at a more abstract level, they are similar and arise from the same criticisms.

For Lawson, economics has sought respectability via a reliance on mathematical modeling based on a successionist view of causation: "whenever x arises do y and event z will occur."[13(p5)] These models have tried to quantify all relevant factors, viewed these as operating in closed systems while giving scant attention to the assumptions about reality made in the models.[13] There has been a consistent lack of success of these models in predicting and identifying the causes of significant market events, such as stock market crashes.[13]

For Pawson and Tilley,[15] crime prevention programs have sought respectability via esteemed methods using closed-systems methods and successionist reasoning, such as the randomized controlled trial and quantitative meta-analysis. Reliance has been made on quantitative data, conceptualized in a simplistic manner, without attention to underlying assumptions about reality. Use of these methods has failed to yield generalizability of the benefits of effective programs in open systems and provided little insight into the complexities of what causes programs to be more or less effective.[15]

Epidemiological studies have historically been based principally on data collected on individuals and/or examined frequency and correlation rather than causation.[31] Attention has been drawn to the simplistic views of causation in health inequalities and epidemiological research.[32] More sophisticated epidemiological research has attempted to incorporate data on populations more overtly, most notably multilevel modeling. However, by a continued reliance on a relatively small number of quantified variables (albeit in large populations), the ability to discern what causes outcomes of interest (as opposed to correlates) and predict or change outcomes at the individual level is limited. Although some epidemiologists have now moved to examine causative mechanisms,[33] there is a continued pursuit of the identification of a small number of elusive pivotal explanations for data patterns,[14] underpinned with little theory[34] or sophisticated sense of causation.[14]

Hence, in each of these areas, to limited success, research has used an overly simplified and closed-systems view of reality that simultaneously relies heavily on quantification and avoids addressing the views of causation and reality that underpin inquiry. What are the lessons of this for nursing research? Although knowledge can be discovered of correlates and pattern regularities, this is of more limited practical utility than knowing what causes phenomena of interest and how to change these. Complex realism advocates that the complex causes of how and why changes in health or social factors occur need to be understood. This type of knowledge is prescriptively more useful. Understanding how, for example, dimensions of context (such as social and physical environments) and characteristics of the individual (including age, race, and sex) interact to influence health is an important step to designing interventions to improve health.

Complex realism-driven research has been applied in nursing care settings to understand the complex causes of racial discrimination[35] and practice change.[36,37] Briefly, this involves understanding how factors in the individual and the workplace setting interact to causally influence key behaviors, such as a nurse's practice. Tolson,[37] for example, drew on CR to inform a critical pathway for complex service evaluation and practice change in healthcare settings. Wilson and McCormack[36] used the approach to facilitate understanding of outcomes in local contexts and then to promote change. These studies use different data collection methods (ie, qualitative and quantitative data[37]) and data about different dimensions of the settings researched. For example, Wilson and McCormack[36] examined a nursing unit's culture via survey and participant observation before further clarifying questions and contradictions in the data with key informant interviews. However, both draw on CR to support the argument that the phenomenon they are researching is complex, is likely to be affected by the interplay of individual *and* contextual factors, and that understanding causes of variations in practice is key and should be prioritized over describing patterns of practice. In nursing research, these studies draw attention to the need to progress beyond measuring outcomes or examining correlates or superficial causes to identify the deeper and wider causes of outcomes (Figure 17-1).

Complex realism has application to areas of nursing in which understanding the nature and effects of interactions between individuals, health systems, and settings is important (Table 17-1). These represent some of the most important issues facing nursing and society including knowledge translation in practice settings, chronic disease management, and promoting health in the community and home. Because of current patterns in healthcare, moving to a more sophisticated understanding of the factors affecting key phenomena in these areas will be vital in the coming decades.

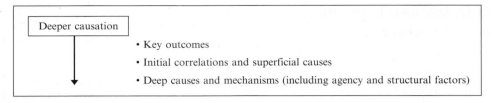

Figure 17-1 *Critical realist approach to deeper causation levels.*

Understanding and Improving Interventions

Why are cardiac rehabilitation programs so variable in effectiveness?[38]

Why do mandatory arrest policies for domestic violence increase violence?[39]

How can health be improved in areas of high social deprivation?[40]

Behavioral interventions and programs are important strategies to influence patterns of behavior. Neighborhood watch, mass-media health promotion campaigns, and cardiac rehabilitation programs are all examples of such initiatives. These are highly complex and multifaceted interventions that are very different from the tablets studied in pharmaceutical trials.[41]

Yet, in terms of evaluation, behavioral interventions are often evaluated on the basis of using the same successionist/closed-systems views of causation and methods (frequently randomized controlled trial) as trials of medications.[17] As a result, findings do not examine the influence of context,[28] often lack replicability of effect,[15] and cannot explain why any variability occurs.[38] As an alternate approach, CR-driven research directs researchers to understand "what works for whom, when and why"[15] and explore the complex ways in which interventions interact with people, professionals, and settings to cause different outcomes.

Complex realism-driven approaches around the evaluation of interventions have been used to examine nursing practice settings,[36,37] health behaviors,[38] and area-based health promotion.[42] This work draws mostly

TABLE 17-1	Possible Areas of Complex Realism-Driven Research in Healthcare		
Area	**Nursing issue**	**Desired outcome**	**Phenomena of interest**
Knowledge translation	Consistently low rates of evidence-based practice	Practice in accordance with best evidence/ clinical guidelines	Disciplines (S) Organizational characteristics (S) Local experts (S, HS) Clinical settings (S) Individual personality type, attitudes, beliefs, and knowledge (I)
Chronic disease management	Low compliance and ineffective self-management	Effectiveness of chronic disease management	Social capital, values, and norms (S) Health system characteristics (HS) Health services (HS) Professional interactions (S, I) Social support (S, I, HS) Caregivers (S, I, HS) Patient values, knowledge, embodiment, and attitudes (I)
Public health	Declining population health	Improved health-promoting and decreased health-harming opportunities and behaviors	Social capital, values, and norms (S) Places and communities (S) Health and social services (HS) Public attitudes, values, knowledge (I)

Abbreviations: HS: health system; I: individual; S: setting.

TABLE 17-2	**Understanding Interventions in Context**

1. Identify program/intervention/policy of interest
2. Specify key outcome and mediating behaviors
3. Explore and/or measure key outcomes and behaviors
4. Explore how program/intervention/policy of interest is causally linked to key outcomes and behaviors (ie, *mechanisms of effect*)
5. Explore how contextual factors affect mechanisms of effect
6. Identify key mechanism-context synergies linked to different outcomes and behaviors

Adapted from Pawson and Tilley.[15]

on the work of Pawson and Tilley[15] (Table 17-2), whose approach is to examine the effectiveness of interventions in a manner that is context acknowledging, focused on deep complex causation, and is prescriptively useful. The primary unit of study is likely to be a particular change-focused entity, such as a program, an intervention, or a policy. Although evaluations of these programs in the health sphere of ten measure "hard outcomes" such as mortality or morbidity, CR-driven approaches are appropriate when the outcome(s) of interest are determined by or are themselves behavioral. This grounds the program in open systems.

Pawson and Tilley[15] conceive behaviors in such systems as complex outcomes, produced from the ways in which programs come together with people to generate new choices and capacities. The power of the program is therefore not inherent in the program, people, or places, but in the ways the program works (mechanisms) for people in different contexts.

How then to do this empirically? Although conceptually examining these mechanisms would seem appropriate, doing so is challenging. Mechanisms can be inactive under some circumstances and have a large effect on an outcome with only a correspondingly small change in the mechanism. Moreover, mechanisms and contexts are likely to be in a degree of constant flux. It is easier to capture and measure outcomes because underlying mechanisms are difficult to conceptualize, identify, and explore.

Some argue that it is best to examine mechanisms using qualitative research[15,38]; others argue that "clues" to the nature and effects of mechanisms are accessible through analytical statistics.[26] Irrespective of competing claims, either or both can be used legitimately as long as the intention is to examine clues regarding complex causation.[12] However, relying solely on qualitative accounts (particularly of those directly involved in a program) runs the risk of ascribing primacy to subjective accounts. Conversely, relying on quantification may lead to important non-quantifiable or unexpected mechanisms to be missed.

The utility of CR arises from its constructive perspective regarding success and failure. Irrespective of whether programs have the desired effect, learning can occur on how the intervention works (or fails to) that can be used to improve effectiveness.

A small number of studies have examined nursing issues that use CR in this way. Bauld and Judge[42] and Bonner[43] describe the benefits of using a CR-driven evaluation approach to the evaluation of health action zones in the United Kingdom. These zones refer to community-wide projects in which local stakeholders work particularly closely together to address the health of local populations. A critique is therefore made of traditional experimental approaches to evaluation that fail to capture the complex dynamics of programs, populations, and settings—the understanding of which is essential to explaining program effects.[42]

Clark et al[38] examined variations in outcomes after cardiac rehabilitation, identifying that the mechanisms of effect of these programs were principally social and body related rather than related to program content or didactic information. Programs did not work through the information they provided about risk factor reduction but through patients' social experiences of the program and other participating patients and by affecting their embodied experiences of exercising. Programs generated considerable camaraderie among participants and this increased motivation and self-efficacy around exercise, particularly when patients experienced pushing their body to extremes they had not envisaged would be possible even prior to their cardiac event. However, exercise changes were not maintained if patients who experienced positive changes after rehabilitation (ie, these mechanisms were activated) did not then identify a context in which they could continue to exercise safely.

More recently, variations of this CR-driven approach to evaluation have been used to guide systematic reviews.[44] In this usage, it is the nature of key mechanisms that is seen to be more important in determining program effectiveness than the content or supposed objective characteristics of the intervention. Complex realist-driven systematic review examines family-based interventions across different fields, using the same key mechanisms.[44] Hence, name-and-shame policies in the disparate areas of pedophilia, property tax nonpayment, and television license evasion share a similar underlying mechanism that can be meaningfully analyzed, although the outcome behavior in each area is clearly different.[20]

With regard to future applications in nursing research, the mainstream evaluation of interventions remains dominated by randomized control trials and other variations of experimental methods. Yet, there is an emerging recognition that behavioral interventions related to health promotion or disease management require approaches that produce more than a dichotomous answer to the question of "does this work?" to examine the effects of context, implementation, and user perceptions and reactions in different sites. Efficacy is no longer viewed as being determined by a small number of dimensions of programs but by the complex interactions between people, places, and programs.

Areas of contemporary nursing research amenable to this approach relate to chronic disease management programs (eg, in relation to diabetes and heart disease), health services access, and promoting health improvement in vulnerable populations. In each of these areas, although knowledge exists about what actions should be employed in leading to effective management or better health, current approaches yield disappointingly inconsistent results while there is little understanding or generation of evidence as to how current approaches could be improved.

Toward Integrative Programs of Nursing Research: Understanding Biopsychosocial Pathways

What are the links among experiences of the body, biology, and behavior?[45]

Based on an emergent ontology, CR views biological matter as being necessary to the existence of psychosocial entities and structural phenomena. Emergent ontology suggests that causally important phenomena arise out of a combination of factors within and between different domains. Hence, biological factors (genetics, production of neurological chemicals, environment exposure) can combine to cause changes in the psychological domain (depression, anxiety, hostility). The influence of these factors coming together can also be modified by social circumstances (isolated spatial environment, lack of family network, partner support). The effects of this can be social (apathy, reduced social networks, aggression) or physical (reduced physical activity, violence to partner). Separate to all of this are people's experiences of both external (other people, services, places) and internal (such as views and experiences of the body) phenomena. In terms of complexity, this reflects the

so-called "butterfly effect" in which small changes in one factor could cause a much larger effect in a different domain.[14] In and between these systems, there is neither chaos nor order but complexity.[46]

This simplified account conveys the interdependency and complexity of these different systems that are familiar to practicing nurses but are very challenging to research. Many approaches to nursing have advocated that the discipline be based on philosophies that recognize the biological, social, and psychological dimensions of health, illness, and healing,[47] dimensions of human experience such as embodiment, the multiple determinants of health,[23] and the need to examine causal interactions between the individual and his or her environment. However, examining links in research among biological, social, and psychological factors is challenging. Few researchers are expert across these domains and measurement difficulties abound. Complex realism, however, offers a common approach through which researchers from different disciplines can work together with common language and approach to understand biopsychosocial phenomena. Consequently, although this area of CR inquiry is in its early stages, it offers great potential to nursing. First, biologists are comfortable with a vocabulary that makes references to mechanisms, outcomes, and environmental effects. With advances in gene mapping and increasingly large data sets and causally focused data-mining techniques, it is conceivable that researchers will be able to explore the sophisticated pathways that causally link genetics, biology, behavior, and psychosocial variables. As yet, there have been few attempts based on CR to address these multiple levels. To show the potential of research in this area, we discuss a recently funded CR project in the area of women's health.

Although it has been postulated that postpartum depression is linked to hormonal changes, no hormonal causes have been established.[48] Psychosocial predictors of postpartum depression have been identified including life stress, lack of social support, and socioeconomic disadvantage.[49] However, in CR terms, these may not be the actual causes of depression. Although depression before pregnancy predicts postpartum depression in around 50% of cases, even taking these other factors into account, it is unclear why some women with previous depression do not experience postpartum depression, whereas others do. Postpartum depression, therefore, appears to be the result of a complex and reciprocal interplay of underlying biological, psychological, and social causal factors that produce vulnerability to depression with specific contextual processes/circumstances and expressions of the clinical syndrome varying from woman to woman by context.[50] By examining causes of depression in women stratified by the presence or the absence of depression (ie, by varied outcomes), it is possible to explore how dimensions of context and mediating psychological mechanisms appear to influence mental health. Using semistructured interviews, clues regarding the possible mechanisms linking contextual and personal factors to the depression can be illuminated and investigated using future quantitative and qualitative studies.

Concluding Comments

Understanding complex patterns should be a priority for nursing because it addresses key present and future healthcare challenges. The presence of a sound and articulated ontology is an important element of nursing research. Critical or complex realism offers a stated and unified approach that confronts complexity, acknowledges the importance of both agency and structural factors, and enables nurse researchers to work collaboratively across disciplines and methods. Complex realism is particularly useful for informing research into priority areas related to understanding complexity, improving interventions, and explicating biopsychosocial pathways.

REFERENCES

1. Crotty M. *Phenomenology and Nursing Research*. Melbourne: Churchill Livingstone; 1996.
2. McEvoy P, Richards D. Critical realism: a way forward for evaluation research in nursing? *JAdv Nurs*. 2003;43(4): 411–420.
3. Wainwright SP. A new paradigm for nursing: the potential of realism. *J Adv Nurs*. 1997(26):1262–1271.
4. Hussey T. Realism and nursing. *Nurs Philos*. 2000;1:98–108.
5. Bhaskar R. Facts and values: theory and practice/reason and the dialectic of human emancipation/depth, rationality and change. In: Archer M, Bhaskar R, Collier A, Lawson T, Norrie A, eds. *Critical Realism: Essential Readings*. London: Routledge; 1998:409–443.
6. Bhaskar R. Societies. In: Archer M, Bhaskar R, Collier A, Lawson T, Norrie A, eds. *Critical Realism: Essential Readings*. London: Routledge; 1998: 206–257.
7. Parker J. Social movements and science: the question of plural knowledge systems. In: Lopez J, Potter G, eds. *After Postmodernism: An Introduction to Critical Realism*. London: Athlone Press; 2001: 251–259.
8. Williams SJ. Beyond meaning, discourse and the empirical world: critical realist reflections on health. *Soc Theory Health*. 2003;1(1):42–47.
9. Clark AM. The qualitative-quantitative debate: moving from positivism and confrontation to postpositivism and reconciliation. *J Adv Nurs*. 1998;27(6):1242–1249.
10. Bricmont J. Sociology and epistemology. In: Lopez J, Potter G, eds. *After Postmodernism: An Introduction to Critical Realism*. London: Athlone Press; 2001:100–115.
11. Paley J. Phenomenology as rhetoric. *Nurs Inq*. 2005;12(2): 106–116.
12. Sayer A. *Realism and Social Science*. London: Sage; 2000.
13. Lawson T. *Reorientating Economics*. London: Rout-ledge; 2003.
14. Byrne D. *Complexity Theory and the Social Sciences: An Introduction*. London: Routledge; 1998.
15. Pawson R, Tilley N. *Realistic Evaluation*. Sage: London; 1997.
16. Lawson T. *Economics and Reality*. London: Rout-ledge; 1997.
17. Clark AM, MacIntyre PD, Cruickshank J. A critical realist approach to understanding and evaluating heart health programmes. *Health*. 2007;11(4):513–539.
18. Carpiano RM. Toward a neighborhood resource-based theory of social capital for health: can Bourdieu and sociology help? *Soc Sc Med*. 2006;62(1):165–175.
19. Carpiano R, Daley D. A guide and glossary on post-positivist theory building for population health. *J Epidemiol Community Health*. 2006;60:564–570.
20. Pawson R. *Evidence-based Policy: A Realist Perspective*. London: Sage; 2006.
21. Clark AM, Barbour RS, White M, MacIntyre PD. Promoting participation in cardiac rehabilitation: patients' choices and experiences. *J Adv Nurs*. 2004;47(1):5–14.
22. Archer M. *Realist Social Theory: The Morphogenetic Approach*. Cambridge, England: Cambridge University Press; 1995.
23. Wilkinson R, Marmot M, eds. *Social Determinants of Health: The Solid Facts*. Copenhagen: World Health Organization Regional Office for Europe; 2003.
24. Archer MS, Tritter JQ. *Rational Choice Theory: Resisting Colonization*. London: Routledge; 2000.
25. McEvoy P, Richards D. A critical realist rationale for using a combination of quantitative and qualitative methods. *J Res Nurs*. 2006;11(1):66–78.
26. Pratschke J. Realistic models? Critical Realism and statistical models in the social sciences. *Philsophica*. 2003;73(1):13–38.
27. Olsen W, Morgan J. A critical epistemology of analytical statistics: addressing the sceptical realist. *J Theory Soc Behav*. 2005;35(3):255–284.
28. Clegg S. Evidence-based practice in educational research: a critical realist critique of systematic review. *Br J Sociol Educ*. 2005;26(3):415–428.
29. Fitzpatrick S. Explaining homelessness: a critical realist perspective. *Housing Theory Soc*. 2005;22(1):1–17.
30. Scrambler G, Higgs P. "The dog that didn't bark": taking class seriously in the health inequalities debate. *Soc Sci Med*. 2001;52:157–159.
31. Byrne D. Complex and contingent causation. In: Carter B, New C, eds. *Making Realism Work: Realist Social Theory and Empirical Research*. London: Routledge; 2004.
32. Wainwright SP, Forbes A. Philosophical problems with social research on health inequalities. *Health Care Anal*. 2000;8:259–277.
33. Marmot MG. Status syndrome: a challenge to medicine. *JAMA*. 2006;295:1304–1307.
34. Frohlich K, Mykhalovskiy E, Miller F, Daniel M. Advancing the population health agenda: encouraging the integration of social theory into population health research and practice. *Can J Public Health*. 2004;95:392–395.
35. Porter S, Ryan S. Breaking the boundaries between nursing and sociology: a critical realist ethnography of the theory-practice gap. *J Adv Nurs*. 1996;24(2):413–420.
36. Wilson V McCormack B. Critical realism as emancipatory action: the case for realistic evaluation in practice development. *Nurs Philos*. 2006;7(1):45–57.

37. Tolson D. Practice innovation: a methodological maze. *J Adv Nurs.* 1999;30(2):381–390.

38. Clark AM, Whelan HK, Barbour RS, MacIntyre PD. A realist study of the mechanisms of cardiac rehabilitation. *J Adv Nurs.* 2005;52(4):362–371.

39. Pawson R. Evidence and policy and naming and shaming. *Policy Stud.* 2002;23(3):211–230.

40. Judge K. Testing evaluations to the limits: the case of English Health Action Zones. *J Health Serv Res Policy.* 2000;5:1–8.

41. Oakley A, Strange V, Bonell C, Allen E, Stephenson J, and RIPPLE Study Team. Process evaluation in randomised controlled trials of complex interventions. *BMJ.* 2006;332: 413–416.

42. Adams C, Bauld L, Judge K. *National Evaluation of Health Action Zones.* Report submitted to the Department of Health. Canterbury, England: University of Kent; 1999. PSSRU Discussion Paper No. 1627.

43. Bonner L. Using theory-based evaluation to build evidence-based health and social care policy and practice. *Crit Public Health.* 2003;13(1):77–92.

44. Pawson R. Realist review—a new method of systematic review designed for complex policy interventions. *J Health Serv Res Policy.* 2005;10(suppl 1):S1–S21.

45. Williams S. Medical sociology and the biological body: where are we now and where do we go from here? *Health.* 2006;10(1):5–30.

46. Sawyer R. *Social Emergence: Societies as Complex Systems.* Cambridge, England: Cambridge University Press; 2005.

47. Morton PG, Fontaine DK, Hudak CM, Gallo BM. *Critical Care Nursing: A Holistic Approach.* Philadelphia, PA: Lippincott Williams; 2005.

48. Bloch M, Schmidt P, Danaceau M, Murphy J, Nieman L, Rubinow D. Effects of gonadal steroids in women with a history of postpartum depression. *Am J Psychiatry.* 2000; 157:924–930.

49. Beck C. Predictors of postpartum depression: an update. *Nurs Res.* 2001;50:275–285.

50. Mazure C, Keita G, Blehar M. *Summit on Women and Depression: Proceedings and Recommendations.* Washington, DC: American Psychological Association; 2002.

THE AUTHORS COMMENT | Complex Critical Realism: Tenets and Application in Nursing Research

The article was written to provide a clear and accessible introduction to critical realism as it could be applied to research into nursing phenomena. Hopefully, it crosses that tricky bridge from world of abstract theory and philosophical tenets to the nuts-and-bolts details needed for applied research approaches. Rather than just explain what critical realism is, the paper seeks to explain more how it can be applied in nursing. We hope the article shows why critical realism is especially useful for research into some of the main challenges facing nursing and health in the 21st century.

ALEXANDER M. CLARK
SUE L. LISSEL
CAROLINE DAVIS

Bridging the Gulf Between Science and Action: The "New Fuzzies" of Neopragmatism

CATHERINE A. WARMS, RN, PhD
CAROLE A. SCHROEDER, RN, PhD

Rather than a philosophy, pragmatism is a way of doing philosophy that has major implications for solving disputes involving nursing science, theory, and practice that may otherwise be interminable. Pragmatism weaves together theory and action so that one modifies the other continuously, but both maintain their mutual relevance. Pragmatism emphasizes pluralism and diversity, and depends on an ethical base for determination of what is reasonable. Recently repopularized by the philosopher Richard Rorty and others, pragmatic ideals seem inherent to nursing. We propose that a better understanding of the history and utility of pragmatism will enhance both clinically relevant nursing theory and theoretically relevant nursing practice.

Pragmatism may be the most misunderstood philosophical movement in the history of philosophy. Unlike most philosophy, pragmatism is not based on theoretical notions of truth or falsity, and it refuses to offer a method for discovering truth. Instead, pragmatism is a way of *doing* philosophy. On its most basic level, pragmatism is the theory that the meaning of a proposition or course of action lies in its observable consequences. Moreover, the sum of these consequences constitutes the meaning of the proposition or action. Pragmatism is a method for evaluating philosophical problems by tracing the practical consequences of each question. In the words of William James, "The question is not, "Is that true?" but *"What difference* would it make if that is true?"[1(p112)] For the pragmatist, belief in a truth cannot be separated from intent, performance, and consequences. Considering the immense ethical contradictions inherent in both the theory and practice of nursing, pragmatism may be a way of grounding our work in a new coherence.

The purpose of this article is twofold: (1) to discuss the history of pragmatism as a philosophical movement, and (2) to argue its relevance to the advancement of nursing knowledge and action in a postmodern world. Pragmatism is a way of "doing" philosophy that weaves together theory and action so that they intertwine, each modifying the other, continuously maintaining their mutual relevance.[2] In contrast to the criterion-based conception of reality, which creates a gulf between scientific objectivity and everyday human activity by its continual search for a defined "truth," the pragmatist conception of reality bridges that gap through inquiry that is a continual reweaving of different versions of the truth, one that incorporates new ideas and better explanations in the context of human encounters and activities. Pragmatism may be a means for nursing to abandon stale theoretical and scientific debates that have inhibited our progress toward philosophical and clinical relevance.

Definition: Confusion and Clarification

The words pragmatism and pragmatic have been co-opted into common usage with meanings that have lost their original richness. Today, pragmatic is commonly used to mean practical or utilitarian. This association of pragmatic with practical assumes knowledge must be limited to promote action. But, as conceived by the early pragmatists, action is creative, complex, knowledgeable, and expansive; it is directed toward new applications of knowledge that bridge the gap between the "actual good and possible better."[9(p43)] The tendency for the term to be used only in its most basic sense of "practical" has separated pragmatism from its history and transformed it into a term of disparagement. A person who is considered pragmatic may also be thought atheoretical, narrow minded, and dogmatic. In actuality, in the philosophical sense of the word,

ABOUT THE AUTHORS

CATHERINE A. WARMS was born in Bremerton, WA and attended the University of Washington for all her undergraduate and graduate nursing education. She received a BA in social welfare in 1971, a BSN in 1981, an MN in family nursing in 1986, and a PhD in nursing science in 2002. She has been a Rehabilitation Nurse for more than 20 years and has worked in multiple nursing roles, including inpatient nursing, outpatient nurse practitioner, and research study nurse. Her work focuses on health promotion for people with disabilities and/or chronic conditions, with an emphasis on physical activity, its measurement, and its effect on health in populations with mobility impairments. She currently practices as a care provider with the Rehabilitation Medicine Clinic at University of Washington Medical Center. Her hobbies include gardening, cooking, and reading.

CAROLE A. SCHROEDER was born in the San Francisco Bay Area and grew up in Reno, NV; received her doctorate at the University of Colorado Health Sciences Center; and did postdoctoral study at the University of Washington in health systems before taking a faculty position. She is an Associate Professor Emerita at the University of Washington. She has been a single parent for most of her adult life, an experience that leaves her with a unique understanding of issues of gender, class, power, and privilege. The focus of her scholarship is to promote social justice and decrease inequalities in health and healthcare access. Her key contributions include her theoretical writings, work with vulnerable populations, and teaching approach using the Peace and Power philosophy and methods developed by Dr. Peggy Chinn.

a pragmatic person is very open minded and willing to listen to as many ideas or versions of the "truth" as possible to better solve problems.

History of Pragmatism

Pragmatism began as a uniquely American philosophical movement that appeared near the end of the 19th century, peaked in popularity just before World War II, and then lay dormant for 25 years. In 1977, pragmatism reemerged in a postmodern cloak as neopragmatism, largely because of the efforts of philosophers Richard Rorty at the University of Virginia in Charlottesville, Hilary Putnam at Harvard University in Cambridge, Massachusetts, and Richard Bernstein at the New School for Social Research in New York. As a philosophical movement, pragmatism has been evolutionary in nature, changing with each philosopher who contributes to its tenets. In its earliest stages in the 19th century, pragmatism was popularized by the work of three major philosophers, Charles Sanders Peirce, William James, and John Dewey. We briefly discuss the contributions of each to the development of both pragmatic thought and the pragmatic method below.

Pragmatism was first named by William James (1842–1910) in a lecture given at Berkeley in 1898. In this lecture James presented what he called Peirce's principle of pragmatism, giving Charles Sanders Peirce (1839–1914) credit as originator of the philosophical movement. In 1877, Peirce and several other scientists and philosophers formed the Metaphysical Club in Cambridge, Massachusetts. During discussions with James and others, Peirce began to piece together a method "for making ideas clear."[3(p109)] The earliest versions of pragmatic thought emphasized respect for the views of others and the notion that conversations, not dogma or universal truth, are the basis for developing beliefs.

After James had named this way of "doing" philosophy pragmatism in the Berkeley lecture, Peirce outlined the pragmatic method. This method involved carefully defining conceptual terms and then imagining the practical, ethical, and theoretical consequences of affirming or denying a concept. Unlike previous thought that emphasized definition and preset evaluative criteria, the pragmatic method emphasized that inherent in those *consequences* was the whole of the concept.

Although Peirce has been credited as being the originator of pragmatism, William James popularized the movement. James emphasized that pragmatism was a way of doing philosophy, a method of "settling metaphysical disputes that otherwise might be interminable."[1(p94)] Graduate students in nursing may appreciate James' descriptions of such disputes:

> *Is the world one or many? Fated or free? Material or spiritual? Disputes over such notions are unending. The pragmatic method in such cases is to try to interpret each notion by tracing its respective practical consequences. What difference would it practically make to anyone if this notion were true?*[1(p96)]

James claimed pragmatism to be "anti-intellectualist." He believed rationalism to be pretentious, for pragmatism has no dogmas or doctrines, only method. James also coined the term "cash-value," a term that relates to the worthwhileness of a theory, meaning theories are only worth what they can be used for. He stated, "Theories thus become instruments, not answers to enigmas, in which we can rest. Pragmatism unstiffens all our theories, limbers them up and sets each one at work."[4(p27)] He describes this "work ethic" as the standard for value:

> Pragmatism is willing to take anything, to follow either logic or the senses and to count the humblest and most personal experiences. She will count mystical experiences if they have practical consequences.[1(p111)]

James also tackled the notion of truth, heretically claiming that truths are plastic and made, rather than discovered by using the rigorous methods of science. James' work predated our postmodern relinquishment of the notion of universal truth, handed down by higher authority.

The philosopher John Dewey (1859–1952) was the final member of the founding triumvirate of pragmatism. Dewey was a student of Peirce at Johns Hopkins University in Baltimore and later taught at the University of Chicago and Columbia University in New York. For Dewey, the essential feature of the pragmatic way of knowing was "to maintain the continuity of knowing with an activity which purposely modifies the environment."[5(p216)] For Dewey, reason was the ability to apply prior experience to a new experience, and a reasonable person kept an open mind.

Although denied entry into academic halls because of gender, Jane Addams (1860–1935) was also extremely influential in pragmatic thought. An early social worker and women's suffrage advocate, Addams opened Hull House, a settlement house that was a community service center for the poor in Chicago. She envisioned Hull House as a place of possibility, one where people, working together, could produce meaningful change. She viewed action as integral to life:

> The settlement stands for application as opposed to research; for emotion as opposed to abstraction, for universal interest as opposed to specialization… it is an attempt to express the meaning of life in terms of life itself, in forms of activity.[6(p276)]

Addams' life work exemplified the tenets of pragmatism by her willingness to value humble experiences and disciplinary pluralism, and to examine the ethical and practical consequences of an act.

Richard Rorty, Richard Bernstein, and the Pragmatic Revival

By the 1930s, the popularity of pragmatism appeared to wane. Existentialism, structuralism, Marxism, and psychoanalysis also emerged in the 1930s, and all of these schools of thought competed with pragmatism for public attention. In actuality, pragmatism did not disappear at all, but became so ingrained in the American way of life that its tenets were inherent in all of the major schools of thought and philosophical approaches.

Richard Rorty, a professor of humanities at the University of Virginia, is credited with the recent revival of pragmatism as a way of doing philosophy in the United States. This reemergence of pragmatic thought is popularly referred to as neopragmatism.[7] With the publication of Philosophy and the Mirror of Nature in 1979, Rorty successfully adapted pragmatism to the postmodern environment of the late 20th century:

> The aim … is to undermine the reader's confidence in the mind as something about which one should have a philosophical view, in knowledge as something about which there ought to be a theory and that has foundations and in philosophy as it has been conceived since Kant.[7(pxxxii)]

Rorty used irony to carry on the anti-intellectualist tradition of William James, and developed his own particular version of pragmatism that is tolerant of alternative views and humanistic, "not in the sense of trying to bring about something already defined, an essential human nature, but in the sense of creating something better than what we have known before."[8(p78)]

In 1987, Rorty described 20th century pragmatism as "new fuzziness,"[9] and claimed that pragmatism blurs the distinctions between objective and subjective and fact and value. See Table 18-1 for Rorty's version of pragmatism.[9]

Perhaps the most radical aspect of Rorty's work is a set of moral values, rather than preordained criteria, used by the new fuzzies as the basis for judgment of logic. These values include:

- tolerance
- respect for the opinions of those around us
- willingness to listen
- reliance on persuasion rather than force
- emphasis on communication over agreement or truth.

TABLE 18-1 Rorty and the New Pragmatism

Tenet	Explanation
No theory of truth, instead, an ethnocentric view of truth ("work by our own lights," no better lights to work from).	Humans are responsible only to our selves. Each person will hold as "true" those beliefs we find good to believe.[9(p42)] Ethnocentric view is that there is nothing to be said about truth separate from our own descriptions of procedures of justification.
Distinctions between objective/subjective, rational/irrational, true/false unhelpful.	Beliefs can be agreed upon without being true or rational in the methodological sense. The best way to find out what to believe is to listen to as many suggestions and arguments as possible, contrast our beliefs to proposed alternatives and choose that which offers the best solution or answer for that time, place, and situation—not that which is most true.
Redefine inquiry.	Inquiry is a matter of "continually reweaving a web of beliefs"[9(p44)]—trying out new beliefs as they are suggested and incorporating or discarding them as we see fit. The goal of inquiry is the attainment of an appropriate mixture of unforced agreement with tolerant disagreement in a community which encourages "free and open encounters."[9(p44)]
Pragmatism has an *ethical* base, not an epistemological or metaphysical base.	Pragmatism depends on moral values or virtues for determination of what is reasonable: "tolerance, respect for the opinions of those around us, willingness to listen and reliance on persuasion rather than force."[9(p40)]
Disciplinary diversity is the goal.	All disciplines participate in cooperative human inquiry and all are equally objective if there is unforced agreement. "Fierce competition" between disciplines is vital.[9(p45)]
Redefine progress.	Progress cannot be judged by forward direction but by the fact of richer human activity, the opportunity for humans to do more interesting things and to be more interesting people.

Rorty promotes broad intellectual tolerance and, above all, leaves room for alternative narratives.

> Rorty qualifies as a legitimate heir to the pragmatic tradition by virtue of his implicit focus on a problematic deeply embedded in the American experience: the fact and consequences of plurality in its psychological, social, and political forms.[10(p66)]

The emphases on plurality and tolerance figure prominently in the works of another neopragmatist, Richard Bernstein. Professor of Philosophy at the New School for Social Research, Bernstein declines to identify a pragmatic essence or a set of propositions shared by all pragmatists, because "... there can be no escape from plurality—a plurality of traditions, perspectives, philosophic orientations."[11(p389)] Like Rorty, Bernstein suggests that disciplinary boundaries dissolve so that richer conversations can take place across them. He calls us to

> nurture the type of community and solidarity where there is an engaged fallibilistic pluralism—one that is based upon mutual respect, where we are willing to risk our own prejudgments, are open to listening and learning from other and we respond to others with responsiveness and responsibility.[11(p400)]

Narrative, or dialogue, is the method espoused by Bernstein for encounters between individuals and disciplines. He characterizes a community as "a group of individuals locked in an argument,"[12(p66)] and suggests that a vital pragmatism is "the ongoing process of being locked in argument."[12(p66)] The variety of voices constituting the narratives is the primary basis for vitality. Rather than truth, the reason for inquiry is the *application* and *usefulness* of beliefs held by a discipline.

The history of pragmatism is found in the writings of its founders. Peirce emphasized respect for all viewpoints and conversation as the pathway to developing beliefs. For James, pragmatism was not a philosophy in and of itself, but a way of settling disputes. James believed theories to be instruments, valued only for their utility. James also initiated the important emphasis on pluralism. Dewey added an educator's perspective with his approach to learning as doing, a way of applying experience to life. The neopragmatists Rorty and Bernstein revived the notion of narrative, tolerance for all viewpoints, and truth as what we *choose* to believe. They added an emphasis on communication and free and open encounters as methods to achieve interdisciplinary cooperation in human inquiry. Both philosophers remind us that pragmatism relies on an ethical base of moral values, rather than specific criteria to evaluate the worth of knowledge.

> We should relish the thought that the sciences as well as the arts will always *provide a spectacle of fierce competition between alternative theories, movements, and schools. The end of human activity is not rest, but rather richer and better human activity. We should think of human progress as making it possible for human beings to do more interesting things and be more interesting people, not as heading toward a place which has somehow been prepared for us in the past.*[9(p45)]

Pragmatism and Nursing

> *the usefulness of theory … is ultimately answerable to those whose lives are supposed to be bettered by it.*[13(p263)]

The tenets of pragmatism are not new to nursing. Nursing has always attended to the cash value or the worthwhileness of nursing theories to achieve desired results in clinical nursing. Clearly, nurses are interested in doing what works. Donaldson (1995) posits that nurse scholars and scientists who intend to build the discipline of nursing "keep in mind that the centrality and value of this knowledge will be determined by the nurse pragmatist."[14(p6)] For Donaldson, a nurse pragmatist is willing to use any existing theory or knowledge relevant to the situation, "spanning distinct philosophies, paradigms, and disciplines."[14(p6)] For nursing science to be relevant, it must have utility, usually for the achievement of mutually determined clinical outcomes. For Donaldson, a nurse pragmatist is a nurse in practice, "one who is caring for patients and requires a useful knowledge base from which to make applications to "do" nursing."[14(p10)] Donaldson's discussion of the nurse pragmatist emerges from the early pragmatists' assertions of theories as instruments, learning by doing, and the notion of valuing interdisciplinary knowledge.

Although pragmatism seems embedded in the ideals and reality of nursing practice, it also has great utility for furthering the long-standing debates regarding nursing theory and research. In the following sections, we offer four noteworthy examples from the nursing literature that seem to use pragmatic ideals to solve problems in nursing science.

In a 1992 article, Schumacher and Gortner[15] discuss recent shifts in philosophy that replace the tenets of traditional, positivistic science with so-called scientific realism. Shumacher and Gortner move away from the old view that universal laws apply to all situations regardless of circumstance, to a view of science and research that takes into account the context of the phenomena under discussion. Discussing causality, they assert that the notion of causation in "human science is complex, multifaceted, and possibly multidirectional."[15(p7)] At the same time, they defend the traditional notion of causality, stating it is required to make science clinically relevant and because clinicians need to know "the likely consequences of certain events under given conditions."[15(p7)] This approach is pragmatic, illustrating a pluralistic approach that solves problems using ideas from both traditional positivistic science and scientific realism. Schumacher and Gortner weave their ideas into a conception of nursing science that they believe is relevant and useful for nursing. Our task in nursing becomes one of encouraging free and open encounters while listening to as many conversations as possible to discern the utility of Schumacher and Gortner's ideas for nursing.

Utility is also foremost in the 1995 treatise from Ford-Gilboe et al on the pragmatics of science in nursing.[16] The authors discuss the postpositivist, interpretive, and critical paradigms and the use of qualitative and quantitative methods. They conclude that combining strategies across paradigms enhances the value of a study. Ford-Gilboe et al, like Schumacher and Gortner, seem to believe that "good" nursing science is pragmatic. They expand their argument for a pragmatic nursing science by advocating the critical paradigm as an appropriate perspective for advancing nursing knowledge.[17] Under the umbrella of the critical paradigm, the authors propose methods for the purpose of accomplishing a "critical agenda"[17(p13)] to create knowledge that will be persuasive for the purpose of producing change. They emphasize respect for the opposing opinions and reliance on persuasion rather than force, both moral values inherent in pragmatism.

Missing from pragmatist writings is a comprehensive analysis of the inescapable power dynamics inherent in the process of communication. Henderson opens the conversation in nursing with a presentation of participatory action research as a research method that may reduce power hierarchies between researcher and researched.[18] She describes consciousness raising as a method that precedes other forms of data collection, for it is the format in which research takes place: "By engaging in critical and liberating dialogues, individuals uncover the hidden distortions within themselves that help to maintain an oppressive society."[18(p63)]

Critical and liberating dialogues, similar to Rorty's notion of free and open encounters, are both based in ethical notions of unshackled communication and tolerance for diversity. The ideals of feminism and critical theory could advance pragmatic tolerance by addressing power imbalances that create rifts between the researcher and the researched. The tolerant pragmatist would not object to this agenda as long as she can evaluate its value in the given situation.

Boyd also presents a structure for nursing research that is congruent with pragmatist ideals.[19] Boyd uses multiple approaches to research and emphasizes the utility of each approach for specific types of situations depending on context. Her ideas are pragmatic in their respect for pluralism and notions of theories as instruments. Boyd portrays nursing encounters as opportunities for communication and for constructing theories that will be useful in future encounters. For Boyd, nursing becomes a mutual search for both meaning and action, by "adding a research agenda to one's nursing work merely provides for the communication of what is learned so that other nurses, other patients may profit from it."[19(p20)]

Boyd's approach to nursing science is an example of a willingness to use the "humblest and most personal experiences"[1(p111)] to create a knowledge that is tolerant, inclusive, and contextual in nature.

 ## Nursing at the Crossroads

In a discussion of shifting paradigms in the fields of bioethics and health law, Wolf[20] describes these fields as standing at a crossroads between

the well trod road of conversations among experts, governed by top-down theory ... abstract pronouncements, inattentive to differences ... (and) a new more complex path, wide enough to accommodate multiple proposals and critiques as to method, willful attention to feminist, race-attentive and other contributions ... teeming with people.[20(p415)]

Nursing stands at that same crossroads. The struggle for nursing science to find itself, to be able to name a tradition or paradigm into which nursing knowledge belongs, has proven interminable and impractical. As nursing science evolves into the millennium, an enhanced willingness to use knowledge from other disciplines and share that knowledge with all disciplines seems to be emerging in nursing.[21] As professional nursing matures, we welcome the fact that our old fascination with long-standing debates regarding appropriate methodologies and methods of inquiry in nursing seems to be waning. Pragmatism is an approach that holds promise for developing innovative and useful nursing knowledge in the future, and we would do well to heed Peirce's words: "The willful adherence to a belief and the arbitrary forcing of it upon others, must both be given up and a new method of settling opinions must be adopted."[3(p10)]

Writing on pragmatism and feminism, Seigfried[13] discusses the interrelationship of theory and practice in words that seem particularly relevant for nursing.

emancipatory theory arises out of practice as much as it reflects back on it. It is a tool for directing practice, not a privileged insight into reality. As a tool it is instrumental to an outcome desired, rather than a hegemonic imposition of a predelineated order. Therefore, theories should be capable of revision as outcomes surpass or undercut expectations ... The usefulness of theory, therefore is ultimately answerable to those who lives are supposed to be bettered by it.[13(p263)]

Nurse-philosopher Dr. Sally Gadow (unpublished poem, 1995) says words similar to those of Seigfried in a more poetic form:

Musings on Theory

Theory speaks as if a theorist's words are more
    true, more important,
than the words a particular patient and nurse
    will say with each other
      in their experience together.

Ambiguity is the possibility for a different
    meaning: ambiguity is freedom.
Can theory have a different meaning?
Can theory emancipate instead of coerce, open
    instead of closing the door to meanings?
Can there be a critical theory?

I think so—if a theory is just another story,
    one meaning among many,
    without authority,
always surpassed by the stories each
    nurse and patient compose in their
    situation together.*

Pragmatism is proposed as one way of assisting nursing to emerge from the old constraints of modernism, and begin to act on what is known, rather than act upon what has been told. No longer concerned only with the truth or falsity of a proposition or situation, nurses can begin to ask the pragmatists' question, "*What difference* would it make if this were true?" Pragmatism is a way of doing philosophy that weaves together theory and action, each continuously modifying the other and maintaining their mutual relevance.[2] Considering the immense ethical contradictions inherent in the theory and practice of nursing, pragmatism may be a means for nursing to move toward a higher level of philosophical and clinical relevance.

REFERENCES

1. James W. Pragmatism's conception of truth. In: Menand L, ed. *Pragmatism: A Reader*. New York: Vintage Books: 1997:94–131. (Original work by James written in 1907).

2. Mahowald MB. So many ways to think. An overview of approaches to ethical issues in geriatrics. *Clin Geriatr Med.* 1994;10(3):403–418.

3. Peirce C. The fixation of belief. In: Houser N, Kloesel C, eds. *The Essential Peirce: Selected Philosophical Writings, Vol. 1 (1867–1893)*. Bloomington: Indiana University Press; 1992:109–123. (Original work by Peirce written in 1877).

4. James W. Pragmatism. In: Burckhardt F, ed. *The Works of William James: Pragmatism*. Cambridge, MA: Harvard University Press; 1975:20–30. (Original work by James published 1904).

5. Dewey J. Theories of knowledge. In: Menand L, ed. *Pragmatism: A Reader*. New York: Vintage Books; 1997: 205–218. (Original work by Dewey written in 1916).

6. Addams J. A function of the social settlement. In Menand L, ed. *Pragmatism: A Reader*. New York: Vintage Books; 1997:273–286. (Original work by Addams written in 1899).

7. Menand L, ed. An introduction to pragmatism. In: *Pragmatism: A Reader*. New York: Vintage Books: 1997: i-xxxiv.

8. Kolenda K. *Rorty's Humanistic Pragmatism*. Tampa: University of South Florida Press; 1990.

9. Rorty R. Science as solidarity. In: Nelson J, Megil A. McCloskey D. eds. *The Rhetoric of the Human Sciences: Language and Argument in Scholarship and Public Affairs*. Madison: University of Wisconsin Press. 1987: 38–52.

10. Hall DL. *Richard Rorty: Prophet and Poet of the New Pragmatism*. Albany, NY: State University of New York Press; 1994.

11. Bernstein RJ. Pragmatism, pluralism and the healing of wounds. In: Menand L. ed. *Pragmatism: A Reader*. New York: Vintage Books; 1997:382–401. (Original work by Bernstein written in 1988).

12. Bernstein, RJ. American pragmatism: The conflict of narratives. In: Saatkamp J. ed. *Rorty and Pragmatism*. Nashville. TN: Vanderbilt University Press; 1995:54–68.

13. Seigfried C. *Pragmatism and Feminism*. Chicago: University of Chicago Press: 1996.

14. Donaldson SK. Nursing science for nursing practice. In: Omery A, Kasper C, Page G, eds. *In Search of Nursing Science*. Thousand Oaks. CA: Sage Publications; 1995:3–12.

15. Schumacher K, Gortner S. (Mis)conceptions and reconceptions about traditional science. *Adv Nurs Sci.* 1992;14(4): 1–11.

16. Ford-Gilboe M, Campbell J, Berman H. Stories and numbers: coexistence without compromise. *Adv Nurs Sci.* 1995; 18(1):14–26.

17. Berman H, Ford-Gilboe M, Campbell J. Combining stories and numbers: A methodologic approach for a critical nursing science. *Adv Nurs Sci.* 1998;21(1):1–15.

18. Henderson D. Consciousness raising in participatory research: Method and methodology for emancipatory nursing inquiry. *Adv Nurs Sci.* 1995;17(3):58–69.

19. Boyd C. Toward a nursing practice research method. *Adv Nurs Sci.* 1993;16(2):9–25.

20. Wolf S. Shifting paradigms in bioethics and health law: The rise of a new pragmatism. *Am J Law Med.* 1994;20(4): 395–414.

21. Moody L. The quest for nursing science. In: Woody LE. ed. *Advancing Nursing Science through Research*. Newbury Park, CA: Sage Publications; 1990:15–46.

---

* Courtesy of Dr. Sally Gadow © 1995.

THE AUTHORS COMMENT

Bridging the Gulf Between Science and Action: The "New Fuzzies" of Neopragmatism

This article began as a class project for a course on the philosophy of nursing science taught by Carole Schroeder, my first attempt to write a scholarly paper after more than 20 years of practice as a nurse clinician. My need to find a way to bridge my own gulf between my past nursing practice and my hope for a relevant nursing science was clearly addressed by Rorty's writings and the philosophic tenets of neopragmatism that Dr. Schroeder presented in class. Together, we built upon the original class project by merging the ethical basis for pragmatism with the notion of emancipatory theory emerging from and reflecting back on nursing practice. This article presents an approach for development of nursing knowledge in the 21st century that argues for disciplinary postmodernity, diversity, free and open conversations, and tolerance of ambiguity. We hope that by adopting a neopragmatic approach to philosophy, nursing science will evolve beyond truth seeking and instead will find a way to interweave theory and action by developing knowledge that is ultimately "answerable to those whose lives are supposed to be bettered by it."

CATHERINE A. WARMS
CAROLE A. SCHROEDER

An Analysis of Changing Trends in Philosophies of Science on Nursing Theory Development and Testing

MARY CIPRIANO SILVA, RN, PhD, FAAN
DANIEL ROTHBART, PhD

The effects of changing trends in philosophies of science on nursing theory development and testing are analyzed. Two philosophies of science—logical empiricism and historicism—are compared for four variables: (a) components of science, (b) conception of science, (c) assessment of scientific progress, and (d) goal of philosophy of science. These factors serve as the basis for assessing trends in the development and testing of nursing theory from 1964 to the present. The analysis shows a beginning philosophic shift within nursing theory from logical empiricism to historicism and addresses implications and recommendations for future nursing theory development and testing.

Both philosophy of science and nursing theory are in a state of transition. At times this transition is characterized by contradictory, divergent, and confusing points of view that lead to probing questions about the nature of science in general and nursing theory and science in particular. What are the goals and components of science? How should science be conceptualized and scientific knowledge assessed? Have nursing theory development and testing kept pace with changing trends in philosophies of science?

The goal of this analysis is to show the influences of changing trends in philosophies of science on nursing theory development and testing and to encourage dialogue among nurses about the future directions of nursing theory.

Philosophies of Science

Since the 1940s, two major schools of philosophical thought have influenced philosophy of science: logical empiricism (1940s-1960s) and historicism (1960s to the present). The most influential proponents of logical empiricism (the orthodox view) included Braithwaite (1953), Ayer (1959), Nagel (1961), Scheffler (1963), Hempel (1965, 1966), and Rudner (1966). These proponents understood the nature of scientific knowledge as an application of logical principles of reasoning.

Although the logical empiricist view dominated the study of philosophy of science for more than two decades, a wave of criticism began in the early 1960s. Logical empiricism was subjected to intense philosophical scrutiny, revolving around the general contention that the orthodox view became too purified in its idealistically formal approach to science. In providing logical rigor and formalization to the nature of scientific knowledge, logical empiricism removed itself from the actual practice of working scientists; the orthodox view approached logic more closely than it did science according to critics. These critics began to reexamine the actual practices of scientists, the patterns of reasoning, and the sociological influences during a historical era. The history of science became an essential element of any adequate philosophical analysis, prompting a new philosophy of science known as historicism.

Major historicists include Hanson (1958), Kuhn (1962, 1970), Lakatos (1968), Toulmin (1972), Laudan (1977), and Feyerabend (1978). Although Kuhn is the best known of these historicists, based on the influential work *The Structure of Scientific Revolutions* (1962, 1970), his philosophical proposals have been widely criticized by other historicists, and Kuhn himself (1977) has had second thoughts about certain aspects of this work.

Therefore, to draw the distinctions between logical empiricism and historicism, it is desirable to focus on the work of Laudan rather than Kuhn. The reasons are threefold: (1) Laudan's works represent the forefront of philosophy of science today; (2) his views are largely shared by other historicists; and (3) his works have gone almost unnoticed by nurse theorists and researchers.

To show fundamental differences regarding theory development, testing, and assessment between logical empiricism and Laudan's version of historicism, these two philosophies are compared for four

ABOUT THE AUTHORS

MARY C. SILVA was born and raised in the small town of Ravenna, OH. She earned a BSN and an MS from Ohio State University and a PhD from the University of Maryland. She also undertook postdoctoral study at Georgetown University in healthcare ethics. The focus of her scholarship and key contributions to nursing has been in philosophy, metatheory, and healthcare ethics. She is a Professor Emerita, at George Mason University, Fairfax, VA. When not working, she attends foreign films, the Shakespeare Theatre, and fine and performing arts events. DANIEL ROTHBART received three degrees in philosophy: a BA in 1972 from Fairleigh Dickinson University, an MA in 1975 from the State University of New York at Binghamton, and a PhD in 1978 from Washington University in St. Louis. He is Professor of Philosophy and Conflict Analysis and Resolution in the Department of Philosophy at George Mason University, Fairfax, Virginia. Dr. Rothbart has lectured on medical ethics and philosophy of science throughout both the United States and Europe. He was appointed a visiting research scholar at the University of Cambridge in England a few years ago. He has published articles, chapters, and a book titled *Metaphor and the Growth of Scientific Knowledge*. He has been a member of the faculty at George Mason University since 1979.

significant variables: (1) the components of science, (2) the conception of science, (3) the assessment of scientific progress, and (4) the goal of philosophy of science. Table 19-1 summarizes the basic differences between logical empiricism and historicism. These comparisons show the shifting trends within philosophy of science. From this table one can also surmise implications for the emergent development of new nursing theory.

Components of Science

The components of science, as defined by logical empiricists, are well documented in both the philosophical literature and the nursing literature. Logical empiricists attempt to understand science in terms of theories and the relationships among the components of a theory. A scientific theory is intended to systematically unify all the diverse phenomena of a particular discipline. The unification is achieved by encompassing descriptions of phenomena within an abstract set of statements known as a deductive system.

A deductive system is composed of three major components that are arranged in descending order of abstractness. First, the system's most abstract statements are its assumptions, which introduce the theory's basic concepts through the use of theoretical terms. Secondly, from these theoretical assumptions, propositions are deduced as part of the second level of abstraction. Together these assumptions and propositions systematically organize the entities and processes that presumably "lie behind" the observable phenomena. To complete the theory it is necessary to bridge these principles to empirical generalizations. Toward this goal, bridge principles, still within the second level of abstraction, indicate how the theoretical entities and processes relate to empirical phenomena. Without

TABLE 19-1	**A Comparison of Logical Empiricism and Historicism on Four Parameters of Science**	
Parameters	**Logical Empiricism**	**Historicism**
Components of science	Concepts, theoretical assumptions, empirical generalizations	Concepts, scientific theories, research traditions
Conception of science	Science as product	Science as process
Assessment of scientific progress	Accept theories as probably true Reject theories as probably false	Number of solved problems within a discipline
Goal of philosophy of science	Logical explanation of nature of scientific knowledge	Historical explanation of the nature of scientific knowledge

Note: Although this table highlights the major differences between two philosophies of science, there are some shared views. For example, historicists primarily define science as a human process, but they also examine the products of solved scientific problem.

these principles no empirical explanations or prediction would be possible and the system would be immune to empirical testing. Thirdly, these bridge principles in turn produce empirical generalizations within the lowest level of abstraction. In summary, the components of a scientific system, according to logical empiricists, are a set of statements that are systematically unified within a deductive system and that link theoretical concepts to empirically observable properties through the use of bridge principles (Braithwaite, 1953).

In contrast to the logical empiricists who attempt to understand science in terms of theories, historicists like Laudan (1977) attempt to understand science in terms of research traditions, each of which includes many theories. Although theories are seen by logical empiricists to be specific, short-lived, stable in formulation, and testable, historicists believe research traditions to be global, long-lived, and changeable within the boundaries of an acceptable ontological commitment.

By definition, a research tradition is a broadly based foundation of many theories and is an accepted way of viewing the fundamental phenomena within a discipline. It provides a global backdrop from which theories are constructed and evaluated through a set of guidelines for identifying the fundamental objects of a particular research tradition. Laudan does recognize, however, that the domains of science are not always clear; thus, classification of knowledge into a particular research tradition may be ambiguous. Every discipline has several research traditions, as illustrated by the nursing research traditions of holism and particularism.

According to Laudan (1977), three specific components make up a research tradition: (1) specific theories, (2) ontological commitments, and (3) methodological commitments. Some of the specific theories within a given research tradition are new and others are modified versions of older theories that "fit" within the tradition. The function of any theory is to solve scientific problems within the discipline, from the perspective of the research tradition's, ontological commitments. If, for example, one ontological commitment of a research tradition is holism, various theories within this research tradition might address the problem of how to view the person as a holistic being without looking at parts.

In addition to specific theories and ontological commitments, the third component, methodological commitments, is also essential for a research tradition. Methodological commitments define the legitimate methods of inquiry and experimental procedures that are inseparably linked to a research tradition's ontology. To follow the logic of the above example, would not the case study method of inquiry better preserve the ontological commitment to holism than the elemental design method of inquiry with its built-in reductionism?

The components of a scientific system, according to historicists like Laudan, are multiple research traditions, each containing theories that produce a set of ontological viewpoints and methods of inquiry that are not only essentially compatible with the research tradition but also capable of solving problems within it.

Conception of Science

Based on this comparison of the components of science for logical empiricism and historicism, it is apparent that the two schools assume very different views about what science means. Logical empiricists do not understand science in terms of the human activities of working scientists (e.g., experimenting and compiling data). Instead, they conceive of science only in terms of the results of these activities. The term *science* refers only to a product; i.e., a set of statements that purportedly constitute the body of scientific knowledge. The product includes scientific terminology and definitions, propositions, hypotheses, theories, and laws. This conception of science as product rests on the philosophical goal of articulating the logical foundations of scientific knowledge (Rudner, 1966). Within this viewpoint, it is important to recognize that logical empiricists are not interested in how scientific hypotheses are conceived but rather in how they can be sufficiently supported by empirical evidence. Their emphasis is one of theory validation, not theory discovery (Rudner, 1966).

In contrast, historicists understand science as a process of human behavior and thought exhibited by practicing scientists. Historicists would be interested in different questions. What reasoning patterns do practicing scientists use to accept or reject a theory? To what extent are scientists influenced by the theory's empirical findings in contrast to the theory's logical elegance in such a decision? How do external factors such as religious convictions influence the scientist's decision-making judgments?

To the historicist, every facet of the scientific process is subject to philosophical examination, including the process of explaining how fruitful theories are conceived by practicing scientists. With greater understanding of this process, historicists hope to develop models for future theory construction. Within this scientific viewpoint, valid data for theory construction include:

■ The psychological factors of individual scientists

■ The social forces on the community of scientists at a particular time

■ The overall historical environment, especially the "nonscientific" influences on scientists.

Assessment of Scientific Progress

The assessment of scientific progress within the logical empiricist tradition rests on the ability to justify a scientific theory by examining the requirements for the theory's truth and the conditions of its falsehood. If a scientist can demonstrate the truth of a theory, the scientist has acquired scientific knowledge.

Certain criteria identify theory as false or true. Generally, if a theory's predictions are repeatedly disconfirmed, the logic of testing requires a rejection of the problematic dimensions of the theory, assuming that the observations are correct (Hempel, 1966). But logical empiricists have more difficulty explaining the method of proving that a theory is true. According to the logic of theory testing, no finite number of experiments can conclusively prove that a theory is true. If a theory passes many severe tests, it is only empirically confirmed; that is, the theory's probability of truth has increased. Therefore, to logical empiricists, scientific progress is assessed by the degree of probability that the theory is true, based on the number and severity of empirical tests it passes.

In addition, logical empiricists consider theoretical reduction an important scientific goal. In theoretical reduction, one theory can be absorbed by or reduced to some other inclusive theory. The philosophical advantage of reduction lies not only with the simplicity of fewer theoretical concepts and laws but also with the insight into the ultimate character of reality (Nagel, 1961).

For historicists, the question of whether philosophy of science should try to explain when, if ever, a theory is true or false is the subject of considerable debate. Many agree with Laudan (1977), who argues that philosophy should not search for distinguishing characteristics of true theories, primarily because practicing scientists rarely evaluate theories in terms of truth or falsity. The history of science includes many instances in which a theory was accepted even though it contained scientific anomalies or produced false experimental predictions. Conversely, some theories have been rejected even though they received the most empirical confirmation. Thus, Laudan argues that questions about truth are essentially irrelevant to scientific progress. The relevant element is the theory's problem-solving effectiveness; a theory's progress is defined by the degree to which it solves more scientific problems than its rivals. As stated by Laudan, "*the solved problem—empirical or conceptual—is the basic unit of scientific progress*" (Laudan, 1977, p. 66).

Historicists such as Laudan find reductionism counterproductive to the goal of solving scientific problems. Research traditions should not be seen as competitors trying to mutually undermine each other rather as collaborators toward the goal of solving scientific problems. This process of synthesizing research traditions, thus expanding them, is called the "integration of research traditions," according to Laudan (1977). Two ways in which this integration may occur are described:

1. One research tradition can be grafted onto another without any major modifications in the components of either.
2. Two or more research traditions may each sacrifice fundamental elements that have been refuted while combining their remaining elements in a new way.

An important scientific motivation for integrating research traditions is the goal of explaining different dimensions of the same phenomena under study. For example, in nursing, the integration of divergent research traditions from biology, psychology, and sociology can account for the ontological perspective that individuals are biopsychosocial beings, which is common in nursing. This pattern of conjoining fundamental perspectives from different traditions is common when scientists develop new interdisciplinary fields of study to account for previously unexplained scientific problems. The integration of research traditions and corresponding theories is shown in Figure 19-1.

Laudan's analysis of integration departs significantly from the logical empiricist contention that science progresses through the elimination of theories by reduction. But the process of integration does not involve elimination by reducing one tradition to another, because both traditions retain their identity. Integration aims at extracting the progressive components of each tradition in a way that produces solutions to previously unsolved problems.

Goal of Philosophy of Science

According to logical empiricists, the ultimate goal of philosophy of science is to present a formalized account

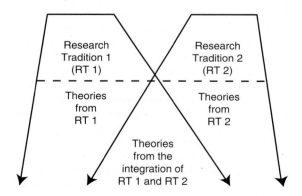

Figure 19-1 *A conceptualization of the integration of research traditions and corresponding theories within historicism.*

of the nature of scientific knowledge. This includes an application of logical principles to questions about the nature of science, since logic provides the eternal principles for relationships between scientific statements. By examining these relationships, the foundation of science is intended to systematically reveal the logical requirements for all scientific knowledge.

Historicists share with logical empiricists the belief that the philosopher's task is to construct a general account of the nature of scientific knowledge. But for historicists like Laudan, such a task must conform to the human elements of scientific evolution and growth. To meet this goal, historicists engage in studies of the actual activities, behavior patterns, and reasoning processes of working scientists. The belief is that philosophy of science must show how science, as it is actually practiced, can yield knowledge about the world. Such examination of the actual practice of scientists is used by historicists as evidence against logical empiricism, because the growth of scientific knowledge seems at times to be aided by illogical and nonrational decision making. It is believed that illogical processes can contribute to create growth of knowledge within a discipline.

 ## Nursing Theory Development and Testing

Since 1964, nurse scholars have become more aware of the influences of philosophy—in particular philosophy of science—on the development of nursing theory. A review of significant and representative nursing theory literature within three time periods shows the status of nursing theory in regard to logical empiricist and historicist trends in philosophy of science.

1964 to 1969

An important influence on nursing theory development during the 1960s was support given by the Division of Nursing of the U.S. Department of Health, Education, and Welfare (now the Department of Health and Human Services) to nursing schools to sponsor programs on the nature and development of nursing science. An analysis of metatheoretical papers from the proceedings of two such conferences—the Symposium on Theory Development in Nursing (1968) held at Case Western Reserve University in 1968 and the Conference on the Nature of Science in Nursing (1969) held at the University of Colorado in 1969—gives insight into how nurse scholars and others during the late 1960s conceptualized the derivation of nursing knowledge.

In 1968, Dickoff and James (1968) presented a version of their position paper on a theory of theories,

introducing the idea that significant nursing theory must be situation producing. Although they modified the orthodox view about the purpose of theory—that is, they postulated that theory could be capable of both more than and less than prediction—they, nevertheless, explicitly stated their faithfulness to the logical empiricist tradition. They forthrightly spoke of their work as a broader interpretation of the writings of such philosophers as Nagel (1961) and Hempel (1965, 1966). The language they used to describe theory supports logical empiricism. They spoke of concepts, propositions, set; they assessed scientific progress in terms of truth; and they insisted on a product orientation to science (i.e., production of desired situations).

In 1969, Abdellah (1969) discussed the nature of nursing science. Although no mention was made per se of the writings of philosophers who supported logical empiricism, Abdellah's views of what constitutes a scientific theory were nevertheless consistent with their writings; that is, terms must be operationally defined and preferably observable and quantifiable. Postulates are validated by testing deductions, which either helps to confirm the theory or leads to modifications of the postulates. Abdellah concludes that the reward of nurse scientists for their efforts is the discovery and affirmation of truth. Thus, as with Dickoff and James (1968), the criterion for the assessment of scientific progress is an increase in scientific truths.

Other writings (Dickoff, James, & Widenbach, 1968a, 1968b) related to nursing theory development and testing during the late 1960s all tended to have a logical empiricist perspective, with the exception of Leininger's (1969) introductory comments to the Conference on the Nature of Science in Nursing, which offered an ethnoscience research methodology to the discovery of scientific knowledge. This approach stresses the viewing of behavior from the subject's perspective rather than the researcher's. This accommodation to subjectivism is more compatible with historicism than with the objectivism of logical empiricism.

1970 to 1975

In the first half of the 1970s, two major trends in nursing theory occurred:

1. Metatheoretical formulations relevant to nursing theory and testing within the logical empiricist tradition were developed to a high degree by such investigators as Jacox (1974) and Hardy (1974).

2. A number of conceptual frameworks for nursing were published; for example, the work of Rogers (1970), King (1971), Orem (1971), and Roy (1974).

According to Jacox (1974), the goal of science is the discovery of truths, and the purpose of scientific theory is description, explanation, and prediction of part of our empirical world. In discussing theory construction, Jacox uses the language of the logical empiricists, including concepts, propositions, axioms, and theorems. Hardy (1974) is even more oriented to the formal logic underlying logical empiricism, discussing nine possible relationships that can exist between concepts and presenting a diagrammatic and matrix presentation of a situation that shows (1) the concepts, (2) the sign of the relationship between concepts, and (3) the nature of the relationships between concepts.

These two articles represented a culmination of the metatheoretical notions about logical empiricism in nursing theory. The irony, of course, is that at the time these and similar reports were making a profound impact on the derivation of theory in nursing, the logical empiricist viewpoints espoused in them were being strongly repudiated by a growing number of philosophers of science. In other words, nursing's theoretical link to philosophy of science was, from the historicist perspective, about a decade behind the times.

The irony continues in regard to the second trend—the publication of a number of important conceptual frameworks for nursing. Several conceptual frameworks published in the early 1970s were essentially devoid of any explicit linkage to philosophy of science (King, 1971; Orem, 1971). This is in no way meant to diminish the quality or significance of these seminal works but only to point out that a situation existed in which the most influential nursing literature on theory construction and testing followed rather than preceded the derivation of the conceptual frameworks, apparently because the metatheoretical movement in nursing was, for the most part, a separate movement from the conceptual framework movement.

1976 to Present

Since 1976, the following trends have occurred:

1. A continued and relatively stable commitment to logical empiricism, although a beginning trend toward historicism is apparent;

2. A revision of several conceptual frameworks for nursing and the introduction of some new frameworks; and

3. A questioning of the adequacy of strictly quantitative research methods to test nursing theory deductions.

The relatively stable commitment to logical empiricism is reflected in the current writings of several nurse authors (Chinn & Jacobs, 1983; Fawcett, 1983; Menke, 1983; Walker & Avant, 1983). However,

there are some new trends. For example, in 1979 when Newman (1979) introduced a new theory of health, the viewpoint was one of logical empiricism. However, in a recent work, a shift in her thinking is evident. Reflecting the thoughts of Kuhn (a historicist), Newman defines science as "a process of knowing, a process of challenging, and a continuing revolution" (Newman, 1983, p. 387). This emphasis on process (not product) and revolution (not logic) is a noticeable shift in viewpoint from logical empiricism to historicism.

In a recent publication, Hardy (1983) also extensively cited Kuhn in discussing nursing theory. The primary emphasis is on metaparadigms; however, Hardy also seems to agree, at least implicitly, with Kuhn's definition of the development of scientific knowledge as both nonrational and noncumulative. This represents a marked shift in viewpoint from the 1974 Hardy article, which, of all the metatheoretical articles, represented the most rigorous and logically structured formulations in support of logical empiricism. These contradictions in the works of Hardy and other metatheorists are indicative of the pull between orthodox and new ideas in philosophy of science and in nursing theory development and testing.

Although several other nurse authors (Carper, 1978; MacPherson, 1983; Meleis, 1983; Menke, 1983; Munhall, 1982) briefly address Kuhn's *The Structure of Scientific Revolutions* (1962; 1970), with the exception of Meleis (1983) they do not discuss Kuhn's more recent writings or mention Laudan's work, which represents the forefront of philosophy of science today. However, Laudan's work is briefly mentioned in an article by Watson (1981) and cited in the bibliographies of books by Parse (1981) and Chinn and Jacobs (1983). Although this attention to the work of Laudan is scant, it is encouraging because it begins to bring the development of nursing theory knowledge in line with current trends in philosophy of science.

The second trend occurring between 1976 and the present is the expansion and revision of the works of those nurse authors who in the early 1970s had developed conceptual frameworks for nursing. For example, first editions of books and other publications were rewritten, expanded, or revised by Orem (1980), King (1981), Roy (1981), Roy and Roberts (1981), and Rogers (1980). Several of these nurse theorists, in an attempt to bring their works more in line with what the nurse metatheorists of the mid-1970s were espousing—logical empiricism—revised their works to explicitly identify such elements as concepts and propositions that are inherent in the orthodox viewpoint.

Thus, an interesting situation has been created: While these nurse theorists have been updating trends in philosophy of science as espoused in the nursing literature of the mid-1970s, those who espoused these views have begun to question them and some no longer espouse them. This is not to say that individuals should not alter their viewpoints but to point out again the seeming separateness of the metatheoretical and conceptual framework movement in nursing and the effect of this separateness on perpetuating traditional or singular viewpoints about philosophy of science.

Two other conceptual frameworks were developed in books published in 1976 by Paterson and Zderad and in 1981 by Parse. Neither book has received much attention in the nursing literature, although there is some evidence that this is changing (Chinn & Jacobs, 1983; Fitzpatrick & Whall, 1983). Could it be that both of these books have a strong existential-phenomenological perspective that, until recently, was out of the mainstream of the thinking of orthodox nurse scientists about philosophy of science? The underlying assumptions these three authors hold about the nature of science are much more in keeping with nontraditional views about philosophy of science than with traditional views. In particular, they see science as process; they envision a strong link between the theory's ontological commitment and its methodological commitment; and they place little emphasis on precise, logical formulations.

The third trend is a shift in emphasis from quantitative to qualitative research methods to test nursing theory deduction. In the late 1970s, nurse scholars (Silva, 1977) began to question the limits of quantitative research methods because they too often sacrificed meaningfulness for rigor. Out of this questioning, articles suggesting alternative approaches to logical empiricism began to appear in the nursing literature (Munhall, 1982; Oiler, 1982; Omery, 1983; Swanson & Chenitz, 1982; Tinkle & Beaton, 1983; Watson, 1981). These approaches were sought because of the inadequacy of logical empiricism to deal with certain phenomena in nursing, in particular, those phenomena dealing with humanism and holism. By exploring alternative philosophies of science and research methodologies that are compatible, it seems possible to study these phenomena in a more meaningful and creative way and, in so doing, to help bridge the gaps among philosophies of science, nursing theory, and nursing research. Historicism is one of the alternative philosophies that holds promise in helping to bridge these gaps.

Implications and Recommendations for the Future

Since every scientific theory is tied to some philosophical framework as the basis for understanding and assessing theory, it is important for the theorists within a given discipline to be aware of the discipline's philosophical orientation. Therefore, nursing

theorists should continue to explore the philosophical underpinnings of their discipline in order to integrate the latest advances in nursing theory development and testing with a coherent philosophical foundation.

This review of the trends in nursing theory from 1964 to the present shows not only that nursing theory is presently in a state of transition, but also that many of the changes in nursing theory reflect a reorientation of the underlying philosophy of the discipline. This is evident in the beginning metatheoretical shift away from a strongly empirical and logical orientation to theory construction reminiscent of logical empiricism and toward a more holistic and humanist approach more in line with historicism. There are several implications for nursing theory development and testing:

- Laudan dismisses as counterproductive the logical empirical goal of reducing one theory to another. Rather than trying to restrict the range of possible theories, Laudan encourages theory expansion through a process of integrating components from different research traditions, which results in a multidimensional understanding of the phenomena. Based on this historicist orientation, there should not be a single, conceptual framework for nursing. This orientation suggests, rather, the expansion of nursing theory through the integration of progressive components of the various existing nursing conceptual frameworks, which results in multiple frameworks. This process should be a cooperative endeavor and, if adhered to, should encourage a cooperative rather than a competitive attitude among nurse scholars. In the future some of the conceptual frameworks for nursing may be integrated so that the unimportant elements are sacrificed and the important elements are combined in a new way.

- The historicist's conception of science as a human process, rather than a product of some endeavor, suggests that nursing theory should always be understood as a stage in its evolution and growth. Although nursing theory is experiencing shifts in its evolution, the result of the transition will not be some final and static body of knowledge. Like any scientific discipline, nursing theory construction will never culminate in some static set of eternal truths but will represent one episode in its evolving history.

- Historicism strongly encourages a careful study of the actual practices, belief systems, and external factors influencing a community of scientists within a given discipline. This has a direct bearing on the type of data relevant for any theory construction. Thus, data for nursing theory development and testing will include the common practices of nurse clinicians, the social and psychological factors affecting the profession of nursing, the widely held beliefs of the community of nurses, and the reasoning patterns of individual nurse theorists. A result of integrating these data will be a nursing theory that more explicitly addresses the human dimensions of nursing and the practitioners of nursing.

■ Scientific progress for Laudan reduces to the number of solved problems within a discipline. Therefore, the assessment of progress in nursing theory development and testing will be less rigid and more practical than suggested by a logical empiricist orientation. That is, there will be less emphasis on truth and error as the criteria for assessing scientific progress and more emphasis on the actual solution to nursing care problems. This shift should help to bridge the gap between those persons who are primarily nurse scholars and those who are primarily nurse clinicians. The clinician, of course, is in an ideal position to both understand and assess whether, and to what degree, a nursing care problem has been solved. Within this framework, the nurse clinician should be highly valued as an integral part of the process of nursing theory development and testing.

Based on the changing trends in philosophies of science and nursing theory, four recommendations are made:

1. Creation of liaisons between departments of nursing and departments of philosophy to help nurse scholars, theoreticians, researchers, and clinicians stay abreast of changes in philosophy of science;

2. Establishment of closer, cooperative working relationships among nurse metatheorists, theoreticians, researchers, and clinicians with a common goal of solving problems of significance in nursing;

3. Exploration of innovative, qualitative methods for testing nursing theory that are in keeping with the historicist tradition; and

4. Continued and explicit emphasis in nursing theory courses on the interrelationships among philosophies of science, nursing theory, and nursing research.

If the above recommendations are implemented, they should help to establish and maintain an open dialogue, which portends a healthy and promising future for the advancement of nursing science.

REFERENCES

Abdellah, F. G. (1969). The nature of nursing science. *Nursing Research, 18,* 390–393.

Ayer, A. J. (1959). Editor's introduction. In A. J. Ayer (Ed.), *Logical positivism* (pp. 3–28). New York: Free Press.

Braithwaite, R. B. (1953). *Scientific explanation: A study of the function of theory, probability and law in science.* London: Cambridge University Press.

Carper, B. A. (1978). Fundamental patterns of knowing in nursing. *Advances in Nursing Science, 1*(1), 13–23.

Chinn, P. L., & Jacobs, M. K. (1983). *Theory and nursing: A systematic approach.* St. Louis: C. V. Mosby.

Conference on the Nature of Science in Nursing (1969). *Nursing Research, 18,* 388–411.

Dickoff, J., & James, P. (1968). A theory of theories: A position paper. *Nursing Research, 17,* 197–203.

Dickoff, J., James, P., & Wiedenbach, E. (1968a). Theory in a practice discipline: Part I. Practice-oriented theory. *Nursing Research, 17,* 415–435.

Dickoff, J., James P., & Widenbach, E. (1968b). Theory in a practice discipline: Part II. Practice-oriented research. *Nursing Research, 17,* 545–554.

Fawcett, J. (1983). Hallmarks of success in nursing theory development. In P. L. Chinn (Ed.), *Advances in nursing theory development* (pp. 3–17). Rockville, MD: Aspen Systems.

Feyerabend, P. (1978). *Against method: Outline of an anarchistic theory of knowledge.* London: Verso.

Fitzpatrick, J. J., & Whall, A. L. (1983). *Conceptual models of nursing: Analysis and application.* Bowie, MD: Brady.

Hanson, N. R. (1958). *Patterns of discovery: An inquiry into the conceptual foundation of science.* London: The Syndics of the Cambridge University Press.

Hardy, M. E. (1974). Theories: Components, development, evaluation. *Nursing Research, 23,* 100–107.

Hardy, M. E. (1983). Metaparadigms and theory development. In N. L. Chaska (Ed.), *The nursing profession: A time to speak* (pp. 427–437). New York: McGraw-Hill.

Hempel, C. G. (1965). *Aspects of scientific explanation and other essays in the philosophy of science.* New York: Free Press.

Hempel, C. G. (1966). *Philosophy of natural science.* Englewood Cliffs, NJ: Prentice Hall.

Jacox, A. (1974). Theory construction in nursing: An overview. *Nursing Research, 23,* 4–13.

King, I. M. (1971). *Toward a theory for nursing: General concepts of human behavior.* New York: John Wiley & Sons.

King, I. M. (1981). *A theory for nursing: Systems concepts, process.* New York: John Wiley & Sons.

Kuhn, T. S. (1962). *The structure of scientific revolutions.* Chicago: The University of Chicago Press.

Kuhn, T. S. (1970). *The structure of scientific revolutions* (2nd ed.). Chicago: The University of Chicago Press.

Kuhn, T. S. (1977). Second thoughts on paradigms. In F. Suppe (Ed.), *The structure of scientific theory* (pp. 459–482). Urbana, IL: University of Illinois Press.

Lakatos, I. (1968). Changes in the problem of inductive logic. In I. Lakatos (Ed.), *The problem of inductive logic* (pp. 315–417). Amsterdam: North-Holland.

Laudan, L. (1977). *Progress and its problems: Toward a theory of scientific growth.* Berkeley, CA: University of California Press.

Leininger, M. M. (1969). Nature of science in nursing. *Nursing Research, 18,* 388–389.

MacPherson, K. I. (1983). Feminist methods: A new paradigm for nursing research. *Advances in Nursing Science, 5* (2), 17–25.

Meleis, A. I. (1983). A model for theory description, analysis, and critique. In N. L. Chaska (Ed.), *The nursing profession: A time to speak* (pp. 438–452). New York: McGraw-Hill.

Menke, E. M. (1983). Critical analysis of theory development in nursing. In N. L. Chaska (Ed.), *The nursing profession: A time to speak* (pp. 416–426). New York: McGraw-Hill.

Munhall, P. L. (1982). Nursing philosophy and nursing research: In apposition or opposition? *Nursing Research, 31,* 176–177, 181.

Nagel, E. (1961). *The structure of science: Problems in the logic of scientific explanation.* New York: Harcourt Brace & World.

Newman, M. A. (1979). *Theory development in nursing.* Philadelphia: F. A. Davis.

Newman, M. A. (1983). The continuing revolution: A history of nursing science. In N. L. Chaska (Ed.), *The nursing profession: A time to speak* (pp. 385–393). New York: McGraw-Hill.

Oiler, C. (1982). The phenomenological approach in nursing research. *Nursing Research, 31,* 178–181.

Omery, A. (1983). Phenomenology: A method for nursing research. *Advances in Nursing Science, 5*(2), 49–63.

Orem, D. E. (1971). *Nursing: Concepts of practice.* New York: McGraw-Hill.

Orem, D. E. (1980). *Nursing: Concepts of practice* (2nd ed.). New York: McGraw-Hill.

Parse, R. R. (1981). *Man-living-health: A theory of nursing.* New York: John Wiley & Sons.

Paterson, J. G., & Zderad, L. T. (1976). *Humanistic nursing.* New York: John Wiley & Sons.

Rogers, M. E. (1970). *An introduction to the theoretical basis of nursing.* Philadelphia: F. A. Davis.

Rogers, M. E. (1980). Nursing: A science of unitary man. In J. P. Riehl & C. Roy (Eds.), *Conceptual models for nursing practice* (2nd ed.) (pp. 329–337). New York: Appleton-Century-Crofts.

Roy, C. (1974). The Roy adaptation model. In J. P. Riehl & C. Roy (Eds.), *Conceptual models for nursing practice* (pp. 135–144). New York: Appleton-Century-Crofts.

Roy, C. (1981). *Introduction to nursing: An adaptation model.* Englewood Cliffs, NJ: Prentice Hall.

Roy, C., & Roberts, S. L. (1981). *Theory construction in nursing: An adaptation model.* Englewood Cliffs, NJ: Prentice-Hall.

Rudner, R. S. (1966). *Philosophy of social science.* Englewood Cliffs, NJ: Prentice Hall.

Scheffler, I. (1963). *The anatomy of inquiry: Philosophical studies in the theory of science.* New York: Knopf.

Silva, M. C. Philosophy, science, theory: Interrelationships and implications for nursing research. *Image, 9,* 59–63.

Swanson, J. M., & Chenitz, W. C. (1982). Why qualitative research in nursing? *Nursing Outlook, 30,* 241–245.

Symposium on Theory Development in Nursing (1968). *Nursing Research, 17,* 196–222.

Tinkle, M. B., & Beaton, J. L. (1983). Toward a new view of science: Implications for nursing research. *Advances in Nursing Science, 5*(2), 27–36.

Toulmin, S. (1972). *Human understanding* (Vol. 1). Princeton, NJ: Princeton University Press.

Walker, L. O., & Avant, K. C. (1983). *Strategies for theory construction in nursing.* Norwalk, CT: Appleton-Century-Crofts.

Watson, J. (1981). Nursing's scientific quest. *Nursing Outlook, 29,* 413–416.

THE AUTHORS COMMENT | An Analysis of Changing Trends in Philosophies of Science on Nursing Theory Development and Testing

The ideas for this article arose when Dr. Silva was introduced to logical empiricism as the accepted mode of scientific inquiry, which she found limiting. Because every discipline has more than one point of view that changes with time, Dr. Silva asked Dr. Rothbart what major shifts had occurred in the philosophy of science during the decade before publishing this article. In reviewing writings from nursing, Dr. Rothbart revealed that nursing had a somewhat outdated philosophic emphasis on logical empiricism. He went on to describe historicism and the profound effect it could have on constructing nursing theory and research methods. Although philosophy of science has continued to change, the historicist views of Kuhn, Laudan, and others continue to influence how nursing and other disciplines practice their science.

MARY C. SILVA
DANIEL ROTHBART

The Advocate-Analyst Dialectic in Critical and Postcolonial Feminist Research

Reconciling Tensions Around Scientific Integrity

SHERYL REIMER-KIRKHAM, RN, PhD

JOAN M. ANDERSON, RN, PhD

With increased attentiveness to social justice and the social and economic inequities that shape health, well-being, and health care access, nurse researchers, particularly those positioning their work as emancipatory, negotiate the dialectic of analysis and advocacy. Drawing on postcolonial feminism, we explore this dialectic and associated ramifications for scientific integrity. Staying true to critical foundations shifts the focus from advocacy as "speaking on behalf of" to rigorous reflexive analysis that decenters dominant discourses to open up the possibility for those who have been marginalized to exercise human agency and work alongside researchers toward social justice for all. **Key words:** *advocacy, critical inquiry, feminism, postcolonial, research methodology, rigor, scientific integrity, social justice*

The topic of advocacy is now central in many nursing research discourses, particularly those formulated from a critical perspective. Structural constraints have become more clearly understood, with increasing recognition that attentiveness to social justice and the social and economic inequities that shape health, well-being, and access to health care is a key aspect of competent and effective nursing practice. The works of critical and feminist scholars (eg, see references 1–4) have directed us to examine reciprocity, intersubjectivity, reflexivity, and the coconstruction of knowledge as key features of a critical research process, to more fully understand the complex context of health, well-being, and health care. Alongside this, the development of qualitative research methods problematized the presumption of objectivity and "truth" for all research endeavors and provided frameworks for evaluation of the scientific quality of critical and interpretive research. As critical research methodologies have taken hold, we (as researchers employing postcolonial feminist research) have become increasingly aware of tensions that can arise from concurrent commitment to rigorous analysis and the advocacy that characterizes much of today's critical nursing inquiry. This tension, particularly as it relates to scientific integrity, has arisen in our work on the topics of social justice and equity as we have explored the social determinants of health, including access to health care, and analyzed the social context of health, illness, and healing in various population groups.

The authors recognize that the generation of knowledge is not a neutral enterprise; we are mindful that the labeling of research as concerned with equity and social justice, might preselect research study participants who have been historically disadvantaged and thereby generate expectations that findings will contribute to the amelioration of human distress. Even the consent forms that are constructed for research, that state specifically the benefits to be derived from such research, may set up stakeholders' expectations about the outcomes of the research. Although as "analyst," we can never predict outcomes before we conduct our studies, we might unwittingly position ourselves as "advocates" to speak for those whom we construct as disadvantaged, and whom we might characterize as "vulnerable." In other words, advocacy for a particular group might precede the doing of the research, with unexamined ideologies and beliefs driving the research process. These issues, foremost in our minds for some time now, are explored in this article. The purpose of this article was therefore to engage in a reflexive discussion about the advocate-analyst dialectic in critical and postcolonial feminist research, and how we might reconcile related tensions around scientific integrity.

We ask, if one begins with preconceived notions about inequities in health and health care, might one construct the research question and interpret findings to support certain conclusions? And, might this undermine scientific integrity, as we have defined it

ABOUT THE AUTHORS

SHERYL REIMER-KIRKHAM is an Associate Professor in the School of Nursing at Trinity Western University, Langley, where she is Director of the graduate nursing (MSN) program and teaches healthcare ethics, health policy, and qualitative research. With her roots and early nursing career in Winnipeg, she completed her post-RN BSN at the University of Victoria and her MSN and PhD at University of British Columbia. She was awarded a 2010 Award of Excellence in Nursing Research by the College of Registered Nurses of British Columbia (CRNBC). Her research program focuses on pluralism, health inequities, and social justice in healthcare and nursing education. With colleagues, she has explored applications of postcolonial feminism and other critical theories to nursing scholarship. Her current funded research project examines religion, spirituality, culture, gender, and place in home healthcare. She is a founding member of TWU's Religion in Canada Institute and Institute of Gender Studies, and the Critical Research in Health and Health Inequities Unit at University of British Columbia.

JOAN M. ANDERSON is a Health and Social Scientist. She received a bachelor's degree in nursing from McGill University, and a masters of science in nursing, and a PhD in sociology both from the University of British Columbia. Dr. Anderson is currently a Professor Emerita at the University of British Columbia in Vancouver, Canada. Funded by the Canadian Institutes of Health Research (CIHR) and the Social Sciences and Humanities Research Council of Canada (SSHRC), she has conducted extensive research in the areas of culture, gender, migration, health, and inequities in health and healthcare through the lens of postcolonial inquiry and, more recently, critical humanism. With colleagues in academic and clinical settings, she has engaged in knowledge translation research with health professionals at the point of care, administrators, and policy makers. A commitment to social justice in health and healthcare, the mentoring of colleagues and graduate students locally and nationally, writing, knowledge translation and other forms of dissemination of research, and consultation remain important dimensions of her active scholarship. In her spare moments, she enjoys the outdoors.

from a postcolonial and critical inquiry perspective? When one is invited into a community to conduct participatory research, one might ask, "Why was *I* invited in the first place? Is it because of my scientific abilities, or might I be perceived as someone who *will speak on behalf of the community (as an advocate)?* What are the expectations of community participants of the research outcomes? And, what if the research findings run counter to people's expectations?" It is the (sometimes unspoken) tension between analysis[*] and advocacy[†], and the uncompromising need for scientific integrity, that we interrogate in this article.

In tackling the aforementioned questions, we begin by situating our discussion and our reliance on postcolonial feminist inquiry against the backdrop

of contemporary discourses on critical perspectives. We draw on several examples where we have experienced a pull between advocacy and analysis to elucidate the nature of tensions that arise in relation to scientific integrity. With this discussion, we seek insight into the interface between critical social justice and advocacy, and how claims of advocacy may support or threaten the very nature of scientific integrity. We are cautious about how we use the term "advocacy" recognizing that this process sets up unequal power relations between advocates and those for whom they speak. We argue that, above all, getting to the root causes of social inequities—social justice—is what is needed to restore human dignity to those who have been inequitably treated. With this in mind, we turn to an examination of the advocate-analyst dialectic in current critical discourses.

Situating the Advocate-Analyst Dialectic in Current Critical Discourses

In recent decades, we have seen a remarkable expansion of nursing research with criticalist aims,[6–12] a trend that is shared with other health and social

---

[*] By "analysis" we refer to rigorously exacting a method of science designed to address a clearly differentiated area for investigation. Analysis encompasses processes such as comprehending, examining, synthesizing, evaluating, and theorizing. The analyst moves between an examination of the component parts, and their relationship within the "whole," in a systematic and predictable fashion for the purposes of understanding, evaluating, and making resultant recommendations.

[†] We reference Webster's definition of advocacy as "active support; especially the act of pleading or arguing for something."[5] A central concern raised in this article is the risk of slipping into a colonizing speaking on behalf of "other."

sciences research. The ultimate ends of this type of research, sometimes referred to as "emancipatory" research,[13,14] is liberation from oppressions, in particular those oppressions that lead to inequities in access to health care services and health disparities. Broadly put, critical inquiry is committed to social justice, often employing language such as praxis, social change, or advocacy to connote this orientation toward social justice. Building on nursing's long legacy of emancipatory knowing—exemplified in historical figures such as Florence Nightingale and Lillian Dock; and derived from the evolution of critical social theories such as those developed by Karl Marx, Max Weber, members of the Frankfurt School including Jurgen Habermas, and other theorists such as Paulo Freire, and Foucault; and most directly the women's movement—a growing number of nurse scholars have in the latter half of the 20th century aligned centrally with critical perspectives.[13] With the expansion of nursing doctoral programs in the last 20 years that examine the philosophical foundations of nursing science and propose shifts in nursing, health care, and society to address entrenched health disparities and other social injustices in the purview of nursing, nurses are taking seriously the dual role of critiquing the status quo and imagining an equitable society. Reflecting this growing awareness of social justice in qualitative health research more broadly, Denzin and Lincoln posit that qualitative research has evolved from interpretive roots to embrace a commitment "up front to issues of social justice, equity, nonviolence, peace, and universal human rights. We do not want a social science that says it can address these issues if it wants to. For us, that is no longer an option."[15(p13)]

Sharing this commitment to praxis are many forms of participatory, community, and action research methods that often draw on theories such as poststructuralism, postcolonialism, feminism, critical social theory, and neo-Marxism. Although there are points of connection, such as those deriving from epistemological claims and notions about relations of power, each perspective is distinct.[‡] For example, some postcolonial and Black feminist scholars turn a critical gaze on postmodernism and an all-encompassing "critical perspective." Finding herself, as she puts it, on the outside of postmodern discourse, looking in, bell hooks had this to say: "It is sadly ironic that the contemporary discourse [meaning postmodernism] which talks the most about heterogeneity, the decentered subject, declaring breakthroughs that allow recognition of Otherness, still directs its critical voice primarily to a specialized audience that shares a common language rooted in the very master narratives it claims to challenge."[17(p25)] We would echo a similar perspective today. Postmodernism, poststructuralism, and other critical discourses, we would argue, are for the most part located within Eurocentric theorizing, which is at the center, with postcolonial theories, Black feminist scholarship, and Aboriginal and decolonizing epistemologies on the margins.

The Postcolonial Feminist Lens: Central Tenets

In this article, we focus, in particular, on postcolonial feminist theory. This theory *calls for the inclusion of voices silenced in the social production of knowledge* and disrupts the history of the categorization of people according to their presumed race. It analyzes how historical and racialized relations have contributed to structural inequities along the axes of race, class, gender, and other social relations. These social relations have structured, and continue to structure, life opportunities (eg, see references 18 and 19). A distinctive and grounding element in postcolonial feminism is that of exposing and countering marginalizing practices and relations of power rooted in colonizing histories. In the process of doing so, the analytic method is one of linking individual experience with the social forces that structure that experience, in essence, oscillating one's focus between the micropolitics and the macrostructures of relations of power. To do so effectively, the researcher critiques taken-for-granted assumptions, analyzes discourses and structures that support the status quo, and also turns a critical eye upon self (self-reflexivity). Mainstream discourses are decentered to create space for subaltern voices and epistemologies. Like other critical methods, relationality, respect, and collaboration mark research relationships. Taken together, these methodological principles underline postcolonial feminist's social justice orientation. Social justice, as a 3-dimensional concept requiring a combination of redistribution, recognition, and parity of participation *depending on particular context and situation,*[19,20] is brought about by various means conceived as a dialectic between analytic scholarship and action-oriented activism and advocacy (ie, theory and action).[§]

[‡]We have written elsewhere about the commonalities and distinctions within the broad and diverse family of critical perspectives.[16]

[§]Some caution must be taken in putting forward this type of conception to avoid reinforcing dualisms. Emphasizing the (interdependence) dialectic between politics (or action) and science, Harding explains: "We need not—indeed, must not—choose between "good politics" and "good science," … for the former can at least sometimes produce the latter, and the latter, at least in some cases, requires the former."[21(p30)]

Exemplifying the Advocate-Analyst Dialectic

Tensions in navigating the advocate-analyst dialectic have been a feature of many of the research studies we have engaged in, both as research supervisors of different graduate theses and as researchers in various research projects. We have learned over the years that even though research questions and approaches might be clearly articulated prior to setting out for the field, the pull between "researcher as analyst" and "researcher as advocate" surfaces as we navigate the terrain of rapport-building with research participants, and as we adhere to the principles of feminist inquiry and interviewing. It is a fine balance between maintaining the analytic stance of a researcher, with a certain detachment, and slippage into advocacy, as we enter into a research participant's personal and social space. Yet, enter this space we must, if we are to do rigorous inquiry and apply good science—herein lies the challenge. Our sense of obligation to those who have allowed us to enter into their lives can be a strong force in tipping the balance toward advocacy; it is for this reason that critical reflexivity is crucial as we engage in such encounters.

Furthermore, we need to be cognizant that our own a priori agendas—stemming from our theoretical commitments and/or our social locations and the agendas of stakeholders such as funders or policy makers—might potentially shortcut analytic processes and, ultimately, threaten the scientific integrity of our work. On the basis of such experiences, we have frequently, in various research contexts, pondered the dialectic between advocacy and analysis. To illustrate the advocate-analyst tensions that can arise, we refer to several examples from our research.

Researcher Positionality and Its Influence on Advocate-Analyst Dialectic

Demonstrating how one's theoretical orientation might shape research, we draw on research where we have applied the theoretical lens of cultural safety[22,23] (grounded in postcolonial assumptions regarding the historical legacy and ongoing oppressive structures of neocolonial relations) to the analysis of hospitalization and help-seeking experiences of diverse ethnocultural communities (Canadians of European, Chinese, and South Asian descent). Browne et al sum up cultural safety, developed in the bicultural context of New Zealand, as aiming "to counter tendencies in health care that create cultural risk (or *unsafety*)—those situations that arise when people from one ethnocultural

group believe they are demeaned, diminished or disempowered by the actions and the delivery systems of people from another culture."[24(p169)] We approached our research assuming that the concept of cultural safety would provide an appropriate analytic framework for examining the experiences of immigrant and indigenous populations. In a sense, our *a priori notions about different groups* had positioned us as advocates for those groups whom we considered to be most susceptible to experiencing inequities in health care delivery, given their historical location. Yet, as we were to find out through rigorous analysis of the data, and the examination of structural constraints, *in context,* and at *the intersection* of various social relations, we came to understand that cultural safety is relevant not only for groups that have been historically marginalized but for anyone.[25] Vulnerability is not a static or preexisting category belonging only to certain individuals affiliated with particular "marginalized" groups; rather vulnerability can be situational and dependent upon the negotiation or micropolitics of power in any given situation.[18,26] Likewise, advocacy needs to be problematized as a concept located in unspoken power relations between researchers and research participants situated within histories of colonial relations, with the very real potential of undermining the agency and resilience of research participants. This rereading against the "script" of cultural safety reflects a process of resisting theoretical imposition through rigorous analysis.

As with theoretical allegiances, we have also felt the premature pull to advocacy based on our individual gendered, classed, and racialized social positions. We may claim to enter into research from a scientifically neutral position, yet there are no value-free positions. Research is an intensely political process, with no one coming from an apolitical position. One's positioning is often at the root of the very questions one asks, and how one chooses to address them. Our own experiences, for example, of being from groups historically racialized or otherwise marginalized, and how these factors interact on life opportunities to become determinants of one's physical and psychological health, may, unwittingly, lie behind our work in the area of social and health inequities. Although this history and these factors may not be in the forefront of our consciousness, they have shaped us in particular ways. Likewise, our affiliations with the academy and our gendered, raced, and classed positionings serve as lenses through which we engage in scholarship. passions and personal experiences indeed drive us to advocate, for example, for equity in health and health care, and access to health care for immigrants and Aboriginal populations. Memories of a grandmother who could not speak English, or of poignant forms of racism, operate as subtexts in our everyday lives. Our starting point can be shaped by these experiences.

For example, in our research we have insisted on including different language groups in research studies. As we reflect on this, we suspect that there are many reasons for this. For example, this can be read as "doing good science." Knowledge is always partial and incomplete but is even more incomplete if some voices are shut out of the discourse. How can knowledge be credible if some voices are excluded? But we cannot leave it at that. As we reflect on our own positionality, we recognize our deep-seated belief and commitment to giving voice to those who have been silenced through history, as grounded not only in science but also in our personal histories and narratives. We use this example to show the complexity of the issue.

Although extending our research beyond English-speaking participants can be seen as "doing good science," we would argue that scientific integrity is also compromised when our ideologies are not held up to scrutiny, but are instead taken up and used to drive research so as to produce certain outcomes. Such would be the case, for example, if we were to decide *a priori* that *all* people who do not speak English are underserved or oppressed, and overlook the complex context in which they experience health and illness. Hence, we argue for continuing critical reflection in our work to bring to explicit clarity the deep-seated beliefs that, inadvertently, might shape the ways in which we approach analysis and arrive at conclusions from our data. It was this kind of critical reflection that led us, in one of our earlier manuscripts,[25] to highlight that *those seen as privileged within our society can be made vulnerable through illness and aging.*

So, we argue that although we cannot avoid our positionality, we can critically reflect on it to know ourselves, so to speak, and what drives us, and to always hold this up as a mirror for reflexivity. However passionate we are about the work we do, it does not entitle us to abandon the rigors of science. For example, we cannot fall into the trap that the "immigrant or the Aboriginal person is always oppressed" and allow this to drive our research agenda. Collins'[27] insights prompt us to recognize that the so-called marginalized, oppressed person can also be an oppressor, depending on context. We must therefore formulate research questions and engage in inquiry that allow us to examine, rigorously, the contexts of people's lives, and the broader social processes that shape human experience. In fact, *because* we are acutely aware of our own positionality, we are particularly vigilant to ensure that passion does not trump science. Thus, although one might be driven to ask certain research questions based on one's sociopolitical location, it is scientific rigor, not preconceived ideology, that crafts the position of advocacy. We do not deny that we come with certain presuppositions, but through critical reflection, we try to be aware of our biases and reflexively hold them up to scrutiny in our analytic work.

Stakeholder Agendas

Stakeholder agendas, whether those of funding agencies, decision-makers, community members, or research participants, may also pressure researchers to move prematurely from analysis to advocacy. We have been in research situations where people indicated they volunteered to participate because they hoped our research would bring about certain ends (eg, improved resources for spiritual-care services in one study). Such situations speak to the ways researchers can be pulled toward advocacy, particularly, when conducting research informed by critical perspectives. We have come to question whether such predicaments are inherent to critical inquiry—and in part, perhaps that is so. But, more often, such dilemmas derive from lack of clarity in regard to methodological principles, resulting, ultimately, in threats to scientific integrity. In response to this question, we now discuss how we might reconcile the tensions around scientific integrity and advocacy from critical and postcolonial feminist perspectives.

 ## Reconciling Tensions Around Scientific Integrity

Scientific integrity, at its base, has to do with the ethical and rigorous conduct of research, regardless of paradigm or methodology. Clearly, it involves the classic protection of participants' rights and meeting accepted standards for "rigor" in academic research. Generally, breaches in scientific integrity have been reported to fall most frequently into the areas of unethical treatment of research participants, fabrication and/or falsification of data, plagiarism, and failure to disclose conflict of interest.[28] Scientific integrity encompasses the "goodness" and trustworthiness of research in the broadest sense, with attention to dimensions such as intellectual and moral integrity.

In their précis on integrity in scientific research, the Institute of Medicine emphasizes a broad interpretation of scientific integrity: "Because of the complexity, variability, and nature of scientific inquiry, the concept of integrity in research can be elusive, and its value cannot be easily assessed or measured."[29(p16)] Our interest in the notion of scientific integrity here encompasses the value of integrity in our engagement with all stakeholders in the research process and the rigorous analysis of data. Put simply, scientific integrity is evaluated on the basis of being "true" or consistent to one's research method. It follows that adherence to the methodological principles should be of utmost interest to a critical researcher.

For a critical researcher, including those drawing on postcolonial feminism, methodological principles that serve as benchmarks for determining the worth and validity of emancipatory knowing/knowledge are put forward by Chinn and Kramer[13]: (i) sustainability—how well the envisioned social change survives and thrives; (ii) social equity—a demonstrable elimination or reduction of conditions that create disadvantage for some and advantage for others; (iii) empowerment—the growing ability of individuals and groups to exercise their will, have their voices heard, and claim full human potential; and (iv) demystification—making things that were formerly hidden from understanding visible and openly disclosed. When anchored to these methodological requirements for scientific integrity, we gain new insights regarding our involvement in advocacy and analysis as researchers. In our earlier work, we have articulated a method for postcolonial feminist research[30-32] that offers reference points for scientific rigor to the degree that one stays "true" to these methodological principles in the research endeavor.

From a postcolonial feminist perspective, we see the fundamental importance of embracing rigorous inquiry—regardless of whether we use qualitative, quantitative, or mixed methods—to clearly elucidate the social organization of health disparities and social injustices in ways that carry credence in academic and community settings. We recognize that the postcolonial scholar runs the risk of having her work marginalized and dismissed as serving the interests of particular groups; it is therefore imperative for us to demonstrate the rigor of our analyses. So, at this point in our scholarship, we take the position that postcolonial feminist research *as a legitimate form of critical inquiry and knowledge generation holds to standards of scientific integrity similar to other critical perspectives*. We recognize, however, that our knowledge and perspectives are always evolving and, in time, we may develop other "yardsticks" for judging the scientific integrity of our work.

We take the stance that all research can lead to advocacy; the biomedical scientist can be as much of an advocate as the social scientist or health researcher who works within the tradition of a critical perspective. For example, the results of research about smoking and cancer, or pesticides and cancer, have led to advocacy for certain groups, and some of the scientists who do this research are strong advocates for groups that are at risk. Ecofeminists, such as Vandana Shiva,[33,34] who is a physicist, philosopher, and feminist, demonstrate to us that science and advocacy can go hand in hand. In fact, rigorous science is often a precursor of advocacy. Critical inquiry, in particular postcolonial feminist inquiry, needs to be based on data that are unassailable because it may provoke controversy and contested conclusions.[35] Importantly, the

call for unassailable data is not to argue for a value-free science or knowledge in some objective, reified sense, but, rather, to recognize fundamental tenets of rigorous scholarship.

 ## Re-examining the Advocacy and Analysis Dialectic: Toward Critical Social Justice

So far, we have attempted to elucidate the types of tensions a researcher informed by critical and postcolonial feminism might encounter in regard to the dialectic processes of advocacy and analysis. Here, we move to a closer reexamination of the advocacy-analysis dialectic. We argue that although the topic of social justice is now relatively commonplace in nursing,[36] the call for critical social justice from a postcolonial feminist perspective provides one angle for refocusing on advocacy.

As illustrated in the earlier examples, both of us have experienced situations where the premature pull to advocacy could have undermined scientific integrity while we seek to reconcile science with praxis. The philosophical frameworks and corresponding methodological commitments of postcolonial and other critical inquiry typically place high value on deep engagement and reciprocity with participants and giving voice to marginalized perspectives and indigenous knowledges, resulting in rich knowledge generation. This same engagement and "giving voice" inherently results in the heightening of these incongruities between advocate and analyst roles. Although concerned with people whose voices have been marginalized and who have had to survive inequitable social relations, to say that one is conducting research to promote social justice and equity does not inherently mean you are "speaking for" a certain group. Nor does it mean using *a priori* notions of oppression, for example, as an analytic framework for the data.[37] As researchers working from a postcolonial feminist perspective, we are well aware of oppressive structures within society, yet we guard against seeing oppression everywhere in our data, lest our research simply becomes about "getting the proof." Oppression is not the starting point of inquiry; rather we start with everyday experience and work backwards, as it were, to analyze how social forces such as oppression shape these everyday experiences. We argue that rather than constructing analysis and advocacy as distinct or perhaps even contradictory processes, we need to hold up for questioning what we mean by advocacy, and whether advocacy paradoxically emphasizes the researcher's "superior" social location in relation to the research participant—that is, the researcher "has the power" to speak on behalf of the other, reinscribing colonizing relations in the process. The methodology of postcolonial feminism, with its obvious imperative of decolonizing research processes,[38] cautions us in promoting advocacy uncritically.

In reflecting on some of the central tenets of postcolonial theorizing, we have often drawn upon Homi Bhabha's words, "it is from those who have suffered the sentence of history—subjugation, domination, diaspora, displacement—that we learn our most enduring lessons for living and thinking."[39(p172)] An interpretation of Bhabha would suggest to us that engagement in the research *enterprise is not about speaking for others,* but, instead, *learning from voices that have been silenced.* What is called for, then, is not speaking on behalf of those constructed as "oppressed" and "vulnerable" as associated with advocacy, or using the familiar notion of empowerment as if we had power to give to others, but recognition of human agency, individual responsibility, engagement, and analysis. Social justice, from a postcolonial feminist perspective, calls for an engagement with voices that have not been listened to, to bring these voices to the forefront.[(19,20,40)] It is about writing in the notion of human agency, and exploring the tensions between agency and structural constraints located in histories of colonization. The emphasis is on unmasking the taken-for-granted, and producing new knowledge that allows us to address social structures and correct inequitable social relationships. As we noted elsewhere, "Postcolonialism is one of the critical theories that provides a theoretical lens that allows access to the everyday experiences of marginalization, as structured by the micropolitics of power and the macrodynamics of structural and historical nature,"[32(p2)] thus fostering a "paradigmatic shift of thinking inclusively about other oppressions, such as age, sexual orientation, religion and ethnicity."[27(p225)] We suggest that it may not be advocacy per se that is required, as much as social justice that addresses the complex historical, economic, social, and political processes shaping the micropolitics of power and injustices, and that puts forward the strategies that are needed to mitigate them. From a postcolonial feminist perspective, *speaking on behalf of the other* is seen as a reproduction of colonial relations; empowerment comes through the processes of finding one's voice, articulating one's perspectives, and engaging as a person of equal worth with those who have been "privileged" by their social location.[20] So, it is not that those with privilege advocate for the "oppressed" Other; rather through the processes of dialogic engagement, researcher and research participant engage in reflexive discourse to explicate *oppressive structures* that influence health and well-being and plan ways to move forward to address them. Quoting Bishop who writes about research in the Maori context:

> *Researchers are repositioned in such a way to no longer need to seek to give voice to others, to empower others, to emancipate others, to refer to others as* subjugated voices, *but rather to listen and participate … in a process that facilitates the development in people as a sense of themselves as agents and of having an authoritative voice …. A Kaupapa Maori approach to research … challenges colonial and neocolonial discourses that inscribe "otherness."[(cited in 41,p14)]*

A point to be reiterated here is that, from a postcolonial feminist perspective, the purpose of research and scholarship is not to serve particular "interest groups"; rather, the agenda is to unmask historically embedded, taken-for-granted social structures that support the status quo, that positioned people in particular ways, and that are major determinants of health and well-being. These deep-seated historical relations and their reproduction in everyday life are among the root causes of social and economic inequities. To this extent, postcolonial feminist scholarship applies to everyone, as we are all positioned in history. The discipline of nursing has a moral, ethical, professional, and social responsibility to understand and address inequitable social relations, to provide competent, effective, and efficient nursing care.

Concluding Comments

As critical methods gain momentum within nursing, it is timely to reflect on the dialectic of advocacy and analysis. We have mulled over this dialectic for several years, and we hope that this manuscript will engage others in a continuing dialogue. We anticipate that subsequent conversations will extend this critical analysis of the advocate-analyst dialectic, perhaps with a resignification of the very notions of scientific integrity itself, and whether it might be constructed differently through a postcolonial feminist, decolonizing lens. Undoubtedly, the most important point to be made here from a postcolonial feminist perspective is that the advocate-analyst dialectic enables the decentering of dominant discourses and promotes rigorous reflexive analyses that open up the possibility for those who have been marginalized through their historical positioning to speak for themselves. In so doing, they can exercise their human agency and work alongside researchers toward social justice for all.

REFERENCES

1. Oakley A. Interviewing women: a contradiction in terms. In: Roberts H, ed. *Doing Feminist Research*. London, UK: Routledge and Kegan Paul; 1981:3061.

2. MacPherson KI. Feminist methods: a new paradigm for nursing research. *Adv Nurs Sci*. 1983;5(2):17–25.

3. Campbell JC, Bunting S. Voices and paradigms: perspectives on critical and feminist theory in nursing. *Adv Nurs Sci*. 1991;13(3):1–15.

4. Anderson JM. Reflexivity in fieldwork: toward a feminist epistemology. *Image J Nurs Scholarsh*.1991;23(2):115–118.

5. *Webster's Online Dictionary*. http://www.websters-online-dictionary.org/definition/advocacy. Accessed April 19, 2010.

6. Allen D. Nursing and oppression: "the family" in nursing texts. *Feminist Teacher* 1986;2(1):15–20.

7. Canales MK. Othering: toward an understanding of difference. *Adv Nurs Sci*. 2000;22(4):16–31.

8. Cheek J, Rudge T. Been there done that? Consciousness raising, critical theory and nurses. *Contemp Nurse*. 1994;3(2):58–63.

9. Diekelmann N. Reawakening thinking: is traditional pedagogy nearing completion? *J Nurs Educ*. 1995; 34(5):195–196.

10. Drevdahl D. Diamond necklaces: perspectives on power and the language of "community." *Res Theory NursPract*. 1998;12(4):303–317.

11. Thompson J, Allen D, Rodriquez-Fisher L, eds. *Critique, Resistance, Action: Working Papers in the Politics of Nursing*. New York, NY: National League for Nursing Press; 1992.

12. Thorne S, Hayes V, eds. *Nursing Praxis: Knowledge and Action*. Thousand Oaks, CA: Sage; 1997.

13. Chinn P, Kramer M. *Integrated Theory and Knowledge Development in Nursing*. Philadelphia, PA: Mosby Elsevier; 2008.

14. Rose J, Glass N. The importance of emancipatory research to contemporary nursing practice. *Contemp Nurse*. 2008; 29(1):8–22.

15. Denzin N, Lincoln Y. Introduction. The discipline and practice of qualitative research. In: Denzin N, Lincoln Y eds. *The Sage Handbook of Qualitative Research*. 3rd ed. Thousand Oaks, CA: Sage; 2005:1–32.

16. Reimer-Kirkham S, Varcoe C, Browne A, Khan K, Lynam J, Anderson JM. Critical inquiry and knowledge translation: exploring tensions. *Nurs Philos*. 2009;10(3):152–166.

17. hooks b. *Yearning: Race, Gender, and Cultural Politics*. Boston, MA: South End Press; 1990.

18. Anderson JM. Lessons from a postcolonial-feminist perspective: suffering and a path to healing. *Nurs Inq*. 2004;11(4):238–246.

19. Reimer Kirkham S, Browne A. Toward a critical theoretical interpretation of social justice discourses in nursing. *Adv Nurs Sci*. 2006;29(4):324–339.

20. Anderson JM, Rodney P, Reimer-Kirkham S, Browne AJ, Basu Khan K, Lynam MJ. Inequities in health and healthcare viewed through the ethical lens of critical social justice: contextual knowledge for the global priorities ahead. *Adv Nurs Sci*. 2009;32(4):282–294.

21. Harding S. A socially relevant philosophy of science. *Hypatia*. 2004;19(1):25–47.

22. Ramsden I. *Kawa Whakaruruhau: Cultural Safety in Nursing Education in Aotearoa*. Wellington, New Zealand: Nursing Council of New Zealand; 1991.

23. Ramsden I. Cultural safety in nursing education in Aotearoa (New Zealand). *Nurs Prax N Z*. 1993;8(3): 4–19.

24. Browne A, Varcoe C, Smye V, et al. Cultural safety and the challenges of translating critically-oriented knowledge in practice. *Nurs Philos*. 2009;10(3): 167–179.

25. Anderson JM, Perry J, Blue C, et al. "Rewriting" cultural safety within the postcolonial and postnational feminist project: toward new epistemologies of healing. *Adv Nurs Sci*. 2003;26(3):196–214.

26. Reimer Kirkham S. The politics of belonging and in-tercultural health care provision. *West J Nurs Res*. 2003;25(7): 762–780.

27. Collins PH. *Black Feminist Thought: Knowledge, Consciousness, and the Politics of Empowerment*. Boston, MA: Unwin Hyman; 1990.

28. Merlo D, Vahakangas K, Knudsen L. Scientific integrity: critical issues in environmental health research. *Environ Health*. 2008;7(suppl 1):S9. http://books.nap.edu/openbook.php?record_id=10430& page=16. Accessed January 6, 2010.

29. Institute of Medicine. Integrity in scientific research: creating an environment that creates reasonable conduct. 2002. http://books.nap.edu/openbook.php?record_id=10430&page=16. Accessed January 6, 2010.

30. Anderson JM. Toward a post-colonial feminist methodology in nursing research: exploring the convergence of post-colonial and Black feminist scholarship. *Nurse Res*. 2002;9(3):7–27.

31. Khan K, McDonald H, Baumbusch J, Reimer Kirkham S, Tan E, Anderson J. Taking up postcolonial feminist methodology in the field: working through a method. *Womens Stud Int Forum*. 2007;30(3):228–242.

32. Reimer Kirkham S, Anderson JM. Postcolonial nursing scholarship: from epistemology to method. *Adv Nurs Sci*. 2002;25(1):1–17.

33. Shiva V, ed. *Close to Home: Women Reconnect Ecology, Health and Development*. London, UK: Earth-scan Publications Ltd; 1994.

34. Shiva V. *Biopiracy: The Plunder of Nature and Knowledge*. Cambridge: Southend Press; 1997.

35. Charmez K. Grounded theory in the 21st century: applications for advancing social justice studies. In: Denzin N, Lincoln Y, eds. *The Sage Handbook of Qualitative Research*. 3rd ed. Thousand Oaks, CA: Sage; 2005:507–536.

36. Boutain D. Social justice in nursing: a review of the literature. In: De Chesnay M, Anderson B, eds. *Caring for the Vulnerable: Perspectives in Nursing Theory, Practice, and Research*. 2nd ed. Mississagua, ON, Canada: Jones & Bartlett; 2008:39–52.

37. Lather P. *Getting Smart: Feminist Research and Pedagogy With/in the Postmodern*. NewYork, NY: Routledge; 1991.

38. Tuhawai Smith L. *Decolonizing Methodologies: Research and Indigenous Peoples*. London, UK: Zed Books; 2002.

39. Bhabha H. *The Location of Culture*. London, UK: Routledge; 2004.

40. Browne AJ, Tarlier D. Examining the potential of nurse practitioners from a critical social justice perspective. *Nurs Inq*. 2008;15(2):83–93.

41. Denzin N, Lincoln Y, Smith LT. *Handbook of Critical and Indigenous Methodologies*. Thousand Oaks, CA: Sage; 2008.

THE AUTHORS COMMENT | **The Advocate-Analyst Dialectic in Critical and Postcolonial Feminist Research: Reconciling Tensions Around Scientific Integrity**

For over a decade—initially in our doctoral advisor/student relationship, and then as colleagues conducting research together—we talked about the struggles of doing social justice work and balancing advocacy with scientific integrity. We found that with the increased attention to social justice and health inequities, along with critical and participatory research methods, there is often a tendency (even a push) to speak on behalf of "other." Reflexivity has alerted us to the potential tensions inherent in critical inquiry of taking an ideological approach to social justice work. We hope that this article will foster dialogue on how to take up social justice in a rigorous way to build the knowledge required, and to create the possibility for the expression of voice and the exercise of human agency by those who have been marginalized through their social positioning

SHERYL REIMER-KIRKHAM
JOAN M. ANDERSON

Validity and Validation in the Making in the Context of Qualitative Research

MIRKA KORO-LJUNGBERG, PhD

In this article, I focus on two ways of conceptualizing validity and validation, by using reductionist and (e)pistemological approaches, respectively. I question some common understandings of reductionist validation and describe an (e)pistemological standpoint that provides an alternative to reductionist views. In addition, I argue that validity and validation, as concepts, are tools rather than reflections of truth. Furthermore, fallibility, which is embedded in all views of validity and validation, can be compensated with pluralism, as well as acceptance, coexistence, and collaboration with the Other. **Key words:** *epistemology, qualitative methods, general, validity.*

In this time of increased accountability, "Bush science" (Lather, 2004, p. 19) and "gold standards" (Nespor, 2006, p. 119) have rendered strategic awareness and the discussions around validity more important than ever. The boundaries and goals of current discussions on validity and "state methodology" (Nespor, 2006, p. 118) are dangerous and bothersome for many. To work against hegemony and corporate ideologies, one must observe how various positions operate in the discourses surrounding validity. Lather (as cited in Wright, 2006) suggests that the direction in validity discussions should be from the ground up, so researchers will acknowledge the messiness related to the concept of validity. At the same time, it is important for researchers to consider alternatives to normalizing discourse by providing counterstories and complementary accounts of validity and by questioning assumed categories of validity (see Lather, 2006).

Various researchers (eg, Angen, 2000; Denzin & Lincoln, 2000; Hesse-Biber & Leavy, 2004; LeCompte, Millroy, & Preissle, 1992; Lincoln & Guba, 1985; Schwandt, 1997) have discussed diverse ways of conceptualizing validity in situated research approaches, and some, such as Agar (1986), have even replaced the term *validity* with *credibility*. Guba and Lincoln (1981) similarly referred to credibility and *transferability*. Numerous definitions, labels, and attempts to characterize and understand validity indicate that a unified definition of the concept is missing. Gergen and Gergen (2000) labeled this continuous linguistic and conceptual discussion a validity crisis in qualitative research.

However, in this article, my purpose is not to dismiss or deny the existence of a validity concept, which I think is "inaccurate yet necessary" (Spivak, 1997, p. xii); rather, my intention is to elaborate on how the label of validity and its identifiers function, are understood, and are used. I do not promote the unquestioned uses of any, including (e)pistemological validation, but I intend to continue the dialogue (see Angen, 2000) to work against dualism by promoting pluralism. I situate my conceptual discussion in the field of qualitative research even though I believe that many of my arguments could be transferred to other research approaches as well.

Mishler (1990) defined validation as a process through which trustworthiness of observations and interpretations are evaluated. In addition, Mishler emphasized the social construction of knowledge during the ongoing validation process, as well as the roles of cultural and linguistic practices in shaping validation. Angen (2000) proposed that even though validity as truth should be abandoned, validity might be viewed "as a process of validation, and evaluation of trustworthiness taking place within a human community" (p. 392). Similarly, I prefer to use the term *validation* instead of *validity* for several reasons. First, validation highlights the diverse ways of making, conducting, and even legitimizing research. Second, it illustrates the active role and agency of knowers. Furthermore, when it is assumed that various ways of conceptualizing validity and validation can coexist, it becomes important to identify genuine differences among these conceptualizations. However, to identify differences, one must first presuppose some common criteria for recognizing issues that relate to validity. We should

Author's Note: An earlier version of this article was presented at the American Educational Research Association conference in San Francisco, April 2006.

ABOUT THE AUTHOR

MIRKA KORO-LJUNGBERG is an Associate Professor of Qualitative Research Methodology at the University of Florida. She received her doctorate from the University of Helsinki, Finland. Prior to joining the faculty at the University of Florida, she conducted research as a visiting scholar at the University of Georgia. Her research focuses on the conceptual and theoretical aspects of qualitative research and participant-driven methodologies. Her work has been published in various research journals including *Educational Researcher, Field Methods, International Journal of Qualitative Studies in Education, Qualitative Inquiry, Qualitative Research, Qualitative Health Research*, and *Social Science & Medicine*.

begin by looking for similarities, which, in turn, will enable us to identify the ways in which difference and epistemological variation become meaningful.

Ultimately, the assumptions of validity and validation in many contexts are linked to theory, epistemology, technique, and the ways in which research interacts with practice. In this article, to mark the separations between transcendental epistemology (having access to transcendence, knowing what is True or Real, a priori Goodness and Beauty, assumptions of absolutism) and nontranscendental epistemology (meaning is located within the context of this world, in social and everyday experiences), I use Thayer-Bacon's (2003) term *(e)pistemology* to separate different uses and meanings associated with the term *epistemology*. Thayer-Bacon defined relational (e)pistemologies as "theory that insists that knowers/subjects are fallible, that our criteria is corrigible [capable of being corrected], and that our standards are socially constructed, and thus continually in need of critique and reconstruction" (p. 7). Reality cannot be separated from the subject, and knowing is a process instead of a product or an object. As a result, socially constructed epistemology is open to criticism and revision. In essence, when Thayer-Bacon's perceptions of standards are applied to the discussions on validity, every definition or each conceptualization of validity (including those that are most accepted and cited) is discursive, limited, and based on a particular argumentation structure (see Brinberg & McGrath, 1985; Maxwell, 1992) and thus represents only limited perceptions and evolving understandings.

Reductionist Validation in the Making

Reductionist views of validity and the criteria embedded in valid research processes are commonly based on epistemological or methodological exclusionism. Historically, many reductionist views on validity can be linked to the beliefs of a realistic truth theory and the correspondence theory of truth as defined by Campbell and Stanley (1966) and Cook and Campbell (1979). By reductionism, I mean an approach that promotes singularity based on a priori selection criteria or process. Furthermore, a reductionist view implies that particular criteria—for example, related to an external evaluation by the experts of the field or methodological specificity—grant trustworthiness, value, and legitimacy to research.

In the field of qualitative research, Merriam (1995), for example, proposed that the rigor of qualitative research is found in three interrelated areas: (a) internal validity, which describes the connection between study findings and a belief of reality (which in qualitative research is constructed or interpreted); (b) external validity, which explains the extent to which the findings could be applied to other situations (reader or user generalizability); and (c) reliability, the extent to which the same findings can be found again. Merriam further states that findings in qualitative research are never static; rather, it is more important to ask whether the findings of the study are consistent with data collected. Despite the fact that Merriam questions whether validity and reliability can be transferred directly from quantitative research to qualitative research, she promotes a particular set of external criteria for validity that can be verified or constructed outside the knowers themselves.

Other researchers have proposed alternative definitions and consequential techniques that characterize many qualitative studies by ensuring validity through triangulation, audit trails, peer reviews, and member checking (e.g., Creswell, 1998; Lincoln & Denzin, 1994; Michrina & Richards, 1996). However, it can be argued that the above techniques also rely on factors, elements, and reference points outside the research and beyond the researcher. For instance, if triangulation is used to emphasize how various perspectives, methods, and investigators enable more truthful representations of reality, an externalization and objectification of data and the research process might take place. Similarly, even though an audit trail requires researchers to document the entire research process in detail, describe the choices researchers have made, and illustrate the values and beliefs associated with research, it remains for the readers and the research community to decide whether the research is actually valid.

Anderson and Herr (1999) suggested that outcome validity and process validity are two essential types of validity that are interconnected. They entertain the idea that a well-conducted study will produce an answer to the research question. This positioning assumes a particular connection between theory and research questions and proposes that research questions serve as a vehicle to describe and construct a meaningful relationship between existing literature and lived experiences. However, it can be argued that Anderson and Herr's concepts of validity are ultimately based on transcendental epistemology; the belief in Truth; and a consequential, accurate representation of reality in which it is assumed that there exist right, singular, or accurate answers to research questions. Anderson and Herr do not take into account that researchers might find multiple, situated, contextual, and even conflicting answers to their research questions that can all be considered true depending on different epistemologies, theoretical perspectives, individual and collective experiences, discourses, values, and beliefs.

Kirk and Miller (1986) explained that validity becomes a meaningful concept only in relation to a theoretical perspective. A theoretical perspective and the key concepts closely associated with it shape the research process and produce knowledge. In addition, epistemological goals linked with particular theoretical perspectives also influence how validity within a study should be evaluated (see Smith & Deemer, 2000). Heikkinen, Kakkori, and Huttunen (2001) argued that validity is constructed discursively; therefore, it is equally important to consider how various epistemologies affect research differently and how they lead to a variety of values associated with trustworthy and valid research. Similarly, Creswell and Miller (2000) proposed that both paradigmatic assumptions and the employed lens(es) (of the researcher, study participants, and people external to the study) influence how validity will be approached. Creswell and Miller also suggest that from a systematic paradigm perspective, validity is established through triangulation (researcher lens), member checking (participant lens), and audit trail (external lens), whereas researcher reflexivity, collaboration, and peer debriefing would better suit a critical paradigm and the researchers operating within it. However, when Creswell and Miller choose to define validity through accurate representation of participants' realities, assuming there is one accurate representation, they again refer to Truth as knowledge and to the conditions in which knowledge can be justified by true beliefs. By doing so, Creswell and Miller reduce the definition of validity to the accurate representation of reality.

From another reductionist perspective, appropriate and epistemologically consistent methods can increase the validity of situated research approaches.

Situated research approaches refer, in this context, to the study designs that investigate, for example, patients' perceptions of their health and individuals' experiences of their well-being in particular sociopolitical and economic contexts. Furthermore, epistemological-methodological consistency during the research process implies a connection between a theoretical perspective of phenomenology and phenomenological analysis methods, such as Moustakas's (1994) phenomenological analysis. From this perspective, epistemologically appropriate methods (*i.e.*, those methods that produce knowledge consistent with the selected epistemological perspective) produce knowledge that is consistent with the epistemological goals and purposes of the research. It can be argued that epistemological-methodological consistency is a desirable goal in its own right and can assist researchers in methodological decision making and design choices.

However, epistemological-methodological reductionism has its limitations, especially when it is assumed that only one appropriate method exists for a particular epistemological project. Moreover, the selection of suitable methods is often based on external resources such as literature, research training, or consultation with other researchers. As a consequence, the responsibility for regarding validity and validation of one's research can be overlooked and externalized by referring, for example, to invalid instruments or the insufficient use of methods.

Reductionist views of validity and the correspondence theory of truth have many proponents. For example, Puolimatka (2002) proposed that qualitative research loses its credibility by giving up the correspondence theory of truth. He believes that an epistemological criterion for truth only describes some conditions through which truth may emerge or exist, but it does not define truth itself, which Puolimatka sees as a serious limitation. However, a single, realistic truth and a transcendental criterion for validity become problematic if researchers do not believe in truth as a stable, definable, and foundational concept. Thayer-Bacon (2003) argued that many philosophers have moved away from the truth correspondence theory because universal truth is impossible to define and achieve. Therefore, it seems reasonable to consider (e)pistemological conceptualizations of validity simultaneously with transcendentally based assumptions.

 ## (E)pistemological Validation in the Making

Thayer-Bacon (2003) proposed that from a relational (e)pistemological perspective, reality cannot be separated from the subject, and fallibility must be compensated through plurality. In addition, when knowing is viewed as a process and it focuses on the subject, not on the object, the concepts (such as validity) that evaluate different and appropriate ways of knowing must be also viewed from the knowers' perspectives. When knowing is viewed as a situated and plural process, it allows researchers to accept various ways and purposes of knowing and communication, such as prediction, description, emancipation, or deconstruction (Habermas, 1971). Carspecken (1996) argued that validity requires the consensus of a cultural group, and this consensus is based on the structures of human communication. Truth claims and validity cannot be conveyed to other persons without the structures of communication. Moreover, Carspecken (1996) contended that when researchers understand the essential role of validity in normal human communications, researchers are "able to formulate the special requirements that a social researcher conducting formal inquiries into social processes must employ to produce a trustworthy account" (p. 58).

Thayer-Bacon (2003) added that researchers cannot discount the concept of epistemology as it holds power over people's lives, but we can address and dissolve the dualism it creates. Validation would then include the ways in which the knowers build assertions warranted by their individual, collective, and spiritual experiences within social worlds, as well as the ways in which they engage in dialogue about their assertions with their environment. Scheurich (1996) also promoted dissolving dualism in relation to validity. He argued that the dualistic regularity shaping validity discussions in different paradigms needs to be unmasked and new forms of validity that construct validity as perspectival and complex need to be established.

Next, I discuss three assumptions about validation from the (e)pistemological perspective that might assist researchers when engaging in a validity and validation dialogue that moves away from dualism and exclusivism.

First Assumption: Interconnectedness Between Reality and Subjects

It can be argued that the process of validation refers to the connection between findings and reality, and that reality cannot be separated from the subject. This means that research findings cannot be distinct from the subject or knower (e.g., researcher, participant, community, and readers who are connected to their social and natural worlds), and knowers cannot act as spectators in knowledge construction. This position implies that qualitative health researchers cannot assume objective roles or distance themselves from knowledge production or from study participants when conducting research. Rather, all knowers

(researchers and study participants) are constructing reality by living it, and they are equally engaged in the construction of this knowledge. Furthermore, "Reality is nonrational, it is where things *happen*" (Thayer-Bacon, 2003, p. 59). For example, participants' descriptions of their health problems cannot be rationalized; instead, they are described and constructed within an experimental space in which participants act and live at the moment.

Similarly, Anderson and Herr (1999) referred to the interconnectedness between reality and subjects by referring to the concept of catalytic validity,[1] which illustrates the degree to which the "research process reorients, focuses, and energizes participants toward knowing reality in order to transform it" (p. 16), and democratic validity, which emphasizes the role of collaboration among the knowers. Study participants are seen as active collaborators and coconstructors of knowledge rather than as objects of research.

In the process of validating a particular construction of reality, the information regarding a knower's positivities, subjectivities, values, beliefs, and operating discourses and their connectedness to the research act itself become not only essential but also problematic. In situated research approaches, this could mean that the validation of research would heavily rely on the knowers and their clear articulation of applicable knowledge interests, as well as the knowers' ability in demonstrating how knowledge interests shape the research process. It would also call for in-depth and detailed descriptions of the knowers' dialogue with the environment, which, in turn, would portray the context and place where things happen and knowledge is constructed. For example, researchers document how they interact with participants, what kind of discourses shape those interactions, and what events lead to particular knowledge construction. In addition, validation viewed from this perspective requires various degrees of reflexivity, openness, and epistemological awareness from researchers.

When interconnectedness between reality and subjects is assumed, the criteria for validation that relies on individuals or experts outside the context of the immediate study, or anyone who is not a subject in the knowledge production, seem irrelevant and objectifying. Instead, it could be argued that the purpose of an audit trail or member checking, for example, is to highlight our ability to communicate with one another, in a sense creating the reality of our lives by engaging in a continual dialogue that, layer by layer, shapes our lives. New conversations documented in research evoke new realities, and the frequency and intensity of our conversations play an important role in the continual construction of reality. Therefore, during the validation process, subjective realities are modified and social meanings are communicated and thus, need to be reported. However, it must be acknowledged that negotiation, change, and modified meanings are sometimes not possible, allowed, or even desirable.

Ideally, the interconnectedness between reality and subjects places the subjects within particular and personal realities, creating a position that should avoid exploitation and misuse through agency and self-activation. However, sometimes exploitation cannot be avoided, and misuses occur outside and inside a researcher's awareness, world-views, and intentions. Knowers, who are also subjects of knowledge production, make ethical and moral decisions regarding their acts and whether particular assertions are worth making, as well as what the implications of making certain assertions or collecting particular evidence are. Both researchers and study participants make decisions about disclosures, questions, probes, and their impact on current and future interactions. Furthermore, it is ethically and morally important for knowers to question why a particular study is conducted, who benefits from it, and how they benefit.

Second Assumption: Knowledge as a Process

For James (1909/1977), "what really *exists* is not things made but things in the making" (p. 117). Similarly, from the (e)pistemological perspective of validation, knowledge is a process of making, instead of a final product. Furthermore, knowledge is constructed in the "process of socialization into a particular 'form of life'" (Mishler, 1990, p. 435). To know means that we acknowledge our relatedness—we are actively connected as knowers to Others (eg, individuals, texts, contexts, and cultures) and to various ways of knowing, including the spiritual, material, and natural worlds (see Thayer-Bacon, 2003).

From this point of view, it is essential to use and illustrate primary data and the knowers' interpretations of data, as well as how the data and interpretations change or become problematic during the research process. Similarly, the accessibility and openness of knowledge construction become essential not only during data collection but also during data analysis. In academic writing, for example, this might mean more accessible texts, clear process descriptions, illustrative footnotes, and direct data access.

When validation focuses on the process of knowledge production, it also acknowledges creativity, openness to difference, and infinity. These conditions emphasize the fallibility of assertions and leave knowing open-ended, inviting alternative knowings, which, in turn, promote social dialogue, new understandings, and alternative areas of future research. However, the fallibility of assertions can also create uncertainty and possible confusion, especially among novice researchers. It can be bothersome that the research report or academic writing does not conclude with one Truth; rather, it invites various other truths and realities. Then again, according to Richardson (2000), openness leads to other texts and knowledges and will also move knowers toward intertextuality and connectedness.

Openness and infinity also refer to the knowers' propensity for approaching and moving toward the unknown, for contesting boundaries and questioning taken-for-granted assumptions (see Lather, 1993). A researcher's openness to difference and the Other (other theories, values, beliefs, methods, data, and interpretations) enables and requires criticism/questioning through self-reflection by considering the historical conditions and discursive formations that shape produced assertions and evidence. Furthermore, assertions and evidence should be continuously placed under scrutiny during their generation.

Third Assumption: Pluralism

According to Thayer-Bacon (2003), "fallibilism entails pluralism" (p. 70); therefore, social beings are limited by their involvement and embodiment, and thus no one can claim privilege. The only way to overcome one's limitedness is through connectedness and collaboration. By relating to Others, individuals can expand their thinking and become more accepting of diversity. In addition, it is valuable to accept, consider, and ultimately use a range of points of view, theories, perspectives, world-views, and material conditions to improve our ability to search for multidimensional evidence and alternative justifications for knowledge claims. For example, multilayered texts, multivocality (as a type of data representation), and various forms of social activation and engagement support, as well as illustrate, the close collaboration between knowers and their communities.

Furthermore, Thayer-Bacon (2003) encouraged the researcher to pay close attention to alternative and (w)holistic ways of knowing, such as Buddhism, Native American's Great Spirit, Dream, and Holy Wind, which are built on a relationship between man and nature. For example, Buddhists and Native Americans emphasize the role of spirituality in describing one's experiences. According to Thayer-Bacon, spirituality, stories, and metaphors assist Buddhists and Native Americans in moving away from dualism toward a holism that can only be experienced. The purpose here, however, is not to deny dualism but to acknowledge that there is more than dualism. This idea, applied to validity, implies that there exists more than valid or invalid, good or bad, and well- or ill-executed research. "Nonduality is not something we can understand conceptually or intuitively, it is something we must experience" (Thayer-Bacon, 2003, p. 86).

Moving Toward Unthinkable Validity and Validation

It is important to move away from validity as a set of a priori criteria for well-established and well-conducted research. I argue that validity in qualitative research that can be generalized across contexts is always escaping and never complete because of various situational elements and differences in study designs and the sociopolitical influences that shape one's research. Instead, validity is in its making.[2] Qualitative health researchers need to engage in the validation, continuous establishment, and questioning of the validity of their studies. Researchers need to ponder how they will establish knowledge claims, prioritize data, connect with participants, use themselves as instruments of research, and how they communicate their findings to various audiences. In addition, it is crucial to portray validity and validation as possibilities and processes that enable scholars to establish various knowledge claims rather than to execute an objective evaluation of truth or demonstration of the researchers' fixation on transcendental truth. The legitimacy of validity and validation "lies in the natural world, which is a contingent, ever-changing world in which we are active participants" (Thayer-Bacon, 2003, p. 48). This means that all validity and validation definitions are limited and partial, and it is through their coexistence that the fields of science and research can change and grow. Dominant and narrow conceptions of validity and validation need to be questioned, allowing and welcoming alternative perspectives. The more we know about particularities and other conceptualizations of validity and validation, the more informed we will be when making decisions regarding validity and validation in our projects, as well as the research studies we read.

It is essential to highlight the fallibility associated with validity and validation, as it is assumed that any created criteria, standards, and conditions are subject to error. In addition, validity and validation are always partially misleading, inaccurate, and changing. A priori standards or universal criteria for validity or validation applicable to all discourses are impossible. I believe that it is time to stop legitimating validity and validation with reference to a metadiscourse and acknowledge its connections to politics and hegemony. Moreover, it is equally important to recognize that all definitions and conceptualizations of validity and validation are contextualized constructions (even the most popular and accepted ones), which are always limited, partial, and located within particular discourses (see Brinberg & McGrath, 1985; Maxwell, 1992). These discourses are shaped by significantly different moral codes and ethical practices, and ultimately there exists more than one defensible code of ethics.

Moreover, there should be no unified science and no unified validity criteria that limit, control, and surveil the possibilities of theories and the creativity of knowers. Sparkes (2001) proposed that qualitative validity criteria that replicate, parallel, or diversify criteria from quantitative research, as well as criteria that question the entire conceptualization of validity, could coexist. This coexistence would allow for the constant making and remaking of the validation and legitimatization of research. In addition, Lather (2006) referred to the question of validity as "a 'limit-question' of research, one that repeatedly resurfaces, one that can neither be avoided nor solved" (p. 52). In another context, Lather (1993) compared validity to simulacra (a copy without original) that is always escaping itself. Thus, the goal of researchers, in the process of validation, might include disabling existing binaries, such as good research and bad research and science and nonscience, as well as the separation between knowers and the known, by referring to the situated theories, experiences, and testimonies of ourselves and those who we accept and trust. The validity of the validity question in qualitative research can be found in the persistent process of making it (Kvale, 1996). Validity and validation, as concepts, are tools rather than reflections of Truth. Researchers can only hope "for temporary alliance and agreements, and truths that satisfy our corrigible standards" (Thayer-Bacon, 2003, p. 71). The process of searching for similarities, recognizing privilege, and the constant making of validity keeps the concept itself always unthinkable, on the move, in flux, and open to the Other—ways of knowing, living, experiencing, and researching.

NOTES

1. The concept *catalytic validity* has been earlier introduced by Patti Lather (1986).

2. The discussion in the last section of this article can be applied to the concepts of validity and validation; thus, I will use both terms interchangeably.

REFERENCES

Agar, M. (1986). *Speaking of ethnography.* Beverly Hills, CA: Sage.

Angen, M. (2000). Evaluating interpretive inquiry: Reviewing the validity debate and opening the dialogue. *Qualitative Health Research, 10,* 378–395.

Anderson, G., & Herr, K. (1999). The new paradigm wars: Is there room for rigorous practitioner knowledge in schools and universities? *Educational Researcher, 28*(5), 12–21, 40.

Brinberg, D., & McGrath, J. (1985). *Validity and the research process.* Newbury Park, CA: Sage.

Campbell, D., & Stanley, J. (1966). *Experimental and quasi-experimental designs for research.* Chicago: Rand McNally.

Carspecken, P. (1996). *Critical ethnography in educational research.* New York: Routledge.

Cook, T., & Campbell, D. (1979). *Quasi-experimentation: Design and analysis issues for field settings.* Chicago: Rand McNally.

Creswell, J. (1998). *Qualitative inquiry and research design: Choosing among five traditions.* Thousand Oaks, CA: Sage.

Creswell, J., & Miller, D. (2000). Determining validity in qualitative inquiry. *Theory Into Practice, 39(3),* 124–130.

Denzin, N., & Lincoln, Y. (Eds.). (2000). *Handbook of qualitative research* (2nd ed.). Thousand Oaks, CA: Sage.

Gergen, M., & Gergen, K. (2000). Qualitative inquiry: Tensions and transformations. In N. Denzin & Y. Lincoln (Eds.), *Handbook of qualitative research* (2nd ed., pp. 1025–1046). Thousand Oaks, CA: Sage.

Guba, E., & Lincoln, Y. (1981). *Effective evaluation.* San Francisco: Jossey-Bass.

Habermas, J. (1971). *Knowledge and human interests* (J. J. Shapiro, Trans.). Boston: Beacon.

Heikkinen, H., Kakkori, L., & Huttunen, R. (2001). This is my truth, tell me yours: Some aspects of action research quality in the light of truth theories. *Educational Action Research,* 9(1), 9–24.

Hesse-Biber, S., & Leavy, P. (Eds.). (2004). *Approaches to qualitative research: A reader on theory and practice.* New York: Oxford University Press.

James, W. (1977). *A pluralistic universe.* Cambridge, MA: Harvard University Press. (Original work published 1909)

Kirk, J., & Miller, M. (1986). *Reliability and validity in qualitative research* (Vol. 1). Beverly Hills, CA: Sage.

Kvale, S. (1996). *Interviews: An introduction to qualitative research interviewing.* Thousand Oaks, CA: Sage.

Lather, P. (1986). Issues of validity in openly ideological research: Between a rock and a soft place. *Interchange,* 17(4), 63–84.

Lather, P. (1993). Fertile obsession: Validity after poststructuralism. *Sociological Quarterly,* 34(4), 673–693.

Lather, P. (2004). This is your father's paradigm: Government intrusion and the case of qualitative research in education. *Qualitative Inquiry, 10*(1), 15–34.

Lather, P. (2006). Paradigm proliferation as a good thing to think with: Teaching research in education as a wild profusion. *International Journal of Qualitative Studies in Education,* 19(1), 35–57.

LeCompte, M., Millroy, W., & Preissle, J. (Ed.). (1992). *The handbook of qualitative research in education.* San Diego, CA: Academic Press.

Lincoln, Y., & Denzin, N. (1994). The fifth moment. In N. Denzin & Y. Lincoln (Eds.), *Handbook of qualitative research* (Vol. 1, pp. 575–586). Thousand Oaks, CA: Sage.

Lincoln, Y. S., & Guba, E. G. (1985). *Naturalistic inquiry.* Beverly Hills, CA: Sage.

Maxwell, J. (1992). Understanding and validity in qualitative research. *Harvard Educational Review,* 62(3), 279–300.

Merriam, S. (1995). What can you tell from an N of 1? Issues of validity and reliability in qualitative research. *PAACE Journal of Lifelong Learning,* 4, 51–60.

Michrina, B., & Richards, C. (1996). *Person to person: Fieldwork, dialogue, and the hermeneutic method.* Albany: State University of New York Press.

Mishler, E. (1990). Validation in inquiry-guided research: The role of exemplars in narrative studies. *Harvard Educational Review,* 60(4), 415–442.

Moustakas, C. (1994). *Phenomenological research methods.* Thousand Oaks, CA: Sage.

Nespor, J. (2006). Morphologies of inquiry: The uses and spaces of paradigm proliferation. *International Journal of Qualitative Studies in Education,* 19(1), 115–128.

Puolimatka, T. (2002). Kvalitatiivisen tutkimuksen luotettavuus ja totuusteoriat [The validity of qualitative research and theories of truth]. *Kasvatus [Finnish Journal of Education],* 33(5), 465–473. Richardson, L. (2000). Writing: A method of inquiry. In N. Denzin & Y. Lincoln (Eds.), *Handbook of qualitative research* (2nd ed., pp. 923–948). Thousand Oaks, CA: Sage.

Scheurich, J. J. (1996). The masks of validity: A deconstructive investigation. *International Journal of Qualitative Studies in Education,* 9(1), 49–60.

Schwandt, T. (1997). *Qualitative inquiry: A dictionary of terms.* Thousand Oaks, CA: Sage.

Smith, J., & Deemer, D. (2000). The problem of criteria in the age of relativism. In N. Denzin & Y. Lincoln (Eds.), *Handbook of qualitative research* (2nd ed., pp. 877–896). Thousand Oaks, CA: Sage.

Sparkes, A. (2001). Myth 94: Qualitative health researchers will agree about validity. *Qualitative Health Research, 11,* 538–552.

Spivak, G. (1997). Translator's preface. In J. Derrida (Ed.), *Of grammatology* (pp. ix-lxxxvii). Baltimore, MD: Johns Hopkins University Press.

Thayer-Bacon, B. (2003). *Relational "(e)pistemologies."* New York: Peter Lang.

Wright, H. (2006). Qualitative researchers on paradigm proliferation in educational research: A question-and-answer session as multi-voiced text. *International Journal of Qualitative Studies in Education,* 19(1), 77–95.

THE AUTHOR COMMENTS Validity and Validation in the Making in the Context of Qualitative Research

This article was written to work against simple definitions and postpositivist notions of validity in qualitative research. I believe that to reflect the diverse theoretical and methodological practices characterizing qualitative research today, the definitions of validity should take into account epistemological diversity and multiple ways of knowing (many of which are still to come). Rather than focusing on externally evaluated correspondence with Truth, I view validity in qualitative research as an ongoing process that is closely related to researchers' epistemological positionings. This approach to validity and validation also requires researchers to take responsibility of their research differently and to reflect on their knowing and epistemological decision making throughout the research process.

MIRKA KORO-LJUNGBERG

The Cocreating Environment
A Nexus Between Classical Chinese and Current Nursing Philosophies

JOAN E. DODGSON, RN, PhD, MPH

Although nursing theorists have incorporated some concepts from Asian wisdom traditions (Buddhism, Confucianism, and Daoism) into their works, the ways that these traditions might inform Western nursing philosophies, praxis, and ethics is underdeveloped in the professional literature. These differences have been more extensively explored in disciplines other than nursing (psychology, philosophy, and education).[1-3] In the scholarly nursing literature, areas of cross-cultural fertilization do exist. This literature has focused on explaining Chinese values[4,5] and exploring a Chinese understanding of the Western nursing metaparadigm concepts.[6-8] Chinese nursing scholars, many of whom have received graduate education in the West, have begun a dialogue in the professional literature that incorporates modifications to Western nursing theories reflecting their Asian contexts and traditions.

The professional nursing (English language) literature about the Chinese concept of person, written by Chinese scholars, has focused on conveying the very basic concepts of Confucianism and Daoism. Framed as identifying Chinese values, several authors have given basic definitions of Confucian appropriateness (*yi*) within relationships, the Daoist goal of maintaining health through harmonious balancing (*jing*), and the contextual nature of all things (*wanwu*), common to both Confucian and Daoist perspectives.[7-12] This literature is needed and important in developing cross-cultural understandings; however, it does not go far enough in discussing the underlying philosophical assumptions of these traditions. It is only through analyzing how fundamentally the Chinese and Western philosophies differ that mutual understandings may be developed.

Wong and colleagues have broadened the cross-cultural discourse by exploring the Chinese understanding of concepts central to nursing (ie, caring, holism)[7,8] and describing a Chinese definition of nursing.[12,13] Pang and colleagues[13] interviewed 254 nurses in China to determine how they would describe nursing (*huli*). Themes found were focused on the dynamic nature of all things (*wanwu*) and optimizing actions within the act of nursing (*huli*). These are worthy first

steps in drawing distinctions and finding common ground, but they are only first steps.

Over the past 100 years, a variety of social and cultural circumstances have led nursing scholars in North America, Great Britain, and Australia to predominate within the international development of nursing theory and philosophy. As a result, most professional publishing (journals and textbooks) and conferences use the English language. This has led to an abundance of conceptual thinking in nursing, being framed by Western philosophy, particularly the philosophy of science. International students seek graduate nursing education in North American universities, to assist in their country's development of nursing; this continues the hegemony of Western nursing theories and philosophies. The time has passed, when nurses, along with other professionals, could work within the global community and maintain a dominant Western worldview.[14]

The hegemony of Western conceptual understandings about the nature and goals of nursing practice is evidenced by the extent to which the global discourse is framed in these ethnocentric conceptual understandings. Although areas of congruence exist between the Chinese and Western conceptions of the nature of nursing, a fundamental dissonance resonates between the 2 because of very different epistemological, ontological, and ethical perspectives. Understanding these differences is essential to a meaningful nonethnocentric dialogue within our discipline and profession.

The purpose of this article is to briefly describe the Daoist and Confucian philosophies, which permeate Chinese culture, and to compare and contrast these perspectives with Western nursing thinking in the unitary-transformative paradigm. My thesis is that a nexus or convergence of conceptualizations occurs between these 2 very different perspectives in their mutual understanding of the primacy of a cocreative environment. To set the stage for this discussion, an overview of the development of conceptual thinking in nursing is presented, followed by a comparative analysis of ways the environment, the self, and the relationship between the 2 are understood from each philosophical tradition.

From J. E. Dodgson, The cocreating environment: A nexus between classical Chinese and current nursing philosophies.
Advances in Nursing Science, *2008, 31(4), 356–364. Copyright © 2008 Wolters Kluwer Health | Lippincott Williams & Wilkins.*
Reprinted by Permission of Lippincott Williams & Wilkins.

ABOUT THE AUTHOR

JOAN E. DODGSON is Associate Professor at the College of Nursing & Health Innovation, Arizona State University. She began her nursing career as an LPN in a major medical center and has continued to be challenged by the scope and depth of the issues driving the discipline's knowledge development. As she has moved from critical care to perinatal health promotion and from hospital-based to community-based practice and research, the thematic trajectory of her work has remained steeped in social justice and intercultural teaching/learning and understandings. Her contribution to nursing that is central in her work is the facilitation of cross-cultural understandings through a variety of avenues.

Background

The development of philosophy within nursing has been slow but continuous. As a relatively new scholarly discipline, just 50 years old—a mere beginning when compared with the discipline of philosophy—nursing has struggled conceptually to find language and foundational assumptions that encompass all that nurses do and are. The earliest theorists, including Florence Nightingale, identified the main concerns of nurses to be the person, the environment, and the relationship between them. Subsequently, these concepts, along with caring and the act of nursing, have been formalized into the metaparadigm concepts of the discipline.

The taxonomy of paradigmatic perspectives suggested by Newman et al,[15] frames this comparative discussion. These authors conceptualized 3 categories with paired terms (ie, particulate-determinist, integrative-interactive, and unitary-transformative). The first term used represents the operative paradigmatic understanding of phenomena; the second word is the process used to create knowledge within the paradigm. Initially, nursing theorists based their work on the positivist perspective (particulate-deterministic paradigm) common to the Western medical model. It is a paradigm reflecting traditional Western philosophies (ie, philosophies of Plato, Aristotle, and Descartes) and Newtonian physics, which are characterized by duality (ie, separation of mind and body, categorizing and separating phenomena into parts) and causal deterministic relationships.[16] Nursing scholars using this perspective focus on identifying and understanding parts (particulates) of the phenomena they study, and not a contextualized phenomenological whole. Causal (deterministic) explanations are considered the building blocks of knowledge and the determinant of truth.[16] Knowledge created by determining causal explanations is preferred over other types of knowledge in this worldview. Although most basic sciences have moved beyond this paradigm, it was their traditional perspective for the 19th century and a major portion of the 20th century.

Striving for legitimacy, particularly from our medical colleagues, most nursing theorists and scholars of the 1960s to 1990s attempted to define nursing in this compartmentalized linear language, also used in the medical literature. Although this language and structure had a comfortable familiarity, as most nurses had spent the majority of their education in basic science courses, this conceptual perspective did not adequately reflect the contextual and temporal reality of nursing praxis. It created gaps between the experience of nursing practice and the conceptualizations about the experience of nursing practice.[17] Unfortunately, this discordance has continued to be an issue for many within the field, who have been educated within the positivist (particulate-deterministic) and/or postpositivist (integrative-interactive) paradigms.[15]

The second paradigmatic category, the interactive-integrative, is postpositivist (postmodern) perspectives adapted from the social and physical sciences. Systems theory, which has been widely used in nursing, falls into this category. The interactive-integrative paradigmatic approach is the most frequently observed paradigm in nursing research, because it focuses on interactions within a social context consisting of interactive phenomena, which more accurately reflects the contextualized environment, particulate-deterministic paradigm, nurses work within. However, this paradigm continues to incorporate the notion of duality by separating parts of the whole context, separately focusing on examining the relationships among the parts and the resultant interactions. For example, a human body is viewed as a whole but the mind and body can be studied separately. The mind and body affect each other and are parts of the whole, while remaining distinctly different entities. This conception continues the Cartesian mind-body duality, which is incongruent with Asian perspectives that emphasize an indivisible phenomenological holism.

The unitary-transformative paradigm is the third and final paradigm in this taxonomy. The theorists working within this paradigm have developed bodies of work that can best be called philosophies of nursing praxis and research. Dualistic thinking and relating are not relevant to this worldview.[18] In the mid-1980s, several seminal works in nursing grounded in existential (Heideggerian) phenomenological and deconstructionist (ie, Derrida) perspectives highlighted the complex, contextual, and cocreative nature of nursing praxis. The most widely known theorists working within these traditions are Benner[19] and Parse.[20] Other nursing theorists informed by recent paradigm shifts within the physical (ie, relativity, quantum theory, and Chaos theory) and social sciences (constructivism and naturalistic inquiry) elaborated the transformative and irreducibly interrelated nature of nursing praxis for both the client and the nurse.[17,20-22] The body of nursing philosophical and theoretical work that comes out of these conceptual shifts occurring in the 20th century has been termed the unitary-transformative paradigm in the professional literature.[15,18] The unitary-transformative perspective is not yet a mainstream thinking in nursing. However, it has resonated with many Asian nurses, who have used these conceptual approaches in their graduate education and to frame their research,[7,9,10,23] suggesting the possible congruencies between this nursing paradigm and classical Chinese philosophy, which still informs current Chinese cultural norms and understandings. Both similarities and profound differences occur when comparing these 2 philosophies.

Comparative Analysis

The wisdom of classical Chinese philosophy (ie, Daoism and Confucianism) offers insights into the nature of context, the person, and personal relationships directly relevant for practicing nurses and nurse educators internationally. To begin a dialogue about these insights and their usefulness for current nursing philosophy and praxis, 3 concepts commonly addressed with the nursing literature holism, the nature of the self, and the nature of personal relationships within a holistic context are discussed from the classical Chinese philosophical perspective. In choosing to compare and contrast the classical Chinese philosophy with the unitary-transformative nursing perspective related to these 3 themes, it is hoped that a deeper mutual and meaningful understanding will be possible that may lead to continued dialogue.

The Holistic Nature of the Environment

A holistic worldview of the environment encompassing one's context socially, culturally, and environmentally, is foundational within both classical Chinese philosophy and the unitary-transformative paradigm in nursing. Drawing on a variety of 20th century conceptual perspectives ranging from existential phenomenology to chaos theory, nursing theorists working within the unitary-transformative paradigm have defined *holism* as unity. Although theorists define holism within their own conceptual scheme, their definitions share the underlying assumption that the world in which one lives can not be broken down or separated into parts, rather the interconnectedness of all things is fundamental and instrumental in understanding the self and others. All theorists working in this paradigm view change as an ongoing and dynamic process. The transitions that occur over time are seen as a normal and expected course of things. The inherent ever-present nature of change is incorporated into their theoretical assumptions. These assumptions are congruent with the classical Chinese perspective.

According to Newman et al, within the unitary-transformative paradigm, "a phenomenon is viewed as a unitary, self-organizing field embedded in a larger self-organizing field. It is identified by pattern and by interaction with the larger whole."[15(p4)] The use of the term "self-organizing" within this definition implies a telos not evident in the classical Chinese perspective. Assumptions fundamental to the Abrahamic traditions can be found in most theories of nursing theorists/philosophers working in the unitary-transformative paradigm. These underlying assumptions are not found in classic Chinese traditions, and they include notions of a transcendent God and a personal soul, which have a relationship commonly termed "the one-behind-the-many."[24] Although this nursing paradigm is not centered on the causally determined and dualistically compartmentalized perspective, as the other 2 nursing paradigms, it is not completely free of Western transcendent notions of the one-behind-the-many, which are common to Abrahamic traditions and the cultures in which they predominate. These distinctions are elaborated in greater detail in subsequent sections.

Within classical Chinese perspectives, the conceptualization of holism is process oriented with a correlative continuity among all things (*wanwu*). This correlative nature refers to the inherent mutual relationality occurring in any particular context and the assumption that multiple points of view coexist at all times. It is not a view that privileges the truth of the-one-behind-the-many, rather it is a relational truth of "the-one-among-the-many."[24] Understanding this distinction is fundamental to understanding why Westerners frequently misunderstand the Chinese conceptions of truth, ethics, and contextualized relationships.[2,14,25,26] Another way to describe a correlative continuity among all things (*wanwu*), is to use the familiar Daoist depiction of yin and yang as circle with black and white elements, which illustrates how apparent opposites enable each other to exist and are complementary aspects of a holistic process.[25,26]

The Chinese conception of a contextualized environment has been termed a focus-field distinction by Ames and Hall.[25] The *field* refers to the totality of the particular context and the *focus* refers to that part of the field one is attending to at any point in time, which may change at any time. Change is understood to be a constant. Holism is inherent within the focus/field, as parts can not be separated out, highlighting the plurality of vantage points within the perceptual horizon and the infinite possibilities inherent within it. Multiple valid vantage points exist within the field; it is a pluralistic approach that does not privilege one view over others (ie, the-one-behind-the-many).[25,26] The description of a contextualized environment as a focus/field is not unique to the Chinese perspective; it has also been described in the works by phenomenologist, existentialist, and pragmatist. Perhaps this accounts for the similarities found between the unitary-transformative and the classical Chinese philosophical perspectives related to the contextualized environment.

Other similarities found between the classical Chinese and unitary-transformative nursing perspectives, center around their mutual emphasis on the inherent nature of change. For example, Parse uses a specific language of gerund pairs (eg, connecting-separating, enabling-limiting) within her philosophy/theory to denote the dynamic and changing nature of all things.[20] Newman views change as continual and moving toward ever higher levels of growth.[17] Change is assumed.

These similarities have provided enough mutually understood ground for collaborative research and teaching to occur internationally; however, the similarities may also blind international colleagues to the fundamental differences that remain between these 2 perspectives.[2,14,17] Mutual understanding is necessary to have a dialogue, the pitfalls come when one is not attentive to and aware of the range of possible misunderstandings. Transcendent notions are so deeply embedded in Western culture and so deeply not present in classic Chinese traditions that they remain unseen too often within both cultures.[14]

The Nature of the Self

These 2 ecological perspectives differ on how the self is situated in relation to the holistic context or focus/field. The unitary-transformative nursing paradigm comes out of the Western Abrahamic traditions, which are substantive and essentialistic in nature.[26] "There is perception of the universal in the particular, which is a concrete manifestation of the universal. The particular becomes symbolic of the universal."[15(p48)] Self-determination and individualistic goal setting remain; agency has priority over situation. The self is viewed as substantive, being with a set persona that grows and develops within a specific context. Although interdependency and cocreativity enable transformations to occur through intimate connections with the environment that are assumptions setting this paradigm apart from others in nursing, the understanding of the self remains fundamentally defined by individualism. "Wholeness is the bedrock of our reality. We have been, are and will be whole in our being and relationships with others."[27(p228)]

Within the Chinese tradition there is no self (whole in our being), independent of the relationships constituting one's life. The classical Chinese view of self is neither substantive nor essentialistic.[25(p20)] The self is a "dynamic pattern of personal, social and natural relationships."[24(p39)] The various roles (daughter, mother, and employee) define the self and the interactions most appropriate within that relational context as described in the Confucian Analects.

The Master said:

> In serving your father and mother, remonstrate with them gently. On seeing that they do not heed your suggestions, remain respectful and do not act contrary. Although concerned, voice no resentment.[28(p93)]

The Master said:

> As a younger brother and son, be filial (xiao) at home and deferential (di) in the community, be cautious in what you say and then make good on your word (xin); love the multitude broadly and be intimate with those who are authoritative in their conduct (ren).[28(p72)]

No specific single individual with a set persona is seen in this worldview rather a relational self whose responsibility is to maintain appropriate relationships with others and within specific contextual environments so that particular circumstances have optimal harmony (he) by creating balance. There is a priority of situation over agency (de) in this tradition[25(p58)] and a lack of ontological knowing (wuzhi).[24(p40)] In other words, "a human being is not something we are: it is something that we do and become."[25(p49)] The Chinese self is relational not essentialistic, as is the Western notion of self.[25(p24)] The Chinese notion of self is constituted by roles and inherent relationships; there is no individualistic notion of self that is separated from contextualized particularities.

On a continuum with the Western conception of the rugged individualist at one end and classical Chinese notion of the relational self anchoring the other, the self defined by the unitary-transformative nursing paradigm would be at least midway and perhaps closer to the classical Chinese perspective. The definitions of self found within the unitary-transformative perspective acknowledge the interdependent mutual cocreation of relationships, coming closer to the Chinese relational self than other philosophical perspectives, but retaining the individualistic notion of self apart from the environmental context. These areas of conceptual congruence suggest the possibility of exploring mutual commonalities and meaningful dialogue. The differences between the classical Chinese and unitary-transformative nursing perspective are key to understanding the mutual gap in understanding that may exist between these worldviews. Although originating from different philosophical and cultural traditions, the primacy of relationships in both paradigms is a mutual commonality (ie, nexus) where a meaningful cross-fertilization might occur if accompanied by mutual respect of differences.

The Nature of Person-Environment Relationship

Conceptualizations of the nature of the person in their environment are similar between the 2 paradigms, yet, the underlying assumptions are fundamentally different. This situation presents opportunities, as well as challenges, that may not be readily apparent because of the tacit understandings involved. These subtleties may affect the dialogue and the nature of nursing praxis. The unitary-transformative and classical Chinese philosophical understandings of this relationship are discussed and compared.

The Unitary-Transformative Perspective

Within the unitary-transformative paradigm, personal relationships are dynamic mutual interactions that are context dependent within the unitary-transformative nursing paradigm.[17,20] Context matters, the environment affects the person and the person affects the environment. A mutual flow exists that is ever-changing and requires awareness of this change if a nurse is to be effective.

Pattern, the dynamic relatedness among all things (*wanwu*), is viewed as defining and refining element of the whole, revealing that which is meaningful.[29] An interpenetration of specific fields creates the diversity within the unified field.[15(p4)] The nurse's role is to develop an understanding of the client-environment pattern (field) through interactions and then to cocreate a healing unified field with the client. Scholars working in this paradigm have differing perspectives on the mutual process of dynamic relatedness among all things (*wanwu*). A brief overview of the range in conceptual diversity follows.

Margaret Newman has termed this transformative process of mutual and creative unfolding as expanding consciousness.[30] She has used the self-organizing-disorganization-reorganization process elaborated in Chaos theory to inform her thinking on the ever-transforming nature of all things (*wanwu*). "Understanding the individuality of rhythm and timing in relationship is important in establishing the relevancy and

effectiveness of nursing practice."[29(p229)] Transformation only occurs in a positive direction. She has diagramed this process as an upwardly swirling continuous circle.

Parse[20] describes the environment as contextual, dynamic, and cocreated. She views the human project as a continuum of human becoming facilitated by dynamic relatedness with the environment. "Human becoming is a unitary phenomenon that refers to the human's co-creation of rhythmical patterns of relating in mutual process with the universe."[20(p31)] Her work relies heavily on the existential works of 20th century European philosophers and the American pragmatist, John Dewey. Her work is grounded in the reality of experiences with the world and emphasizes the processional nature of all things.

Jean Watson's continued the development of the philosophy of caring in nursing, which is holistic and dynamically situated contextually, has led her to view caring as the moral imperative organizing self and the environment.[22] Caring actions during all interactions are fundamental to her perspective, which has a strong metaphysical component. "We are spirit made whole; non-manifest to manifest field, connected to and belonging to the infinity of cosmos and the universe, before separating as individuals and other entities."[22(p111)]

Each of these philosophies/theories recognizes the centrality of personal relationships within the environment, as does the classical Chinese perspective. It is through the active participation of individuals that relationships are facilitated and outcomes may be influenced. Recognition of the equal importance of multiple viewpoints within any context (ie, plurality) is another commonality. However, differences exist. The classical Chinese perspectives are pluralistic in nature, recognizing that the self is among the many without any conception of the monotheism of Western transcendental metaphysics.[25(p32-33)] Although deeply spiritual in nature, classical Chinese wisdom traditions do not contain any conceptions of a God that transcends human existence, as do the Abrahamic traditions.[26] Many the works done from the unitary-transformative perspective maintain an assumption of the transcended deity, rooted in Abrahamic traditions. For example, Watson grounds her theory on work by the Talmud ethicist, Levinas[22]; Parse formulates her ontological base within the Abrahamic tradition.[20] Although Newman specifically states it is not her intention to incorporate a particular spiritual orientation in her work, she acknowledges her work is congruent with many of the religious traditions of the world.[17(p94)]

The Chinese Perspective

The goal of the Confucian tradition is to become an authoritative person (*ren*), which encompasses all personal attributes (cognitive, aesthetic, moral, and spiritual). Authoritative in this context does not imply any sense of authority, rather a wisdom developed intentionally. The authoritative person is one who has developed a deep understanding (*zhi*) of context and uses this wisdom to grow (*sheng*) appropriate (*yi*) noncoercive relationships (*wuwei*) with others.[25(pp47–51)] This growth process or way of becoming human is an aesthetic project, qualitative in nature, and particular by necessity, because the nature of personal relationships is always contextual. Appropriateness (*yi*) is always dependent on the contextual particulars; it is a relational not relativistic perspective.

Within the Daoist focus/field understanding of context human becoming is a cocreative process aimed at optimizing relationships with all things (*dao*) at any point in time.[24(p16)] The *dao* is "a way of becoming consummately and authoritatively human."[26(p46)] This perspective values the "insistent" particularity within each context (*de*) while requiring attention to both the focus and field—"the inseparability of the one and the many in continuity and multiplicity" (*Tang Junyi*).[24(p33)] This particularity provides the possibility of mutual growth through "making the most of one's ingredients" using cocreative processes.[24] "It is the person who is able to broaden the way, not the way that broadens the person."[28(p190)] Mutual cocreation of a harmonious balance (*jing*) with all things (*wanwu*) is possible through optimizing within in any context. This interactive and correlative perspective on personal relationship is also inherently transformative. Each interaction transforms those participating to some extent. It is the Daoist goal to transform all within the context in such a way that outcomes are optimized for each and for all at the same time.

 ## Conclusion

By comparing and contrasting classic Chinese perspectives of person, environment, and the relationship between the two with the unitary-transformative nursing paradigm, areas of commonality have been highlighted. These commonalities create a nexus that needs further exploration and conceptual development. Within the described nexus, nursing scholars working from each of the 2 philosophical traditions can dialogue in ways that have common meanings. It is easy to assume, when some areas of common meanings exist, that the more tacit understandings supporting these common meanings are mutually understood. Too often, this is not the case, misunderstandings occur because the deeper more fundamental philosophical orientations are not evident. Although this nexus opens opportunities for greater mutual understanding, it can not be overstated that fundamental epistemological, ontological, and ethical differences also exist within the 2 traditions. This article was a beginning effort to explore some of the fundamental distinctions that underlie these different philosophical orientations, which on the surface may seem to have so much in common.

REFERENCES

1. Bond MH. *Beyond the Chinese Face.* Oxford: Oxford University Press; 1991.
2. Nisbett RE. *The Geography of Thought.* New York: Free Press; 2003.
3. Watkins DA, Biggs JB. *Teaching the Chinese Learner: Psychological and Pedagogical Perspectives.* Hong Kong: The University of Hong Kong Press; 2001.
4. Chao Y. Nursing's values from a Confucian perspective. *Int Nurs Rev.* 1995;42(5):147–149.
5. Chen Y. Chinese values, health and nursing. *J Adv Nurs.* 2001;36(2):270–273.
6. Kao HS, Reeder FM, Hsu M, Cheng S. A Chinese view of the Western nursing metaparadigm. *J Holist Nurs.* 2006;24(2):92–101.
7. Pang SMC, Arthur DG, Wong TKS. Drawing a qualitative distinction of caring practices in a professional context: the case of Chinese nursing. *Holist Nurs Pract.* 2000;15(1):22–31.
8. Wong TKS, Pang SMC. Holism and caring: nursing in the Chinese health care culture. *Holist Nurs Pract.* 2000;15(1):12–21.
9. Chen Y. *A Taoist Model for Human Caring: The Lived Experiences and Caring Needs of Mothers With Children Suffering From Cancer in Taiwan.* Denver, CO: University Of Colorado Health Sciences Center; 1988.
10. Lu L. A preliminary study on the concept of health among the Chinese. *Couns Psychol Q.* 2002;15(2):179–189.
11. Pang SM, Sawada A, Konishi E, et al. A comparative study of Chinese, American and Japanese nurses' perceptions of ethical role responsibilities. *Nurs Ethics.* 2003;10(3):295–311.
12. Wong TKS, Pang SMC, Wang CS, Zhang CJ. A Chinese definition of nursing. *Nurs Inq.* 2003;10(2):79–80.
13. Pang SMC, Wong TKS, Wang CS, et al. Towards a Chinese definition of nursing. *J Adv Nurs.* 2004;46(6):657–670.
14. Melby CS, Dodgson JE, Tarrant M. The experience of western expatriate nursing educators teaching in Eastern Asia. *J Nurs Scholarsh.* 2008;40(2):176–183.
15. Newman MA, Sime AM, Corcoran-Perry SA. The focus of the discipline of nursing. *Adv Nurs Sci.* 1991;14(1):1–6.
16. Rutty JE. The nature ofphilosophyofscience, theory and knowledge relating to nursing and professionalism. *J Adv Nurs.* 1998;28(2):243–250.
17. Newman MA. *Transforming Presence: The Difference That Nursing Makes.* Philadelphia, PA: F.A. Davis; 2008.
18. Newman MA, Smith MC, Pharis MD, Jones D. The focus of the discipline revisited. *Adv Nurs Sci.* 2008;31(1):E16–E27.
19. Benner P. *From Novice to Expert.* Upper Saddle River, NJ: Prentice-Hall; 1984.
20. Parse RR. *The Human Becoming School of Thought.* Thousand Oaks, CA: Sage Publishing; 1998.
21. Rogers ME. *An Introduction to the Theoretical Basis of Nursing.* Philadelphia, PA: FA Davis; 1970.

22. Watson J. *Caring Science as Scared Science*. Philadelphia, PA: F. A. Davis Company; 2005.

23. Chan C, Ho PSY, Chow E. A body-mind-spirit model in health: an Eastern approach. *Soc Work Health Care*. 2001;34(3/4):261–282.

24. Ames RT, Hall DL. *Daodejing: making this life significant*. New York: Ballantine Books; 2003.

25. Ames RT, Rosemont H. Introduction. In: Ames RT, Rosemont H, eds. *The Analects of Confucius: A Philosophical Translation*. New York: Ballantine Books; 1999:1–65.

26. Hall DL, Ames RT. *Thinking From the Han*. Albany, NY: The State University of New York Press; 1998.

27. Newman MA. Experiencing the whole. *Adv Nurs Sci*. 1997;20(1):34–39.

28. Confucius. *The Analects of Confucius: A Philosophical Translation*. Ames RT, Rosemont H, trans. New York: The Ballentine Publishing Group; nd/1999:395.

29. Newman MA. The rhythm of relating in a paradigm of wholeness. *Image J Nurs Sch*. 1999;31(3):227–230.

30. Newman MA. *Health as Expanding Consciousness*. New York: National League of Nursing; 1994.

THE AUTHOR COMMENTS

The Cocreating Environment: A Nexus Between Classical Chinese and Current Nursing Philosophies

I had the wonderful opportunity to teach at the University of Hong Kong for three years, which provided an extensive experience of submersion into a culture very different than my own. This experience brought up many more questions than answers about the differences between Western and Asian ways of thinking and operating in the world; it provided the impetus for my studies related to the issues that I discuss in this paper. I continued my exploration of these differences while a member of the nursing faculty at the University of Hawaii in Manoa by studying East-West comparative philosophies with Drs. Roger Ames and Chung-ying Cheng (Philosophy Department). Unfortunately, Western notions have dominated the nursing discipline; however, in the 21st century, we can no longer justify this hegemonic view. Developing mutually meaningful conversations between Asian and Western nurses are essential to advancing the disciple and to global health and well-being, in ways we have yet to discover.

JOAN E. DODGSON

CHAPTER 23

Scientific Inquiry in Nursing: A Model for a New Age

HOLLY A. DeGROOT, RN, PhD, FAAN

Despite the acknowledged need for widespread and rapid scientific advancement in nursing, little systematic attention has been paid to the progenitor of research, the individual investigator. The nature of scientific problem solving as the fundamental process of research practice is explored, and a model of scientific inquiry is proposed. Variables in the model are discussed in relation to their potential effect on the inquiry process, and strategies that facilitate the practice of research are identified.

Concern with the growth of nursing science has received full attention from nursing scholars over the past decade. The need for nursing as a foundation for nursing science and professional growth has been repeatedly acknowledged by contemporary nursing authors (Donaldson & Crowley, 1978; Hardy, 1983). Roy (1983) considers theory development as the number one priority for this decade. Current economic pressures have added unprecedented urgency to this scientific quest as health care policy makers and administrators demand research verification of nursing's disciplinary contribution.

Theory development literature in nursing has largely focused on theory construction (Dickoff, James, & Weidenbach, 1968; Jacox, 1974; Meleis, 1985), the nature of nursing's scientific advancement (Hardy, 1983; Newman, 1983), and the identification of conceptual and methodological deficiencies (Batey, 1977; Gortner, 1977; Jacobsen & Meininger, 1985). Despite agreement that creative strategies are required to resolve these theoretical inadequacies (Caper, 1978; Oiler, 1982), surprisingly little attention has been paid to the process and practice of scientific inquiry with the individual investigator as the unit of analysis. An understanding of the nature of scientific activity and the factors that influence individual inquiry and research practice is essential if nursing is to exercise its fullest intellectual power for theory development.

The Nature of Scientific Activity

Science has been characterized as a "creative and imaginative human activity" (Goldstein & Goldstein, 1978, p. 4) and as a form of contemplative wisdom

(Weiskopf, 1973). Bronowski observes that "all science is the search for unity and hidden likenesses" (Bronowski, 1965, p. 14). As the method of inquiry employed in this quest, the research process is virtually indistinguishable from what Bigge (1982) calls reflective thinking. This is "a reflective process within which persons either develop new or change existing tested generalized insights or understanding. So construed, reflective thinking combines both inductive—fact gathering—and deductive processes in such a way as to find, elaborate and test hypotheses" (Bigge, 1982, p. 105).

It is clear that the research process and the reflective thinking process constitute parallel attempts directed toward problem solving. Polanyi (1962) distinguishes between two phases of problem solving: an initial stage of perplexity and a subsequent stage of taking action directed toward dispelling the perplexity. Polanyi summarizes the four well-known stages of discovery in problem solving: (a) stage of preparation, during which a problem is initially recognized; (b) stage of incubation, which is an unconscious preoccupation with the problem; (c) stage of illumination, characterized by the tentative discovery of a possible solution; and (d) stage of verification, during which the solution withstands tests of practical reality. Implicit in this notion of scientific activity as a process of reflective thinking and of problem solving is the fundamental relationship of both to creativity. Bronowski (1965) asserts that while science is involved in a search for hidden likenesses, creativity is the discovery of hidden likeness.

Creativity can be viewed as a five-step process that is triggered by identifying or sensing a problem (Mackinnon, 1970). The first stage is called the period of preparation, during which experience, cognitive skills, and problem-solving techniques are acquired.

From H. A. DeGroot, Scientific inquiry in nursing: A model for a new age. Advances in Nursing Science, April 1988, 10(3), 1–21. Copyright © 1988. Reproduced with permission of Lippincott Williams & Wilkins.

ABOUT THE AUTHOR

HOLLY A. DeGROOT is the founder of Catalyst Systems, LLC, Novato, CA, a nurse-owned and nurse-operated firm dedicated to evidence-based staffing decisions in healthcare. As founder of Catalyst, Dr. DeGroot has developed the largest objective database of its type on nursing workload and staff utilization patterns. In addition, she has created a family of patient classification measures and staffing methodologies for virtually every inpatient and outpatient clinical area where patient care is provided. She has been closely involved in regulatory and legislative issues involving nurse staffing throughout the United States, frequently providing expert testimony and advice on related topics. Dr. DeGroot has worked in several administrative, faculty, and research positions throughout her career and also serves as faculty in the graduate program in Nursing Administration and Informatics at the University of California, San Francisco. Born in Pittsburgh, PA, Dr. DeGroot has spent the majority of her life in northern California, where she enjoys swimming, reading, traveling, and writing.

The second stage, or period of concentrated effort, is often accompanied by frustration that results from unsuccessful attempts to solve the problem. Next comes a period of withdrawal, which is akin to the incubation stage of problem solving. In this stage the problem and its possible solutions are considered on a conscious as well as subconscious level. This stage is characterized by what Worthy (1975) has termed "fruitful obsession." The fourth stage, or moment of insight, is accompanied by a feeling of exhilaration that comes from the sudden discovery of a solution to the problem. Worthy calls this "aha thinking," which results in intuitive leaps and sudden insights related to problem solution. The last step in the creative process, the period of verification, is characterized by the elaboration of the newly created insight or solution and its subsequent testing, refinement, extension, and evaluation. The attainment of this fifth and final step in the creative process forms the foundation and the starting point for further creative activities. That this creative process bears a striking resemblance to the problem-solving and reflective thinking processes of scientific activity, as outlined earlier, is central to the discussion of scientific inquiry.

Since scientific problem solving necessarily involves an individual's contribution to the creative process, characteristics of creative persons and their work are also important to consider. Creativity in individuals has been associated with divergent thinking, intelligence, commitment or involvement, and a preference for complexity from which simplicity and order may be derived (Nicholls, 1983). The willingness to take risks (Albert, 1983) and to use imagination and intuition (Yukawa, 1973) are other fundamental characteristics of creative individuals. Introversion, playfulness, and a well-developed sense of humor also figure heavily with these individuals (Worthy, 1975).

Characteristics of the outcomes or products of creative problem solving (e.g., research findings and theories) have also been identified (MacKinnon, 1970). Originality and the ability of the solution to actually solve an existing problem are key characteristics. In addition, the solution must be "produced," which implies development, refinement, and communication of the problem solution. Additional criteria have relevance if nursing theory is considered to be the creative "product." These criteria are that the creative outcome or theory contains truth and beauty and that it contributes to the quality of human existence. It has also been observed that creativity can be generated as much by the nature of the problem as by the person attempting to solve it (Albert, 1983; Yukawa, 1973). Creative problem solving has beneficial psychological effects on others who are exposed to the process by encouraging and engaging them in more imaginative and creative activity. Although creativity alone does not ensure successful problem solving, it is a vital ingredient for the theoretical complexity of knowledge generation in human sciences. It should be remembered that less than successful problem solving can be equally rich in stimulating creative scientific problem solving because it forces the consideration of alternative possibilities (Yukawa, 1973).

Phases of Inquiry

It is clear from this discussion that the quintessence of scientific inquiry is creative problem solving conducted through the research process. Scientific inquiry thus comprises at least four interrelated phases: (a) formulation of the research problem, (b) method selection, (c) method implementation, and (d) communication of findings. Each of these phases shares common characteristics that have implications for a model of scientific inquiry. Although these phases are typically presented as the orderly and normative approach to inquiry, it has been pointed out that the actual research process has little resemblance to such a rational model (Martin, 1982). The inquiry process has been aptly described as a series of dilemmas that can be neither solved nor avoided (McGrath, 1982).

Problem Formulation

The pivotal point for a system of scientific inquiry is the research problem, question, or hypothesis, for it reflects all that came before and directs all research activity that will follow. Kerlinger goes a step further, calling the research problem or hypothesis the "working instrument of theory" (Kerlinger, 1973, p. 20). The research problem (a term to be used alternatively with "research question" or "research hypothesis," denoting the same or similar entity) is a highly subjective construction. As such, it is an intensely personal and intimate creation because of its contextual and historical proximity to the very essence of its creator. Not surprisingly, Polanyi calls research problems "intellectual desires" (Polanyi, 1962, p. 152), noting that in any scientific controversy personal attacks rather than scientific arguments are the norm because intellectual passions, not reason, are truly at odds.

Since the formulation of a research question is a creative effort based on imagination, ingenuity, and insight (Polit & Hungler, 1983), the research results stemming from it ultimately reflect the intellectual power of the question and, undeniably, the researcher. Research problem selection is closely related to personal values (Kaplan, 1964; Tucker, 1979) and actually discloses the direction of human will and intuition (Noddings & Shore, 1984). Runkel and McGrath observe that as a researcher attempts to formulate the research problem, "he begins with his own previous way of thinking about things; he seeks help in organizing his complexities from literature and colleagues; finally, he is inevitably affected by his own personal experience as he interacts with the world" (Runkel & McGrath, 1972, p. 13). Not surprisingly, this characteristic of subjectivity is inherent in the other phases of inquiry as well.

Selection of Methods

Although Kaplan (1964) acknowledges at least four distinct usages of the term "methodology," only the fourth is inclusive enough for a discussion of the process of scientific inquiry. This definition incorporates specific techniques and procedures as well as abstract philosophical imperatives. Kaplan asserts that the use of this expanded meaning allows for the inclusion of a wide range of activities, including concept delineation, hypothesis formation, observation and measurement, and model and theory construction, as well as explanation and prediction. The advantage of such a definition is that it treats all tools that a researcher has at his or her disposal (including the conceptual and the concrete) and the research implementation phases, such as data collection and analysis, as interrelated components of inquiry. Conceived in this way, factors influencing problem formulation directly or indirectly influence all phases of inquiry.

The implications of this expanded and integrated view of research methodology are not universally appreciated. At the very least, authors agree that the methods are dictated by the research question (Kerlinger, 1973; Kaplan, 1964; Runkel & McGrath, 1972; Wilson, 1985). However, there seems to be tacit endorsement of a greater rationality and objectively of method selection than actually exists. For example, some authors (Polit & Hungler, 1983) subscribe to a design selection hierarchy, usually with experimental designs at the top and nonexperimental approaches clearly at the bottom. This view implies that the selection of design methodology is based primarily on whether the research can meet the three requirements for a true experiment, namely, the ability for manipulation, control, and randomization. If these requirements can be met by the proposed study, the choice of methods is clear. If researchers are somehow unable to meet these requirements for experimentation, they are at once relegated to the realm of nonexperimental methodology. Kerlinger (1973) goes as far as to categorize nonexperimental methods as "compromise designs," consigning them rather casually to the bottom of the design hierarchy. Unfortunately this stance serves to create a methodological double bind: Methods are purportedly dictated by the question, but it is less desirable to ask questions that must be answered by "lower-order" designs and methods.

Brink and Wood (1983) propose a similarly straightforward and deductive approach to method selection based on the level of the research question. These levels are a function of existing amounts of knowledge related to the phenomena of interest. These authors also suggest that selection of methods may be based primarily on the existence of valid and reliable measures. Little attention is given to other factors that may influence the selection of research methods.

Method Implementation and Communication of Findings

How methods are implemented through the use of data collection techniques and analytical strategies is affected by the same subjective considerations inherent in problem formulation and method selection phases of inquiry. There is a wide range of methodological possibilities open to experimental and non-experimental approaches, with choices to be made at each juncture. Whether one decides to use open-ended interview *v* standardized questionnaire, grounded theory *v* hermeneutic interpretation, analysis of covariance (ANCOVA) techniques *v* multiple regression correlation (MRC), or a convenience *v* a stratified random sample is influenced by a combination of interrelated factors. Even the communication of research findings is similarly influenced as choices are made about which journal to submit the results to, what information should be included in the report, how conservative or liberal the interpretations will be, and what the theoretical implications of the findings are.

Despite the rigorous assertions that method selection and implementation are primarily rational processes, some authors concede the influence of subjective factors on these phases of inquiry (Martin, 1982; Kuhn, 1970; Luria, 1973; Polkinghorne, 1983). These include factors such as disciplinary norms, personal research style, funding realities, and other value-laden considerations. Tucker (1979) points out that scientific activity is essentially a process involving a series of value decisions to be made by the researcher and that perhaps the largest number of these decisions is made in relation to methodological issues. Polkinghorne goes one step further, asserting that "particular methods do not operate independently of a system of inquiry" and in fact "the use of a method changes only as a researcher uses it in different systems of inquiry"

(Polkinghorne, 1983, p. 6). This perhaps is the most important point of all, for it posits the inextricable relationship between each phase of inquiry and the subjective factors that necessarily influence each phase.

A Model of Scientific Inquiry

The model proposed here is fundamentally a systems/process model applied to a human system of inquiry (see Figure 23-1). As such, the system comprises six interrelated influencing variables, subdivided into four intrapersonal factors and two extrapersonal factors (Table 23-1). The six factors are assumed to be in constant and mutual interaction, and when there is a change in one variable the other variables are affected. There are four basic phases to the inquiry process, and each phase is influenced by the six variables. Accordingly, the cumulative effect of the variables on the system as a whole is greater than the sum of the influence of the individual variables.

The system is characterized by continual change and is directed toward growth and increasing sophistication. In addition, it operates according to the principal of equifinality (Von Bertalanffy, 1968), which asserts that the same final or end state can be achieved from different beginnings and by different paths or routes. Even though there is never a final state in the research process for the researcher, this proposed inquiry system accepts and encourages individual differences throughout the practice of research,

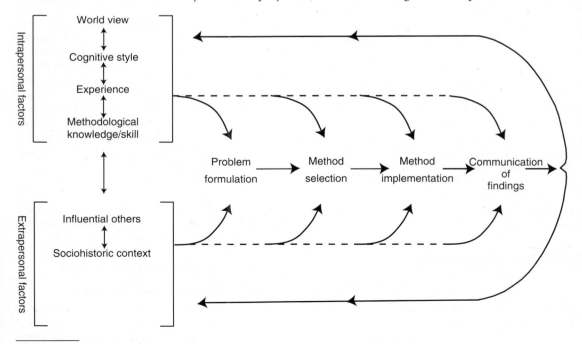

Figure 23-1 *A model of scientific inquiry.*

TABLE 23-1	Major Factors Influencing Scientific Inquiry in Nursing

Intrapersonal Factors

World view
  Nature of human beings
  Nature of knowledge and truth
  Nature of nursing science
Cognitive style
Experience
  Life experience
  Professional nursing experience
  Research experience
  Theoretical experience
Methodological knowledge and skill

Extrapersonal Factors

Influential others
  Individual
  Institutional
Sociohistorical context

since each path chosen can get equally close to the "truth." The six factors or influencing variables are not intended to represent all intrapersonal or extrapersonal possibilities. Rather they should be viewed as a major class of variables that operate in addition to other factors such as personality, intelligence, or other values and beliefs. In addition, individual investigators vary in their awareness of the existence and nature of these variables as well as in the relative degree of influence any one factor may exert on the inquiry process.

Intrapersonal Factors

World View

The first personal variable that influences the process of inquiry is called world view, which consists of the researcher's general philosophical orientation, or world view, of the nature of human beings, the nature of knowledge and truth, and the nature of nursing science. Beliefs about human nature are fundamental to the development of the researcher's theoretical learnings, to the delineation of appropriate research questions, and, ultimately to the selection of research methodology. Relevant beliefs about human nature include such considerations as whether human beings are considered to be rational or irrational, whether human behavior is predetermined, and what the basis is for motivation of behavior. For example, are human motivations primarily conscious or unconscious? Is

human behavior dictated by the need for growth or by the deprivation humans feel? Research questions generated will differ sharply, depending on whether human beings are viewed as highly self-directed individuals constantly striving for self-actualization *v* individuals who are at the mercy of their subconscious and who are constantly suppressing the primal urges the subconscious seeks to satisfy. Tucker points out that these latter beliefs as espoused by Freud and others, for example, have very specific implications for research methodology as well. He reminds us that the belief that one cannot ask a person directly about his or her thoughts and feelings provided the primary impetus for the development of popular psychological methods that employ unobtrusive and often deceptive testing techniques (Tucker, 1979).

Other beliefs related to a researcher's world view include how human beings are perceived in relation to their environment. For example, are people viewed as primarily passive reactors to events that impinge on them, or are they seen as proactive or mutually interactive with the environment? Does the human boundary end at the skin, or does the human field extend, as Rogers (1970) insists, beyond the skin to actually merge with the environmental field? Other perceptions that contribute to a researcher's world view relate to the multidimensionality of human beings. Are people seen as the popularized "biopsychosocial" beings, or are they seen as "biopsychosocial-spiritual-cultural" being? The very nature of the research questions would be altered by these two alternative views in that they would contain a very different constellation of variables and possible methodological implications.

These beliefs form the basis for establishing theoretical congruence, or the degree to which prevailing theories comfortably conform to one's world view. For example, if one believed that human beings were passive reactors to their environment and that behavior is motivated by the desire to avoid discomfort, it is unlikely that a systems perspective or symbolic interaction-based method would be very appealing. In this way beliefs about human nature delimit the realm of theoretical possibility in the practice of research.

Beliefs about the *nature of knowledge and truth* also affect a researcher's world view and thus the process of inquiry. Two major competing schools of thought best illustrate the diversity of these beliefs. Logical positivism, later known as the received view, asserts that objective, axiomatic truth exists that is discoverable and able to be verified by hypothetico-deductive methods (Suppe, 1977). Only certain methods that are objective and produce sense data can appropriately demonstrate this truth with any certainty, and only that knowledge derived in this manner counts as true scientific knowledge. The received view, as the dominant contemporary conception of science, conflicts sharply with what Polkinghorne (1983) calls the postpositivist view. A postpositivist conception of scientific knowledge and truth has evolved in reaction to the rather obvious limitations of the received view, especially for the human sciences. This view holds that the pursuit of knowledge and truth is necessarily historical, contextual, and theory laden. It claims no access to certain truth or knowledge but rather accepts certain knowledge to be "true" if it withstands practical tests of reason and utility. In this way, although knowledge may be useful, it is still fallible. Postpositivism does not cling to any one method of science and in fact encourages the use of the most appropriate method for the particular research question. Polkinghorne notes that "those methods are acceptable which produce results that convince the community that the new understanding is deeper, fuller, and more useful than the previous understanding" (Polkinghorne, 1983, p. 3).

The received view, or logical positivist approach to science, conforms closely to the correspondence norms of truth (Kaplan, 1964). What constitutes truth is the degree of correspondence between facts and their related theories and the degree to which propositions can be verified or shown to be false. Truth can be achieved only when it is shown that a proposition cannot be falsified. The received view also relies, in part, on the coherence theory of truth and its appreciation of theoretical aesthetics and logical simplicity in content and form. The postpositivist view, on the other hand, aligns itself with the pragmatic theory of truth, which emphasizes practical utility in problem solving and the degree of community consensus about that utility.

In the conduct of research positivism lends itself to reductionistic observables that must be quantified and verified, while postpositive concerns can be deductive or inductive in nature and can use either quantitative or qualitative strategies. It is clear that whether a researcher has positivist or postpositivist leanings and consciously or unconsciously subscribes to one theory of truth over another, these beliefs have a major effect on the formulation of the research question and the methodological strategy chosen. Thus it is unlikely that a researcher steeped in positivistic principles would ever ask a research question requiring the existential research methods of hermeneutic analysis.

A researcher's world view is also shaped by his or her beliefs about the *nature of nursing science*. Whether or not one believes that nursing is a "science of human health and behavior across the life span" (Gortner, 1983, p. 5) and is specifically concerned with "the diagnosis and treatment of human responses to actual or potential health problems" (American Nurses' Association, 1980, p. 9) has ultimate implications for the types of events, states, and situations perceived to be problematic. Although client, nursing, environment, and health

have all been considered phenomena central to nursing (Fawcett, 1978), one might disagree as to the emphasis that one component has in relation to another or on whether some or all of these concepts must be included in a theoretical formulation for nursing. For example, Stevens (1979) de-emphasizes the environmental aspects, while Fawcett (1978) states that at least one or more of the four concepts must be present if the theory is to be called a nursing theory. Flaskerud and Halloran (1980) insist that the concept of nursing must always be included in any theoretical formulation for it to be considered nursing theory, while Conway (1985) believes the inclusion of nursing is inappropriate.

Whether nursing science is believed to conform more to a human science model (postpositivist) or to a natural science model (positivist) also has implications for the formulation of research problems. As a human science nursing must take into account various characteristics of the human realm. For example, the systemic character of human phenomena and the unclear nature of their boundaries are important to consider (Polkinghorne, 1983). The former necessitates investigating the whole rather than its individual parts, while the latter implies acceptance of indistinct conceptual boundaries. The process nature of the human realm must also be taken into consideration, as it signifies continual growth and repatterning over time. This implies the use of longitudinal or time series designs to fully explicate our phenomena of interest (Metzger & Schultz, 1982).

Fundamental to human sciences is the additional awareness that our perceptions about human phenomena are limited by our perceptions as human being. Total objectivity is an unattainable ideal because "there is no absolute point outside phenomena from which to investigate. Moreover, the knowledge gained in the investigation changes the character of what has been investigated" (Polkinghorne, 1983, p. 263). It also is not possible to directly access the human realm by direct observation. Rather, it must be observed indirectly through our interpretation of human behavioral expressions. This is an important point, since one of the major forms of human expression is through language. This implies that access to human phenomena is rightly obtained from written or oral expressions, for example. Credibility is thus established for subjective data collection methods that include interviews and questionnaires. A natural science mode, however, dictates a hypothetico-deductive approach to research with reliance on objective quantitative methods.

This notion of nursing as a human science—one modeled after a natural science—also has implications for expectations regarding nursing's scientific advancement. Some authors (Hardy, 1983; Newman, 1983) propose carte blanche acceptance of Kuhn's model for scientific growth, even though Kuhn clearly indicates that the model was developed for natural sciences (Kuhn, 1970). Expecting periods of normal science that will be periodically interrupted by scientific revolutions is perhaps unrealistic for nursing as a human science (Meleis, 1985). It may, in fact, lead to erroneous conclusions about scientific progress and, worse yet, hopelessly distort nursing's future direction. Kuhn points out that the rigid pattern of education for normal activity in the natural sciences "is not well designed to produce the man who will easily discover a fresh approach" (Kuhn, 1970, p. 166). It might well be that alleged patterns of revolution in natural science exist only because there is no other way for creative change to occur or for discoveries to be incorporated in such severely structured disciplines. It is clear that an investigator's fundamental beliefs about the nature of human beings, the nature of knowledge and truth, and the nature of nursing science contribute mightily to the definition of a research problem and ultimately to its solution.

Cognitive Style

It has long been observed that individuals have a preferred style of problem solving (Bloom & Broder, 1950) and that this style is a major factor in successful problem solving (Shouksmith, 1970). These cognitive styles "represent a person's typical modes of perceiving, remembering, thinking and problem solving" (Messick, 1970, p. 188). As such, cognitive styles exert a major influence on both the identification of a research problem and the ultimate approach to a solution.

In his theory of experiential learning, Kolb (1981) conceives of learning as a four-stage cycle that includes observations and reflections, formation of abstract concepts and generalizations, testing of implications of concepts and new situations, and concrete experience. Four kinds of abilities are required if this process is to be effective. Concrete experience (CE) is characterized by open, unbiased involvement, while the second ability, reflective observation (RO) involves considering experiences from many perspectives. Abstract conceptualization (AC) involves formulation and integration of concepts into logical and sound theories, and active experimentation (AE) reflects the ability to apply these theories in decision making and problem solving. These abilities can be considered polar opposites on two bisecting dimensions with CE and AC on either end of one continuum and AE and RO as opposites on the other. Kolb points out that the most sophisticated and highly evolved ability, that of creative insight, actually involves synthetic interaction between these abstract and concrete dimensions. In addition, individuals appear to develop cognitive styles that generally emphasize some abilities over others, and those abilities remain remarkably stable over time. It can be demonstrated, however, that styles tend to become somewhat more reflective and analytical as an individual gets older.

Through his research Kolb identifies four cognitive styles. *Convergers* operate predominantly between abstract conceptualization and active experimentation, with an aptitude toward practical application of ideas. These persons approach problems in a hypothetico-deductive way, focusing on a single solution to a problem, often preferring to deal with nonhuman entities. The opposite of convergers are *divergers,* whose abilities lie in concrete experience and reflective observation. These people are "idea generators" who have strong and active imaginations and who are able to connect many unrelated but specific instances into a meaningful whole. Divergers are social and aesthetic in orientation and are often drawn to the humanities and the liberal arts. *Assimilators* operate predominantly in the abstract conceptualization and reflective observation modes and thus show great strength in inductive reasoning and theory formulation. These people are drawn to the logical and the abstract, with little attention to the need for practical application. *Accommodators,* operating on the opposite dimension from assimilators, are adept at concrete experience and active experimentation. These are action-oriented, risk-taking individuals who are often involved in implementation of an idea or a study. Accommodators are highly adaptive to changing situations and use the trial and error approach to problem solving.

These cognitive styles provide a useful way to conceive of general learning and problem-solving styles in individuals. Kolb (1981) warns against strict stereotyping, however, noting that research on cognitive style has consistently demonstrated how diverse and complex these processes actually are in real life. For example, cognitive function will vary in an individual according to the cognitive domain or situational demand.

The four cognitive styles described by Kolb (1981) can be related to inquiry norms in an academic discipline as well. Natural sciences and mathematics generally fall into the abstract-reflective quadrant; science-based professions are abstract-active; and social professions are more concrete-active. The concrete-reflective quadrant is characteristic of humanities and social sciences. Interestingly, in one study of a single university setting described by Kolb (1981), nursing fell into the abstract-active quadrant (converger), while in a much larger study nursing students and faculty fell into the concrete-reflective (diverger) category.

Kolb also proposes a typology of knowledge structures and inquiry processes in academic disciplines, suggesting that "forms of knowledge in different fields can be differentially attractive and meaningful to individuals with different learning styles" (Kolb, 1981, p. 245). That convergers would be drawn to or flourish in science-based empirical disciplines devoted to discrete analysis and conformance to correspondence norms is not surprising, nor is the attraction that the humanities and social science hold for divergers who profess to humanism, norms of coherence, and the conduct of research by historical analysis, field study, or clinical observation. That individuals with various cognitive styles would be attracted to nursing is also not surprising given the acknowledged complex and multifaceted nature of nursing's domain of interest. Certain cognitive styles are undoubtedly drawn to some scientific inquiry strategies more than others. For instance, the assimilator style might prefer theory generation using grounded theory methodology (Glaser & Strauss, 1967), while the accommodator style might choose involvement in clinical trials or intervention studies. A researcher whose predominant style is that of a converger might choose to be involved in theory-testing physiological research with animal subjects, while divergers might be drawn to phenomenological studies. Cognitive style appears to be a variable with major influence in a model of scientific inquiry.

Experience

The role of personal experience in scientific inquiry should not be underestimated. Both *life experience and professional nursing experience* provide fertile ground for problem awareness to grow. Problem identification and formulation of the research question become the fruit of that experience. Evidence of the verification or refutation of theories in the real world is also provided by this experience. Theories that work well are easily identified, while theories that fall short can be revised, extended, or discarded. Anomalous cases become readily apparent, as do continuing perplexities that remain unexplained by existing theories. One's sense of substantive significance stems from this experience, and intuition serves as a guide to the problems that have the most personal and professional meaning.

Prior *research experience* is also an important aspect of this variable, for it is through this experience that investigators learn which questions are able to be answered by current methods, which research approaches have worked in the past, and which ones have not. Experience also teaches what research needs to be conducted in the future and how it might best be accomplished. It also tells researchers whether prior research endeavors fit well enough with what Luria (1973) calls their research style. If prior research experience has been satisfactory and successful, an attempt will be made to replicate aspects contributing to that success, whether substantive or methodological in nature. While research success teaches investigators to utilize similar problem-solving strategies in the future, less than successful research is often as instruc-

tive because of the demand for increasingly novel and creative approaches in subsequent studies.

Theoretical experience is another type of experience that affects the process of inquiry. One aspect of this experience relies upon the existing knowledge base in a substantive area and the researcher's individual perception of that knowledge base. Theoretical experience allows the researcher to identify the existing gaps in knowledge and the significant areas that remain unexplored or unexplained. Individual researcher perception is important in this type of experience, for it is that perception that drives interest in unexplored domains. Scientific advancement depends on theoretical experience over time because of the necessarily progressive nature of research questions based on prior studies. Insight gained from long-standing familiarity with theoretical issues is of inestimable value and contributes to the overall level of understanding about the phenomenon of interest. This level of understanding in turn affects the content and level of subsequent research questions.

A second aspect of theoretical experience relates to the degree to which the researcher has been open to various theoretical approaches and intellectual strategies related to the exploration of the research problem area. If the researcher remains intellectually open to diverging and opposing views, the quality of theoretical understanding will be affected even though initial theoretical orientation may be maintained. Obviously the greater the clarity of understanding of the problem area the greater the possibility of significant answers. This type of intellectual exploration also allows for greater problem tension to exist, which in turn results in greater efforts to resolve the problems (Polyani, 1962). Bruner (1966) points out that it is precisely this dialectical tension between the concrete and the abstract that allows for creativity in problem solving.

Methodological Knowledge and Skill

The level and type of methodological knowledge and skill possessed by a researcher have a major influence on the process and product of scientific inquiry. Since the seeds of the answer lie in every research question (Mackinnon, 1970) and it is asserted that researchers have a preferred style of problem solving (Kolb, 1981), it is natural that researchers pose research questions that they will be able to answer. Kaplan calls this the "law of the instrument" and observes that "it comes as no particular surprise to discover that a scientist formulates problems in a way which requires for their solution just those techniques in which he himself is especially skilled" (Kaplan, 1964, p. 28). He also points out that the cost of becoming an expert in any one research area results in what can be called a "trained incapacity." That is, the more expert one becomes in something the harder it is to solve a problem any other way. Maslow agrees, asserting that "it is tempting, if the only tool you have is a hammer, to treat everything as if it were a nail" (Maslow, 1966, pp. 15–16).

It would seem that the relationship of methodological skills to the formulation of the research question and the process of inquiry for a single investigator study is closer than is often admitted. This limitation may be easier to overcome in larger studies with more than one investigator or over many studies, each conducted by different investigators. Capitalizing on the methodological strengths of multiple investigators to study complex nursing phenomena allows for greater theoretical possibilities through the use of multiple research methods. Polkinghorne points out that multiple methods allow more to be learned about a research problem than could be discovered from any one procedure or method alone (Polkinghorne, 1983).

Extrapersonal Factors

Two classes of extrapersonal variables are proposed to relate to the process and practice of scientific inquiry: influential others and the sociohistoric context.

Influential Others

Two major types of influence on scientific inquiry are inherent in the variable of influential others: individual and institutional. Individual influences are initially conveyed primarily by mentors and other professors in graduate school, the primary wellspring of research values and training for the budding nursing scientist (Tinkle & Beaton, 1983). Here, individual faculty methodological preferences and research values are made known implicitly or explicitly, and disciplinary norms are passed on (Kuhn, 1970). Expectations regarding appropriate methods of scientific inquiry are embedded in each experience and are reinforced at every juncture. It is the prevailing "faculty view" that determines the ultimate breadth and depth of curricular exposure to various research strategies, and it is faculty expertise that delimits actual research opportunities for students. It is here in graduate research training that a nursing scientist's individual research style is born (Luria, 1973).

While the acquisition of disciplinary norms is unquestionably important, the notion implies existing disciplinary consensus on what those norms actually are. Nursing has not quite come to such a conscious consensus, although there is no evidence of the consistent use of diverse research methods to study nursing's complex phenomena (Jacobsen & Meininger, 1985). When disciplinary research norms

are not collectively shared, Toulmin points out that "theoretical debate in the field becomes largely—and unintentionally—methodological and philosophical; it is directed less at interpreting particular empirical findings than at debating the general acceptability (or unacceptability) of rival approaches, patterns of explanation and standards of judgment." (Toulmin, 1972, p. 380). The result is, of course, adamant assertions about one method over another, and the student scientist may be forced early on to align with one camp or another. Thus the norms that are acquired become not disciplinary but methodological and evaluative in nature. Kaplan calls this the "myth of methodology" and warns that "by pressing methodological norms too far, we may inhibit bold and imaginative adventure of ideas. The irony is that methodology itself may make for conformism—conforming to its own favored reconstructions" (Kaplan, 1964, p. 25). Polkinghorne (1983) points out that overall conceptual capacity, or what he calls "conceptual instruments," is also acquired by researchers in their graduate research training. However, he also notes that the unfortunate tendency is for these conceptual abilities to remain relatively unimproved throughout one's research career, even though the scientist may be exposed to diverse inquiry strategies throughout his or her research life. This notion lends support to the considerable influence of faculty norms on student scientists and to the relative strength of the other variables in the model of scientific inquiry as well.

Institutional influences, whether local, regional, or national in origin, also affect the process of scientific inquiry in a similar manner. Institutional norms function as operational imperatives for disciplinary activity in a given setting. Faculty researchers are thus expected, to some degree, to conform to these institutional norms, thus ensuring personal and professional prestige and survival. For example, on a large health science campus where the received view dominates the general conception of science, the faculty and student research in a school of nursing must reflect quasi conformance to these norms to exist at all. In the absence of such conformity university and extramural funding for the school and its research-related activities would be virtually impossible to secure. However, serious scientific repercussions can result when methodological conformity becomes the unquestioned status quo. Thompson (1985) warns that nurse researchers may not even be aware of the extent to which their research questions are prejudiced by the prevailing view. Martin (1982) notes the related influence of resource availability on the selection of the research problem, choice of methodology, and, less commonly, the interpretation of research findings. It is essential to recognize these theoretical and methodological prejudices and the extent to which they enable or disable nursing's scientific progress.

Luria reminds us that "research in a university is free to the extent that the university itself is free" (Luria, 1973, p. 82). The same can be said for research in a school of nursing. Diverse faculty research expertise and activity are characteristic of research climates that are intellectually free. It has also been observed that "the progress of science, good science, depends on novel ideas and intellectual freedom" (Feyerabend, 1981, p. 165). Innovative inquiry and methodological diversity among faculty beget similar opportunity and ability in student scientists. It is upon this foundation of scientific inquiry that the most important advancements in nursing science will be made.

Sociohistorical Context

Sociohistorical influences also affect the process of scientific inquiry in two significant ways. First, significant research problems are often sociohistorically defined and prioritized, thus affecting health policy decisions and funding levels. One obvious example is the current and intense research interest in the causes, cure, and treatment for acquired immune deficiency syndrome (AIDS). This disease has existed in less virulent forms throughout the world for a long time. However, it was the sudden and virulent occurrence of AIDS in western urban population centers, predominantly in otherwise healthy young males, that prompted research interest and subsequent funding by virtue of its threat to public health. Other examples of sociohistorically defined research problem areas include the current focus on quality of life issues, such as stress and coping, as well as the management of chronic illness. These current research concerns are a natural focus in a society that has conquered communicable disease and has extended the human life span. As the aging population grows, so also grows involvement in gerontological health concerns and research problems ultimately related to controlling or decreasing health care expenditures for the elderly.

The second way that the sociohistorical context affects the conduct of inquiry is a function of the idiosyncratic relationship of research style to disciplinary fashion (Luria, 1973). Kaplan wryly observes that "the pressures of fad and fashion are as great in science, for all its logic, as in other areas of culture" (Kaplan, 1964, p. 28). Contemporary scientific fashion alone has the power to dictate substantive focus, theoretical perspective, and methodological approach. For individuals and disciplines in search of academic prestige or research funding, the pressures and priorities of fashion often prove too great to resist. These influences may have the intended effect of stimulating creativity and the solution of significant problems, or they may serve to stultify research activity and to make it less creative than usual.

It is clear from this discussion that the intrapersonal factors of world view, cognitive style, experience, and methodological knowledge and skill as well as the extrapersonal factors of influential others and sociohistorical context together exert a major influence on the progress of scientific inquiry. In the proposed model the process of scientific inquiry is thus depicted as evolutionary emergent, fueled by continual feedback and ultimately directed toward growth and self-actualization. In this way individual research programs develop and progress throughout a scientific career.

Implications for Nursing Science

Several assumptions are fundamental to a discussion of the implications of the model of scientific inquiry for nursing. It will be helpful to state them explicitly:

- The model of scientific inquiry is a reasonable representation of reality.
- As such, the model can be considered to be an existing disciplinary norm for research problem solving in nursing.
- The demand for methodological diversity is implicit in this model or norm because of the complex and multifaceted nature of nursing phenomena and the nature of the individual inquiry process.
- The progress or success of nursing science must be judged by the degree to which the most significant disciplinary problems are actually solved.

These assumptions carry certain implications for nursing science. For example, that this model can be viewed as a norm of nursing science implies ultimate respect for the individual researcher's personal process of problem formulation and resolution. Actions that enhance this personal process ultimately will positively affect the development of nursing theory and science, while actions that interfere or interrupt this process will adversely affect the developing science.

Creativity

The assumption of methodological diversity implies certain mandates for student scientists, their graduate school professors and mentors, and for schools of nursing and other institutions. It has been established that science, at its best, demands the highest degree of creativity in problem solving. Nursing science, in its quest for rapid scientific advancement, is bound even closer than usual to this "constraint of creativity."

Creativity coupled with sound methodological expertise is the rightful key to scientific progress. It is hypothesized that a creative scientist using a creative process and operating in a creative situation or climate is more likely to produce research results or theories that answer significant disciplinary questions. Fortunately there are several ways to enhance this creativity, beginning (for the purposes of this article) in doctoral study.

Creativity flourishes in a climate of intellectual freedom and open exploration. Creative problem solving must begin with self-exploration and self-knowledge. Student scientists should be provided with planned opportunities or activities designed for systematic, philosophical self-exploration so that one's world view can be explored and made known. This would contribute to more conscious decision making related to theoretical alignment, research methods, and the like. Opportunities to share and to discuss one's world view with peers and professors are also fundamental to scientific self-acceptance and acceptance of others. This obviously contributes to an academic atmosphere of openness and intellectual freedom.

Intuition

Intuition is ultimately associated with creativity and must be actively encouraged through the use of intuition-acknowledging and enhancing techniques. Students' exploration of their own pattern of receptivity and creativity should be part of every doctoral curriculum, as well as exposure to the processes of other creative thinkers. Faculty should share their own intuitive and creative processes freely, acknowledging the starts, stops, and detours inherent in the process. Other intuition-enhancing techniques can be employed throughout the educational experience as well. These include providing initial problem contexts or situations and encouraging students to explore the research problem, reformulating it in a manner appropriate to their experience and insight. Involvement in heuristic arguments, exercises in induction, and reasoning by analogy or metaphor all are activities directed toward increasing intuitive and receptive ability (Noddings & Shore, 1984). Ignoring the relationship of intuition to creativity or stifling its natural inclination exacts a terrible price from nursing theory development. To avoid the widespread underuse of such an obvious personal and professional resource implies ultimate acceptance of intuition as a legitimate partner to scholarly creativity and successful scientific enterprise. That intuition and creativity have "female" connotations should not worry those seeking scientific status, for it is relevant only to the observation that female scientists may be superior scientific problem solvers.

Cognitive Style

Assessment of personal cognitive style is also a highly useful strategy for beginning scientists so that existing abilities can be strengthened and weaker ones identified for possible intervention. Although there are obvious advantages and disadvantages to matching cognitive style of students and faculty, it has been proposed that the benefits of matching might be more related to the purpose of the student-faculty relationship (Claxton & Ralston, 1978). If the relationship is *instrumental*, or for the purpose of learning particular skills, as in a research residency or mentor relationship, matching cognitive styles may be productive. If the purpose of the relationship is *developmental* and aimed at developing critical thinking skills, for example, then a mismatch of cognitive style might be more productive because of the exposure to diversity in thinking. Cognitive style assessment would provide useful baseline information upon which later decisions about course work, mentor relationships, research strategies, and the like might be made. The important point is that the assessment process should be a purposive activity within the doctoral curriculum.

Another important consideration related to cognitive style is the degree to which reflective thinking processes are enhanced or encouraged. Although creative and intuitive processes are important to scientific problem solving, critical thinking and analytical ability are equally important (Bigge, 1982). Inherent in reflective thinking is the ultimate balance between the cognitive and affective domains, the rational or analytical intuitive modes, the abstract and concrete levels of thinking, and, finally, the deductive and inductive approaches. Ideally these abilities would exist in exquisite balance in each researcher, but a more realistic focus would be to develop these abilities in each individual as much as possible. Fortunately many of the strategies directed toward enhancing intuition, creativity, and scientific problem solving also serve to improve reflective thinking abilities. Obviously if student scientists are to have adequate opportunity to refine these thinking skills in doctoral study, a faculty similarly skilled must be available to model and engage the students in appropriate exercise. If students are afforded the chance to increase skill in both analytical and intuitive modes, the gaps and flaws in existing theoretical conceptualizations will be easier to see and to overcome. Encouraging such creative yet critical thinking skills is the obvious antidote for nursing education's "long history of squelching curiosity and replacing it with conformity and a non-questioning attitude" (Meleis, 1985, p. 37).

Methodological Diversity

Because the demand for methodological diversity is based as much on researcher characteristics as on the phenomenon of interest, opportunities for exposure to all types of research methods are essential. Thus a faculty must be carefully constructed so that quantitative and qualitative expertise exist side by side. This does not imply that a university cannot develop a research reputation for excellence in certain methodological strategies or theoretical orientation, merely that it should not gain it at the expense of other approaches. If faculty with varied philosophical orientation, cognitive styles, and methodological expertise are not available, then students are forced to match their process of inquiry to that of the available faculty. This can result in rather dire and sometimes dramatic consequences if a gross mismatch exists. At the outset the basic assumptions of the model of scientific inquiry are violated. Since the research problem that is formulated may not be a product of that intensely personal interactive process, there may be less investment in the research problem (Bigge, 1982). With decreased personal investment there may be diminished intellectual desire to solve the problem. When this natural obsession with one's problem is lost, so is what Polanyi calls "the mainspring of all inventive power" (Polanyi, 1962, p. 127). Once this power is lost, the research problem is essentially relegated to the routine, and it becomes a chore instead of an exciting process of discovery. One wonders if the plethora of one-shot studies in nursing is in part a function of the lack of investment in the research problem.

When prevailing scientific attitudes and norms directly conflict with the intellectual-intuitive orientations of the researcher or student scientist and no safe haven for one's methodological learnings exists, interest is lost and so is another opportunity for scientific advancement. Jacox warns that "we have to be careful not to catch students and others who express these alternative views of science in our own somewhat narrower interpretations of science and theory. We must be cognizant that students may be in some jeopardy from faculty not knowledgeable or not accepting of emerging alternative views of science" (Jacox, 1981, p. 20). When it comes to the degree of faculty influence on a student scientist's process of inquiry, it is wise to take heed of Feyerabend's advice: "The hardest task needs the lightest hand or else its completion will not lead to freedom but to a tyranny much worse than the one it replaces" (Feyerabend, 1981, p. 167).

Nursing scientists are a scarce national resource and as such their scholarly productivity must be promoted whenever possible. The ultimate success of nursing science depends wholly on the ability to answer significant disciplinary questions. A creative research effort at all levels of theory building is required to accomplish this formidable task. This demands the existence of an intellectual climate most conducive to creative scientific problem solving and must allow a full array of cognitive and methodological possibilities for use by nursing's budding scientists. This climate should be responsive to individual differences in cognitive style, methodological preference, and the like but should simultaneously foster a fundamental appreciation for divergent approaches and styles.

Admittedly the costs of creating such a climate might appear to be high initially. In the extreme, widespread and epistemological anarchy and methodological revolution might result. At the very least it will require renouncement of scientific conformism, a return to individualism, and acceptance of methodological relativism. In either case the investment will yield a critical mass of highly committed and creative nursing scientists who are intrigued by nursing's scientific complexities and who are fully engaged in finding their solutions. In addition, an increasingly diverse pool of applicants will be attracted to doctoral study in nursing because of the increasing disciplinary consonance with a wide range of philosophical and intellectual possibilities. This can only further enhance the ability to address all levels of theory development.

Once the tremendous force of nursing's unclaimed creative potential is unleashed, a new age of inquiry in nursing science will be born. This new age of inquiry will be characterized by the generation of sophisticated methodological strategies suited to the complexities of a human science, the existence of sound theoretical formulations, and the general societal acknowledgment of nursing's sizable contribution to human welfare. A renewed sense of professional pride will prevail and nursing's scientific competence will be rightly judged by the ability to solve the discipline's most significant problems.

REFERENCES

Albert, R. S. (Ed.). (1983). *Genius and eminence: The social psychology of creativity and exceptional achievement.* Oxford, England: Pergamon Press.

American Nurses' Association (1980). *Nursing: A social policy statement.* Kansas City: Author.

Batey, M. V. (1977). Conceptualization: Knowledge and logic guiding empirical research. *Nursing Research, 26*(5), 324–329.

Bigge, M. (1982). *Learning theories for teachers* (4th ed.). New York: Harper & Row.

Bloom, B., & Broder, C. (1950). *The problem solving process of college students.* Chicago: University of Chicago Press.

Brink, P., & Wood, M. (1983). *Basic steps in planning nursing research, from question to proposal* (2nd ed.). Monterey, CA: Wadsworth.

Bronowski, J. (1965). *Science and human values.* New York: Harper & Row.

Bruner, J. (1966). *The process of education.* New York: Atheneum.

Carper, B. A. (1978). Fundamental patterns of knowing in nursing. *Advances in Nursing Science, 1*(1), 13–23.

Claxton, C., & Ralston, Y. (1978). *Learning styles: Their impact on teaching and administration.* Washington, DC: The American Association for Higher Education.

Conway, M. (1985). Toward greater specificity in defining nursing's metaparadigm. *Advances in Nursing Science, 7*(4), 73–81.

Dickoff, J., James, P., & Weidenbach, E. (1968). Theory in a practice discipline: Part I—practice oriented theory. *Nursing Research, 17* (5), 415–435.

Donaldson, S. K., & Crowley, D. M. (1978). The discipline of nursing. *Nursing Outlook, 26*(2), 113–120.

Fawcett, J. (1978). The relationship between theory and research: A double helix. *Advances in Nursing Science, 1*(1), 49–62.

Feyerabend, P. (1981). How to defend society against science. In I. Hacking (Ed.), *Scientific revolutions.* London: Oxford University Press.

Flaskerud, J. H., & Halloran, E. J. (1980). Areas of agreement in nursing theory development. *Advances in Nursing Science, 3* (1),1–7.

Glaser, B., & Strauss, A. (1967). *The discovery of grounded theory: Strategies of qualitative research.* New York: Aldine.

Goldstein, M., & Goldstein, I. (1978). *How we know: An exploration of the scientific process.* New York: Plenum Press.

Gortner, S., & Nahm, H. (1977). An overview of nursing research in the United States. *Nursing Research, 26,* 10–33.

Gortner, S. (1983). The history and philosophy of nursing science and research. *Advances in Nursing Science, 5*(2), 1–8.

Hardy, M. (1983). Metaparadigms and theory development. In N. L. Chaska (Ed.), *The nursing profession: A time to speak* (pp. 427–435). New York: McGraw-Hill.

Jacobsen, B., & Meininger, J. (1985). The design and methods of published nursing research: 1956–1983. *Nursing Research, 34,* 306–311.

Jacox, A. (1974). Theory construction in nursing: An overview. *Nursing Research, 23*(1), 4–13.

Jacox, A. (1981, June). *Competing theories of science.* Paper presented at the 1981 Forum on Doctoral Education in Nursing, Seattle, WA, June 1981.

Kaplan, A. (1964). *The conduct of inquiry.* New York: Harper & Row.

Kerlinger, F. (1973). *Foundations of behavioral research* (2nd ed.). New York: Holt, Rinehart & Winston.

Kolb, D. (1981). Learning styles and disciplinary differences. In A. Chickering (Ed.), *The modern American college* (pp. 232–255). San Francisco: Jossey-Bass.

Kuhn, T. S. (1970). *The structure of scientific revolutions* (2nd ed.). Chicago: University of Chicago Press.

Luria, S. E. (1973). On research styles and allied matters. *Daedalus, 102*(2), 75–84.

Mackinnon, D. (1970). Creativity: A multifaceted phenomenon. In J. D. Roslansky (Ed.), *Creativity* (pp. 19–32). Amsterdam: North-Holland.

Martin, J. (1982). A garbage can model of the research process. In J. McGrath, J. Martin, & R. Kulka (Eds.), *Judgment calls in research* (pp. 17–39). Beverly Hills, CA: Sage.

Maslow, A. H. (1966). *The psychology of science: A reconnaissance.* South Bend, IN: Gateway Editions.

McGrath, J. E. (1982). Dilemmatics: The study of research choices and dilemmas. In J. McGrath, J. Martin, & R. Kulka (Eds.), *Judgment calls in research* (pp. 69–102). Beverly Hills, CA: Sage.

Meleis, A. I. (1985). *Theoretical nursing: Development and progress.* Philadelphia: J.B. Lippincott.

Messick, S. (1970). The criterion problem in the evaluation of instruction: Assessing possible, not just intended extremes. In M. Wittrock & D. Riley (Eds.), *Evaluation of instruction: Issues and problems.* New York: Holt, Rinehart & Winston.

Metzger, B., & Schultz, S. (1982). Time series analysis: An alternative for nursing. *Nursing Research, 31*(6), 375–378.

Newman, M. A. (1983). The continuing revolution: A history of nursing science. In N. L. Chaska (Ed.), *The nursing profession: A time to speak* (pp. 385–393). New York: McGraw-Hill.

Nicholls, J. G. (1983). Creativity in the person who will never produce anything original or useful. In R. S. Albert (Ed.), *Genius and eminence: The social psychology of creativity and exceptional achievement* (pp. 265–279). Oxford, England: Pergamon Press.

Noddings, N., & Shore, P. (1984). *Awakening the inner eye intuition in education.* New York: Teachers College Press.

Oiler, C. (1982). The phenomenological approach in nursing research. *Nursing Research, 31*(3), 178–181.

Polanyi, M. (1962). *Personal knowledge.* Chicago: University of Chicago Press.

Polit, D., & Hungler, B. (1983). *Nursing research: Principles and methods* (2nd ed.). Philadelphia, J.B. Lippincott.

Polkinghorne, D. (1983). *Methodology for the human science systems of inquiry.* Albany, NY: State University of New York Press.

Rogers, M. E. (1970). *A theoretical basis for nursing.* Philadelphia: F.A. Davis.

Roy, S. C. (1983). Theory development in nursing: Proposal for direction. In N. L. Chaska (Ed.), *The nursing profession: A time to speak* (pp. 453–465). New York: McGraw-Hill.

Runkel, P., & McGrath, J. (1972). *Research on human behavior: A systematic guide to method.* New York: Holt, Rinehart & Winston.

Shouksmith, G. (1970). *Intelligence, creativity and cognitive style.* New York: Wiley Interscience.

Stevens, B. (1979). *Nursing theory: Analysis, application, evaluation.* Boston: Little, Brown.

Suppe, F. (1977). *The structure of scientific theories* (2nd ed.). Chicago: University of Illinois Press.

Thompson, J. (1985). Practical discourse in nursing: Going beyond empiricism and historicism. *Advances in Nursing Science, 7*(4), 59–71.

Tinkle, M. B., & Beaton, J. L. (1983). Toward a new view of science: Implications for nursing research. *Advances in Nursing Science, 5*(2), 27–36.

Tucker, R. (1979). The value decisions we know as science. *Advances in Nursing Science, 1*(2), 1–12.

Toulmin, S. (1972). *Human understanding* (Vol. 1). Oxford, England: Clarendon Press.

Von Bertalanffy, L. (1968). *General system theory.* New York: George Braziller.

Weiskopf, V. (1973). Introduction. In H. Yukawa (Ed.), *Creativity and intuition: A physicist looks east and west* (J. Bester, trans.). Tokyo: Kodansha International.

Wilson, H. S. (1985). *Research in nursing.* Menlo Park, CA: Addison-Wesley.

Worthy, M. (1975). *Aha! A puzzle approach to creative thinking.* Chicago: Nelson Hall.

Yukawa, H. (1973). *Creativity and intuition: A physicist looks at east and west* (J. Bester, trans.). Tokyo: Kodansha International.

THE AUTHOR COMMENTS | Scientific Inquiry in Nursing: A Model for a New Age

This work arose from an intensely passionate intellectual process that kept me in its grips for the first 2 years of doctoral study at the University of California, San Francisco. Coursework in theory development, the philosophy of science, and research methods challenged my assumptions about the research process, forcing a reflective process unlike any I had ever experienced. To understand my role as a budding nurse scientist and how I might best contribute to nursing's knowledge base, I struggled with the question, "How does science really happen?" and, more to the point, "What factors truly affect the conduct of research?" It seemed reasonable that insight into the many influences and pressures I was facing in defining my own research interests would be crucial to the resolution of these issues in my career. Fortunately, the new understanding I gained led to the creation of the model for scientific inquiry in nursing and a sense of peace about my career decisions.

HOLLY A. DeGROOT

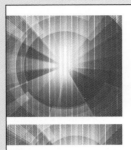

Epistemology is a major area of study within philosophy. Epistemology means the study of knowledge and the kind of evidence that warrants accepted knowledge. This unit focuses on nursing epistemology, including ideas about how evidence and practice come together to make important statements about our disciplinary knowledge. Transformations in the way we think about nursing knowledge and theory can be tracked historically across seminal thinkers, from Florence Nightingale to Hildegard Peplau to Martha Rogers to present-day scholars.

In addition, 30 years ago, Barbara Carper initiated an important change in nursing epistemology that is still being realized today. Writings about the roles of professional and personal knowledge, aesthetics, and critical reflection in knowledge development indicate there is a movement toward greater epistemological diversity than what currently may be warranted as evidence in practice. The context of practice is a central consideration for inventing new approaches to theory generation. In addition, Porter's chapter highlights the context of research in knowledge development. He challenges us to strengthen our standard epistemology and expand warrantable evidence for practice by inserting empirics—through creative research approaches—into other patterns of knowing. Nursing knowledge production in the 21st century will require innovative thinking as well as resistance of domination by biomedical discourse.

QUESTIONS FOR DISCUSSION

- Has nursing epistemology evolved beyond what Nightingale envisioned?

- Has nursing epistemology evolved beyond what Carper envisioned?

- What should be warranted as *evidence* for practice?

- What are the critical dimensions of nursing knowledge?

- What does innovative thinking mean in relationship to nursing knowledge development?

24 | Fundamental Patterns of Knowing in Nursing

BARBARA A. CARPER, RN, EdD, FAAN

It is the general conception of any field of inquiry that ultimately determines the kind of knowledge the field aims to develop as well as the manner in which that knowledge is to be organized, tested and applied. The body of knowledge that serves as the rationale for nursing practice has patterns, forms and structure that serve as horizons of expectations and exemplify characteristic ways of thinking about phenomena. Understanding these patterns is essential for the teaching and learning of nursing. Such an understanding does not extend the range of knowledge, but rather involves critical attention to the question of what it means to know and what kinds of knowledge are held to be of most value in the discipline of nursing.

Identifying Patterns of Knowing

Four fundamental patterns of knowing have been identified from an analysis of the conceptual and syntactical structure of nursing knowledge (Carper, 1975). The four patterns are distinguished according to logical type of meaning and designated as: (a) empirics, the science of nursing; (b) esthetics, the art of nursing; (c) the component of a personal knowledge in nursing; and (d) ethics, the component of moral knowledge in nursing.

Empirics: The Science of Nursing

The term *nursing science* was rarely used in the literature until the late 1950s. However, since that time there has been an increasing emphasis—one might even say a sense of urgency—regarding the development of a body of empirical knowledge specific to nursing. There seems to be general agreement that there is a critical need for knowledge about the empirical world, knowledge that is systematically organized into general laws and theories for the purpose of describing, explaining and predicting phenomena of special concern to the discipline of nursing. Most theory development and research efforts are primarily engaged in seeking and generating explanations which are systematic and controllable by factual evidence and which can be used in the organization and classification of knowledge.

The pattern of knowing which is generally designated as "nursing science" does not presently exhibit the same degree of highly integrated abstract and systematic explanations characteristic of the more mature sciences, although nursing literature reflects this as an ideal form. Clearly there are a number of coexisting, and in a few instances competing, conceptual structures—none of which has achieved the status of what Kuhn (1962) calls a scientific paradigm. That is, no single conceptual structure is as yet generally accepted as an example of actual scientific practice "which include[s] law, theory, application, and instrumentation together … [and] … provide[s] models from which spring particular coherent traditions of scientific research" (Kuhn, 1962, p. 10). It could be argued that some of these conceptual structures seem to have greater potential than others for providing explanations that systematically account for observed phenomena and may ultimately permit more accurate prediction and control of them. However, this is a matter to be determined by research designed to test the validity of such explanatory concepts in the context of relevant empirical reality.

New Perspectives

What seems to be a paramount importance, at least at this stage in the development of nursing science, is that these preparadigm conceptual structures and theoretical models present new perspectives for considering the familiar phenomena of health and illness in relation to the human life process; as such they can and should be legitimately counted as discoveries in the discipline. The representation of health as more than the absence of disease is a crucial change; it permits health to be thought of as a dynamic state or process which changes over a given period of time and varies according to circumstances rather than a static either/or entity. The conceptual change in turn makes it possible to raise questions that previously would have been literally unintelligible.

ABOUT THE AUTHOR

BARBARA A. CARPER is Professor Emerita and former Associate Dean for Academic Affairs at the College of Nursing, University of North Carolina--Charlotte. Dr. Carper received her baccalaureate degree from Texas Woman's University and her MEd and EdD from Columbia University Teacher's College. She also earned a Clinical Certification in Anesthesia from the University of Michigan in 1962. She spent 1981 through 1982 at Harvard University as a Visiting Scholar in Medical Ethics. Her areas of expertise include ethics and nursing theory development. One of her legacies to nursing is her widely cited, critiqued, and admired publication Fundamental Patterns of Knowing. Retirement now allows Dr. Carper to enjoy traveling with her husband, as well as to be active in the community and on the local Hospice Ethics Committee.

The discovery that one can usefully conceptualize health as something that normally ranges along a continuum has led to attempts to observe, describe and classify variations in health, or levels of wellness, as expressions of a human being's relationship to the internal and external environments. Related research has sought to identify behavioral responses, both physiological and psychological, that may serve as cues by which one can infer the range of normal variations of health. It has also attempted to identify and categorize significant etiological factors which serve to promote or inhibit changes in health status.

Current Stages

The science of nursing at present exhibits aspects of both the "natural history stage of inquiry" and the "stage of deductively formulated theory." The task of the natural history stage is primarily the description and classification of phenomena which are, generally speaking, ascertainable by direct observation and inspection (Northrop, 1959). But current nursing literature clearly reflects a shift from this descriptive and classification form to increasingly theoretical analysis which is directed toward seeking, or inventing, explanations to account for observed and classified empirical facts. This shift is reflected in the change from a largely observational vocabulary to a new, more theoretical vocabulary whose terms have a distinct meaning and definition only in the context of the corresponding explanatory theory.

Explanations in the several open-system conceptual models tend to take the form commonly labeled functional or teleological (Nagel, 1961). For example, the system models explain a person's level of wellness at any particular point in time as a function of current and accumulated effects of interactions with his or her internal and external environments. The concept of adaptation is central to this type of explanation. Adaptation is seen as crucial in the process of responding to environmental demands (usually classified as stressors), and enables an individual to maintain or reestablish the steady state which is designated as the goal of the system. The development models often exhibit a more genetic type of explanation in that certain events, the developmental tasks, are believed to be causally relevant or necessary conditions for the normal development of an individual.

Thus, the first fundamental pattern of knowing in nursing is empirical, factual, descriptive and ultimately aimed at developing abstract and theoretical explanations. It is exemplary, discursively formulated and publicly verifiable.

Esthetics: The Art of Nursing

Few, if indeed any, familiar with the professional literature would deny that primary emphasis is placed on the development of the science of nursing. One is almost led to believe that the only valid and reliable knowledge is that which is empirical, factual, objectively descriptive and generalizable. There seems to be a self-conscious reluctance to extend the term knowledge to include those aspects of knowing in nursing that are not the result of empirical investigation. There is, nonetheless, what might be described as a tacit admission that nursing is, at least in part, an art. Not much effort is made to elaborate or to make explicit this aesthetic pattern of knowing in nursing—other than to vaguely associate the "art" with the general category of manual and/or technical skills involved in nursing practice.

Perhaps this reluctance to acknowledge the esthetic component as a fundamental pattern of knowing in nursing originates in the vigorous efforts made in the not-so-distant past to exorcise the image of the apprentice-type educational system. Within the apprentice system, the art of nursing was closely associated with an imitative learning style and the acquisition of knowledge by accumulation of unrationalized experiences. Another likely source of reluctance is that the definition of the term art has been excessively and inappropriately restricted.

Weitz (1960) suggests that art is too complex and variable to be reduced to a single definition. To conceive the task of esthetic theory as definition, he says, is logically doomed to failure in that what is called art has not common properties—only recognizable similarities. This fluid and open approach to the understanding and application of the concept of art and aesthetic meaning makes possible a wider consideration of conditions, situations and experiences in nursing that may properly be called esthetic, including the creative process of discovery in the empirical pattern of knowing.

Esthetics Versus Scientific Meaning

Despite this open texture of the concept of art, esthetic meanings can be distinguished from those in science in several important aspects. The recognition "that art is expressive rather than merely formal or descriptive," according to Rader, "is about as well established as any fact in the whole field of esthetics" (Rader, 1960, p. xvi). An aesthetic experience involves the creation and/or appreciation of a singular, particular, subjective expression of imagined possibilities or equivalent realities which "resists projection into the discursive form of language" (Langer, 1957). Knowledge gained by empirical description is discursively formulated and publicly verifiable. The knowledge gained by subjective acquaintance, the direct feeling of experience, defines discursive formulation. Although an esthetic expression requires abstraction, it remains specific and unique rather than exemplary and leads us to acknowledge that "knowledge—genuine knowledge, understanding—is considerably wider than our discourse" (Langer, 1957, p. 23).

For Wiedenbach (1964), the art of nursing is made visible through the action taken to provide whatever the patient requires to restore or extend his ability to cope with the demands of his situation. But the action taken, to have an esthetic quality, requires the active transformation of the immediate object—the patient's behavior—into a direct, nonmediated perception of what is significant in it—that is, what need is actually being expressed by the behavior. This perception of the need expressed is not only responsible for the action taken by the nurse but reflected in it.

The esthetic process described by Wiedenbach resembles what Dewey (1958) refers to as the difference between recognition and perception. According to Dewey, recognition serves the purpose of identification and is satisfied when a name tag or label is attached according to some stereotype or previously formed scheme of classification. Perception, however, goes beyond recognition in that it includes an active gathering together of details and scattered particulars into an experienced whole for the purpose of seeing what is there. It is perception rather than mere recognition that results in a unity of ends and means which gives the action taken an aesthetic quality.

Orem speaks of the art of nursing as being "expressed by the individual nurse through her creativity and style in designing and providing nursing that is effective and satisfying" (Orem, 1971, p. 155). The art of nursing is creative in that it requires development of the ability to "envision valid modes of helping in relation to 'results' which are appropriate" (Orem, 1971, p. 69). This again invokes Dewey's (1958) sense of a perceived unity between an action taken and its result—a perception of the means and the end as an organic whole. The experience of helping must be perceived and designed as an integral component of its desired result rather than conceived separately as an independent action imposed on an independent subject. Perhaps this is what is meant by the concept of nursing the whole patient or total patient care. If so, what are the qualities that enable the creation of a design for nursing care that eliminate or would minimize the fragmentation of means and ends?

Esthetic Pattern of Knowing

Empathy—that is, the capacity for participating in or vicariously experiencing another's feelings—is an important mode in the esthetic pattern of knowing. One gains knowledge of another person's singular, particular, felt experience through empathic acquaintance (Lee, 1960; Lippo, 1960). Empathy is controlled or moderated by psychic distance or detachment in order to apprehend and abstract what we are attending to, and in this sense is objective. The more skilled the nurse becomes in perceiving and empathizing with the lives of others, the more knowledge or understanding will be gained of alternate modes of perceiving reality. The nurse will thereby have available a larger repertoire of choices in designing and providing nursing care that is effective and satisfying. At the same time, increased awareness of the variety of subjective experiences will heighten the complexity and difficulty of the decision making involved.

The design of nursing care must be accompanied by what Langer refers to as sense of form, the sense of "structure, articulation, a whole resulting from the relation of mutually dependent factors, or more precisely, the way the whole is put together" (Langer, 1957, p. 16). The design, if it is to be esthetic, must be controlled by the perception of the balance, rhythm, proportion and unity of what is done in relation to the dynamic integration and articulation of the whole. "The doing may be energetic, and the undergoing may be acute and intense," Dewey (1958) says, but "unless they are related to each other to form a whole," what is done becomes merely a matter of mechanical routine or of caprice.

The esthetic pattern of knowing in nursing involves the perception of abstracted particulars as distinguished from the recognition of abstracted universals. It is the knowing of a unique particular rather than an exemplary class.

The Component of Personal Knowledge

Personal knowledge as a fundamental pattern of knowing in nursing is the most problematic, the most difficult to master and to teach. At the same time, it is perhaps the pattern most essential to understanding the meaning of health in terms of individual well-being. Nursing considered as an interpersonal process involves interactions, relationships and transactions between the nurse and the patient-client. Mitchell points out that "there is growing evidence that the quality of interpersonal contacts has an influence on a person's becoming ill, coping with illness and becoming well" (Mitchell, 1973, p. 49–50). Certainly the phrase "therapeutic use of self" which has become increasingly prominent in the literature implies that the way in which nurses view their own selves and the client is of primary concern in any therapeutic relationship.

Personal knowledge is concerned with the knowing, encountering and actualizing of the concrete, individual self. One does not know *about* the self; one strives simply to *know* the self. This knowing is a standing in relation to another human being and confronting that human being as a person. This "I-Thou" encounter is unmediated by conceptual categories or particulars abstracted from complex organic wholes (Buber, 1970). The relation is one of reciprocity, a state of being that cannot be described or even experienced—it can only be actualized. Such personal knowing extends not only to other selves but also to relations with one's own self.

It requires what Buber (1970) refers to as the sacrifice of form—i.e., categories or classifications—for a knowing of infinite possibilities, as well as the risk of total commitment.

> Even as a melody is not composed of tones, nor a verse of words, nor a statue of lines— one must pull and tear to turn a unity into a multiplicity—so it is with the human being to whom I say You .... I have to do this again and again; but immediately he is no longer You. (Buber, 1970, p. 59)

Maslow (1956) refers to this sacrifice of form as embodying a more efficient perception of reality in that reality is not generalized nor predetermined by a complex of concepts, expectations, beliefs and stereotypes. This results in a greater willingness to accept ambiguity, vagueness and discrepancy of oneself and others. The risk of commitment involved in personal knowledge is what Polyani calls the "passionate participation in the act of knowing" (Polyani, 1964, p. 17).

The nurse in the therapeutic use of self rejects approaching the patient-client as an object and strives instead to actualize an authentic personal relationship between two persons. The individual is considered as an integrated, open system incorporating movement toward growth and fulfillment of human potential. An authentic personal relation requires the acceptance of others in their freedom to create themselves and the recognition that each person is not a fixed entity, but constantly engaged in the process of becoming. How then should the nurse reconcile this with the social and/or professional responsibility to control and manipulate the environmental variables and even the behavior of the person who is a patient in order to maintain or restore a steady state? If a human being is assumed to be free to choose and chooses behavior outside of accepted norms, how will this affect the action taken in the therapeutic use of self by the nurse? What choices must the nurse make in order to know another self in an authentic relation apart from the category of patient, even when categorizing for the purpose of treatment is essential to the process of nursing?

Assumptions regarding human nature, McKay observes, "range from the existentialist to the cybernetic, from the idea of an information processing machine to one of a many splendored being" (McKay, 1969, p. 399). Many of these assumptions incorporate in one form or another the notion that there is, for all individuals, a characteristic state which they, by virtue of membership in the species, must strive to assume or achieve. Empirical descriptions and classifications reflect the assumption that being human allows for prediction of basic biological, psychological and social behaviors that will be encountered in any given individual.

Certainly empirical knowledge is essential to the purposes of nursing. But nursing also requires that we be alert to the fact that models of human nature and their abstract and generalized categories refer to and describe behaviors and traits that groups have in common. However, none of these categories can ever encompass or express the uniqueness of the individual encountered as a person, as a "self." These and many other similar considerations are involved in the realm of personal knowledge, which can be broadly characterized as subjective, concrete and existential. It is concerned with the kind of knowing that promotes wholeness and integrity in the personal encounter, the achievement of engagement rather than detachment; and it denies the manipulative, impersonal orientation.

Ethics: The Moral Component

Teachers and individual practitioners are becoming increasingly sensitive to the difficult personal choices that must be made within the complex context of modern health care. These choices raise fundamental questions about morally right and wrong action in connection with the care and treatment of illness and the promotion of health. Moral dilemmas arise in situations of ambiguity and uncertainty, when the consequences of one's actions are difficult to predict and traditional principles and ethical codes offer no help or seem to result in contradiction. The moral code which guides the ethical conduct of nurses is based on the primary principle of obligation embodied in the concepts of service to people and respect for human life. The discipline of nursing is held to be a valuable and essential social service responsible for conserving life, alleviating suffering and promoting health. But appeal to the ethical "rule book" fails to provide answers in terms of difficult individual moral choices which must be made in the teaching and practice of nursing.

The fundamental pattern of knowing identified here as the ethical component of nursing is focused on matters of obligation or what ought to be done. Knowledge of morality goes beyond simply knowing the norms or ethical codes of the discipline. It includes all voluntary actions that are deliberate and subject to the judgment of right and wrong—including judgments of moral value in relation to motives, intentions and traits of character. Nursing is deliberate action, or a series of actions, planned and implemented to accomplish defined goals. But goals and actions involve choices made, in part, on the basis of normative judgments, both particular and general. On occasion, the principles and norms by which such choices are made may be in conflict.

According to Berthold, "goals are, of course, value judgments not amenable to scientific inquiry and validation" (Berthold, 1968, p. 196). Dickoff, James and Wiedenbach also call attention to the need to be aware that the specification of goals serves as "a norm or standard by which to evaluate activity … [and] … entails taking them as values—that is, signifies conceiving these goal contents as situations worthy to be brought about" (Dickoff, James, & Wiedenbach, 1968, p. 422).

For example, a common goal of nursing care in relation to the maintenance or restoration of health is to assist patients to achieve a state in which they are independent. Much of the current practice reflects an attitude of value attached to the goal of independence, and indicates nursing actions to assist patients in assuming full responsibility for themselves at the earliest possible moment or to enable them to retain responsibility to the last possible moment. However, valuing independence and attempting to maintain it may be at the expense of the patient's learning how to live with physical or social dependence when necessary; e.g., in instances when prognosis indicates that independence cannot be regained.

Differences in normative judgments may have more to do with disagreements as to what constitutes a "healthy" state of being than lack of empirical evidence or ambiguity in the application of the term. Slote suggests that the persistence of disputes, or lack of uniformity in the application of cluster terms, such as health, is due to "the difficulty of decisively resolving certain sorts of value questions about what is and is not important." This leads him to conclude "that value judgment is far more involved in the making of what are commonly thought to be factual statements than has been imagined" (Slote, 1966, p. 220).

The ethical pattern of knowing in nursing requires an understanding of different philosophical positions regarding what is good, what ought to be desired, what is right; of different ethical frameworks devised for dealing with the complexities of moral judgments; and of various orientations to the notion of obligation. Moral choices to be made must then be considered in terms of specific action to be taken in specific, concrete situations. The examination of the standards, codes and values by which we decide what is morally right should result in a greater awareness of what is involved in making moral choices and being responsible for the choices made. The knowledge of ethical codes will not provide answers to the moral questions involved in nursing, nor will it eliminate the necessity for having to make moral choices. But it can be hoped that:

> The more sensitive teachers and practitioners are to the demands of the process of justification, the more explicit they are about the norms that govern their actions, the more personally engaged they are in assessing surrounding circumstances and potential consequences, the more "ethical" they will be; and we cannot ask much more (Greene, 1973, p. 221).

Using Patterns of Knowing

A philosophical discussion of patterns of knowing may appear to some as a somewhat idle, if not arbitrary and artificial, undertaking having little or no connection with the practical concerns and difficulties encountered in the day-to-day doing and teaching of nursing. But it represents a personal conviction that there is a need to examine the kinds of knowing that provide the discipline with its particular perspectives and significance. Understanding four fundamental patterns of knowing makes possible an increased awareness of the complexity and diversity of nursing knowledge.

Each pattern may be conceived as necessary for achieving mastery in the discipline, but none of them alone should be considered sufficient. Neither are they mutually exclusive. The teaching and learning of one pattern do not require the rejection or neglect of any of the others. Caring for another requires the achievements of nursing science, that is, the knowledge of empirical facts systematically organized into theoretical explanations regarding the phenomena of health and illness. But creative imagination also plays its part in the syntax of discovery in science, as well as in developing the ability to imagine the consequences of alternate moral choices.

Personal knowledge is essential for ethical choices in that moral action presupposes personal maturity and freedom. If the goals of nursing are to be more than conformance to unexamined norms, if the "ought" is not to be determined simply on the basis of what is possible, then the obligation to care for another human being involves becoming a certain kind of person—and not merely doing certain kinds of things. If the design of nursing care is to be more than habitual or mechanical, the capacity to perceive and interpret the subjective experiences of others and to imaginatively project the effects of nursing actions on their lives becomes a necessary skill.

Nursing thus depends on the specific knowledge of human behavior in health and in illness, the esthetic perception of significant human experiences, a personal understanding of the unique individuality of the self and the capacity to make choices within concrete situations involving particular moral judgments. Each of these separate but interrelated and interdependent fundamental patterns of knowing should be taught and understood according to its distinctive logic, the restricted circumstances in which it is valid, the kinds of data it subsumes and the methods by which each particular kind of truth is distinguished and warranted.

The major significances to the discipline of nursing in distinguishing patterns of knowing are summarized as: (a) the conclusions of the discipline conceived as subject matter cannot be taught or learned without reference to the structure of the discipline—the representative concepts and methods of inquiry that determine the kind of knowledge gained and limit its meaning, scope and validity; (b) each of the fundamental patterns of knowing represents a necessary but not complete approach to the problems and questions in the discipline; and (c) all knowledge is subject to change and revision. Every solution of an existing problem raises new and unsolved questions. These new and as yet unsolved problems require, at times, new methods of inquiry and different conceptual structures; they change the shape and patterns of knowing. With each change in the shape of knowledge, teaching and learning require looking for different points of contact and connection among ideas and things. This clarifies the effect of each new thing known on other things known and the discovery of new patterns by which each connection modifies the whole.

REFERENCES

Berthold, J. S. (1968). Symposium on theory development in nursing: Prologue. *Nursing Research, 17*, 196–197.

Buber, M. (1970). *I and thou.* (W. Kaufman, Trans.). New York: Scribner.

Carper, B. A. (1975). Fundamental patterns of knowing in nursing. (Doctoral dissertation, Columbia University Teachers College). *Dissertation Abstract International, 36*, 4941B. (University Microfilms No. 76–7772).

Dewey, J. (1958). *Art as experience.* New York: Capricorn.

Dickoff, J., James, P., & Wiedenbach, E. (1968). Theory in a practice discipline: Part I, Practice-oriented theory. *Nursing Research, 17*, 415–435.

Greene, M. (1973). *Teacher as stronger.* Belmont, CA: Wadsworth.

Kuhn, T. (1962). *The structure of scientific revolutions.* Chicago: University of Chicago Press.

Langer, S. K. (1957). *Problems of art.* New York: Scribner.

Lee, V. (1960). Empathy. In M. Rader (Ed.), *A modern book of esthetics* (3rd ed.). New York: Holt, Rinehart and Winston.

Lippo, T. (1960). Empathy, inner imitation and sense-feeling. In M. Rader (Ed.), *A modern book of esthetics* (3rd ed.). New York: Holt, Rinehart and Winston.

Maslow, A. H. (1956). Self-actualizing people: A study of psychological health. In C. E. Moustakas (Ed.), *The self.* New York: Harper and Row.

McKay, R. (1969). Theories, models and systems for nursing. *Nursing Research, 18*, 393–399.

Mitchell, P. H. (1973). *Concepts basic to nursing.* New York: McGraw-Hill.

Nagel, E. (1961). *The structure of science.* New York: Harcourt, Brace and World.

Northrop, F. S. C. (1959). *The logic of the sciences and the humanities.* New York: World.

Orem, D. E. (1971). *Nursing: Concepts of practice.* New York: McGraw-Hill.

Polanyi, M. (1964). *Personal knowledge.* New York: Harper and Row.

Rader, M. (1960). Introduction: The meaning of art. In M. Rader (Ed.), *A modern book of esthetics* (3rd ed.). New York: Holt, Rinehart and Winston.

Slote, M. A. (1966). The theory of important criteria. *Journal of Philosophy, 63*, 211–224.

Weitz, M. (1960). The role of theory in aesthetics. In M. Rader (Ed.), *A modern book of esthetics* (3rd ed.). New York: Holt, Rinehart and Winston.

Wiedenbach, E. (1964). *Clinical nursing: A helping art.* New York: Springer.

THE AUTHOR COMMENTS | Fundamental Patterns of Knowing in Nursing

The genesis for this article, which was part of my doctoral dissertation, was my perplexity and confusion as an inexperienced teacher regarding what should be included in the nursing curriculum. Both student and teacher became disoriented in a maze of seemingly disparate disarticulated facts. My search for some meaningful guide to a sense of the whole to counteract this fragmentation led me to design a study to qualitatively analyze the types of knowledge that exemplified nursing. The resulting dissertation and article allowed nurses the freedom to begin asking questions about nursing and move beyond the assumptions about the essence of nursing and stimulate new thinking about the discipline. I never anticipated how popular the article would become!

BARBARA A. CARPER

25

Patterns of Knowing: Review, Critique, and Update

JILL WHITE, RN, PhD, RM

Carper's patterns of knowing in nursing have been consistently cited in the nursing literature since they appeared in 1978. The degree to which they represent nursing knowledge in the mid-1990s is explored, and a major modification is suggested—the addition of a fifth pattern, sociopolitical knowing. The article also suggests modifications to the model for nursing knowledge put forward by Jacobs-Kramer and Chinn to enable this model to be used more effectively as a framework for exploring processes of inquiry into nursing knowledge and practice.

In 1978 Barbara Carper[1] published "Fundamental Patterns of Knowing in Nursing" in the first edition of *Advances in Nursing Science*. Based on her doctoral work, the article described her typology of patterns of knowing in nursing. These patterns she named empirics, esthetics, ethics, and personal knowing.

Carper's patterns of knowing have been much cited and commented on, albeit somewhat uncritically, in the writing of nurses over the ensuing years. As with much of nursing's written heritage, there is little connection between the number of citations and the extent of critical development that has taken place. An important exception to this, however, was the work of Jacobs-Kramer and Chinn[2] a decade after Carper's article first appeared. Jacobs-Kramer and Chinn extended Carper's framework by producing a model that elucidated their understanding of the creation and development, the expression and transmission, and the assessment of each of Carper's patterns of knowing. Their intention was for such an elucidation to facilitate the integration of these patterns of knowing in nursing into clinical practice.

The lack of recent dialogue about the patterns themselves or about the model may reflect the decreased interest in the use of models generally in nursing, part of a move from reductionist thinking. The continued citation of both Carper and Jacobs-Kramer and Chinn, however, suggests their work is still being used in teaching.

The "patterns" of Carper[1] and "model" of Jacobs-Kramer and Chinn[2] do provide convenient conceptual organizers for introducing students to different ways of knowing in nursing. The patterns and model can be used to facilitate exploration of nursing practice and to enhance understanding of the rich history of modern nursing writing. They enable the contributions of nurses from the past to be analyzed in terms of the dominant social, political, and philosophical contexts of their time and enable nurses to trace with understanding the cumulative and disparate knowledge development that contributes to the discipline of nursing.

Given that the patterns and the model are still being used in education, it is appropriate that they be reviewed and critiqued within the context of nursing knowledge development in the mid-1990s. This article offers such a review, critique, and update.

In her seminal article "Fundamental Patterns of Knowing in Nursing," Carper[1] identified the following patterns:

- empirics, or the science of nursing;
- ethics, or the moral component;
- the component of personal knowledge; and
- esthetics, or the art of nursing.

In this article the author explores each of these patterns in turn, looking first at what Carper had to say, then at the extension of this pattern within the Jacobs-Kramer and Chinn model, and finally at questions that arise with reference to the current literature and each particular pattern. Table 25-1 summarizes the essential elements of Jacobs-Kramer and Chinn's model of nursing knowledge.

From J. White, Patterns of knowing: Review, critique, and update. Advances in Nursing Science, 1995, 17(4), 73–86.
Copyright © 1995. Reproduced with permission of Lippincott Williams & Wilkins.

ABOUT THE AUTHOR

JILL WHITE was born in Wagga Wagga, a country town in southeast Australia. She grew up viewing healthcare, particularly the hospital, as central to the well-being of the community. However, it was also clear that in the 1950s, the power over illness rested firmly with the doctors and, to a lesser extent, with the nurses, with the virtual exclusion of anyone personally significant to the patient. This, even as a junior Red Cross member, made no sense to her. Making sense of how nurses work together with people in health and illness has become her passion. This led her into nursing, nursing education, and the politics of nursing and healthcare. She is a Professor and Dean at the Sydney Nursing School, University of Sydney. Her life has been significantly enriched by her husband Richard and two terrific children.

Empirics: The Science of Nursing

Carper described empirics as

> knowledge that is systematically organized into general laws and theories for the purpose of describing, explaining and predicting phenomena of special concern to the discipline of nursing …. The first fundamental pattern of knowing in nursing is empirical, factual, descriptive, and ultimately aimed at developing abstract theoretical explanations. It is exemplary, discursively formulated, and publicly verifiable.[1(pp14–15)]

The key element here is that the "ultimate aim" of this knowing is "theory" development. Inherent in theory development is the ontological position that nature has a single or dominant reality commonly experienced and about which one can draw generalizable abstract explanations. This clearly encompasses the traditional view of scientific knowledge with its stance of objectivity and context-free replicability. This view was the dominant one in the nursing research and writing at the time of Carper's doctoral work. However, it is debatable at this time whether this pattern encompasses all research-based knowing, which Jacobs-Kramer and Chinn expressed as "facts, theories, models and descriptions that impart understanding."[2(p132)]

The realist ontological position, whose assumptions allow generalization, may also be seen as

---

TABLE 25-1 | **Summary of Essential Elements: Model of Nursing Knowledge**

Dimension	Empirics	Ethics	Personal	Esthetics
Creative	Describing Explaining Predicting	Valuing Clarifying Advocating	Encountering Focusing Realizing	Engaging Interpreting Envisioning
Expressive	Facts Theories Models Descriptions to impart understanding	Codes Standards Normative-ethical theories Descriptions of ethical decision making	Self: authentic and disclosed	Art-act
Assessment: critical question	What does this represent? How is this representative?	Is this right? Is this just?	Do I know what I do? Do I do what I know?	What does this mean?
Process-context	Replication	Dialogue	Response and reflection	Criticism
Credibility index	Validity	Justness	Congruity	Consensual meaning

Source: Jacobs-Kramer M., Chinn P. Perspectives on knowing: a model of nursing knowledge. *Schol Inq Nurs Pract* 1988;2(2):129–139.

including grounded theory and ethnographic research, which generate generalizable abstractions. However, the relativist position of the interpretive paradigm as represented by phenomenology, for example, also seeks to provide "descriptions that impart understanding" but would not be consistent with Carper's definition of having an ultimate aim of developing abstract theoretical explanations that could be "systematically organized into general laws and theories."[1(p14)]

It is therefore suggested that the definition of the empirical pattern of knowing needs to be modified to accommodate the relativist ontological positions of knowledge development using methodologies such as phenomenology. If not modified, nursing needs to acknowledge the limitations of this definition in encompassing empirical knowing that seeks not to generalize, but rather through interpretation or description to put before the reader context-embedded stories whose purpose is to enrich understanding.

The inclusion of the word "understanding" by Jacobs-Kramer and Chinn[2] within the aim of the empirical pattern of knowing may be confusing; "understanding" is more commonly associated with the aim of research within the interpretive paradigm. The ontological position of the interpretive paradigm embraces the notion of multiple realities that cannot be generalized and puts this paradigm outside Carper's definition of this pattern of knowing. As discussed later, interpretive and critical research is encompassed more appropriately elsewhere.

Jacobs-Kramer and Chinn's model suggests that the pattern of empirics is expressed through "facts, theories, models and descriptions."[2(p132)] This expressive dimension may be extended to include the common mode of expression and transmission via books for academic theoretical instruction and professional journals for stimulation of professional debate.

Jacobs-Kramer and Chinn's[2] assessment dimension asks the critical questions, "What does this represent?" and "How is it representative?" The process of assessment is by replication, and the index of credibility they suggest is validity—that the knowledge can be demonstrated to be what it is thought to be. The assessment dimension is dealt with in their article in a brief paragraph that makes it somewhat difficult to fully grasp the intent of the critical questions; a critical question, one would assume, inquires about the relationships between the variables under study and the generalizability of the relationships.

In the case of grounded theory, a critical question would be the relationship to the core concepts of the other concepts and the nature of these relationships. The process of judging the trustworthiness of the results would require both sufficient detail to enable

replication and application and the seeking out and offering up to professional debate of the findings. As Kuhn said, "There is no standard higher than assent of the relevant community."[3(p94)] The remaining process for ascertaining credibility is the "fit" of the new knowledge with the extant knowledge in the area at the time.

It is within this assessment dimension that the case for empirics, not including work using the interpretive or critical paradigm, gains credence. Here, clearly, the standards of credibility are not related to validity, replication, or relationships between variables or categories. If the empirical pattern were to be expanded to accommodate knowledge created through interpretive or critical work, an entirely new assessment would be required with different critical questions, processes, and credibility indices.[4] Possible modifications to the pattern of empirics within the model of nursing knowledge are proposed in Table 25-2.

Ethics: The Moral Component

"The fundamental pattern of knowing identified here as the ethical component of nursing is focused on matters of obligation or what ought to be done."[1(p20)] In exploring this pattern Carper acknowledged the important place of knowledge of norms and ethical codes: "The examination of the standards, codes, and values by which we decide what is morally right should result in a greater awareness of what is involved in making moral choices and being responsible for the choices made."[1(p21)]

However, Carper goes on to caution that the complexity of the ethical issues in modern health care practice means that "moral choices to be made must be considered in terms of specific actions to be taken in specific concrete situations."[1(p21)] In extending this caution, Carper represents one of the earliest nursing writers to speak of the situational and relational importance of moral decision making, which has become fundamental to the ethic of care now so prevalent in the nursing literature.

There has been a plethora of publications in the area of moral knowing. Principal among these are the works of Benner,[5,6] Benner and Wrubel,[7] Bishop and Scudder,[8,9] Cooper,[10,11] and Watson.[12,13] Not directly within nursing but highly relevant are the works of Gilligan,[14,15] Noddings,[16] Pellegrino,[17,18] and Zaner.[19,20]

Much of this work has its origins in Gilligan's[14] critique of Kohlberg's[21] hierarchy of moral decision making. Gilligan challenged Kohlberg's contention that believing in "the primacy and universality of individual rights" was the highest form of moral development and that this represented a morally superior

TABLE 25-2	Empirics: Essential Elements	
Dimension	**Original Model[2]**	**Modifications**
Creative	Describing Explaining Predicting	Describing Explaining Predicting
Expressive	Facts Theories Models Descriptions to impart understanding	Facts Theories and models described in books and professional journals Descriptions that indicate relationships
Assessment: critical question	What does this represent? How is it representative?	What relationships were found? Under what conditions do these relationships hold?
Process-context	Replication	Replication and application Professional debate Fit with extant knowledge
Credibility index	Validity Reliability	Validity Reliability

position to Kohlberg's penultimate stage, which embodies a "very strong sense of being responsible to the world."[14(p444)] Gilligan suggested that the focus on individual justice is a predominantly male orientation, whereas women more commonly adopt the contextual, relational, care orientation that focuses on social and moral good.

Moss[22] provided an excellent exploration of the impact of Gilligan's work over the past 15 years, particularly in relation to nursing. Together with Moss, Bishop and Scudder,[9] Benner,[6] and Watson[12,13] suggested that the moral ideal of doing what is good (that is, adopting a caring orientation), rather than that which is just, will most fruitfully be revealed through the exploration of practice rather than simply through reference to "rule-books." This, they suggested, will happen through processes of reflection, discussion, and storytelling of life and nursing practice.[6,9] Bishop and Scudder made a particularly salient point for nurses within this discussion by questioning the notion that moral decision making is about "solving" dilemmas at all: "One way in which the moral sense differs from traditional nursing ethics is that it directs us to moral dilemmas which cannot be solved but must be lived with and, when possible, ameliorated."[9(p124)]

Zaner, with reference to physicians but equally applicable to nursing, suggested "Moral life is essentially communal at its root, and it is mutuality (in all its complex forms), not autonomy, that is foundational. Nowhere is this more plainly evident than in the contexts of clinical situations dealing with ill persons."[20(p292)] Zaner went on to say that "autonomy and rights"

inhibit moral decision making within health care, which requires, foundationally, cooperation and collaboration.

Cooperation is also emphasized in the work of Gadow[23] on existential advocacy. She reinforced the importance of collaboratively making "the effort to help persons become clear about what they want to do, by helping them discern their values in the situation and on the basis of that self examination, to reach decisions which express their reaffirmed, perhaps recreated, complex of values."[23(p44)] Gadow put this effort forward as a moral ideal, not duty, norm, or prescription. It is a moral enterprise through situated engagement.

Jacobs-Kramer and Chinn[2] focused on justice in their assessment dimension of this pattern. An expansion of the assessment dimension is required to accommodate an ethic of care as well as an ethic of justice. Thus, potential modifications to the ethical pattern of knowing are listed in Table 25-3.

The discussion about ethics shows how intimately linked the patterns of moral and personal knowing are. Moral knowing requires fundamentally an authentic interpersonal involvement for its development.

Personal Knowing

The pattern of personal knowing is concerned with "the knowing, encountering and actualizing of the concrete individual self. One does not know *about* self; one strives simply to *know* the self. This knowing

TABLE 25-3	Ethics: Essential Elements	
Dimension	**Original Model[2]**	**Modifications**
Creative	Valuing Clarifying Advocating	Valuing the moral idea of caring Critically appraising values Existential advocacy[23] Sensitizing to other value positions Fostering articulation of everyday notions 　of good[6]
Expressive	Codes, standards Normative theories Descriptions of decision making	Codes, standards Normative theories Observation Storytelling to explore embedded notions 　of good
Assessment: critical 　question	Is it right? Is it just?	Is it good? Is it just? Is it right? Does it embody caring?
Process-context	Dialogue	Dialogue Critical reflection Collaborative values elaboration
Credibility index	Justness	Justness Goodness Caring Congruence with personal values of patient

is a standing in relation to another human being and confronting that human being as a person."[1(p18)] The pattern of personal knowing develops when the nurse approaches the patient not as an object or category of illness, but strives instead "to actualize an authentic personal relationship between two persons."[1(p19)] This pattern requires the nurse to allow the person who is the patient-client to "matter." It involves engagement as opposed to detachment.

Mayeroff, whom Carper[1] cited as a source for her notion of personal knowing, saw a special feature of caring for a person as being "able to understand [the person] and his world as if I were inside it."[24(p42)] For Mayeroff relationship is about reciprocity, about helping the other "grow" and through this, growing oneself. However, Mayeroff's words harbor subtle paternalism: "I want it to grow in its own right ... and I feel the other's growth as bound up with my own sense of well-being."[24(p8)] Such a position mitigates against genuine reciprocity.

Mayeroff's reciprocity was elaborated on and refined in the works of Watson[12] in describing her concept of "transcendental moment," by Taylor[25] in her exposition of the "ordinariness" of nursing, in Morse's[26] work on nurse-patient relationships, and in Moch's[27] exploration of "personal knowing," and

probably most well known within nursing is Benner's[5] seminal work *From Novice to Expert*. Benner's notion of involvement and engagement was further developed collaboratively with Tanner[28] on intuition and with Wrubel[7] on the primacy of caring.

The idea of "being-with," of presence, of letting the person matter and being open to help that person make meaning out of his or her experience, is an essential feature of nursing practice. Without this knowing of self that allows an openness to the knowing of another person, nursing is only technical assistance, not involved care. In Carper's words, "It is concerned with the kind of knowing that promotes wholeness and integrity in the personal encounter, the achievement of engagement rather than detachment, and it denies the manipulative, impersonal orientation."[1(p20)]

In the model of nursing knowledge described by Jacobs-Kramer and Chinn,[2] the pattern of personal knowing is seen as being created by "experiencing the self—encountering and focusing on self while realizing the realities and potentialities."[2(p135)] It also involves "experiencing, encountering and focusing."[2(p135)] These are not easy concepts to grasp. Carper herself said of this pattern that it "is the most problematic, the most difficult to master and to teach. At the same time, it is

TABLE 25-4	Personal Knowing: Essential Elements	
Dimension	Original Model[2]	Modifications
Creative	Encountering Focusing Realizing	Encountering, focusing, and realizing through practice and through art, literature, poetry, and storytelling
Expressive	Self: authentic and disclosed	Self: authentic and disclosed
Assessment: critical question	Do I know what I do? Do I do what I know?	Do I know what I do? Do I do what I know?
Process-context	Response and reflection	Reflection informed by the response of others and our reflection on our response to the life-world of other
Credibility index	Congruity	Congruity

perhaps the pattern most essential to understanding the meaning of health in terms of individual well-being."[1(p18)]

The creation of personal knowing may be enhanced through the use of art, poetry, literature, and storytelling in an endeavor to more truly "understand [the person] and his world as if I were inside it."[24(p42)] An example of this is poetry about childbirth that helps the midwife "see" inside the patient's world; poems such as Sharon Doubiago's "South American Mi Hija" (in Chester[29]) show the intensity that can allow the soul to grow, whereas stories such as Anais Nin's "Birth" (in Chester[29]) illuminate the potential for the soul to shrivel if a woman is not supported by the right kind of caring. Poems such as "Sunshine Across Living Centre" in Krysl and Watson[30] help nurses "see" the humanity of nurse and patient in interaction. The expressive dimension is the self as authentic (privately known) and disclosed (revealed to others): "Personal knowledge is expressed as ourselves, through the self."[2(p135)]

The assessment of this pattern comes through the "focus on the self as privately known and expressed to others. Assessment of self is a process carried out by the self through a rich inner life."[2(p135)] The critical questions involve exploration for congruence between knowing what we do and doing what we know, between the authentic and disclosed self. The process through which this assessment is made is the reflection and response of others to us, which we reflect on in turn. Agan put it succinctly by suggesting that "credibility of this type of knowing is determined through *individual reflection that is informed by the responses of others* [italics added]."[31(p70)] The credibility index is therefore congruence with the authentic and disclosed self.

Although the volume of literature in this area has provided much clarification and extension of the notion of personal knowing, the "essential elements" identified by Jacobs-Kramer and Chinn[2] are still pertinent. An elaboration could include, within the creative dimension, some examples of the means by

which "encountering, focusing and realizing" might be facilitated (eg, poetry, art, literature, and storytelling) and within the process-context dimension, reflection informed by the response of others (see Table 25-4).

 ## Esthetics: The Art of Nursing

Carper suggested that the delay in explicating the esthetic pattern of knowing is associated with nursing's attempt to see itself as scientific and to "exorcise the image of the apprentice-type education system."[1(p16)] This delay has certainly been overcome, and there has been intense interest in this pattern recently. The pattern had its beginnings in the works of many early nursing writers. Wiedenbach[32] suggested that esthetic practice is making "visible through action" the nurse's perception of what the patient needs. Orem[33] spoke of the "creativity and style in design" of the provision of care. Orem also mentioned as necessary in artful practice the ability to "envision" models of helping with regard to the appropriate outcomes. Benner[5] was foremost in the development of the notion of perceiving the whole of a situation, without reference to rational processes, in her work on expert nursing practice. The concept of "intuitive" knowing developed by Benner and Tanner,[28] Rew,[34] and Agan[31] (and mentioned earlier as part of personal knowing) is an important component of perceiving and envisioning.

The design of the art-act combines all patterns of knowing in its esthetic form—it is all of and more than the other patterns: "The design, if it is to be esthetic, must be controlled by the perception of balance, rhythm, proportion and unity of what is done in relation to the dynamic integration and articulation of the whole."[1(p18)]

Carper named "empathy" as an important mode in the esthetic pattern of knowing; however, there is currently debate in the nursing literature over the appropriateness of this concept for nursing. Morse,

Bottorff, Anderson, O'Brien, and Solberg suggested that "empathy was uncritically adopted from psychology and is actually a poor fit for the clinical reality of nursing practice."[35(p273)] They recommended exploration of other communication strategies that have been devalued, such as sympathy, pity, consolation, compassion, and commiseration. To these Taylor[25] might add affiliation, fun, and friendship.

Whatever the definitional outcome, the basic requirement of effective and authentic interpersonal engagement remains. This is highlighted in the recent Australian work of Taylor[25] and in the innovative work of Lumby[36] in her development of a critical feminist methodology for exploring nursing.

According to Jacobs-Kramer and Chinn,

> Esthetic knowledge finds expression in the art-act of nursing. Like personal knowledge, the expression of esthetic knowledge is not in language. We can unfold our art and retrospectively recollect and write about its features, and we can record it using electronic media, but the knowledge form itself is not what we write or record. The knowledge form is the art-act [italics added].[2(p137)]

They then proceeded to raise an important issue, albeit indirectly, that experience is an important component of esthetic knowing:

> As practice contexts are encountered, processes within the creative dimension of esthetics are initiated. Through the process of engagement, interpreting, and envisioning, "past" knowledge is enfolded into esthetics, and clients are uniquely cared for. As caring processes continue, new knowledge merges.[2(pp137–138)]

In putting forward experience as a necessary condition to esthetic practice, it may be necessary to include this context-specific experience as part of the creative and generative dimension, suggested by Jacobs-Kramer and Chinn as including "engaging, interpreting and envisioning." The addition of experience, particularly context-specific experience, suggests that these acts are cumulative, aligning with Benner's[5] position that expertise is context specific and not a transferable skill.

In exploring the assessment dimension within Carper's model of knowledge, Jacobs-Kramer and Chinn followed her inclusion of notions of esthetic appreciation from other art forms. They suggested that the critical question is, "What does this mean?"

> Criticism requires empathy and an intent to fully appreciate what the actors meant to convey. As the art-act is criticized, credibility is discerned by reaching for consensus— a full and rich understanding of the art-act that brings together the perspectives of a community of co-askers who construct and confer meanings.[2(p137)]

Table 25-5 presents the essential elements for the esthetic pattern.

The major point of Jacobs-Kramer and Chinn's model development appears to be the unfolding of a story that suggests that each pattern may be seen by "examination of the art-act that integrates all knowledge patterns as expressed in practice … [as it] provides a comprehensive, context-sensitive means for enfolding multiple knowledge patterns."[2(p138)] This, they suggested, leads nursing away from "a quest for structural truth and towards a search for dynamic meaning."[2(p138)]

The model and its exposition of essential elements provide critical questions that may structure

TABLE 25-5   Esthetics: Essential Elements

Dimension	Original Model[2]	Modifications
Creative	Engaging Interpreting Envisioning	Cumulative experience by engaging, interpreting envisioning and including the "artful enfoldment" of all other patterns
Expressive	Art-act	Art-act
Assessment: critical question	What does this mean?	What does this mean?
Process-context	Criticism	Exhibition and criticism Recognition as authentic to other nurses
Credibility index	Consensual meaning	Consensual meaning

our process of inquiry, processes by which the inquiry might take place, and credibility indices to which claims of rigor may be addressed. If it is to be useful in the process of our practice-based inquiry, the model must adequately account for all patterns of knowing and their appropriate processes of inquiry.

Sociopolitical Knowing: Context of Nursing

The patterns and inquiry processes in Jacobs-Kramer and Chinn's[2] model appear adequate to the description of the nurse-patient relationship and the persons of the nurse and the patient. What appears to be missing is the context—the sociopolitical environment of the persons and their interaction. This represents a fifth pattern of knowing essential to an understanding of all the others.

The other patterns address the "who," the "how," and the "what" of nursing practice. The pattern of sociopolitical knowing addresses the "wherein." It lifts the gaze of the nurse from the introspective nurse-patient relationship and situates it within the broader context in which nursing and health care take place. It causes the nurse to question the taken-for-granted assumptions about practice, the profession, and health policies.

Sociopolitical knowing may be conceptualized as including understandings on two levels: (1) the sociopolitical context of the persons (nurse and patient), and (2) the sociopolitical context of nursing as a practice profession, including both society's understanding of nursing and nursing's understanding of society and its politics.

The sociopolitical context of the persons of the nurse-patient relationship fundamentally concerns cultural identity, for it is in culture that "self" is intrinsically located. This cultural location influences each person's understanding of health and disease causation, language, identity, and connection to the land. Such understanding goes well beyond Carper's[1] or Mayeroff's[24] notion of personal knowing. It is related to deeply embedded historical issues of connection to and dislocation from land and heritage.

Chopoorian suggested that "nursing ideas lack an archaeology of the social, political, and economic worlds that influence both client states and nursing roles."[37(p41)] She claimed that unequal class structure, power relationships, and political and economic power produce sexism, racism, ageism, and classism, which in turn affect health and result in illness. Chopoorian continued, "Nursing practitioners continually confront the human responses to the underlying social dynamics of poverty, unemployment, undernutrition,

isolation and alienation precipitated through the structures of society."[37(pp40–41)]

Violence, drug dependence, and diabetes are examples of responses to what are inherently political rather than simply personal problems, and nurses' efforts to deal with them require nurses to articulate what they see resulting from societies' structures. Stevens suggested that nurses must provide a "critique of domination within fundamental social, political and economic structures and the analysis of how domination affects the health of persons and communities."[38(p58)] This effect includes the position and visibility of nursing in policy planning and decision making about health issues.

To have a voice in these decisions, nurses must both be articulate about what they know and do and be recognized by others as having something to contribute to debate. Nurses must have an understanding of the gatekeeping mechanisms within the political arena and their function. It is a paradox that when people are involved with nurses and nursing as patients or as concerned friends, the contribution of nurses is prized. Why then is it so quickly forgotten when these same people are influencing health care decisions? Diers and Fagin[39] suggested that the reason is visible in the metaphors the public associates with nursing, which include nurturance, dependence, and intimacy. These images are often reminders of personal pain and vulnerability, the natural reaction to which is suppression. To resurface an understanding of nursing is to resurface the context and all that is associated with it. Nurses must find a way of helping people remember, when they are well and politically able, what they knew of nursing when in crisis. Nurses must find the intersections between the health-related interests of the public and nursing and must become involved and active participants in these interests.

A sociopolitical understanding in which to frame all other patterns of knowing is an essential part of nursing's future in an increasingly economically driven world. Nurses must explore and expose alternative constructions of health and health care, find means of enabling all concerned to have a voice in this care provision, and develop processes of shared governance for the future. Table 25-6 illustrates how the sociopolitical dimension might be added to the model of knowing.

As Chinn said of nursing in the next century, "it is time to construct critical analyses of our present that are informed by the ethical and political ideals that we seek. It is time to begin to envision what our future nursing might be like and to create knowledge and skills that we need to begin to make it happen."[40(p56)] Understanding the context of nursing practice is fundamental to this endeavor. Appreciation and exploration of all the patterns of knowing in nursing and their

TABLE 25-6 Sociopolitical Knowing: Essential Elements

Dimension	Characteristics
Creative	Exposing and exploring alternate constructions of reality
Expressive	Transformation Critique
Assessment: critical question	Whose voice is heard? Whose voice is silenced?
Process-context	Critique and hearing all voices
Credibility index	Shared governance, enlightenment Movement toward equity

interactions can contribute to the future articulation and development of nursing practice and nurses' place in determining the future of nursing practice and of health care.

REFERENCES

1. Carper B. Fundamental patterns of knowing in nursing. *ANS.* 1978;1(1):13–23. Reprinted with permission from Aspen Publishers, Inc. © Copyright 1978.

2. Jacobs-Kramer M, Chinn P. Perspectives on knowing: a model of nursing knowledge. *Schol Inq Nurs Pract.* 1988;2(2):129–139. Used by permission of Springer Publishing Company, Inc., New York 10012.

3. Kuhn T. *The Structure of Scientific Revolutions.* Chicago, Ill: University of Chicago Press; 1970.

4. Sandelowski M. Rigor or rigor mortis: the problem of rigor in qualitative research revisited. *ANS.* 1993;16(2):1–8.

5. Benner P. *From Novice to Expert: Excellence and Power in Clinical Nursing Practice.* Menlo Park, Calif: Addison-Wesley; 1984.

6. Benner P. The role of experience, narrative, and community in skilled ethical comportment. *ANS.* 1991;14(2):1–21.

7. Benner P, Wrubel J. *The Primacy of Caring: Stress and Coping in Health and Illness.* Menlo Park, Calif: Addison-Wesley; 1989.

8. Bishop A, Scudder J, eds. *Caring, Curing, Coping.* University, Ala: University of Alabama Press; 1985.

9. Bishop A, Scudder J. *The Practical, Moral and Personal Sense of Nursing.* Albany, NY: State University of New York Press; 1990.

10. Cooper M. Reconceptualizing nursing ethics. *Schol Inq Nurs Pract.* 1990;4(3):209–218.

11. Cooper M. Principle-oriented ethics and the ethic of care: creative tension. *ANS.* 1991;14(2):22–31.

12. Watson J. *Nursing: Human Science and Human Care.* Norwalk, Conn: Appleton-Century-Crofts; 1985.

13. Watson J. The moral failure of the patriarchy. *Nurs Outlook.* 1990;28(2):62–66.

14. Gilligan C. In a different voice: women's conception of self and morality. *Harvard Educ Rev.* 1979;47:481–517.

15. Gilligan C. *In a Different Voice.* Cambridge, Mass: Harvard University Press; 1982.

16. Noddings N. *Caring—A Feminine Approach to Ethics and Moral Education.* Berkeley, Calif: University of California Press; 1984.

17. Pellegrino E. Being ill and being healed. In: Kestenbaum V, ed. *The Humanity of the Ill.* Knoxville, Tenn: University of Tennessee Press; 1982.

18. Pellegrino E. The caring ethic. In: Bishop A, Scudder J, eds. *Caring, Curing, Coping.* University, Ala: University of Alabama Press; 1985.

19. Zaner R. How the hell did I get here? In: Bishop A, Scudder J, eds. *Caring, Curing, Coping.* University, Ala: University of Alabama Press; 1985.

20. Zaner R. *Ethics and the Clinical Encounter.* Englewood Cliffs, NJ: Prentice Hall; 1988.

21. Kohlberg L. *The Philosophy of Moral Development.* San Francisco, Calif: Harper & Row; 1981.

22. Moss C. Has Gilligan's "Different Voice" made a difference? In: *Nursing Research: Scholarship for Practice.* Geelong, Victoria, Australia: Deakin Institute of Nursing Research, Deakin University; 1992.

23. Gadow S. Existential advocacy: philosophical foundation of nursing. In: Spicker S, Gadow S, eds. *Nursing: Images and Ideals: Opening Dialogue with the Humanities.* New York, NY: Springer; 1980.

24. Mayeroff M. *On Caring.* New York, NY: Harper & Row; 1971.

25. Taylor B. Enhancement of the nursing encounter through a shared humanity. In: *Nursing Research: Scholarship for Practice.* Geelong, Victoria, Australia: Deakin Institute of Nursing Research, Deakin University; 1992.

26. Morse J. Negotiating commitment and involvement in the nurse-patient relationship. *J Adv Nurs.* 1991;16:455–468.

27. Moch S. Personal knowing: Evolving research and practice. *Schol Inq Nurs Pract.* 1990;4(2):155–165.

28. Benner P, Tanner C. Clinical judgment: how expert nurses use intuition. *Am J Nurs.* 1987;87:23–31.

29. Chester L, ed. *Cradle and All.* Boston, Mass: Faber & Faber; 1989.

30. Krysl M, Watson J. Existential moments of caring: facets of nursing and social support. *ANS.* 1988;10(2):12–17.

31. Agan RD. Intuitive knowing as a dimension of nursing. *ANS.* 1987;10(1):64–70.

32. Wiedenbach E. *Clinical Nursing: A Helping Out.* New York, NY: Springer-Verlag; 1985.

33. Orem D. *Nursing: Concepts of Practice*. New York, NY: McGraw-Hill; 1971.

34. Rew L. Intuition and decision-making. *Image J Nurs Schol*. 1988;20(3):150–154.

35. Morse J, Bottorff J, Anderson G, O'Brien B, Solberg S. Beyond empathy: expanding expressions of caring. *Adv Nurs*. 1992;17:809–821.

36. Lumby J. *A Woman's Experience of Illness: The Emergence of a Feminist Method for Nursing*. Geelong, Victoria, Australia: Deakin University; 1993.

37. Chopoorian T. Reconceptualizing the environment. In: Moccia P, ed. *New Approaches in Theory Development*. New York, NY: National League for Nursing; 1986.

38. Stevens P. A critical social reconstruction of environment in nursing: implications for methodology. *ANS*. 1989;11(4): 56–68.

39. Diers D, Fagin C. Nursing as a metaphor. *N Engl J Med*. 1981;309(2):116–117.

40. Chinn P. Looking into the crystal ball: positioning ourselves for the year 2000. *Nurs Outlook*. 1991;39(6):251–256.

THE AUTHOR COMMENTS | Patterns of Knowing: Review, Critique, and Update

Having been a teacher of nursing theory at a graduate level for some time, I used Carper's work as a conceptual framework for structuring an understanding of research and theory in nursing. However, I became progressively uncomfortable with what I perceived as an absence of "place" for understanding indigenous health practices and other sociopolitical health-related issues. Nursing's apparent invisibility and lack of power within healthcare was also missing.

After class one day over coffee, I "doodled" on a napkin, and those doodles became the bones of this article. Although written some time ago, I believe sociopolitical issues in healthcare are now of even greater relevance in a world dominated by uncritical globalization, juxtaposed with significant indigenous health issues, disparity of access to healthcare and education, and religious and cultural intolerance.

JILL WHITE

Mediating the Meaning of Evidence Through Epistemological Diversity

DENISE TARLIER, PhD, NP(F)

*N*ursing's disciplinary recognition of 'multiple ways of knowing' reflects an epistemological diversity that supports nursing praxis. Nursing as praxis offers a conceptual way to explore what it is about the interface of practice, knowledge and evidence in nursing that distinguishes us as a discipline. I suggest that the relationship between evidence and knowledge is defined and mediated by the same epistemological diversity that supports nursing as praxis. Just as the meaning and truth-value of evidence is evaluated from within the body of existing disciplinary knowledge, new evidence may prompt an evaluation of the meaning and truth-value of extant nursing knowledge. Nursing practice that relies on scientific evidence as a singular basis of practice knowledge is susceptible to exploitation by the diverse agendas operating within an ideology of evidence-based practice and the healthcare system. Mediating the meaning of evidence for nursing practice through acknowledgment of the diverse epistemologies that underpin nursing knowledge will contribute to a disciplinary-specific definition of what constitutes evidence for nursing, and will better direct how evidence is integrated into a disciplinary body of knowledge.

A disciplinary existential angst amongst nurses drives us to identify, define, rationalize and sometimes defend what nursing is and what nurses do. As a discipline, nurses are adamant that nursing—in theory—offers a unique perspective on health-care. In practice, nurses *know* that what they do for patients 'makes a difference', but have difficulty articulating *how* they know what they 'do'. That is, a fundamental disconnect exists between knowing what nursing is and being able to explicate the source of nursing knowledge. This disconnect has implications for understanding what constitutes evidence for nursing practice. Nursing as praxis offers a conceptual way to explore what it is about the interface of practice, knowledge and evidence in nursing that distinguishes us as a discipline.

Nursing's disciplinary recognition of 'multiple ways of knowing' reflects an epistemological diversity that supports nursing praxis. Evidence, in the traditional positivist scientific sense that underpins modern health science (Scott-Findlay and Pollock 2004), is merely one source of nursing knowledge and not necessarily privileged over other ways. It is fundamental to the development of nursing knowledge, but is not in itself a sufficient basis for all practice knowledge. Epistemological diversity is necessary to define, evaluate and value what constitutes evidence for nursing practice. Examining how nursing's epistemological diversity sustains praxis will explicate how nursing as a discipline mediates the meaning of evidence in a healthcare system where evidence may have different meanings for different disciplines, and where the term 'evidence-based practice' has taken on ideological proportions.

Epistemological Diversity: A Nursing Tradition?

Nursing as a discipline has always embraced multiple and diverse epistemologies. Historically, acknowledgment of our diverse epistemological bases has been expressed in a variety of ways, but explicit recognition of nursing's diverse epistemologies has not taken place. Carper (1978) is credited as the first nursing scholar to describe what has since become commonly referred to as nursing's multiple ways of knowing (Fawcett et al. 2001), which she originally described as four fundamental patterns of knowing in nursing: empirical, ethical, aesthetic and personal knowing. Many others have built on Carper's seminal work, conceptualizing and writing about nursing's multiple ways of knowing in varying ways but with essentially the same two theses: (a) nursing practice is complex

ABOUT THE AUTHOR

DENISE TARLIER was born and grew up on the West Coast of Canada, in North Vancouver, British Columbia. She completed a diploma in general nursing in 1982 at the British Columbia Institute of Technology, followed by a certificate program in Operating Room Nursing in 1986, and a BSN from the University of British Columbia in 1992. She was drawn to working with Canada's remote northern Aboriginal populations. To better prepare for the demands of this complex clinical nursing role, she completed the diploma program in Outpost and Community Health Nursing at Dalhousie University in 1996 and, subsequently, successfully challenged the American Academy of Nurse Practitioners (AANP) Family

Nurse Practitioner certification examination in 1998, a time when nurse practitioner roles were just beginning to be recognized and formalized in Canada. After practicing in remote communities for several years, she returned to school (yet again) and completed an MSN (2001) and a PhD (2006) at the University of British Columbia. Dr. Tarlier is currently an Assistant Professor in the School of Nursing at Thompson Rivers University in Kamloops, British Columbia, where the focus of her scholarship continues to be guided by a strong clinical practice orientation to primary healthcare, rural and remote health services, aboriginal health issues, and primary care and nurse practitioner nursing roles.

and holistic, thus nursing knowledge relies on more than a singular source of knowing (Jennings and Loan 2001); and (b) the singular source of knowledge represented by empirics is insufficient to account for all nursing knowledge (Nagle and Mitchell 1991).

The concept of multiple ways of knowing in nursing is patently the same concept as epistemological diversity. Examining how various scholars, both in nursing and in related social sciences, have written about the concept of epistemological diversity substantiates this claim. The review presented here is brief and by no means inclusive, as comprehensive historical reviews already exist in the literature (e.g. Johnson and Ratner 1997; Meleis 1997).

In 1988, Jacobs-Kramer and Chinn extended Carper's (1978) work by presenting a model integrating the four patterns of knowing identified by Carper. These scholars later expanded on and further refined the model they proposed (Chinn and Kramer 1999). In the epilogue to their 1999 textbook, Chinn and Kramer described how their thinking about knowledge development had shifted over the years to better accommodate patterns of knowing—or epistemologies—that could not be accommodated appropriately within the empirical pattern, demonstrating a deliberate rebuttal of empirics as a singular epistemology for nursing knowledge. Most recently, Fawcett et al. (2001) used Carper's original work as the basis of a critical treatise on the interface of nursing theories and evidence-based practice, which once again affirmed 'the diverse patterns of knowing [that] constitute the ontological and epistemological foundations of the discipline of nursing' (p. 117).

Nursing scholars Nagle and Mitchell (1991) approached epistemological issues in terms of theoretical

and paradigmatic diversity. These authors concluded, 'it is myopic and naïve to suggest that a single-paradigm approach can adequately fulfill nursing's mandate' (p. 22). Their conclusion was remarkably similar to that offered by Schwandt (1990). Schwandt, a social scientist, addressed epistemological diversity in terms of ontologies and methodologies. He concluded that any one particular epistemological-methodological coupling is insufficient on its own to represent the nature of truth in the context of the social sciences, and recognized the complex contextual issues that influence disciplinary epistemologies.

Wolfer (1993), another nursing scholar, used an 'aspects of "reality"' (p. 141) framework based on a philosophy of mind/body/spirit to illustrate how different types of problems require different epistemologies, and also different ontologies. He characterized the different epistemologies in terms of body, mind and transcendental ways of knowing. While this approach is evocative of the traditional reductionist approach based on Cartesian dualism (Capra 1982), Wolfer asserted that all three ways of knowing are needed to provide holistic care. He claimed that his framework offered 'a way of looking at the reality of nursing which "sees" different types of knowledge, theory and research as complementary rather than competitive or exclusionary' (p. 145).

In 1995, White suggested modifying Jacob-Kramer and Chinn's (1988) model of Carper's (1978) work to be inclusive of interpretive and critical ontologies and epistemologies. White added sociopolitical knowing as a fifth pattern to accommodate her modifications, recognizing that Carper's original definition of the empirical pattern excluded the relativist positions White proposed. Sociopolitical knowing was presented as an integrating pattern 'essential to understanding all the others' (p. 83). The basis of White's claim was that sociopolitical knowing represented the contextual knowledge within which all other nursing knowledge was situated.

Johnson and Ratner (1997) described the nature of nursing knowledge in terms of ontology, epistemology and practical utility. Empirical and interpretive epistemologies are equally privileged in these scholars' conceptualizations of knowledge, thus furthering the claims made by earlier nursing scholars. Johnson and Ratner concluded that nursing practice knowledge is highly complex and 'multifarious' (p. 19).

Most recently, physicians Upshur, VanDenKerkhof and Goel (2001) proposed a conceptual model of evidence that has patent similarities to both Carper's (1978) work and the conceptualizations of knowledge presented by Johnson and Ratner (1997). Upshur, VanDenKerkhof and Goel's (2001) model privileges information derived through both quantitative and qualitative methods of inquiry. Evidence is recognized as being mediated between context and method. While Upshur, VanDenKerkhof and Goel addressed the concept of evidence rather than knowledge, it is clear that the model they proposed is founded on diverse epistemologies and a radically broad conceptualization of empiricism that encompasses interpretive methods, philosophy and political theory. Whether or not this conceptualization of empiricism ultimately withstands critique, the model itself represents a notable break with the status quo in medicine; a discipline traditionally grounded in a biomedical, empirical epistemology.

The short review presented here illustrates some of the different ways in which scholars in the social science and health disciplines have characterized the epistemological underpinnings of practice knowledge. The differences between the characterizations may be largely explained by the temporal context at the time of writing: the presented works span two decades during which the dominant postpositivist view was continually challenged by emerging paradigms such as constructivism and critical theory. Through this evolutionary process, scholars first recognized and then worked toward situating and refining diverse epistemologies relative to existing and emerging philosophies.

Nursing Praxis

Despite the different approaches taken by various scholars, each article presented in the preceding review explored essentially the same concept: the complexities of holistic practice call for multiple and diverse ways of knowing. That is, multiple and diverse

sources of knowledge necessarily underpin nursing practice knowledge. Defining 'epistemology' as a 'theory of knowledge' (Mautner 1996, p. 174), it is reasonable to think of and refer to these ways of knowing as diverse epistemologies. Nurse scholars have—over at least the past 20 years—recognized nursing's diverse epistemologies as fundamental to nursing as a complex and holistic practice. Moreover, a reciprocal, conscious, reflective bond between epistemology and practice is the basis of nursing as praxis (Jones 1997; Thorne 1997).

Praxis articulates nursing practice that is complex, holistic, reflective, and both grounded in and supportive of dynamically integrated knowledge, theory and practice (Jones 1997; Thorne 1997; Chinn and Kramer 1999). 'Praxis is theory and practice that are inter-related, integrated, and dialectical in nature. Inherent within praxis is reflection both on and in practice' (Jones 1997, p. 126). Holmes and Warelow (2000) claim that nurses must 'critically reflect upon their practices in order to elaborate the implicit and often complex theories and attitudes, by which it is established, developed and sustained' (pp. 179–80). Praxis describes practice that is continuously infused by nurses' critical reflection on and integration of diverse elements of practice. Thus, praxis implies practice that transcends what knowledge alone would support. The reciprocal integration of knowledge with practice in itself adds a dimension that elevates the whole of practice beyond the mere sum of its parts.

There has been a tendency in the nursing literature to reflect upon nursing practice as dualistic in nature: is nursing an art or a science? (Bishop and Scudder 1997). Dichotomizing nursing practice in this way is based in and reflects a positivistic, biomedical, reductionist ontology in that practice is being reduced to discrete parts. Such a dichotomy fails to represent the holistic and complex nature of nursing as praxis and is problematic because it fosters the possibility of viewing practice in 'either/or' terms, that is, practice as either a science or an art (Jones 2001). Some nursing scholars have recognized the inherent dangers of subscribing to this dichotomy and have suggested various alternative ways of conceptualizing practice: as a practical science (Johnson 1991), as practice (Bishop and Scudder 1997), as phronesis (Benner 2000; Flaming 2001), and even as pragmatism (Warms and Schroeder 1999).

I suggest that despite these alternative conceptualizations, the notion of practice as dichotomous persists; not merely within nursing but in how other health disciplines and society view nursing. For example, the tendency to dichotomize practice is at the root of what nursing scholars discuss as visible vs. invisible nursing practice (e.g. Rafael 1999). The persistence of such a dichotomous conceptualization of practice reflects just how deeply ingrained a biomedical, reductionist ontology and epistemology are in western society and within nursing (Jones 2001). This dominant paradigm has made it difficult for a discipline that aspires to recognition as a science (as nursing does) to openly admit to holding diverse other epistemologies. Thus, although nursing has recognized 'multiple ways of knowing' for almost 25 years, acknowledgment of these has remained within nursing and in these somewhat nebulous terms, rarely claimed outright as being diverse epistemologies.

Dichotomizing nursing practice (and thereby creating the 'either/or' dilemma) allows the possibility that the practice of nursing is purely a science.[1] Viewing practice as a science in turn supports the possibility that scientific evidence alone may be sufficient for practice knowledge. That is, that evidence derived through a singular, positivistic epistemology provides an adequate evidence base for nursing practice. Scott-Findlay and Pollock (2004) claim,

> Within the evidence-based practice paradigm, the implication of giving the authority for practice to the scientific evidence, in other words, the research findings (an inherently narrow implicit definition of evidence), is that other influences in the decision-making process (e.g. clinical practice knowledge) get lower value or priority' (p. 95).

Thus, evidence or knowledge arising through other epistemologies, or ways of knowing, are less valued, and by implication, the 'art' of nursing is devalued (Wolfer 1993; Mitchell 1999; Flaming 2001; Rycroft-Malone et al. 2004). Some nursing scholars have adamantly decried the implicit devaluation of the art of nursing: 'Neither science of a basic nature nor the "creative use" of basic scientific knowledge will provide the tools necessary for the art of nursing' (Johnson 1991, p. 11). Without the art, the integrated, synchronous character of praxis is lost, and nursing practice is indeed at risk of becoming merely that part of practice that can be supported by scientific knowledge alone.

The diverse epistemologies privileged by nursing as a discipline are central to Johnson and Ratner (1997) and enable praxis. Paradoxically, praxis demands epistemologies that are sufficiently broad (Flaming 2001) to support all of its complexities. The foregoing review of scholarly works suggests that empirical ways of knowing alone are insufficiently broad to support nursing praxis. However, the positivist scientific

tradition that dominates western approaches to healthcare (Harman 1996; Scott-Findlay and Pollock 2004) continues to privilege empirical epistemologies as the singular means to acquire, evaluate and determine the evidence that constitutes knowledge.

Issues of Evidence

Issues of what is considered evidence and how evidence is related to knowledge have become a focus of controversy in nursing, reflecting debate in the health disciplines generally (Madjar and Walton 2001; Dobrow, Goel and Upshur 2004). The controversy has been bitter at times and has led to polarization within disciplines (Greenhalgh and Worrall 1997, e.g. Charlton 1997; Shahar 1998; Mitchell 1999). Debate is based in the way evidence was formally defined by the Evidence-Based Medicine Working Group in their landmark 1992 paper. This group of medical practitioners and academics proposed what they referred to as an evidence-based approach to the practice of medicine, defining the primary sources of evidence as randomized controlled trials (RCTs) and meta-analyses of RCTs. Despite a later effort to partially ameliorate this definition (Sackett et al. 1996), the original definition eventually grew into the hierarchy of levels of evidence that underpin the concept of evidence-based medicine (EBM).

Evidence, according to the proponents of EBM, is judged in relation to a hierarchy of evidence that is based on study design and rigor (Centre for Evidence-Based Medicine 2001; Madjar and Walton 2001; Upshur 2001; Dobrow, Goel and Upshur 2004), and grounded in a positivist, reductionist ontology and epistemology (Upshur, VanDenKerkhof and Goel 2001). While at least four different hierarchies of evidence have been developed (Upshur 2003), each of these clearly places a higher value on quantitative research findings from RCTs and systematic reviews of RCTs (Madjar and Walton 2001; Upshur 2003; Scott-Findlay and Pollock 2004; Dobrow, Goel and Upshur 2004), and information derived from other sources is accordingly assigned lesser value (Rycroft-Malone et al. 2004). Findings from qualitative studies do not qualify as evidence in this schema. Moreover, not only are qualitative findings excluded from the hierarchy of evidence, but there is also an implicit suggestion that such excluded findings represent a challenge or threat to 'real' evidence.

In contrast, many nursing scholars have recognized that the definition of evidence espoused by the proponents of EBM is too narrow and exclusive to support the complexities of nursing practice (Estabrooks 1998; Kitson, Harvey and McCormack 1998; Fawcett et al. 2001; Madjar and Walton 2001; Rycroft-Malone et al. 2004). These scholars have been adamant in their

---

[1]Practice as a science is to be differentiated from practice that is based in part on science, which implies that practice is also based in part on something other than science (such as the art of practice) and nursing science, which implies that nursing creates its own science.

insistence that nursing as a discipline adopt a broader definition of evidence, one that recognizes the influence of context on the application of evidence in practice (Scott-Findlay and Pollock 2004) and considers qualitative research findings.

The call within nursing for a more inclusive understanding of evidence has begun to echo in the recent literature of other health disciplines. For example, the model of the taxonomy of evidence presented by physicians Upshur, VanDenKerkhof and Goel (2001) recognizes qualitative research findings as a form of evidence. In a study that investigated the utilization of social science research knowledge, Landry, Amara and Lamari (2001) found that behavioral and contextual factors were the most significant influences on research knowledge, suggesting that the existence of evidence alone was insufficient cause for uptake and use.

However, an inclusive definition of evidence is problematic. As the definition of evidence expands, the issue of what constitutes evidence becomes more ambiguous (Scott-Findlay and Pollock 2004). Where does one draw the line as to what one is willing to consider as evidence? Some scholars have expressed a willingness to push the meaning of evidence beyond research findings altogether, and have proposed that clinical judgment and experience are forms of evidence (Estabrooks 1998; Rycroft-Malone et al. 2004). For example, Kitson, Harvey and McCormack (1998) define evidence as 'the combination of research, clinical expertise and patient choice' (p. 150). But is a definition of evidence this broad any more useful to nursing practice than a too-restrictive definition? Are all knowledge and all experience to be privileged as evidence?

The Relationship Between Evidence and Knowledge

Upshur, VanDenKerkhof and Goel (2001) recently defined evidence as 'an observation, fact, or organized body of information offered to support or justify inferences or beliefs in the demonstration of some proposition or matter at issue' (p. 93). These writers thus refer to the reality that research findings are seldom presented in research reports as neutral information or facts, but are preassigned some degree of truth-value by researchers, who present their work as an argument in favor of their conclusions—i.e. 'based on the *evidence*.' Additionally, while Upshur, VanDenKerkhof and Goel (2001) claim that their model of evidence is epistemologically 'rooted in empiricism' (p. 93), they recognize management and political theory, social philosophy and Bayesian reasoning as methods of producing evidence, thus expanding the notion of evidence beyond the purely empirical. These writers conclude

that their model of evidence integrates various disciplinary epistemologies, thus ultimately 'enabling a more holistic approach to evidence' (p. 95). However, it is unclear where the boundaries between evidence and knowledge lie in this inclusive model of evidence.

I argue that the ambiguity about what constitutes evidence for nursing practice is based in a fundamental lack of conceptual clarity regarding the language of evidence-based practice (EBP), a problem that has also recently been recognized by other writers (i.e. Scott-Findlay and Pollock 2004). The margins between evidence and knowledge are elusive and overlapping. Scott-Findlay and Pollock have identified the pressing need to address the confusion that exists about the conceptual definitions of evidence and knowledge, in order to break the stalemate that has developed in scholarly debate regarding the nature of EBP for nursing, and allow a way forward.

The definitions offered by Scott-Findlay and Pollock (2004) represent an explicit way to consider the relationship between knowledge and evidence. These scholars make a strong case for differentiating between evidence as a particular form of knowledge (i.e. research findings) and other forms of knowledge (i.e. personal and experiential knowledge) that, while not considered evidence, are critically important influences on the uptake, integration and application of research findings within the context of the broader body of extant knowledge. To maintain this distinction, Scott-Findlay and Pollock propose that *evidence* be defined as exclusively research findings, arguing that this term offers greater clarity and specificity. Notably, these writers do not distinguish between quantitative and qualitative research findings, which is consistent with the diverse epistemological basis of nursing praxis.

Research findings are a tangible form of knowledge that may be shared or transferred among individuals. *Knowledge* implies individuals' broader or more general knowledge, and is defined as being intangible and personal: 'Information in the public domain must first be integrated, transferred, transmitted, or incorporated into the private (or personal) domain before it becomes knowledge' (Scott-Findlay and Pollock 2004, p. 93). Thus, research findings, as information, are taken up into an individual's more generalized body of knowledge through an integrative process. Disciplinary knowledge is therefore by implication structured as an aggregated form of knowledge rather than being a discrete entity unto itself.

I suggest that the relationship between evidence, or research findings and knowledge is defined and mediated by the same epistemological diversity that supports nursing as praxis. Research findings are adapted into a dynamic body of extant knowledge through a selective process that may also imply modification or rejection. The diverse epistemologies that underpin knowledge for nursing praxis are necessary to define, evaluate, contextualize and value research findings from the perspective of nursing and through a disciplinary-specific lens (Thorne 2001).

Johnson and Ratner (1997) offer the following definition of knowledge: 'things perceived or held in consciousness, justified in some way, and therefore regarded as "true"' (p. 4, citing Angeles 1981). The lay understanding of the word *evidence* similarly associates evidence with truth or validity *(Oxford dictionary of current English* 1998). Yet Upshur, VanDenKerkhof and Goel (2001) warn against equating evidence with the truth, saying that it is the defeasible nature of evidence that enables new information to be accommodated in the context of existing beliefs. That is, it is knowledge that imbues evidence (i.e. research findings) with meaning, and thus by extension, nursing disciplinary knowledge that imbues research findings with meaning and truth-value for nursing. To be readily accepted as true, new evidence must exhibit some congruency with what nurses already hold to be true within their existing disciplinary knowledge (Rycroft-Malone et al. 2004).

I suggest that what a discipline might accept as truth and knowledge are also defeasible (McCain 1998), and that defeasibility is the basis of the dynamic nature of knowledge. Thus, knowledge is not a static, manifest body, but a body more in the sense of a body of water: fluid and reactive. Just as the meaning and truth-value of research findings are evaluated from within the body of existing disciplinary knowledge, new research findings may prompt a reevaluation of the meaning and truth-value of existing knowledge.

This process of reciprocal defeasibility addresses the transition in which information, such as research findings, becomes knowledge, or in other words, the process of evaluating the truth-value of new information from a disciplinary perspective. I propose that much of the ambiguity about evidence arises in how we think about this transition. Do we really consider 'information offered' to be evidence? Or is it more likely that by evidence, we mean information that has already been judged as having some truth-value? For instance, evidence as defined by proponents of EBM (Centre for Evidence-Based Medicine 2001) is unquestioningly presented as having truth-value. The truth-value of this evidence is apparent and acceptable to those individuals or disciplines that subscribe to the same ontological and epistemological perspectives in which EBP is grounded; that is, a positivist western scientific perspective. While individuals within nursing may subscribe to such a perspective, it may be (and has been) problematic for nursing as a discipline that subscribes to diverse epistemologies to accept such evidence (i.e. research findings) as sufficient basis for nursing practice.

I will push both Scott-Findlay and Pollock's (2004) and Upshur, VanDenKerkhof and Goel's (2001) definitions of evidence further, and claim that research findings, observations, facts or information are just that, and do not constitute evidence until they have been judged by an individual as being 'true' or 'possibly true.' Information at this stage may more appropriately be conceptualized as 'appeals to evidence' (McCain 1998). Once an appeal to evidence has been evaluated as having truth-value, it becomes evidence, and as evidence, is integrated with existing knowledge. The diverse epistemologies that underpin nursing knowledge provide direction, helping nurses to navigate the process of evaluating the truth-value of information and its subsequent integration into nursing's knowledge base. Upshur, VanDenKerkhof and Goel (2001) claimed that personal belief is the term of measurement of evidence. I propose that disciplinary belief, or the extant body of disciplinary knowledge, is also a term of measurement. The key implication of defining evidence in this way is that the issue of what constitutes evidence becomes subject to (and thus specific to) disciplinary knowledge, rather than the one-size-fits-all definitions of evidence such as the Levels of Evidence (Centre for Evidence-Based Medicine).

While not explicitly recognizing the process of evaluation in their definition of evidence, Upshur, VanDenKerkhof and Goel (2001) imply in their discussion that a process of evaluation occurs, framing the process in terms of analysis, interpretation and mediation of evidence. Other scholars have implicitly addressed the process of evaluating and valuing evidence relative to existing disciplinary knowledge. White (1995) touched on this notion when she stated, 'the remaining process for ascertaining credibility is the "fit" of the new knowledge with the extant knowledge in the area' (p. 76). Fawcett et al. (2001) modified Carper's (1978) ways of knowing by labeling these as theories; they then claimed the theories to be 'diverse ontological and epistemological lenses through which evidence is interpreted and critiqued' (p. 117). Madjar and Walton (2001) discussed the need for clinicians to 'recontextualize such findings and reassess their relevance in a particular situation' (p. 39). Upshur (2001) refers to a conceptually similar process when he states, 'the weighing of evidence is contingent on context' (p. 6), that is, on broader knowledge of the situation.

By defining evidence as research findings that are evaluated as having truth-value according to disciplinary epistemologies, it becomes possible to differentiate between evidence and knowledge. I claim that knowledge represents the sum of what is known and understood through diverse ways of knowing, is regarded as 'true' and therefore holds value. Research findings represent one source of knowledge within a larger body of knowledge. Research data are evaluated in accordance with existing knowledge and judged to be (a) consistent with existing knowledge and having truth-value, therefore accepted as evidence and incorporated into knowledge; (b) inconsistent with existing knowledge but convincingly 'true' and of sufficient value that existing knowledge shifts to allow the new knowledge to be incorporated within existing knowledge (e.g. when research demonstrated that the tradition of preoperative shaving of operative sites was in fact associated with higher rates of postoperative infections); or (c) inconsistent with existing knowledge and having insignificant truth-value, therefore refuted and not accepted as evidence. Thus, existing knowledge, which is based on diverse epistemologies, influences the uptake of research findings and the process though which it is evaluated, reflected upon, valued and recontextualized as evidence; that is, useful nursing knowledge, or knowledge that supports praxis.

The Ideology of Evidence-Based Healthcare

The concept of evidence-based medicine originated within the discipline of medicine just over a decade ago. It is ironic that while 'evidence' itself often takes decades to be accepted into and change healthcare practice (i.e. the research–practice gap), it has taken only 10 years for the concept of evidence-based practice to become firmly entrenched within the healthcare system. Estabrooks (1998) observed that EBM had 'taken on the qualities of a social movement' (p. 18). The entrenchment of EBM and its spread into other disciplines as EBP has occurred despite ongoing controversy within medicine (Dobrow, Goel and Upshur 2004), as well as in disciplines such as nursing (Estabrooks 1998; Mitchell 1999), of the utility of what has been characterized as a 'cookbook' approach to practice. That is to say, the assertion that EBP is a better way to practice has been challenged, both on the premise that EBP itself lacks a convincing body of supporting evidence (Upshur 2003; Dobrow, Goel and Upshur 2004), and also on the grounds that EBP represents prescriptive service based on guidelines and protocols, rather than practice based on disciplinary and professional knowledge and clinical reasoning. Moreover, such prescriptive service lacks relevance when applied to the particularities of practice with individuals (Jones and Higgs 2000). In short, practice is reduced to a science: the 'art' of practice is lost.

So, if not unequivocal evidence, what is driving the uptake of EBP? To find the answer to this question, it is necessary to look beyond the practice of any of the health disciplines and consider the bigger picture of health-care. Stakeholders in health-care include more than practitioners and patients. Nonpractitioner, nonpatient stakeholders such as policy makers, politicians, insurance companies, researchers, pharmaceutical corporations and other suppliers of healthcare products, all have a vested interest (i.e. financial or power) in defining what happens between practitioners and patients. EBP provides a structure that allows these system stakeholders to influence what happens at the practice level (i.e. between patients and practitioners), by influencing disciplinary understandings of what constitutes evidence for practice. The key question in defining EBP becomes not 'what constitutes evidence?' but 'what constitutes evidence for whom and why? Alleged agendas of EBP as a structure of the larger healthcare system include control over clinical decision making between practitioners and patients (Mitchell 1999), redistribution of power (Estabrooks 1998), and control over resource allocation (Jennings and Loan 2001). Other implications of EBP have been identified as loss of autonomous practice and loss of practitioner-client accountability (Mitchell 1999). Within nursing, critics of EBP have pointed out that this approach to healthcare delivery may conflict with other approaches such as patient-centered care (Mitchell 1999; Rycroft-Malone et al. 2004). One basis of this conflict is recognition that the narrow definition of evidence supported by EBP fails to accommodate the inclusive definition of evidence and the range of disciplinary knowledge that influences clinical practice in nursing (Estabrooks 1998; Mitchell 1999; Madjar and Walton 2001).

Paradoxically, research-based evidence is fundamental to the process of uptake and integration of new knowledge into the existing body of knowledge that supports nursing practice. Both the science and the art of nursing benefit when new research-based information is admitted as evidence to nursing's knowledge base. The conflict that surrounds the issue of evidence for nursing is at best superficial and at worst counterproductive to the task of expanding nursing's body of disciplinary knowledge. I claim that the paradox derives from the degree to which the concept of EBP has taken on ideological proportions. Despite Estabrooks's (1998) caution against allowing EBP to 'develop into an ideology' (p. 31), EBP has in fact become an ideology in health-care, driven by health system stakeholders for the purposes described above.

Sustaining Nursing Praxis by Mediating the Meaning of Evidence

I have proposed that epistemological diversity supports nursing praxis, or nursing as a complex and holistic practice. I have shown that a singular epistemology, such as that represented by the prevailing ideological construction of EBP supports, in contrast, a dichotomized conceptualization of nursing as a science. Nursing viewed as a science rather than as praxis would, by definition, privilege scientific evidence in the positivist, western scientific tradition as a singular way of knowing.

Nursing practice that relies on scientific evidence as a singular basis of practice knowledge is susceptible to exploitation by the diverse agendas operating within an ideology of EBP and the healthcare system. Extradisciplinary definitions of evidence, as well as extradisciplinary understandings of what constitutes 'best care' or 'best practice', could be imposed on nursing through the use of EBP as an ideological tool, because nursing, without diverse epistemologies, would have no means of defining, evaluating and valuing research findings in a way that supports and develops nursing knowledge for praxis. Thus, epistemological diversity is both the means by which nursing mediates a disciplinary definition of research-based evidence that serves to sustain praxis, and the basis that enables nurses to critically evaluate alternative sources of knowledge (i.e. non–research-based information).

The mediation of evidence from a disciplinary perspective suggests that it may be difficult to achieve an interdisciplinary consensus concerning the question of what constitutes evidence for health-care. Is consensus necessary or even possible in an interdisciplinary healthcare system? Consensus has implications for interdisciplinary communication and shared meanings in regard to EBP, as well as to other terms such as 'best practice', that are becoming catch-phrases in health-care.

The lack of epistemological and conceptual clarity around evidence (Estabrooks 1998; Scott-Findlay and Pollock 2004) suggests there is still a long ways to go before interdisciplinary consensus is realized. Thorne (2001) suggests that interdisciplinary consensus may not be possible, and urges nursing to define evidence and knowledge in ways that are coherent within nursing's unique disciplinary philosophy. I suggest that the critical first steps in defining evidence and knowledge for nursing are to work toward clarifying the language of EBP (Scott-Findlay and Pollock 2004), to affirm nursing practice as praxis, and to acknowledge the epistemological diversity that sustains praxis. Mediating the meaning of evidence for nursing praxis through diverse epistemologies will contribute to a disciplinary-specific definition of what constitutes evidence for nursing praxis and will explicate how evidence is integrated into a disciplinary body of knowledge.

Nurses need to have faith in how praxis directs us to know the world, and to look first and foremost to developing knowledge in ways that are consistent with the diverse ways in which we know the world (Jones 1997). The soundest strategy for mediating an interdisciplinary understanding of evidence in health-care—and how evidence is used in health-care—is for nurses to clearly articulate what constitutes evidence for nursing. Understanding and appreciating disciplinary differences is possible if the differences are articulated. Interdisciplinary respect may be more valuable over the long-term than interdisciplinary consensus.

Interdisciplinary consensus on what constitutes evidence may not be possible, as the health disciplines tend to subscribe to different epistemologies and therefore different 'truths'. From this perspective, health-care itself, understood as a collective entity, is based on the diverse epistemologies represented by not only the various health disciplines, but also other stakeholders, including the consumers of health-care. Perhaps health-care itself may ultimately be recognized as a form of praxis.

Acknowledgments. I am indebted to Dr Sally Thorne and Dr Angela Henderson at the School of Nursing, University of British Columbia, for their support and guidance in the development of this paper. I would also like to acknowledge the valuable suggestions made by Shannon Scott-Findlay, PhD (c), particularly in reviewing the content pertaining to evidence-based practice and knowledge translation.

REFERENCES

Angeles PA. 1981. *Dictionary of philosophy*. New York: Barnes and Noble.

Benner P. 2000. The roles of embodiment, emotion and lifeworld for rationality and agency in nursing practice. *Nursing Philosophy* 1:5–19.

Bishop AH, and JR Scudder. 1997. Nursing as a practice rather than an art or a science. *Nursing Outlook* 45:82–5.

Capra F. 1982. *The turning point: Science, society, and the rising culture*. Toronto: Bantam.

Carper BA. 1978. Fundamental patterns of knowing in nursing. *Advances in Nursing Science* 1:13–23.

Centre for Evidence-Based Medicine, Oxford. 2001. Levels of evidence and grades of recommendations, http://cebmjr2.ox.ac. uk/docs/levels.html (cited November 2003)

Charlton BG. 1997. Restoring the balance: Evidence-based medicine put in its place. *Journal of Evaluation in Clinical Practice* 3: 87–98.

Chinn PL and MK Kramer. 1999. *Theory and nursing. Integrated knowledge development*, 5th edn. St Louis: Mosby.

Dobrow MJ, V Goel and REG Upshur. 2004. Evidence-based health policy: Context and utilisation. *Social Science and Medicine* 58:207–17.

Estabrooks CA. 1998. Will evidence-based nursing practice make practice perfect? *Canadian Journal of Nursing Research* 30: 15–36.

Evidence-Based Medicine Working Group. 1992. Evidence-based medicine. A new approach to teaching the practice of medicine. *Journal of the American Medical Association* 268: 2420–5.

Fawcett J, J Watson, B Neuman, PH Walker and JJ Fitzpatrick. 2001. On nursing theories and evidence. *Journal of Nursing Scholarship* 33:115–19.

Flaming D. 2001. Using phronesis instead of 'research-based practice' as the guiding light for nursing practice. *Nursing Philosophy* 2:251–8.

Greenhalgh T and JG Worrall. 1997. From EBM to GSM: The evolution of context-sensitive *medicine. Journal of Evaluation in Clinical Practice* 3:105–8.

Harman WW. 1996. The shortcomings of Western science. *Qualitative Inquiry* 2:30–8.

Holmes C and P Warelow. 2000. Nursing as normative praxis. *Nursing Inquiry* 7:175–81.

Jacobs-Kramer MK and PL Chinn. 1988. Perspectives on knowing: A model of nursing knowledge. *Scholarly Inquiry for Nursing Practice* 2:129–39.

Jennings BM and LA Loan. 2001. Misconceptions among nurses about evidence-based practice. *Journal of Nursing Scholarship* 33:121–7.

Johnson JL. 1991. Nursing science: Basic, applied, or practical? Implications for the art of nursing. *Advances in Nursing Science* 14: 7–16.

Johnson JL and PA Ratner. 1997. The nature of knowledge used in nursing practice. In *Nursing praxis: Knowledge and action,* eds SE Thorne and V Hayes, 3–22. Thousand Oaks, CA: Sage.

Jones M. 1997. Thinking nursing. In *Nursing praxis: Knowledge and action,* eds SE Thorne and V Hayes, 125–39. Thousand Oaks, CA: Sage.

Jones M and J Higgs. 2000. Will evidenced-based practice take the reasoning out of practice? *Clinical Reasoning in the Health Professions,* eds J Higgs and M Jones, 307–15. Boston: Butterworth Heinemann.

Kitson A, G Harvey and B McCormack. 1998. Enabling the implementation of evidence-based practice: A conceptual framework. *Quality in Health Care* 7:149–58.

Landry R, N Amara and M Lamari. 2001. Utilization of social science research knowledge in Canada. *Research Policy* 30:333–49.

Madjar I and J Walton. 2001. What is problematic about evidence? In *The nature of qualitative evidence,* eds JM Morse, JM Swanson and AJ Kuzel, 28–45. Thousand Oaks, CA: Sage.

Mautner T. 1996. *The Penguin dictionary of philosophy.* London: Penguin.

McCain RA. 1998. Economic efficiency: A 'reasonable dialog' in economics: Part I, defeasible reasoning. In *Essential principles of economics: A hypermedia text,* williamking. www.drexel.edu/top/prin/txt/EcoToC.html (cited November 2003).

Meleis AI. 1997. *Theoretical nursing: Development and progress,* 3rd edn. Philadelphia: Lippincott.

Mitchell GJ. 1999. Evidence-based practice: Critique and alternative view. *Nursing Science Quarterly* 12:30–5.

Nagle LM and GJ Mitchell. 1991. Theoretic diversity: Evolving paradigmatic issues in research and practice. *Advances in Nursing Science* 14:17–25.

Oxford dictionary of current English. 1998. ed. D Thompson. Oxford: Oxford University Press.

Rafael ARF. 1999. From rhetoric to reality: The changing face of public health nursing in southern Ontario. *Public Health Nursing* 16:50–9.

Rycroft-Malone J, K Seers, A Titchen, G Harvey, A Kitson and B McCormack. 2004. What counts as evidence in evidence-based practice? *Journal of Advanced Nursing* 47:81–90.

Sackett DL, WM Rosenberg, JA Gray, RB Haynes and WS Richardson. 1996. Evidence-based medicine: What it is and what it isn't. *British Medical Journal* 312:71–2.

Schwandt TR. 1990. Paths to inquiry in the social sciences: Scientific, constructivist, and critical theory methodologies. In *The paradigm dialog,* ed. EG Guba, 258–76. Newbury Park, CA: Sage.

Scott-Findlay S and C Pollock. 2004. Evidence, research, knowledge: A call for conceptual clarity. *Worldviews on Evidence-Based Nursing,* Second Quarter: 92–7.

Shahar E. 1998. Evidence-based medicine: A new paradigm or the emperor's new clothes? *Journal of Evaluation in Clinical Practice* 4:277–82.

Thorne SE. 1997. Introduction: Praxis in the con text of nursing's developing inquiry. In *Nursing praxis: Knowledge and action,* eds SE Thorne and V Hayes, ix–xxi. Thousand Oaks, CA: Sage.

Thorne SE. 2001. The implications of disciplinary agenda on quality criteria for qualitative research. In *The nature of qualitative evidence,* eds JM Morse, JM Swanson and AJ Kuzel, 141–59. Thousand Oaks, CA: Sage.

Upshur REG. 2001. The status of qualitative research as evidence. In *The nature of qualitative evidence,* eds JM Morse, JM Swanson and AJ Kuzel, 5–26. Thousand Oaks, CA: Sage.

Upshur REG. 2003. Are all evidence-based practices alike? Problems in the ranking of evidence. *Canadian Medical Association Journal* 169:672–3.

Upshur REG, EG VanDenKerkhof and V Goel. 2001. Meaning and measurement: An inclusive model of evidence in health care. *Journal of Evaluation in Clinical Practice* 7:91–6.

Warms CA and CA Schroeder. 1999. Bridging the gulf between science and action: The 'new fuzzies' of neopragmatism. *Advances in Nursing Science* 22:1–10.

White J. 1995. Patterns of knowing: Review, critique, and update. *Advances in Nursing Science* 17:73–86.

Wolfer J. 1993. Aspects of 'reality' and ways of knowing in nursing: In search of an integrating paradigm. *IMAGE: Journal of Nursing Scholarship* 25:141–6.

THE AUTHOR COMMENTS | **Mediating the Meaning of Evidence Through Epistemological Diversity**

The interdisciplinary perspectives I was exposed to in a first-year PhD course, Topics in Knowledge Utilization, offered by Dr. Carole Estabrooks at the University of Alberta, along with my clinical practice background in primary healthcare, challenged me to better understand how population-based "best" evidence (i.e., evidence according to the hierarchical levels of evidence models) could be made relevant to the contexts of the small, remote, unique aboriginal populations I faced in my practice. I speculated that similar understandings, grounded in clinical practice experience, were also the basis of the apparent disconnect between how researchers and clinicians each understood the uptake and utilization of evidence in practice, and I began writing about the meaning of evidence from a primary healthcare perspective. My understanding of these issues continued to evolve through lively discussions and debate with nursing colleagues in the doctoral student philosophy seminars offered by Dr. Sally Thorne and Dr. Angela Henderson at the University of British Columbia. The article, *Mediating the Meaning of Evidence Through Epistemological Diversity*, took shape in response to my efforts to understand how nurses might best contribute to the development of evidence-based knowledge for nursing practice, within the interdisciplinary team models that increasingly bring together the "disciplines" of research and practice, as well as the traditionally different practice disciplines.

DENISE TARLIER

27

Nursing Epistemology: Traditions, Insights, Questions

PHYLLIS R. SCHULTZ, PhD, FAAN
AFAF I. MELEIS, PhD, DrPS (Hons), FAAN

*E*pistemology is the study of what human beings know, how they come to know what they think they know and what the criteria are for evaluating knowledge claims. Nursing epistemology is the study of knowledge shared among the members of the discipline, the patterns of knowing and knowledge that develops from them, and the criteria for accepting knowledge claims. Three types of knowledge specific to nursing as a discipline are described here: clinical knowledge, conceptual knowledge and empirical knowledge. Different criteria for evaluating each type are suggested.

Nursing epistemology is the study of the origins of nursing knowledge, its structure and methods, the patterns of knowing of its members, and the criteria for validating its knowledge claims. Just as women are aware increasingly that their perceptions, observations and reasoning about the world contribute understandings that are unique, so too nurses, as members of a discipline and profession made up mostly of women, are changing in consciousness as knowledge for and from the practice of nursing continues to grow. This paper explores the epistemology of nursing; it grows out of the belief that, as nurses, our ways of knowing have not yet been fully articulated but that they will emerge if we allow ourselves to see the world through the eyes of practicing nurses and their clients.

The term "epistemology" comes from philosophy, where it is defined as the study of knowledge, or theory of knowledge (Flew, 1984). As a practice discipline and profession, nursing is often described as both an "art" and a "science." Articulating its epistemology is therefore a complex task: The study of nursing knowledge must range from the seemingly intuitive "knowing" of the experienced and expert nurses to the systematically verified knowledge of empirical researchers.

The epistemology of any field of inquiry depends on the nature of the phenomena studied and on the propensities of the inquirers who are developing knowledge in the field. Nursing epistemology, then, is the study of how nurses come to know what they think they know, what exactly nurses do know, how nursing knowledge is structured and on what basis knowledge claims are made.

What is Knowing/What is Known?

For any person, knowing begins with the processes of observation, perception and experience in encountering the world and being in the world. These processes give rise to describing and interpreting phenomena, including anticipating, with some degree of accuracy, what is likely to happen at some future time. It is helpful to think of "knowing" as a process and the knowledge that comes from that process as the product (Benoliel, 1987; Chinn & Jacobs, 1987).

According to Benoliel, "Knowing can be viewed as an individual's perceptual awareness of the complexities of a particular situation and draws on inner knowledge resources that have been garnered through experience in living" (p. 151). It rarely can be expressed through discourse but is experienced through the acts of persons (Benner, 1983; Chinn & Jacobs, 1987). By contrast, knowledge as product is often expressed in some form of communication such as informal conversations, formal oral presentations, written articles and texts or art forms such as paintings, poetry, novels or music.

In a practice discipline, knowing is also working on solutions to problems that are important for the welfare of clients. It includes the ability to identify the questions at the forefront of inquiry in the field, the issues involved in answering these questions, the ways to go about answering the answerable questions and the ways to handle the unanswerable questions. Knowing is also having the wisdom to recognize which questions have top priority, which are secondary and

ABOUT THE AUTHORS

PHYLLIS R. SCHULTZ was born on March 9, 1938. She holds BSN, MN, MA, and PhD degrees from colleges and universities in North Dakota, Georgia, and Colorado and completed postdoctoral studies at the University of California, San Francisco. She is Associate Professor Emerita at the School of Nursing, University of Washington. Her 40-year nursing career included 19 years in various clinical positions, including intensive care, primary care, and community health, coupled with 21 years in higher education at the University of Colorado Health Sciences Center and the University of Washington. Her scholarship focused on examining the theoretical, empirical, and clinical foundations of community nursing and administration as unique practice fields within the nursing domain. She considers her 1987 article "When the client is more than one" key to advancing nursing knowledge in these fields, and she is the coauthor of several review chapters and articles since then that have contributed to the literature in the discipline. Currently, she is learning how to be a long-distance grandmother as well as exploring ways of "being" after a lifetime of "doing."

AFAF I. MELEIS, a nurse and medical sociologist, is currently the Margaret Bond Simon Dean of Nursing at the University of Pennsylvania School of Nursing. She completed her undergraduate nursing education at the University of Alexandria, Egypt (1961), and came to the United States as a Rockefeller Fellow (1962) to pursue her graduate education. She earned an MS in nursing (1964), an MA in sociology (1966), and a PhD in medical and social psychology (1968) from the University of California, Los Angeles. Her scholarship focuses on theory and knowledge development, including her theory on living with transitions, immigrant and international health, and women's role integration and health. She is the author of more than 150 articles and 40 chapters and numerous monographs, proceedings, and books, including the widely used book, *Theoretical Nursing: Development and Progress.* Currently, Dr. Meleis serves as President of the International Council on Women's Health Issues. She has received several national and international awards and honorary doctorates, including the 1990 Medal of Excellence for professional and scholarly achievements, presented by Egyptian President Hosni Mubarak, and an Honorary Professorship from the Department of Health Sciences, the Hong Kong Polytechnic University.

which are trivial; it is recognizing which questions can be answered in the near future and which have to be deferred.

In epistemology, Chisholm (1982) formulated the questions about knowing:

1. "What do we know? What is the extent of our knowledge?"

2. "How are we to decide whether we know? What are the criteria of knowledge?" (p. 50) Chisholm identified three epistemological positions as possible answers to these questions: skepticism, methodism and particularism. Skeptics say that these are unanswerable questions because we cannot answer either set without presupposing an answer to the other. This position is untenable for a practice discipline because we have to take care of real people with real health problems.

By "methodism," Chisholm (1982) meant that to have knowledge is to have a preferred method of inquiry and procedures for recognizing reliable or credible knowledge (i.e., one begins by answering the second set of questions (set 2). Chisholm explicitly identified empiricism as a "type of 'methodism'" (p. 67). Recent debates in nursing about qualitative and quantitative data collection with their corresponding metaphysical and epistemological foundations reflect a type of methodism in nursing (Schultz, 1987). This methodism has led some nurse inquirers to subscribe to science in general and to empiricist science in particular as the preferable epistemological position in nursing.

The allegiance to empiricism can explain some of the sense of separation that has arisen among nurse inquirers who hold different epistemological positions and use different methods of inquiry. Some rely on reflection and reasoning; others elect structured observation and hypothesis testing; still others prefer phenomenological dialogue and reflective interpretation. Academicians tend to insist on knowledge that is formal, orderly, validated and communicable. Practitioners trust knowledge that results in appropriate actions with clients in specific situations. To espouse the methodist's epistemological position is to fail to recognize the legitimacy of these multiple ways of knowing; it is to resist accepting the complexity and holistic character of nursing (Benoliel, 1987; Chinn & Jacobs, 1987; Visintainer, 1986).

By "particularism," Chisholm (1982) meant "We can know and know that we know some particular thing at a particular point in time" (p. 74). This position starts from the premise that there are some things we know, whether or not we agree on the methods and procedures for knowing (Chisholm, 1982; Schultz, 1987). Philosophers begin with rather ordinary, everyday cases of knowledge such as "I know how to drive a car" and "I know that seven plus five equals twelve." Similarly, "I know that the sentence, Some mushrooms are poisonous, is true" (Lehrer, 1974). These three statements can be classified as (a) recounting a practical skill, (b) communicating a conceptual insight and (c) articulating an empirical hypothesis.

As nurses, we begin with particular cases of knowledge from (a) our practice, (b) our theories, or (c) our research. Statements about what we "know" are reflected implicitly or explicitly in the writings of our clinicians, theorists and researchers, for example:

1. The experiences of persons in health and illness are revealed in characteristic patterns. These patterns tend to be repetitive, orderly, predictable, and unified; they reflect organization.

2. Some individuals have health and illness experiences that do not fit the general pattern. Thus another case of what we "know" in nursing is that it is predictable that individuals may be unpredictable in their health and illness experiences.

3. Human health and illness can be perceived and understood through uncovering the meanings that individuals, groups and societies derive from their experiences.

4. The health and illness of persons are interactive with environments.

5. Nursing acts influence the responses of persons in health and illness; nursing and the experiences of persons with health and illness are interactive.

Statements such as these about what we "know" in nursing are what we want to begin with in formulating the criteria of knowledge in our discipline. But before we explore such criteria, we will discuss patterns of knowing revealed in the nursing literature, and those from a study of women (Belenky et al., 1986), which may contribute to our understanding of the types of knowledge in present-day nursing.

 ## Patterns of Knowing in Nursing

The complexity of nursing's epistemology was clearly demonstrated by Carper's (1978) delineation of four fundamental patterns of knowing in nursing: empirics, ethics, esthetics and personal knowledge.

Each of these four patterns has recently been specified epistemologically by Chinn and Jacobs (1987). Here we will elaborate only on personal knowledge, because of our belief in the importance of the practitioner as the knower in nursing's development of knowledge.

Personal knowledge was described by Carper (1978) as self-knowledge, or awareness of the self. This description seems to leave out the knowledge from practice that Benner (1983) termed "practical knowledge," following the reasoning of Polanyi (1964) in his *Personal Knowledge.* For Polanyi, "personal" referred to a characteristic of the knower; "knowledge," to a mental process:

> I regard knowing as an active comprehension of the things known, an action that requires skill ... Comprehension is neither an arbitrary act nor a passive experience, but a responsible act claiming universal validity. (p. xiii)

Thus to know the self is part of comprehending "the things known." Knowing what one knows is also part of comprehending.

Polanyi (1964) distinguished between knowledge as theory and knowledge as practical skill. He termed knowledge that may not be articulated through language as "tacit knowing"; knowledge that is communicable through discourse he termed "explicit knowing." Another way to phrase this distinction is "knowing how" and "knowing that," which Benner (1983) found useful in explaining what expert nurses know. Expert nurses may enter a caring encounter with awareness of the self as therapeutic agent (Carper, 1978) and with a foundation of formal concepts, theories, facts and skills learned in their education (the knowing that). According to Benner (1983), as the encounter, or event, unfolds, they refine, elaborate or disconfirm this "foreknowledge"; the encounter then deserves to be termed "experience" and contributes to the knowing how. These three aspects of personal knowledge—knowing the self, knowing that and knowing how—are the sum of what one knows. All three are brought to the caring situation and are used to identify and solve the problems of the discipline.

Unfortunately, we know very little about personal knowing, especially about knowing the self and knowing how, in part because they can only be articulated retrospectively (Chinn & Jacobs, 1987). The knowing how from practice may, however, be brought to consciousness and made communicable through innovative methods of inquiry such as interpretive, grounded theory or phenomenological research (Benner, 1983; 1985; Pyles & Stern, 1983; Ray, 1987). For example, using a grounded theory approach, Pyles and Stern described the "nursing gestalt," by which expert critical care nurses identify impending cardiogenic shock and prevent untimely death. They learned that novice nurses must work with expert critical care nurses (the Gray Gorilla concept) to acquire their know how for practice. Their findings corroborated those of Benner's (1983) study of the knowledge embedded in clinical practice.

Also, in a study of critical care nursing using phenomenology as method, Ray (1987) discovered that the essence of nursing in critical care involves technological and ethical caring; it is an experiential dialectic between technical competence (doing no harm) and compassion (in response to suffering), which are mediated through ethical choice (preserving autonomy and ensuring justice).

Efforts to bring to consciousness the self-knowledge and knowing how of nursing practice may be aided by examination of women's ways of knowing identified by Belenky et al. (1986). The patterns they discovered were not supposed to be hierarchical, although unfortunately their descriptions appear to be so. In applying their framework to nurses, we will assume that different patterns of knowing exist simultaneously. The five patterns of women's knowing that Belenky et al. identified are silence, received knowledge, subjective knowledge, procedural knowledge and constructed knowledge. Each of the five patterns is explained in the following:

Silence. Persons "experience themselves as mindless and voiceless and subject to the whims of external authority" (p. 16). Belenky et al. add that silent women know at the "gut level" but have not cultivated their capacity for abstract thought; nor do they attempt to articulate why they do what they do. They accept the voices of authority for direction in their work and life because of others' power, not necessarily expertise. Others are "right"; the silent one is "wrong" and "dumb."

According to Colliere (1986) silent nurses may not know how to conceptualize their daily experiences; they follow the voices of others because of fear of others' power. They do not have the language to generalize from what they know so that their knowledge can be communicated. They have learned to be silent. Their work, their patterns of knowing and their knowledge are invisible.

Received knowledge. Persons "perceive themselves as capable of receiving, even reproducing, knowledge from all-knowing external authorities but not capable of creating knowledge on their own" (p. 15). Individuals who use this way of knowing rely on others for the words to communicate what they know. For this type of knower, knowledge is observable; there is no ambiguity in it, and it depends on the expertise of others.

Many nurses have contented themselves with using the words of others to express and guide their knowing. American nurses have used medical knowledge, psychological and sociological knowledge, philosophical knowledge and administrative knowledge to communicate what they know. Following the same pattern, nurses in other countries have used nursing theories developed in the United States to communicate the nature of their practice.

Subjective knowledge. Knowledge is "conceived of as personal, private, and subjectively known and intuited" (p. 15). The subjective pattern of women's knowing reminds us of the debates in nursing today about the usefulness and reliability of experiential knowing (i.e., knowledge from practice). Knowers such as this in nursing offer us their subjective wisdom from their own inner voices, which may enhance our understanding of complex situations, but their knowledge is transient, and not cumulative. Such knowers may find it difficult to articulate the processes that they have gone through in knowing because knowing for them is intuitive, experienced, not thought out and something felt rather than cognitively appraised or constructed.

Procedural knowledge. These knowers depend on careful observation, structured procedures and systematic analyses. In short, they are rationalists. They use objectivity as a measure of what can be known as well as repeated observations under controlled situations for corroboration. They distance themselves from experience in order to know. Though they use subjective awareness to provide insights, they adhere to the idea that objectivity yields the knowledge that is most reliable.

Nurse researchers and academicians are the strongest adherents of this way of knowing. Following strict procedures for inquiry is considered the way to secure reliable knowledge for teaching the principles and practices of nursing and for further inquiry. As we emphasize increasingly research-based practice, clinicians are joining the ranks of the rational, procedural knowers in nursing.

Constructed knowledge. A pattern of knowing in which persons "view all knowledge as contextual, experience themselves as creators of knowledge, and value both subjective and objective strategies of knowing" (p. 15). These knowers integrate the different ways of knowing and the different voices (including the silent voice). To them, "all knowledge is constructed, and the knower is an intimate part of the known" (p. 37).

Nurses who subscribe to this view of knowing see theories as approximations of reality that are ongoing and always in process; their frames of reference are constructed and reconstructed (Visintainer, 1986), and posing questions is as important as attempting to answer questions. These nurses believe that knowing is achieved as much through openness and curiosity and through examination of the assumptions and context within which questions are posed as through adherence to procedures or systematic observation and replication.

For nurses who subscribe to this view of knowing, the development of knowledge is a never-ending process. There are glimmers of certain knowledge if one understands the whole of a situation including formal knowledge of the phenomenon. Experts (i.e., experienced knowers) develop a connected knowing through conversing with each other and through identifying patterns, consistencies and order in the evidence provided by the various ways of knowing (Benoliel, 1987; Schultz, 1987). Their knowledge is corroborated by knowledge from other disciplines.

Types of Nursing Knowledge and Criteria of Credibility

From our reflections on the traditional patterns of knowing in nursing and on women's ways of knowing, we have identified three types of knowledge specific to nursing as a discipline: clinical knowledge, conceptual knowledge and empirical knowledge. Discussed below are their relationships to the different patterns of knowing and possible criteria of credibility for each type.

Clinical Knowledge

Clinical knowledge results from engaging in the gestalt of caring, from bringing to bear multiple ways of knowing in order to solve the problems of patient care. Florence Nightingale knew the needs of the soldiers who fought in the Crimean War because she worked with them day and night; she was able to see the results of limited resources and exposure to the unhygienic environment. She realized that not only were diseases afflicting the soldiers, but the care they failed to receive affected their recovery.

Clinical knowledge is manifested primarily in the acts of practicing nurses; it is individual and personal. Historically, it has often been voiceless except in descriptions of the art of nursing, which have come to be viewed as less important and credible since nursing has been developing formal empirical foundations for practice. Clinicians experience patients' situations and "do" (i.e., they act based on these experiences).

Historically, clinical knowledge has been the product of a combination of personal knowing and empirics. It has usually involved intuition and subjective knowing, although these have tended to be ignored, denigrated or denied (Rew & Barrow, 1987). In the past, the empirical base was often "received empirics" from medicine or the social and behavioral

sciences. Increasingly, however, empirical studies by nurses inform clinical practice. Further, intuition and subjective knowing are regaining their legitimacy as necessary components of humane care (Watson, 1985). The aesthetic and ethical patterns of knowing are also contributing to the development of clinical knowledge in response to the changing needs of persons interacting with technological and organizational environments.

Traditionally, clinical knowledge has been communicated retrospectively, through the publication of articles on specific client problems. These accounts, in national journals of nursing and increasingly in international journals, report individual case descriptions or summaries of multiple cases that provide answers for questions and problems in practice. These published accounts often reflect received knowledge and procedural knowledge and are characterized by prescriptions for practice.

The credibility of clinical knowledge has been based on the usefulness of its communicated wisdom—"It works." This criterion meets the requirement of purposefulness of a practice discipline (Chinn & Jacobs, 1987). Do we need other modes of corroboration? Can the art of nursing yield as reliable and reproducible knowledge as does the "science" of nursing? Should it? Perhaps models of practice, the discovery of patterns within and across clients and testimonials of subjective knowledge might be appropriate criteria for the credibility of clinical knowledge. These are unanswered questions.

Conceptual Knowledge

Conceptual knowledge is abstracted and generalized beyond personal experiences; it explicates the patterns revealed in multiple client experiences in multiple situations and articulates them as models or theories. Concepts are defined, and statements about the relationships among them are formulated. These propositions are supported by empirical and/or anecdotal evidence or defended by inferences and logical reasoning. This type of knowledge is manifested in the works of nurse theorists who seek answers to questions such as, Who is our client? What is it that nurses do that influences persons' health (Meleis, 1985)? These theorists develop comprehensive formulations of the nursing world. They use knowledge from other disciplines but through reflection and imagination evolve perspectives on that knowledge that are unique to nursing. They are influenced by procedures followed in the development of other fields but adhere to procedures supportive of the values and purpose of nursing.

Conceptual knowledge is the product of reflection on nursing phenomena. It emanates from curiosity and evolves from innovation and imagination in inquiry, along with persistence and commitment to the accumulation of facts and reliable generalizations. This type of nursing knowledge requires logical reasoning and comes primarily from individuals who take the position that knowledge is constructed within a context, and its development is a never-ending process.

Empirical knowing has influenced the development of conceptual knowledge in nursing through a dynamic interplay between systematic observation (empirics) and theorizing (reflecting, describing, synthesizing) (Weekes, 1986). The results of an inquirer's own research and that of others are used to support the propositional structure of frameworks or theories. But imagination and risk taking are important in their origination.

Will aesthetic knowing lead to formal conceptualizations of nursing that reflect its art? Will conceptual frameworks and models emerge from ethics as a pattern of knowing to describe this dimension of nursing? The answers to these questions depend on the degree to which nurse inquirers can view multiple ways of knowing as equally valuable in contributing to the mission of nursing.

The credibility of conceptual knowledge rests, in part, on the extent to which nurses find useful models and theories in communicating what they know. Whether or not a particular conceptual formulation holds up to critical appraisal depends also on its coherence and logical integrity—two criteria for evaluating theories (Meleis, 1985; Chinn & Jacobs, 1987).

Conceptual knowledge is often communicated in the form of propositional sentences. Thus it is the propositions and their relationships to each other that are evaluated for credibility. Chisholm's six levels of epistemic preferability illustrate the criteria for evaluating propositional credibility. Schultz (1987) explicated these levels with a proposition exemplifying a nursing knowledge claim:

> Nursing acts influence persons' energy exchange for healing and health. For the person who believes this claim the statement is (1) self presenting to him or her at a particular point in time; (2) the claim has some presumption in its favor because it is not contradicted by other beliefs; (3) the claim is judged to be acceptable because it is not disconfirmed by the set of propositions having some presumption in their favor; (4) the claim is epistemically in the clear because it is not disconfirmed by the set of acceptable propositions and therefore (5) the claim is beyond reasonable doubt. Having met these conditions, the claim is judged to be (6) evident or certain (p. 141).

These are stringent criteria. Since nurses attend to individual experiences as well as to general patterns of experience, we may need to formulate different criteria of credibility for the conceptualization of nursing phenomena.

Empirical Knowledge

Empirical knowledge results from research. By research, we do not mean simply the empiricist approach per se but also historical, phenomenological, interpretive and critical theory approaches (Chinn, 1986). Empirical knowledge is manifest in published reports and is often used to justify actions and procedures in practice. It forms the basis for new studies and thereby contributes to the cumulative body of knowledge of a discipline. It often stimulates theoretical conceptualizations.

Researchers rely, in part, on received and procedural knowledge to inform their inquiries, but the hypotheses they test may originate in subjective knowledge; that is, their experiences with and reflections on nursing phenomena may give rise to hunches that lead to innovative methods or approaches to inquiry. If the empirical inquirer is also a practitioner, self-knowledge and practical knowledge may be brought to bear on the methods of inquiry. It is less clear how the aesthetic or ethical patterns of knowing contribute to the development of empirical knowledge except that usually (a) researchers adhere to ethical precepts in the conduct of their studies and (b) nurse inquirers are turning to the arts and humanities for approaches to systematic inquiry.

Advocates of different types of research approaches and methods have carved out criteria to validate their findings that are congruent with the particular designs and epistemological orientations that they follow (Gortner, 1984; Sandelowski, 1986). For all, however, the credibility of empirical knowledge rests on the degree to which the researcher has followed procedures accepted by the community of researchers and on the logical derivation of conclusions from the evidence without bias or prejudice (Schultz, 1987; Gortner & Schultz, 1987). Of particular importance is whether or not the researcher is cognizant of previous research findings, knowledgeable about the procedures by which they were discovered, and dedicated to basing new research efforts on previous knowledge (Benoliel, 1987).

In addition to the procedural criteria accompanying various research designs and methods, the credibility of empirical knowledge is assessed by the systematic review and critique of research published in annual reviews (Werley & Fitzpatrick, 1983-1986; Fitzpatrick & Taunton, 1987), by consensus conferences focused on corroborating what is known about specific phenomena (e.g., pain) (National Institute of Health, 1987), and by invitational conferences to clarify the state-of-the-art on a topic and suggest new directions to be taken (Duffy & Pender, 1987). The epistemic preferability criteria enumerated above for conceptual knowledge claims may also be useful for assessing the credibility of empirical knowledge claims.

Ultimately credibility criteria must be consistent with nurses' various ways of knowing and types of knowledge. Can criteria be developed to accommodate the epistemological plurality of nursing, its complexity and holism? Is there one set of criteria or are there several? These are unanswered questions, but let us consider the possibility that the criteria for accepting knowledge vary for each type of knowledge.

 ## Conclusion

Throughout this paper, we have deliberately avoided using the concept of "truth." Unfortunately inquirers from differing and contradictory perspectives have a propensity to put forth the view that their way of knowing yields *the* truth rather than *a* truth. Perhaps it is inappropriate to use the language of truth in nursing or in any practice discipline that deals with complex human experiences. Perhaps comprehending the context and patterns of human experiences, adjusted for individual differences, is more appropriate for claiming universal validity (Polanyi, 1964; Visintainer, 1986). Perhaps it is not sufficient to speak of facts alone, rather we should speak of experiences, intuition *and* facts. Perhaps it is not enough to rely on research as the medium for knowledge development; conceptualization and expert knowledge from clinical practice may be equally powerful and credible.

If we agree that there are different ways of knowing, different unknowns to be known, different propensities of knowers for knowing and different aspects to be known about the same phenomenon, then perhaps we can develop appropriate criteria for knowing from what we do know and, then, for knowing what we want to know.

REFERENCES

Belenky, M. F., Clinchy, B. M., Goldberger, N. R., & Tarule, J. M. (1986). *Women's ways of knowing*. New York: Basic Books.

Benner, P. (1983). Uncovering the knowledge embedded in clinical practice. *Image: The Journal of Nursing Scholarship, 15*(2), 36–41.

Benner, P. (1985). Quality of life: A phenomenological perspective on explanation, prediction, and understanding in nursing science. *Advances in Nursing Science, 8*(1), 1–14.

Benoliel, J. Q. (1987). Response to "Toward holistic inquiry in nursing: A proposal for synthesis of patterns and methods." *Scholarly Inquiry for Nursing Practice: An International Journal, 1*(2), 147–152.

Carper, B. A. (1978). Fundamental patterns of knowing in nursing. *Advances in Nursing Science, 1*(1), 13–23.

Chinn, P. L. (1986). *Nursing Research Methodology*. Rockville, MD: Aspen Publications.

Chinn, P. L., & Jacobs, M. K. (1987). *Theory and nursing: A systematic approach* (2d ed.). St. Louis: The C. V. Mosby Company.

Chisholm, R. M. (1982). *The foundations of knowing*. Minneapolis: University of Minnesota Press.

Colliere, M. F. (1986). Invisible care and invisible women as health care-providers. *International Journal of Nursing Studies, 23*(2), 95–112.

Duffy, M. E., & Pender, N. J. (1987). *Conceptual issues in health promotion research*. Indianapolis: Sigma Theta Tau Publications.

Fitzpatrick, J. J., & Taunton, R. L. (1987). Annual Review of Nursing Research (Vol. 5). New York: Springer Publishers.

Flew, A. (1984). *A dictionary of philosophy* (2d Ed.). New York: St. Martin's Press.

Gortner, S. R. (1984). Knowledge in a practice discipline: Philosophy and pragmatics. In C. Williams (Ed.), *Nursing research and policy formation: The case of prospective payment* (pp. 5–16). Kansas City, MO: American Academy of Nursing.

Gortner, S. R., & Schultz, P. R. (1987). Approaches to nursing science methods, *IMAGE: Journal of Nursing Scholarship, 20*(1), 22–24.

Lehrer, K. (1974). *Knowledge*. London: Oxford University Press.

Meleis, A. I. (1985). *Theoretical nursing*. Philadelphia: J. B. Lippincott Co.

National Institute of Health Consensus Development Conference (1987). The integrated approach to the management of pain. *Journal of Pain and Symptom Management, 2*(1), 35–44.

Polanyi, M. (1964). *Personal knowledge: Towards a post-critical philosophy*. New York: Harper Torchbooks.

Pyles, S. H., & Stern, P. N. (1983). Discovery of nursing gestalt in critical care nursing: The importance of the gray gorilla syndrome. *Image: The Journal of Nursing Scholarship, 15*(3), 51–57.

Ray, M. A. (1987). Technological caring: A new model in critical care. *Dimensions of Critical Care Nursing, 6*(3), 166–173.

Rew, L., & Barrow, E. M. (1987). Intuition: A neglected hallmark of nursing knowledge. *Advances in Nursing Science, 10*(1), 49–62.

Sandelowski, M. (1986). The problem of rigor in qualitative research. *Advances in Nursing Science, 8*(3), 27–37.

Schultz, P. R. (1987). Toward holistic inquiry in nursing: A proposal for synthesis of patterns and methods. *Scholarly Inquiry for Nursing Practice: An International Journal, 1*(2), 135–146.

Visintainer, M. A. (1986). The nature of knowledge and theory in nursing. *IMAGE: Journal of Nursing Scholarship, 18* (2), 32–38.

Watson, J. (1985). *Nursing: Human science and human care*. Norwalk, CT: Appleton-Century-Crofts.

Weekes, D. P. (1986). Theory-free observation: Fact or fantasy. In P. L. Chinn, (Ed.). *Nursing Research Methodology*. Rockville, MD: Aspen Publications, 11–22.

Werley, H. H., & Fitzpatrick, J. J. (1983–1986). *Annual Review of Nursing Research* (Vols. 1–4).

THE AUTHORS COMMENT | Nursing Epistemology: Traditions, Insights, Questions

We wrote this article to explore nurses' various ways of knowing and how the knowledge that flows from these ways can provide solutions to the urgent problems germane to client welfare as well as be credible in the larger context of science in practice disciplines. In Schultz's view, it is "an especially good example of careful in-depth reasoning about our discipline." We were challenged to identify what credibility might mean for types of nursing knowledge. Critical to our concerns was a need to legitimize what clinical nurses "know" and to place that type of knowing and knowledge in its rightful place within the discipline. Many of the questions we posed about credibility criteria for different types of nursing knowledge remain unanswered. They await pursuit by nurse scholars in the 21st century.

PHYLLIS R. SCHULTZ
AFAF I. MELEIS

Fundamental Patterns of Knowing in Nursing
The Challenge of Evidence-Based Practice

SAM PORTER, RN, PhD

his article reconsiders the fundamental patterns of knowing in nursing in light of the challenge of narrow empirics in the form of evidence-based practice. Objections to the dominance of evidence-based practice are reviewed, and the reasons for it are examined. It is argued that it is partially the result of weaknesses in the alternative patterns of ethical, personal, and esthetic knowing, the ineffability of which compromises account-ability. This ineffability can be countered only by introducing a wider form of empirics than countenanced by evidence-based practice into all patterns of knowing, to demonstrate their salience and to make their use in practice transparent. **Key words:** *empirics, esthetics, ethics, evidence-based practice, nursing theory, patterns of knowing, personal knowing*

This article addresses the legacy of a seminal article that helped launch *Advances in Nursing Science* so auspiciously, namely Barbara Carper's "Fundamental patterns of knowing in nursing."[1] Carper's article has been cited and discussed times almost innumerable, and her typology of nursing epistemology continues to stimulate and inform. However, the thrust of this article is that the development of evidence-based practice (EBP) and its influence upon nursing has exposed weaknesses in Carper's patterns of knowing that compromise the capacity of her framework to accommodate and counterbalance the very vigorous empirics that EBP entails.

Before embarking on an examination of the nature of EBP and its relationship to patterns of nursing knowledge, it is useful to recapitulate the 4 patterns, as described by Carper. The first, empirics, refers to the science of nursing, and is "empirical, factual, descriptive."[1(p15)] The second is esthetics, the art of nursing. This is the most difficult pattern of knowing to describe succinctly, as it includes a rather confusing list of attributes such as appreciation of patient experience, design of care, and the relationship of the particular to the universal. Personal knowledge "is concerned with the knowing, encountering and actualizing of the concrete, individual self."[1(p18)] In other words, it is the knowledge needed to engage in authentic personal relationships. Finally, ethics is concerned with the moral knowledge of nurses, specifically focusing on "matters of obligation or what ought to be done."[1(p20)]

The Dominance of Empirics

From the outset of its career in nursing discourse, the pattern of empirics has been identified as occupying an overweening position in relation to the other patterns of knowing. Starting with Carper, commentators have identified a continuing tendency to regard it not as one of a number of patterns of knowing, but as nursing knowledge in toto. Thus Carper observed:

> *Few, if indeed any, familiar with the professional literature would deny that primary emphasis is placed on the development of the science of nursing. One is almost led to believe that the only valid and reliable knowledge is that which is empirical, factual, objectively descriptive and generalisable. There seems to be a self-conscious reluctance to extend the term* **knowledge** *to include those aspects of knowing in nursing that are not the result of empirical investigation.*[1(p16)]

This critique of empirics has been repeated by commentators over the years. Thus, a decade after the publication of Carper's paper, Jacobs-Kramer and Chinn[2] argued that this hierarchical approach to the patterns of knowing was counterproductive and that what was needed was a holistic approach to nursing knowledge. A decade after that Stein et al[3] used insights of the

ABOUT THE AUTHOR

SAM PORTER was born and raised in Ireland. He is Chair in Nursing Research, School of Nursing and Midwifery at Queen's University Belfast. He is a qualified RN, has a primary degree in sociology and social policy, and has a PhD on the occupational relationship between nurses and physicians. His main hobby is spending excessive amounts of time in art museums, which he justifies on the grounds that he is preparing a book on the art of caring. In addition to experience as a clinician, he has held university posts in both sociology and nursing. Along with empirical research into care interventions, the main focus of his scholarship is on methodological and theoretical developments from an interdisciplinary perspective, which is reflected in a publications portfolio that includes papers in refereed journals in nursing, midwifery, sociology, political science, public health, economics, medicine, and public administration. His key contribution to the discipline has been to identify how the theoretical developments of other disciplines can illuminate the issues nurses face.

cognitive model of human social behavior to argue that, because knowledge should be seen as an integrative framework, the significance of what they termed episodic and procedural knowledge, as manifested in esthetic and personal knowing, should be afforded equal importance and weight to empirics. Commentators in this century have continued this theme. Thus, Fawcett et al urged "nurse colleagues throughout the world to join us and those who have accurately pointed to the limitations of viewing nursing as a strictly empirical endeavor … to consider what might be gained by recognition and development of ethical, personal, and aesthetic theories."[4(p118)]

The Changing Definition of Empirics

While critical reflections on what has been seen as the unjustifiably privileged position of empirics have remained fairly constant over the years, what has not remained constant is what commentators mean by the term *empirics*. Carper's view on this issue was clear—the gaining of empirical knowledge was not an end in itself, rather its ultimate aim was the development of abstracted theoretical explanations. The generation of general theories through the abstraction of empirical knowledge was required to enable the systematic explanation and prediction of those phenomena that were the concern of nursing.

Since Carper, there have been at least 3 distinct approaches to the relationship between empirical knowledge and theoretical knowledge. The first approach seeks to reinforce the significance of general theory to nursing knowledge and to expand its salience beyond the confines of empirics. Thus, Fawcett et al[4] have sought to argue that theory building should not be associated exclusively with empirics. Because each pattern of knowing is generated and tested by appropriate,

albeit pattern-specific, processes of inquiry, they contend that they can be regarded as types of theory.[4]

In contrast, there has also been an increasing skepticism from a relativist perspective of the role of general theory in nursing knowledge. Thus, White[5] argues that general theory development entails the ontological assumption of a single, commonly experienced reality that can be explained in abstract and general terms. She contends that if nursing knowledge includes the understanding of the "context-embedded stories"[5(p76)] of individuals, then this sort of universal framework is inappropriate. She urges that Carper's definition of empirics should be modified to accommodate more individualistic empirical strategies, such as phenomenology, to include approaches to knowledge that seek to ideographically understand rather than nomothetically explain. This emphasis on the importance of pluralism for nursing knowledge has been taken even further by postmodernist commentators, who have celebrated the variety of approaches that can be accommodated within the rubric of Carper's model.[6]

Empirics as EBP

Distinct from the approaches adumbrated above is a very powerful alternative that seeks to abjure both general and relativist theory. Instead, it involves adherence to a very clear and simple notion of the role of empirical information in the guidance of healthcare actions, one that conceives of a direct relationship between knowledge and action. I refer here to evidence-based practice, defined by its most influential proponents as "the conscientious, explicit, and judicious use of current best evidence in making decisions about the care of individual patients."[7(p71)] The core of EBP is the utilization of information concerning the most effective approaches to care that has been established using the most rigorous methods available, ideally the randomized controlled trial (RCT).[8] The modus operandi of EBP is to ascertain the facts concerning the efficacy of a healthcare intervention under rigorously controlled conditions, which ensure that the effects (or lack thereof) of the intervention under observation can be unequivocally demonstrated. If it is demonstrated that the intervention is efficacious in solving or ameliorating a given healthcare problem under such strict conditions, then it is argued that it should be the intervention of choice when that healthcare problem is encountered by practitioners in their everyday practice.

The simplicity of the logic of EBP challenges both general and relativist theoretical approaches. On the one hand, complex general theories that seek to incorporate factors that lie in the realms of the esthetic or the personal are of little pertinence to this model of explanation, in that it is primarily concerned with that which can be demonstrated to work best in average circumstances. As for ethics, it can be parsed into the formula "effective = good, good = effective." On the other hand, relying as it does on the reliability and validity of its methodological foundations, EBP has little time for relativist theories that argue that the differences between individuals and their contexts make it is impossible to decide before the fact which interventions will be most effective in promoting health. While accepting the need to treat the individual as an individual, for EBP the fundamental causative relationships identified through rigorous research should be the bedrock of clinical decision making in circumstances where similar conditions apply.

 ## Critiques of Evidence-Based Practice

It is hard to overestimate the power of EBP. Starting out in the guise of evidence-based medicine, it has spread to other professional groupings to become one of the most significant developments in healthcare in the last 2 decades.[9] It has particular ramifications for nursing in that it involves an extremely narrow concentration on empirics. Its reduction of healthcare knowledge to the "bald empiricism"[10] of identifiable linear relationships of cause and effect has caused many nursing scholars considerable disquiet. The reason for this disquiet is not difficult to ascertain, given the long-standing suspicion of the dominant position of empirics. With EBP, not only does empirics enjoy a total hegemony, either displacing (as in the case of esthetics and personal knowledge) or incorporating (as in the case of ethics) alternative modes of knowing, it is also itself reduced to a very circumscribed and mechanistic interpretation of empirical knowledge. It is hardly surprising therefore that robust criticisms of EBP have emanated from both the general theoretical and relativist camps.

From supporters of the importance of general theory, one of the most vigorous critiques of the application of EBP has been articulated by Mitchell,[11] who argues that the tenets of EBP are often inimical to those of nursing theory. She contends that nursing has evolved as a theory-driven occupation. The introduction of EBP threatens to sever the linkages between the theories that have been developed to ensure that nurses discharge their societal mandate, and the practices that they perform in their everyday care. Worse, it has the potential to introduce practices that contradict fundamental tenets of the nursing ethos. She cites the example of behavior modification therapy, the efficaciousness of which has been evidentially demonstrated, but the ethos of which transgresses the nursing commitment to a respectful relationship with clients that does not include punishment for noncompliance.

Mitchell's acerbic response to the increasing influence of EBP is shared by a number of prominent nursing theorists, who have unambiguously identified what they see as its significant dangers:

> The current call for evidence-based nursing practice has set the debate in a conventional, atheoretical, medically dominated, empirical model of evidence, which threatens the foundation of nursing's disciplinary perspective on theory-guided practice.[4(p115)]

If we remember how Fawcett et al's[4] argument extended the salience of theory beyond its mutually constitutive relationship with empirical enquiry to encompass all 4 patterns of knowing, we can see the problem that they have with EBP. First, they regard it as yet another example of the unjustified dominance of empirics over other patterns of knowing. Second, they see this dominance being overdetermined by the narrow atheoretical interpretation of empirics that defines EBP In other words, EBP fails to pay even lip service to either the other patterns of knowing or the organizing function of theory.

The attack from the relativist position has been no less vociferous, most notably from postmodernist commentators[9] While the watchword here is not theory but plurality, the critique is very similar Once again, Carper's typology is cited in the argument against EBP, and once again the prime focus of disquiet is EBP's reduction of the variety of patterns involved in Carper's typology down to the single validated epistemology of bald empirics: "It is deeply questionable whether EBM [evidence-based medicine], as a reflection of stratification ... and segmentation, promotes the multiple ways of knowing deemed important within nursing"[12(p45)]

The identification of EBP by general and postmodernist theorists as the common enemy should not be taken to imply a consonance of purpose between the 2 groups. For postmodernists, healthcare occurs "within the parameters in the moment and place."[13] As a consequence, they regard Carper's patterns of knowing as routes to localized solutions. They are as suspicious of general theoretical claims as they are of bald empiricism, regarding the former as "totalizing discourses"[14] which, in their imposition of uniform explanations for unique situations, do violence to the specificities of the particular. It is therefore a remarkable testament to the appeal of Carper's model that both general theorists and postmodernists can incorporate it with such ease into their radically different worldviews.

Explaining the Dominance of Empirics

All of criticism of EBP recounted thus far begs the question as to why it enjoys such dominance in relation to the other patterns of knowing. The most common explanation for this state of affairs lays the blame for it on our medical colleagues. I have already noted Fawcett et al's[4] description of the call for evidence-based nursing practice as being part of a medically dominated debate. In a similar vein, Mitchell[11] talks of EBP as entrapping nurses in the role of medical extenders. From a postmodernist perspective, Holmes et al[12] are even more explicit in their identification of EBP as an example of the colonization of the nursing domain by medical imperialism.

While there is undoubtedly merit to examining the influence of the medical profession in explanations of the rise of EBP within nursing, it is important not to take such an explanation as the whole story. For a start, there is some evidence that nurses are using EBP to tilt the balance of power between them and physicians in their favor. Manias and Street[15] found that medical reliance on the authority of experience is now vulnerable to nursing challenges that are backed up by evidence-based policies and protocols.

More significantly, there is a need to place the rise of EBP in a wider socioeconomic context. At least 2 major trends are at play here. The first is economic and consists largely of the fiscal pressures upon governments and other funders to increase health service efficiencies.[16] The second is cultural and involves the transformation of healthcare clients into informed consumers who are less willing to accept the opinions of healthcare professionals on faith.[17] Thus, Traynor[18] has commented that if the claims of EBP advocates are to be believed, then by challenging the closed shop of medical expertise through the use of systematically gathered and transparently promulgated evidence, evidence-based medicine represents a significant challenge to established medical authority.

Nursing has not been immune to either of these trends. However, while not underestimating the salience of economic forces, I wish to concentrate on the latter, cultural trend, because it is in this arena that nursing has been uniquely challenged. What I wish to suggest is that the manner in which nursing presents its knowledge claims has exacerbated its vulnerability to changing cultural expectations. To be specific, the increasing public distrust of the professional expert[19] is an important factor in explaining why empirics has been so successful to the cost of other patterns of knowing. An explanation of this thesis requires a return to Carper's original paper and the manner in which she formulated the patterns of knowing; specifically the way she distinguished them in terms of public accountability. What is striking is the fact that while empirics is amenable to open processes of refutation and verification, the other patterns are not. She states that "knowledge gained by empirical description is discursively formulated and publicly verifiable."[1(p16)] In contrast, esthetic experience "resists projection into the discursive form of language,"[1(p16)] while the reciprocity required for personal knowing "cannot be described."[1(p20)] Even the value judgments involved in ethical knowing are "not amenable to scientific inquiry and validation."[1(p20)]

I wish to argue that the ineffability of esthetic, personal, and, to a degree, ethical patterns of knowing may at least in part explain their eclipse by empirics in the form of EBP. The simple reason for this is that if they cannot be tested or even described, then it is very difficult to ascertain how, or even if, they are being used. Much of the ideological power of EBP comes from its claim to be able to provide open and transparent evidence to which everyone, including healthcare clients, can have access. This openness of the evidence is portrayed in turn as an example of the democratization of the clinician-client relationship in that it is not based on the esoteric knowledge of the professional to which the client has little or no access, and which therefore limits the layperson's ability to challenge professional decisions about their care.

In contrast, it is very difficult for apologists for patterns of knowing that are claimed not to be amenable to discourse, and therefore public scrutiny, to adopt the same high moral ground. While we may rightly inform clients that empathy and authenticity are core aspects of nursing knowledge, that in itself is not good enough. Gone are the days when professionals could simply make claims about the benign attributes they possessed and expect the laity to accept those claims on face value. As part of the empowerment of our clientele and the attenuation of old-fashioned paternalistic relationships, there is a need to demonstrate the quality of nursing care, not simply to proclaim it. If a particular quality or pattern of knowing cannot be clearly demonstrated, then it is unsurprising that it holds less weight than those patterns of knowing that can be demonstrated. Insofar as ethical, esthetic, and personal knowing are not amenable to discursive challenge by nursing clientele, their influence as modes of nursing knowledge will be compromised.

Evidence of Patterns of Knowing

The dilemma of how to make manifest ways of knowing that deal with "soft" phenomena is one with which nursing theorists have grappled, most notably in attempts to define and measure caring. These attempts are essentially exercises in empirical enquiry, and as such are inevitably reductive in their simplification of the profound and the complex. Put another way, the price of making caring measurable is to bring it within the domain of empirics. Advocates of the assessment of caring, while aware of the dangers of such an approach, are confident of its usefulness: "empirical evidence of caring, captured in an elusive practice world that is unstable, unseen, chaotic, and changing, can be a tangible grasp and glimpse of nursing's contribution to both science, and public health and welfare."[20(p6)] However, while demonstrably robust instruments to measure caring such as that of CARE-Q[21] and CARE/SAT[22] have been successfully used within the limitations described above, attempts at adopting the same sort of approaches specifically in relation to Carper's patterns of knowing have been less successful.

The theoretically oriented approach of Fawcett et al[4] to patterns of knowing led them to map out examples of evidence for each of the patterns. From their pioneering efforts, we can see clearly the problems that such mapping entails. Unsurprisingly, identifying an example of evidence of empirics was unproblematic; it consisted of scientific data. The examples of evidence in relation to ethics were also clear, in that they included standards of practice and codes of ethics. However, when it came to personal knowledge and esthetics, the examples given were far less persuasive. For personal knowing, the example of evidence was autobiographical stories, while the examples for esthetics were esthetic criticism and works of art.

A Philistine Critique of Esthetics

To deal with the last of these patterns first, Fawcett et al's[4] identification of esthetic criticism of the art of nursing as an example of evidence is problematic because esthetic criticism is not in itself evidence; it is a mode of interrogation that may or may not result in evidence. Fawcett et al do not make clear just what would be the product of that criticism. Even more problematic is their assertion that evidence for esthetic theories is manifest "through works of art, such as paintings, drawings, sculpture, poetry, fiction and nonfiction, dance and others."[4(p118)] While works of art may help nurses understand more deeply and

immediately the experiences of those for whom they care, they are tools for education and enlightenment, not evidence that their insights have been operationalized in nurses' interactions with clients. Moreover, the connection between the capacity to paint, sculpt, or dance and the capacity to act empathetically toward patients in day-to-day nursing encounters is tenuous. The ability to perform these activities does not guarantee the ability to nurse well. More reassuringly, the inability to perform these activities does not necessarily indicate an inability to nurse.

To be fair to Fawcett et al,[4] the task of identifying clear evidential examples of a concept as nebulous as esthetic knowing is almost impossible. The problem is that Carper did not express clearly what she meant by esthetics. Moreover, she further obfuscated the issue by asserting that esthetics could not be adequately expressed in language, beginning her discussion about it by citing Weitz's[23] contention that it is too complex and fluid to be definable.

In general terms, Carper describes esthetics as expressive rather than descriptive, directly relating to experience, and therefore wider and more immediate than discourse. Particular aspects of esthetic knowing are, in order of appearance, the ability to:

1. understand the meanings that are being expressed in patients' behavior;
2. synthesize apparently disparate particulars into a meaningful whole;
3. unify means and ends;
4. creatively design and execute plans of care;
5. integrate individual nursing actions into the package of total patient care;
6. empathize with patients; and
7. appreciate that the whole package of care is the result of a dynamic articulation of mutually dependent factors.

Carper also ambiguously refers to the artfulness of manual and technical skills. She concludes this list by stating that esthetic knowing concerns the perception of particulars rather than universals.

It is possible to boil this list down into a number of main themes: the appreciation of and empathy for patients' experience (1 and 6); the aggregation of the particulars of nursing into a meaningful whole (2, 5, and 7); and the capacity to design that holistic care creatively (3 and 4). However, even reduced to 3 headings, it is still not clear why all these functions, which are at best only partially articulated, should be located under the common umbrella of esthetics. Nor is it just a matter of definitional diversity, there is also an implicit contradiction between the claim that esthetics involves the active gathering of particulars into a whole, and Carper's final assertion that esthetics is all about particulars not universals.

The problem of pinning down esthetics is one that has exercised subsequent commentators. Both Jacobs-Kramer and Chinn[2] and White,[5] while concurring about the ineffability of the "art-act" of nursing, developed suggestions as to how it could be assessed subsequently, namely through the lens of art appreciation, the core question to be addressed of the nursing art-act being 'What does this mean?' This is indubitably an extremely important question, the asking of which is the mark of intelligent, humanistic practice. But is it necessarily or even primarily an esthetic question? I wish to suggest that it is not.

Whether we are concerned with understanding the meaning of nursing acts or patients' behaviors, we already have to hand conventional qualitative research strategies that are specifically designed to address such questions. One might recall White's criticism of Carper's notion of empirics on the grounds that it did not include research within the interpretive paradigm such as phenomenology that sought "descriptions that impart understanding,"[5(p75)] to which we might add "that impart understanding of the meanings that health, illness and care have for individual patients and nurses." In short, the question "what does this mean?" is a hermeneutic, not an esthetic question. It follows that the pattern of knowing designed to answer it should likewise be animated by hermeneutic, or more generally, qualitative strategies—empirics by another route.

The conclusion that the gathering of empirical qualitative data is required to gain an understanding of the meanings that people have of health, illness, and care does not sit comfortably with the tenets of EBP, which has traditionally privileged quantitative research, and specifically the RCT, as the superior method of knowledge acquisition.[24] However, nursing researchers have taken the lead in widening the definition of evidence to include qualitative research through, for example, the development of the Joanna Briggs Institute.[25] The success of these efforts to force a reappraisal of the sort of evidence upon which practice should be based reached an important landmark when that paragon of EBP, the Cochrane Collaboration, finally included a chapter on qualitative research in the its 2008 handbook.[26] But we should not get too excited. Notwithstanding this significant breach of the ramparts, the Cochrane dogma still holds the RCT as its exemplary method.[27]

Insofar as promoters of EBP expect us to acquiesce to assertions about the superiority of specific strategies for knowledge attainment, they are asking us to take an approach that is inimical to the concerns of nurses. Rather than fetishizing a particular approach, we need to ask which strategies will best help us understand the particular issues we are addressing, in this case, the hopes, fears, and understandings of those in our care. Empirical knowledge can take many forms and our decision on which form to adopt for any given problem is a pragmatic one.[28] Of course, when one is seeking to discover the functional efficaciousness of a particular intervention, then there are good pragmatic reasons for adopting the strategy of RCTs. However, when asking the question "what does this mean?" the argument for using qualitative strategies is overwhelming, for as Bhaskar observes, "meanings cannot be measured, only understood."[29(p50)] Thus, the adoption of a qualitative empirical approach to demonstrating those areas of nursing knowledge under the rubric of esthetics provides us with a robust counterweight to the quantitative (and therefore deindividuating) impetus of EBP, while staying true to the ethos of understanding meaning that is at the core of Jacobs-Kramer and Chinn's[2] and White's[5] interpretation of this pattern of knowing.

That said, as we saw from Carper's extended list, there is a lot more to the esthetic pattern of knowing than hermeneutics. For example, I fully accept that the arts have much to teach us in developing our sensibilities. To say otherwise would be hypocritical in the extreme, given that I have recently published a paper that uses a 16th-century painting to reflect upon contemporary sexual health promotion.[30] More ironic still, the whole debate presented here was sparked off by my stumbling across an early 15th-century painting of an EBP midwife being punished by God![31] However, even in instances where nursing practice is based on authentically esthetic knowing, this does not obviate the requirement for clear evidence of its benefit to patients. And that requires, in turn, empirical investigation.

 ## The Unbearable Lightness of Being

Objections similar to those made of esthetic knowing are also pertinent to the pattern of personal knowing. Once again, we are faced with the problem of the ineffability of the core concept. As Carper puts it, "One simply does not know *about* the self; one strives simply to *know* the self."[1(p18)] This ineffability is again reflected in the unsatisfactory evidential example given by Fawcett et al, namely "autobiographical stories about the genuine, authentic self."[4(p118)] The problem with this form of "evidence" is its vulnerability to solipsism. While such an autobiographical tale may tell us how the nurse (assuming the author is a nurse) feels herself to have engaged in a genuine and authentic manner, the evidence remains that of the nurse's perspective, a perspective that may or may not be shared by those with whom she interacted.[32] In other words, it is not satisfactory evidence as to whether or not a healthcare encounter has been animated by personal authenticity.

At the risk of being accused of superficiality, I wish to suggest that the way to get around the problem of the will-o'-the-wisp nature of the "genuine" self is once again to approach the problem empirically rather than existentially. Rather than attempting to demonstrate indefinable essences, we should be addressing very definable actions. To use the biblical injunction, by their deeds shall ye know them, and those deeds can be observed and assessed.

This brings us back around to the measurements of caring such as CARE-Q[21] and CARE/SAT,[22] the function of which is to ascertain whether or not healthcare clients believe they have been treated by nurses in a respectful and caring manner. While they may seem prosaic in comparison to the profundities of the self, questions concerning whether clients felt their nurses were prepared to talk to them about their treatment, or whether they responded quickly when called, provide us with clear evidence concerning the authenticity and humaneness of nurse-client interrelations. That clarity, in turn, provides a counterbalance to the data generated by the empirical procedures of EBP, with its exclusive concentration on effectiveness.

 ## The Focus of Ethics

To turn to the last of the patterns of knowing, what I wish to suggest is that Carper's construction of ethics is pitched at such an abstract and nonprescriptive level that it is of limited use in dealing with the issues raised by evidence-based practice. Carper observes that there are no cookbook answers to the manifold, contextually generated moral questions faced by nurses (which implicitly undermines the role of standards of practice as definitive guides). She argues consequently that they will be best prepared to make the moral choices required of them if they have an understanding of ethical codes and of philosophical positions that address what is meant by the good, and what is entailed in the judgment of what is moral. However, she makes no recommendation as to which philosophical positions nurses should concentrate on. The problem with such a liberal position is that it leaves nurses adrift on the stormy seas of moral philosophy, which displays little or no consensus on how to approach its core concept.

The lack of prescription in Carper's description of nurses' ethical knowing does not reflect the fact that nursing knowledge entails very specific ethical assumptions, assumptions that some argue have been violated by what they see as the very mechanistic approach to decision making involved in EBP The moral objection to EBP has been clearly articulated by Mitchell:

> *The very term **evidence** flows from certain assumptions that are not consistent with nursing practices that honor situated freedom, human uniqueness, and client as leader. Nursing's responsibility should be first and foremost to develop and sustain knowledge that honors the client's meanings, realities, possibilities, wishes and choices.[11(p34)]*

While the importance that Mitchell puts upon the uniqueness of the individuals for which nurses care is well-taken, her extrapolation from this that the use of objective evidence is not consistent with the nursing ethic involves a false dichotomy. Most clients' choice is to be cared for by a well-informed practitioner.[33] They want us to be in command of objective evidence because they believe that this will equip us best to help them. This does not negate the client's freedom to choose their modes of care. Deber has identified 2 stages to the process of participative care decisions. The first she terms "problem solving" that "requires that the problem solver have a set of skills and a knowledge base that enable him or her to identify the alternatives and the probability of each outcome."[34(p426)] Clients may or may not have these skills, but practitioners are required to have them. However, knowledge of alternatives does not dictate which actions should be taken. This is decided in the second stage, "decision making," which is the point where clients' wishes and choices come into play in the form of mutually participative discussion. This suggests that we need to conceive of nursing ethics as a combination of the ethics of justice[35] in relation to problem solving and the ethics of care[36] in relation to decision making.

However, identifying the sort of ethics which is appropriate for nurses to adopt is only one stage of the problem. It is also essential that nurses demonstrate through their actions that they adhere to those ethical tenets in practice. We are back to empirics. While the danger of doing violence to the complexities of ethical issues by reducing them to empirical questions is one that should not be underestimated, this does not relieve nurses of the responsibility to make their ethical approaches transparent. Nor is it beyond our ken to develop sensitive and occupation-appropriate tools to enable this. Work by Dierckx de Casterlé et al, for example, has demonstrated the possibility of both combining Kohlberg's ethics of justice with Gilligan's ethics of care[37] and applying the adapted framework empirically to nurses' ethical behavior in practice using both qualitative and quantitative techniques.[38] While we might observe that the model of Dierckx de Casterlé et al is a little too reliant on Kohlberg,[35] and not reliant enough on Gilligan,[36] there is no reason why future theoretical developments could not rectify this imbalance. Indeed, if my arguments are accepted, it is almost an imperative to do so.

To return to the problem of Carper's pattern of ethical knowing, we can draw a number of conclusions from our discussion. First, facing the moral challenge of EBP teaches us that it is not sufficient simply to argue that nurses should be familiar with moral philosophy in the round. Rather, there is a need to focus on and utilize those approaches to moral philosophy that are congruous with the specific ethical concerns of nurses, namely those that help us honor "client's meanings, realities, possibilities, wishes and choices."[11(p34)] Second, there is no necessary contradiction between the use of empirical evidence and the requirement to honor clients' choice. Third, there is a need to make nurses' ethical decisions transparent through empirical interrogation.

Conclusion

The main thrust of this article has been to identify the limitations of Carper's patterns of knowing in nursing that have been exposed by the challenge of evidence-based practice. While critical in nature, I hope it has followed the spirit of Carper's original thesis, which concluded with the following words:

> Every solution to an existing problem raises new and unsolved questions. These new and as yet unsolved problems require, at times, new methods of enquiry and different conceptual structures; they change the shape and patterns of knowing.[1(p22)]

It has been my contention that the "new problem" of EBP requires nurses to change the shape and patterns of knowing to respond to the challenge it represents. The challenge involves its threat to reduce nursing knowledge to a very narrow form of empirics. The power of the challenge lies in the consonance of EBP with prevailing economic, social and cultural trends. In terms of culture, EBP's claim to provide transparent evidence that is open to all, chimes well with the public's increasing distrust of esoteric professional expertise. In contrast, claims that esthetic, ethical and personal knowing are, to greater or lesser degrees, unamenable to scrutiny, means that they fall foul of public expectations for transparent and accountable healthcare. This is an increasingly untenable position for nursing to adopt.

My response to this problem has been to advocate the insertion of empirics into the three other patterns of knowing. In relation to esthetics, I have argued that, to the extent that "what does this mean?" is the key question for this pattern, qualitative research techniques have a major role to play in uncovering the meanings held by nurses and clients. As far as personal knowing is concerned, it is my contention that attempts to make the "genuine self" transparent are doomed to failure. Rather than trying to do so, it is more fruitful to concentrate on how the authenticity of nurses is manifest in practice. Apropos ethics, once again, I argue that this can best be assessed by examining the actions nurses take as a consequence of their ethical decisions.

At this point I should make it clear what I am not saying. I am not claiming that ethical, personal, and esthetic knowing should be replaced by empirics, or even that they should be reparsed into the language of empirics. Still less do I advocate foisting EBP upon them. With the exception of esthetics, where I have argued that some of what has previously gone under its rubric lies better within the domain of qualitative empirical knowledge, this has not been about attempting to reduce or undermine nonempirical patterns. The very important contribution to nursing knowledge these patterns can make, using their own logic and procedures, is accepted. But empirics are needed to show clearly what that contribution is, and where it is missing.

Rather than advocating evidence-based practice, my argument might be described as promoting practice-based evidence. By this I mean that while nonempirical patterns of knowing animate practice, the fact that they do can be established only by empirical means. The role of empirics, then, is demonstrative rather than determinative.

The whole argument here has been cast in rather negative tones, portraying the need to demonstrate empirically the effects of nonempirical patterns of knowing as arising from the challenge of EBP empiricism. But it can be cast in a far more favorable light.

If we aspire to mutually respectful, egalitarian relationships with our clients, then part of that contract involves a requirement for us to be transparent in our dealings with them. The overarching role of demonstrative empirics is to provide such transparency. The accountability that it entails can help us improve the quality of our care, and that in the end is what it is all about.

REFERENCES

1. Carper B. Fundamental patterns of knowing in nursing. *ANS Adv Nurs Sci.* 1978;1(1):13–23.
2. Jacobs-Kramer M, Chinn P. Perspectives on knowing: a model of nursing knowledge. *Sch Inq Nurs Pract.* 1988;2(2):129–144.
3. Stein K, Corte C, Colling K, Whall A. A theoretical analysis of Carper's ways of knowing using a model of social cognition. *Sch Inq Nurs Pract.* 1998;12(1):43–60.
4. Fawcett J, Watson J, Neuman B, Walker P, Fitzpatrick J. On nursing theories and evidence. *Image J Nurs Sch.* 2001;33(2):115–119.
5. White J. Patterns of knowing: review, critique, and update. *ANS Adv Nurs Sci.* 1995;17(4):73–86.
6. Holmes D, Perron A, O'Byrne P. Evidence, virulence, and the disappearance of nursing knowledge: a critique of the evidence-based dogma. *Worldviews Evid Based Nur.* 2006;3(3):95–102.
7. Sackett D, Rosenburg W, Gray J, Haynes R, Richardson W. Evidence-based medicine: what it is and what it isn't. *BMJ.* 1996;312:71–72.
8. Ingersoll G. Evidence-based nursing: what it is and what it isn't. *Nurs Outlook.* 2000;48:151–152.
9. Porter S, O'Halloran P. The postmodernist war on evidence-based practice. *Int J Nurs Stud.* 2009;46:740–748.
10. Mills CW. *The Sociological Imagination.* London, England: Oxford University Press; 1959.

11. Mitchell G. Evidence-based practice: critique and alternative view. *Nurs Sci Q.* 1999;12(1):30–35.

12. Holmes D, Roy B, Perron A. The use of postcolonialism in the nursing domain: colonial patronage, conversion, and resistance. *ANS Adv Nurs Sci.* 2008;31(1):42–51.

13. Koerner JG. Imagining the future for nursing administration and systems research. In: Rolfe G, ed. *Research, Truth, Authority: Postmodern Perspectives on Nursing.* London, England: Macmillan Press Ltd; 2000:133–147.

14. Lyotard J-F. *The Postmodern Condition: A Report on Knowledge.* Manchester, England: Manchester University Press; 1984.

15. Manias E, Street A. Legitimation of nurses' knowledge through policies and protocols in clinical practice. *J Adv Nurs.* 2000;32(6):1467–1475.

16. Muir Gray J. Evidence-based public health. In: Trinder L, Reynolds S, eds. *Evidence-Based Practice: A Critical Appraisal.* Oxford, England: Blackwell; 2000:89–110.

17. Schlesinger M. A loss of faith: the sources of reduced political legitimacy for the American medical profession. *Milbank Q.* 2002;80(2):185–235.

18. Traynor M. The oil crisis, risk and evidence-based practice. *Nurs Inq.* 2002;9(3):162–169.

19. Trinder L. Introduction: the context of evidence-based practice. In: Trinder L, Reynolds S, eds. *Evidence-Based Practice: A Critical Appraisal.* Oxford, England: Blackwell; 2000:1–16.

20. Watson J. Introduction. In: Watson J, ed. *Assessing and Measuring Caring in Nursing and Health Science.* New York, NY: Springer Publishing Co; 2002:3–10.

21. Larson P. Comparison of cancer patients' and professional nurses' perceptions of important nurse caring behaviors. *Heart Lung.* 1987;16(2):187–193.

22. Larson P, Ferketich S. Patients' satisfaction with nurses' caring during hospitalization. *West J Nurs Res.* 1993;15(6):690–703.

23. Weitz M. The role of theory in aesthetics. *JAAC.* 1956;15:27–35.

24. Mantzoukas S. A review of evidence-based practice, nursing research, and reflection: levelling the hierarchy. *J Clin Nurs.* 2008;17:214–223.

25. Pearson A, Wiechula R, Court A, Lockwood C. The JBI model of evidence-based healthcare. *Int JEvid Based Healthc.* 2005;3(8):207–216.

26. Noyes J, Popay J, Pearson A, Hannes K, Booth A. Qualitative research and Cochrane reviews. In: Higgins J, Green S, eds. *Cochrane Handbook for Systematic Reviews of Interventions, Version 5.0.0.* London: The Cochrane Collaboration; 2008. Sections 20–20.6.7, http://www.cochrane-handbook.org.

27. Higgins J, Green S, eds. *Cochrane Handbook for Systematic Reviews of Interventions, Version 5.0.0.* London: The Cochrane Collaboration; 2008. Sections 20-20.6.7, http://www.cochrane-handbook.org.

28. Putnam H. *Pragmatism: An Open Question.* Oxford, England: Blackwell; 1995.

29. Bhaskar R. *The Possibility of Naturalism: A Philosophical Critique of the Contemporary Human Sciences.* 3rd ed. London, England: Routledge; 1998.

30. Porter S, Kelly C. Bronzino's allegory of "Venus and Cupid": an exemplary image for contemporary sexual health promotion? *Int J STD AIDS.* 2009; 20:726–731.

31. Porter S. On the antiquity of evidence-based midwifery and its discontents [Editorial]. *Evid Based Midwifery.* 2009;7(1):3.

32. Gadamer H-G. *Truth and Method.* New York, NY: Continuum; 2004.

33. Neuberger J. Primary care: core values. Patients' priorities. *BMJ.* 1998;317:260–262.

34. Deber R. Physicians in healthcare management: 8. The patient-physician partnership: decision making, problem solving, and the desire to participate. *CMAJ.* 1994;151(4):423–427.

35. Kohlberg L. *Essays on Moral Development, Vol I. The Philosophy of Moral Development: Moral Stages and the Idea of Justice.* San Francisco, CA: Harper and Row; 1981.

36. Gilligan C. *In a Different Voice: Psychological Theory and Women's Development.* Cambridge, MA: Harvard University Press; 1982.

37. Dierckx de Casterlé B, Roelens A, Gastmans C. An adjusted version of Kohlberg's moral theory: discussion of its validity for research in nursing ethics. *J Adv Nurs.* 1998;27:829–835.

38. Dierckx de Casterlé B, Grypdonck M, Cannaerts N, Steeman E. Empirical ethics in action: lessons from two empirical studies in nursing ethics. *Med Health Care Philos.* 2004;7(1):31–39.

THE AUTHOR COMMENTS

Fundamental Patterns of Knowing in Nursing: The Challenge of Evidence-Based Practice

This article emerged from my concern about the increasing gulf between theoretically-oriented and empirically-oriented nursing, which is reflected in the differences of opinion expressed about the benefits of otherwise evidence-based practice. My basic belief and the basic premise of this paper can be summed up in the Kantian aphorism that experience without theory is blind, but theory without experience is mere intellectual play. On the one hand, I accept that evidence-based practice's marginalization of other patterns of knowing has the capacity to subvert the basic tenets of nursing. On the other hand, I argue that those very patterns are weakened by the fact that there is little empirical evidence of their effectiveness. My tentative solution is to propose the development of practice-based evidence that uses empirics to demonstrate the contribution of esthetic, personal, and ethical knowing to the optimization of nursing care.

SAM PORTER

Knowledge Development and Evidence-Based Practice: Insights and Opportunities from a Postcolonial Feminist Perspective for Transformative Nursing Practice

SHERYL REIMER-KIRKHAM, RN, PhD

JENNIFER L. BAUMBUSCH, RN, PhD

ANNETTE S. H. SCHULTZ, RN, PhD

JOAN M. ANDERSON, RN, PhD

Although not without its critics, evidence-based practice is widely espoused as supporting professional nursing practice. Engaging with the evidence-based practice discourse from a vantage point offered by the critical perspectives of postcolonial feminism, the incomplete epistemologies and limitations of the standardization characteristic of the evidences-based movement are analyzed. Critical analysis of evidence is suggested, such that it recognizes the evidence generated from multiple paradigms of inquiry, along with contextual interpretation and application of this evidence. We examine how broader interpretations of evidence might contribute to nursing knowledge development and translation for transformative professional nursing practice, and ultimately to address persistent health disparities within the complex context of healthcare delivery.

Nursing knowledge development is largely understood as generating the evidence required for professional nursing practice. Evidence-based practice (EBP) is currently the primary approach to knowledge uptake for professional practice, and is believed to support efficiency and ensure that practice decisions result in the provision of effective treatment.[1,2] Best practices based on sound research-based evidence are undisputedly needed given the complexity of today's healthcare environments, with their reliance on rapidly evolving technology, corporate priorities with a focus on efficiencies, and diverse sociopolitical milieus characteristic of the broader society.[3] However, there have been wide-ranging critiques of EBP, from concern with the definition and breadth of evidence, to how this approach erodes the autonomy of nursing practice.[4–8]

In this article, we engage with the EBP discourse from another vantage point—that offered by critical perspectives such as postcolonial feminism (PCF)—with the aim of examining how this interpretation of evidence might contribute to knowledge development

and translation for transformative nursing practice, and ultimately to address persistent health disparities within the complex context of healthcare delivery. This effort is not to replace the current discourse on evidence, but rather to add another dimension or analytic perspective. Our interest is both epistemological and pragmatic, as we question: "What is evidence?" "How might evidence be conceptualized within different paradigms of inquiry?" "Can different conceptualizations of evidence complement one another?" Driving these questions is a pragmatic concern that traditional notions of evidence, based in Western science, may not sufficiently address the types of deep-rooted factors underlying health disparities, such as poverty and material life circumstances, nor fully account for the complexities of people's everyday lives that ultimately shape health and illness to a significant extent. For example, we have put forward the argument[9,10] that it is not "culture" in some narrow sense that organizes the ways in which people manage an illness, but rather the complex mediating circumstances

From S.R. Kirkham, J.L. Baumbusch, A.S.H. Schultz, and J.M. Anderson, Knowledge development and evidence-based practice: Insights and opportunities from a postcolonial feminist perspective for transformative nursing practice. Advances in Nursing Science, 2007, 30(1), 26–40.

ABOUT THE AUTHORS

SHERYL REIMER-KIRKHAM is an Associate Professor in the School of Nursing at Trinity Western University, Langley, where she is the Director of the graduate nursing (MSN) program and teaches Health Care Ethics, Health Policy, and Qualitative Research. With her roots and early nursing career in Winnipeg, she completed her post-RN BSN at the University of Victoria and her MSN and PhD at University of British Columbia. She was awarded a 2010 Award of Excellence in Nursing Research by the College of Registered Nurses of British Columbia (CRNBC). Her research program focuses on pluralism, health inequities, and social justice in healthcare and nursing education. With colleagues, she has explored applications of postcolonial feminism and other critical theories to nursing scholarship. Her current funded research project examines religion, spirituality, culture, gender, and place in home healthcare. She is a founding member of TWU's Religion in Canada Institute and Institute of Gender Studies, and the Critical Research in Health and Health Inequities Unit at University of British Columbia.

JENNIFER L. BAUMBUSCH is an Assistant Professor at the School of Nursing, University of British Columbia (UBC). Jennifer's background is in gerontological nursing, and she has held a variety of roles in nursing administration, education, and practice in this area. Since beginning her doctoral studies in 2002, Jennifer has been engaged in an exploration of participatory approaches to knowledge translation. Her doctoral dissertation was a critical ethnography in long-term residential care. Jennifer has been supported during her doctoral studies by the Elizabeth Kenny McCann Doctoral Award, a Killam Doctoral Award, and a Canadian Institutes of Health Research (CIHR) Canada Graduate Scholarship Doctoral Award.

ANNETTE S. H. SCHULTZ is an Assistant Professor at the University of Manitoba, Faculty of Nursing. Her career as a nurse, spanning more than 20 years, has included working clinically in direct patient care positions, conducting policy research focused on the practice of newly graduated RNs for the College of Registered Nurses in British Columbia, and conducting tobacco control research. Her research primarily focuses on tobacco control in the context of healthcare, which draws on her mixed-methods dissertation study on the nurses' role in tobacco control. Future work will include focusing on patients' experiences of tobacco control during healthcare interaction, specifically while in hospitals with "smoke-free grounds" policies. Additionally, future work will explore individual and contextual factors influencing practitioners' engagement in addressing tobacco use. She is a Mentor with the CIHR Strategic Training Program in Tobacco Research and an alumni member of NEXUS: Researching the Social Context of Health Behaviour at the University of British Columbia.

JOAN M. ANDERSON is a health and social scientist. She received a bachelor's degree in nursing from McGill University, and a masters of science in nursing, and a PhD in sociology both from the University of British Columbia. Dr. Anderson is Professor Emerita at the University of British Columbia. Funded by the Canadian Institutes of Health Research (CIHR) and the Social Sciences and Humanities Research Council of Canada (SSHRC), she has conducted extensive research in the areas of culture, gender, migration, health, and inequities in health and healthcare through the lens of postcolonial inquiry and, more recently, critical humanism. She has engaged in knowledge translation research with health professionals at the point of care, administrators, and policy makers. A commitment to social justice in health and healthcare, the mentoring of colleagues and graduate students locally and nationally, writing, knowledge translation and other forms of dissemination of research, and consultation remain important dimensions of her active scholarship. In her spare moments, she enjoys the outdoors.

of their lives. Certain interpretations and use of EBP tend to turn our attention away from these social factors to focus on individualistic models of health with biomedical solutions,[11] in effect bypassing complex problems. Indeed, such complexities may well require that evidence derived from multiple sources, through various modes of inquiry, be considered to support clinical practice.

We begin our engagement with EBP discourses by providing an overview of EBP, and the critiques leveled against it. We then employ the theoretical perspective of PCF as a point of engagement with the EBP movement. Finally, drawing on our programs of research, we apply these insights to a discussion of the reciprocal processes of knowledge development and knowledge translation that serve as a foundation for the transformative knowledge necessary to support professional nursing practice, with the contention that multiple forms of intersecting and complementary evidence are required to address current complexities in health and healthcare.

 ## Précis of Critical Questions About Evidence-Based Practice

The evolution of the EBP movement within healthcare has taken place over the last 3 decades. Reflecting its roots in evidence-based medicine, as envisioned by Sackett,[12]* nursing's equivalent of EBP has been defined as "the integration of best research evidence with clinical expertise and patient values to facilitate clinical decision-making."[13(p4)] Underlying this beginning was the belief that epidemiological and statistical research findings could be useful for influencing the effectiveness of clinical practice.[5,6] The reflection of this origin is present in EBP tools today; for instance, best

practice guidelines usually display a set of criteria—strongly favoring evidence from random clinical trials (RCTs) over other studies[14,15]—regarding validity of research findings.

In tandem with the evolution of EBP, we have witnessed a rise in concern about economics and the costs of healthcare. This concern has resulted in the goal of providing efficient care, in that decisions about healthcare practice often require a cost-benefit analysis component, yet how we define "benefit" is not always clear. Healthcare management's adoption of EBP processes has been used to support resource allocation decisions.[2,7] Economic restrictions have resulted in shifts toward decentralization of governance and the subsequent requirement for management tools related to clinical practice decisions.[4] Therefore, while ensuring that professional practice is based on the latest scientific evidence, the evolution and adoption of the EBP movement has also supported economic restrictions and decentralization of governance, which rests on the values of *effectiveness, efficiency,* and *standardization* of care. As we argue later in the article, we are not quarreling with these notions, *but rather in their interpretation and use,* particularly when these concepts are used as recipes, without attentiveness to context. Although we would all support the notion of efficient care, the complexity of this concept is often overlooked. For care to be efficient, it has to be effective, and for care to be effective, it means that it has to be appropriate to the context.

Nursing, along with other healthcare professionals, has been faced with integrating this approach to EBP into care delivery. The push toward adopting EBP within nursing has met with critical questions; here, we highlight three interrelated positions within the academic dialogue that are particularly germane to our engagement, later in this article, with EBP.

The first position, articulating an epistemological concern, focuses on the limited view of nursing knowledge characteristic of EBP. It is argued that EBP, with its reliance on RCTs and systematic reviews, provides limited guidance to critically consider evidence from the diversity of research methodologies found within nursing literature and other related disciplines relevant for nursing practice.[6,14] Furthermore, other sources of knowing such as personal experience or expert knowledge are de-emphasized in clinical decision making, yet nurses clearly rely on knowledge beyond that which can be empirically verifiable.[16] Included in these "ways of knowing" are Carper's[17] personal, aesthetic, and ethical knowledge. Representing these types of concerns, nurse scholars have argued that the very nature of nursing as relational practice does not lend itself to "highly rationalized frameworks of perception, let alone intervention."[7(p151)]

---

*Sackett defined *evidence-based medicine* as "the conscientious, explicit, and judicious use of current best evidence in making decisions about the care of individual patients. The practice of evidence-based medicine means integrating individual clinical expertise with the best available external clinical evidence from systematic research. By individual clinical expertise, we mean the proficiency and judgment that individual clinicians acquire through clinical experience and clinical practice. Increased expertise is reflected in many ways, but especially in more effective and efficient diagnosis and in the more thoughtful identification and compassionate use of individual patients' predicaments, rights, and preferences in making clinical decisions about their care. By best available external clinical evidence, we mean clinically relevant research, often from the basic sciences of medicine, but especially from patient-centered clinical research into the accuracy and precision of diagnostic tests (including the clinical examination), the power of prognostic markers, and the efficacy and safety of therapeutic, rehabilitative, and preventive regimens."[12(p71)]

The second position raised in nursing literature relates to concerns about the translation of research findings into practice[5] and the relevance of research studies, especially RCTs, which control contextual factors that might be influencing the variable being studied. There is concern that applying context-stripped findings to a context-rich clinical setting makes the application irrelevant. For example, a clinical guideline for pain management may be of limited usefulness when the contexts in which pain occurs are not explored.[16] Underlying such a concern is the ongoing debate regarding the application of evidence to particular or individual circumstances, given the inferential mechanisms of evidential knowledge by which particularities (eg, individual variations) have been averaged out.[16] Research studies, such as random control studies, result in an ability to predict a specific behavior or treatment outcome at a population level. However, what they do not tend to provide is a complete explanation of a behavior or treatment outcome, in particular, an integration of individual variations or contextual factors.

The final position raises concern in relation to nurses' professional practice. Given the complexity of nurses' work environment, nurses need to acquire information or evidence from sources, such as philosophic or aesthetic knowledge, other than research findings to support professional practice.[18] The concern stated here is that EBP tools do not acknowledge or address the reality of nurses' work environment, and so will have, at best, limited utility. Barnes,[4] for example, raises the possibility that this limited utility could well result in the erosion of nurses' autonomy and authority within their current scope of practice. The concern then is that if the practice expectations defined within an evidence-based tool become the norm for practice, these tools will begin to reshape nurses' work. Notably, other scholars[19] tell us that EBP has been embraced within the health professions as a means to improve professional status by making visible their "scientific" knowledge base. These critical issues highlight the complexity of bringing together a narrow view of evidence, such as that traditionally advocated for by EBP, with the realities of nursing practice. While we offer our own critical analysis of EBP later in this article, our response to this concern regarding the erosion of professional practice puts forward a somewhat different interpretation; another way of looking at this is that these tools, in and of themselves, do not address the complexity of patients' lives. We would argue that it not EBP, per se, that risks eroding nurses' autonomy. Rather, autonomy is eroded if nurses use evidence as recipes, without drawing on their professional knowledge and clinical judgment to interpret evidence, and make decisions about *best evidence* in context—this is the core of professional practice.

In summary, although healthcare systems and the profession of nursing have adopted EBP, there are philosophical and practical concerns regarding how EBP is used to guide professional nursing practice. Proponents of EBP refute these concerns as ill-founded misconceptions, and argue that when correctly operationalized, EBP integrates the best research evidence (derived by various research methods) with clinical expertise and patient values to facilitate decision making, implying a thoughtful and critical use of knowledge.[13] Given the complexity of practice and the persistent presence of health disparities, we contend that although the EBP perspective has considerable merit, different ways of looking at evidence are nonetheless needed, not to jettison the work that has been done, but rather to broaden the scope of how evidence is constructed. Furthermore, we would stress that a key issue relates to how nurses interpret and use evidence. The problem arises when evidence is seen as driving clinical decision making, rather than as a tool to be used by the professional nurse as he or she assesses, and makes decisions about best practices within a given context. PCF, we suggest, offers one framework that might help to further our understandings of evidence and EBP. We suggest that rather than replacing evidence generated from a scientific perspective, PCF complements EBP by enriching contextual understandings, and underscoring professional responsibility and accountability to use this knowledge to work toward equitable healthcare for all people. As such, it provides another angle on doing science that reframes our ways of constructing what counts as evidence.

A Postcolonial Feminist Reading of Evidence-Based Practice

Postcolonial theory, joining other critical social theories that have at their core the analysis of relations of power, represents a broad based and rapidly expanding domain of scholarship. Said to have originated in the 1960s and 1970s, led by the influential work of anti-colonial scholars such as Frantz Fanon[20] and Edward Said's *Orientalism*,[21] postcolonial theory deals with the relations and aftermath of the colonial period and ongoing neocolonialism characterized by oppressive tactics, economic and cultural hegemonies, and totalizing global expansions. Postcolonial feminist theory and black feminist theory, particularly that of scholars such as Patricia Hill Collins,[22] bell hooks,[23] Toni Morrison,[24] and Rose Brewer,[25] direct attention to multiple intersecting oppressions, inclusive of gender, class, and *race* oppression to reveal the multiple dimensions of oppression within societies, and the unequal effects of racism on certain groups of people (eg, women and children). Feminist theory also contributes sustained critique of issues of identity, voice and difference, and the politics of representation; and the articulation of clear methodological direction for both research and practice.

A growing body of nursing scholarship informed by postcolonial feminist theories provides rich analyses of the historical, economic, cultural, and social dynamics at play within healthcare (see, for instance, references 9, 10, 26–34) and demonstrate the salience of these perspectives for nursing scholarship. These works not only attempt to examine the complex intersections between different social relations that have a profound impact on the experiencing of health and illness but also hold up to scrutiny taken-for-granted assumptions about different ethnocultural communities. Indeed, like Ahmad,[35] these scholars challenge notions of culture as static and determining, and draw attention, instead, to the context in which cultural meanings are constructed, to issues of racialization, systemic racism, and other forms of oppression. Perhaps, most important, no one form of oppression is privileged, but there is the continuous search to understand how intersections operate in everyday life, and in everyday social encounters. This growing postcolonial feminist scholarship builds on earlier integration of critical theories such as feminist and antiracist theories into nursing, as exemplified by Allen et al,[36] Barbee,[37] Campbell and Bunting,[38] and Webb,[39] and shares the agenda of other nurse scholars committed to pursing social justice through critical analyses of how the social construct of race is employed.[40–44]

Postcolonial feminist theory, with its cogent critique of oppressive structures that tend toward standardization, representation of majority view, and erasing of experiences of racialization, classism, sexism, ageism, and homophobia, expands EBP's scientific discourses to be inclusive of various social relations, and in doing so transforms our notions of science. As both academics and practitioners, we have grappled with the application of postcolonial feminist perspectives to practice, and, in particular, to current management discourses and practices. Recognizing the entrenchment or perhaps the inevitability of these discourses and mechanisms, we seek to examine critically current EBP discourses, and offer alternative interpretations that might equip healthcare workers for professional practice and assist in the creation of practice environments that nurture such practice. In doing so, we are working toward opening up spaces for an enriched dialogue regarding evidence as it is generated and applied in practice, with the understanding that EBP itself is not a single entity but rather can be taken up in various ways to support professional practice.

In our effort to reappraise EBP, we join together the deconstructive and constructive imperatives of postcolonial feminist theorizing. PCF approaches are disruptive and resistive in their primary intent, seeking to uncover theoretical, moral, and political inadequacies through lenses of race, class, gender, age, sexual orientation, and other forms of oppression. Simultaneously, the PCF project opens up new sites for the legitimation of currently delegitimated knowledge,[45] and offers new possibilities for professional practice within current practice environments that have become increasingly restrictive. Salient to our discussion here are those features of PCF that hold up for scrutiny of epistemological claims that derive from and maintain the hegemonic center (in this case, the Western center). Equally valuable in the tenets of postcolonial feminist theorizing is the attention to power relations along a shifting and intersecting variety of axes, including race, religion, gender, and class. Our critique focuses on 3 themes made visible through the PCF lens: the problem of incomplete epistemologies; the shortcomings of uncritical standardization; and the everyday realities of race, class, gender, age, and sexual orientation as they operate within contexts of EBP. Together these themes point to the need for a shift toward a more inclusive, reciprocal approach to knowledge development and uptake.

Incomplete Epistemologies as the Basis for Evidence-Based Practice

A PCF reading reveals how the knowledge upon which EBP is based can, unwittingly, be racialized, gendered, ageist, classist, and homophobic. Notably, a PCF lens does not mean one sets out to criticize science itself, rather we raise questions about *how* science is practiced by those who conduct and fund research to perpetuate racialized, classed, and gendered approaches to study design. Furthermore, we are not arguing against empirical knowledge as foundational to professional practice, but do caution against segregating science from the humanities and social sciences in our knowledge generation and application.

Randomized clinical trials (RCTs) serve as the criterion standard of evidence for EBP.[14,15] However, for various reasons such as the complication of seeking interpretive services and the ethical implications of conducting research with people who might be vulnerable for a variety of reasons, researchers have traditionally conducted RCTs with the most accessible dominant majority populations. Yet, the findings of these studies have routinely been generalized as though they represent a universal experience.[11] Similarly, many of the research instruments, interview questions, and tools used today have been developed by and for the majority population and therefore may not capture the experiences of those marginalized within mainstream society.[11,46] Furthermore, the types of research questions that gain funding have traditionally been reflective of the interests of the dominant majority (eg, cardiovascular disease in white men) rather than the needs of groups that have been marginalized. According to a study by the Global Forum for Health Research, health research continues to reflect the priorities of the rich, with 90% of research funding investigating the diseases of 10% of the world's population.[47] Moreover, current values in the scientific community see the favoring of efficient research approaches that require homogeneous study populations, consequently excluding those who find themselves on the margins.[11,46]

The inclusion in our research of social groups that have been marginalized is an important step in developing knowledge to support nursing practice. However, inclusion alone is not sufficient—the nature of our questions, the research methods we use, and the theoretical lenses informing research carry considerable importance in the types of knowledge that result. Meleis and Im[46] observe that while nursing scholarship has moved to study diverse ethnocultural populations, a culturalist and relativist approach has resulted in knowledge that remains essentialist and incomplete through the application of dichotomous thinking that constructs difference as irrevocable and acontextual. They explain,

> By dividing into dichotomies, we may be maintaining categories that have historically defined each culture and each gender. Dichotomies such as male/female, immigrant/nonimmigrant, and African American/Euro-American have helped us to value interstice patterns and responses, but the dichotomies may be preventing us from recognizing the socio-political forces that inhibit us from changing the status quo.[46(p96)]

To counter these historically embedded incomplete epistemologies, a shift in research agendas is needed, such that researchers not only study cultural knowledge but also situate such knowledge against the historically bound and contextually situated processes and effects of marginalization.

A growing body of evidence from across the globe demonstrates that social inequities in health are widespread, both within and between countries. Whitehead et al[48] note that overall gains in a nation's health frequently mask significant and worsening health outcomes for some population groups (often along lines of gender, geographic region, ethnicity, or socioeconomic characteristics). Many of the causes of inequities in health are social in origin, reflecting income and education disparities, differential exposure to health hazards, and systematic variations in life opportunities

for healthy lifestyle or reasonable access to essential goods and services. As Whitehead et al [48(p313)] explain, "Individual lifestyles are embedded in social and community networks, and in living and working conditions, which in turn are related to the wider cultural and socioeconomic model." How is this convincing body of evidence regarding the crucial influence of social determinants of health taken up in the realm of health policy and healthcare services, including at the point of care? Is this type of evidence amenable to the heavily relied upon tools of EBP? Kemm is cautious in the application of the EBP model to public health policy:

> Taking communities rather than individuals as the unit of intervention and the importance of context means that frequently randomized controlled trials are not appropriate for study of **public health** interventions. Further, the notion of a "best solution" ignores the complexity of the decision making process. **Evidence** "enlightens" policy makers shaping how policy problems are framed rather than providing the answer to any particular problem.[49(p319)]

From a PCF perspective, then, the mediating circumstances of what are often referred to as the "social determinants of health" need to be integrated into our nursing knowledge. This inclusion is particularly urgent in the area of culture and health. Given the rise in diversity and the implications this diversity carries for healthcare delivery, considerable nursing scholarship energy has been invested in describing various cultural beliefs and practices, with the hope of improving healthcare services, and, in turn, health outcomes, for ethnocultural communities. Yet, this focus on the individual as a member of a circumscribed cultural group often overlooks the evidence offered by population-based studies pointing to the root causes of health disparities. Put another way, our knowledge development and concomitant knowledge uptake need to extend beyond "culture" per se as a static determinant of health, to account for the complex intersectionalities with the social, historical, economic, and political forces, in determining health and health outcomes. The individual experience must be linked to the social context.

How this accounting of social determinants of health is accomplished is fraught with its own set of challenges. Deriving from a Western empiricist paradigm reliant on operationalization and measurement of discrete variables, health and social sciences have for some time used race as a variable of study, citing the possibility of identifying, tracking, and eliminating health disparities as reason to do so. Yet, race as a biological category has been contested, and, by and large, discounted as a biologically based and meaningful category. In its place, race has been recast as fluid and socially constructed, varying across time and place as a function of historical circumstance.[50] This latter line of argument resonates with the postcolonial feminist conception of race that acknowledges the salience of the term, not in a reified or essentialized fashion, but as a signifier of social relations. While the collection of health statistics by ethnicity continues, and increases in some contexts,[51] the concurrent trend to identifying more specific indicators for health disparities studies stands to offer improved explanatory capacity regarding the mechanisms behind health disparities. Estroff and Henderson explain,

> When factors such as individual lifestyle and behaviours, cultural beliefs, physiologic measures, geographical location, insurance coverage, education, and income are included in studies, the remaining health differences may be attributed to the effects of racial bias or discrimination.[50(p19)]

Underlying such racial bias/discrimination is the context of broader historic and contemporary social and economic inequality. A PCF reading of EBP thus, necessarily, warns against this type of operationalization of variables such as race (and its metonym, ethnicity).[42] Where race is adopted uncritically as an indicator or a variable, the "evidence" derived may contribute to policy and practice that focuses once again solely on the individual, suggesting in effect that cultural difference accounts for variations in the experience of health and illness. In the process, the scientific use of these social categories inadvertently reinscribes the predominant social approach to racializing groups of people by color or ethnic affiliation.[52] Instead, the nature of evidence needed is that which makes visible the *social* pathways that lead to health disparities.

Future research enterprise, thus, must seek a new level of rigor in conceptualization, expanding research to incorporate the role of power in knowledge development through theoretical frameworks that carry the capacity to uncover injustice and marginalization.[46]

The Limitations of Standardization in the Applications of Evidence-Based Practice

At the level of the pragmatic, a PCF lens also draws our attention to some potential shortcomings stemming from EBP's move toward standardization of patient care, in effect extending the general critique of acontextual application of research findings. By strictly

or uncritically adhering to the tools that bring EBP into practice (clinical pathways, best practice guidelines), rich contextual issues that influence patients' experiences as they move through the healthcare system may be stripped away (eg, important factors that may influence a patient's ability to successfully recover from an acute episode may be overlooked). Thus, while tools such as care maps provide a beginning point for guiding practice, their usefulness is dependent to a large degree upon the nurse's professional judgment based on knowledge of science and the social context of people's lives.

One of the challenges of these tools is the tension between supporting standardization of practice and the corporate agenda versus supporting critical thinking regarding practice decisions.[4, 8, 19, 53] Standardization can support and strengthen a profession's claim to legitimacy as indicated earlier, but it also lays the groundwork for external controls, the imposition of which, suggest Timmerman and Berg,[19] are the very antithesis of professional autonomy and power. Approaching this issue from another vantage point, a PCF lens prompts consideration of the embeddedness of EBP in current organizational discourses, and envisions ways to resist the associated *colonizing* possibilities. Organizational theory has been acknowledged, indeed promoted, as being distinctly Western, with its bent toward expansionism, managerialism, and rationalism.[54] In efforts to foster the development of organizational theory as legitimate "science," proponents have drawn on Enlightenment assumptions of universalism to establish management practices that would apply in all contexts, not unlike "natural law." Building on gender analyses that have unveiled the masculinist propensities of organizational theory, and the falsity of representing organizations as gender and race neutral,[55] a PCF lens offers unique analytic leverage in making visible the influence of *empire* on contemporary ways of knowing and being in the arena of organizational practices. PCF scholars have gone as far as to typify today's organizational practices as "colonial regimes."[56] The deconstructive imperative of postcolonial critique, thus, provides an angle of analysis from the margins as to how managerial concepts such as EBP tend to be taken up as neutral uncontested categories in organizational theory. To hold such concepts up for scrutiny becomes an important contribution, particularly as we ask "who is privileged or advantaged by management practices such as EBP?"

A PCF lens raises questions about when such standardization serves as a force for social justice (eg, in ensuring that all receive equitable care based on empirical knowledge for best practice), and when standardization becomes a force for inequities as its homogenizing bent writes out group histories and individual identities. On the one hand, several authors have argued on behalf of EBP as a mechanism to ensure equitable healthcare for all by the merit of an objective application of "best practices" to all clients, regardless of group affiliation and a healthcare provider's potential propensity to discrimination.[57] On the other hand, the contingencies and particularities, all imbued with relations of power, exposed by postcolonial feminist and other critical theories stand in contrast to the standardization of EBP.[53] To treat all as equals risks the real chance of inequitable treatment where the unique qualities and life circumstances of certain people continue to be overlooked. A postcolonial feminist analysis of EBP, then, while not debunking the notion of EPB, would advocate critical reflection on the concept of "evidence" and the context of people's lives in which such evidence would be used. From a PCF perspective, we bring into focus multiple forms of evidence from different paradigms of inquiry.

To counter the epistemic violence that results from generic applications of incomplete knowledge, a shift is needed as to how evidence itself is established, the types of evidence valued within the clinical setting, and subsequently how evidence is applied. Our concern then lies with a culture of standardized clinical decisions based on a larger healthcare environment of managerialism—particularly where EBP becomes a routinized recipe approach to decision making without attentiveness to context, or a management-imposed method of clinical decision making that diminishes nurses' clinical decision-making processes. In this way, the PCF lens picks up cogent critiques of EBP and extends the analyses more specifically to consider *for whom* the standardization might not "fit."

The Obfuscation of Everyday Realities Such as Racism, Sexism, and Classism

The two proceeding concerns regarding incomplete knowledge development and uncritically applied standardization work in tandem to obscure a world of racialized, gendered, ageist, and classed relations within healthcare. To illustrate, our research has uncovered how a politics of belonging is created as the dynamics of racialization and gender oppressions are negotiated in today's healthcare settings,[10] and how the mechanisms of health reform have disproportionately disadvantaged those in minority positions.[9,58] Commonplace racialized assumptions drawn upon within healthcare (eg, that families from certain ethnocultural groups will care for their elderly) result in overlooking the needs of individuals made vulnerable by the mediating circumstances of their lives, and who often do not speak the languages of healthcare (English; medicalized discourse).[9] Societal discourses—typically taken-for-granted—regarding culture, aboriginality

and egalitarianism as professional mandate similarly shape nurses' encounters with First Nations patients to the detriment of respectful care.[59] Women have been the "workhorses" of healthcare as nurses, care aides, frontline managers, rehabilitative specialists, nutritionists, kitchen staff, and cleaners, yet remain underrepresented in current management decisions and structures. White women, in particular, are in ambivalent positions, as they themselves have lost voice in the corporate discourses of today's healthcare management, but have also been complicit in long-standing patterns of racializing practices.

Through a PCF analysis of the EBP movement, we question whether the priorities and practice environments created by EBP foster critical reflection that acknowledges such everyday realities of privilege and disadvantage, oppression and resistance, within healthcare. Clearly, if we want to create spaces for addressing these relations of power, we must carefully consider the types of practice environments created by the agendas of EBP. Likewise, as far as EBP assumes a "standardized patient" in a homogeneous or universalist sense to whom evidence can predictably be applied, a PCF framing alerts us to the possibility of erasure of individual differences and imposition of dominant mainstream ways. For example, where clinical practice guidelines are invaluable in the case management of HIV/AIDS, experiences of urban First Nations women living with HIV/AIDS speak to the profound shortcomings of existing healthcare services and programs in meeting their needs, given the intersecting realities of poverty, gender positioning, and racialization.[60] Without making visible the context of their everyday lives, healthcare services fall short of addressing their particular needs. Such situations require thoughtful practitioners who bring together evidence from a range of knowledge to apply in patient-oriented and context-specific ways. A PCF approach then draws attention to the pragmatics of the everyday and supports the inclusion of transformative knowledge in order to support nursing practice in the current context of healthcare delivery.

Transforming Practice Through Knowledge Development and Translation: Insights and Opportunities from a Postcolonial Feminist Perspective

In this final section, we consider in further detail the implications of the insights derived through a PCF reading of EBP for knowledge development and knowledge translation, both of which are foundational to transforming nursing practice. What are the lessons we might take from a PCF critique of the current EBP movement for application to knowledge translation efforts? Can the divergent epistemologies of EBP and PCF be brought together in a complementary alignment to expand our sources of evidence upon which to base practice? Some nurse scholars who critique EBP distance themselves from its applications. Given the widespread adoption of EBP, we look for ways to constructively engage with the evidence-based movement, with the assertion that PCF offers another angle by which to understand evidence, thereby enriching the possibilities for knowledge development and translation that open spaces for transformative practice. In this way, we hope to contribute to the EBP discourses in a manner that encourages critical engagement with the notion of evidence, pushing for an expanded understanding of the types of knowledge needed for clinical decision making.

Anderson explains that transformative knowledge is "under girded by critical consciousness on the part of healthcare providers, and … unmasks unequal relations of power and issues of domination and subordination, based on assumptions about 'race,' 'gender,' and class relations."[61(p205)] We take as a starting point that transformative knowledge for practice is dependent upon the interrelated processes of knowledge development and knowledge translation. In the arena of knowledge development, insights from a postcolonial feminist perspective have brought to light the common claims of representative research-derived generalizable knowledge that is, in reality, based on selective populations that often exclude marginalized populations. Great caution must thus be taken in applying this knowledge in a universalizing sense. In response, a PCF lens calls for the inclusion of subjugated knowledge in our knowledge development processes. In addition, the need for empirical evidence to provide a better understanding of the mechanisms of health disparities is also emphasized through a postcolonial feminist analysis of EBP, such that the broader intersecting forces impinging on life opportunities necessary for health—including access to education, housing, income, social networks, and healthcare resources—are identified and addressed. Expanded research agendas will be necessary to fill these gaps.

At its heart, the evidence-based movement draws on a view of science that holds to a hierarchy of evidence that profiles the purported objective, quantifiable outcomes of RCTs, and other measurement-based methods as superior to narrative-based "subjective" methods. Our PCF reading suggests the importance of recognizing the limitations of this trend, and seeking complementary sources of knowledge that bring to light both large-scale phenomena as well as the contingencies and particularities of situated knowledge. We call for what Lather articulates as "a more capacious scientificity of disciplined inquiry."[62(p28)] Such science does not "divest experience of its rich ambiguity because it stays close to the complexities and contradictions of existence."[62(p23)] Notably, an insistence on a broad range of inquiry methods is driven not by allegiance to any methods for the sake of method per se, but rather by recognition of the breadth and depth of knowledge required for transformative practice. That is, a PCF commitment might see research conducted via a range of methodologies, across a range of quantitative and qualitative methods, with the goal of generating knowledge that supports practice in today's complex environments while illuminating the broader social forces (historical, economic, political) that shape how healthcare services are structured and delivered with ultimate implications for health outcomes. Importantly, the call for multiple sources of evidence accumulated in part (giving credence to practice-based and personal knowledge) through a range of disciplined scientific approaches takes a remarkably different stance to knowledge translation, seeing it as an *effort to foster understanding, reflection, and action,* instead of a narrow translation of research into practice.[62]

A postcolonial feminist framing makes clear that narrow applications of procedural knowledge without the incorporation of other ways of knowing and knowledge about the social context of health/illness for the individual healthcare recipient will continue to fall short of providing humanistic, effective, and efficient healthcare. As explained, the EBP movement has largely been taken up in practice through the tools of clinical pathways, best practice guidelines, and care maps. The orthodoxy of EBP suggests a linear approach to clinical decision making; however this is just one way of viewing the applications of professional knowledge. Although some aspects of clinical practice may well be predictable, the complexities of the clinical environment, along with the heterogeneity of people seeking healthcare services, point to the need for a thoughtful practitioner who draws on a variety of knowledge, with the clinical judgment to know *when* and *how* to integrate this knowledge. Moreover, as the feminist perspective cautions against viewing research participants as "objects of study" so too the warning can be taken not to construct the recipients of healthcare as "objects of evidence-based practice." Any efforts at transformative knowledge translation must grapple with this challenge of enhancing nursing practice for individualized, client-appropriate, contextualized care based on the latest knowledge and skill. To illustrate how PCF interpretation of EBP might support transformative nursing practice, we conclude with an example of a knowledge translation project.

Contextualizing Our Position: Reframing Cultural Safety

Providing the impetus for this article and its rereading of the EBP movement is a recently initiated knowledge translation pilot project, *Cultural Safety and Knowledge Uptake in Clinical Settings: A Model for Practice for Culturally Diverse Populations** (nominated principal investigator, J. Anderson funding Canadian Institutes of Health Research), that synthesizes knowledge from the programs of research of a team of investigators in the Culture, Gender, and Health Research Unit at the University of British Columbia (http://www.cghru.nursing.ubc.ca/) and, in a collaborative effort with clinicians, translates this knowledge into practice. Shared themes of these programs of research are culture, social justice, gender, and health, with substantive foci including inequities in access to health and healthcare services; vulnerabilities as structured by various socially constructed classifications (eg, racializing categories and stigmatizing labels) and by certain life transitions and circumstances (eg, poverty, aging, violence, migration, hospitalization, and transition to home); and strategies to reduce inequities and vulnerabilities through innovative approaches to knowledge translation that engage key stakeholders.

Specifically, our exemplar here draws on our experiences in developing and implementing a collaborative approach to knowledge translation (J. Baumbusch et al. unpublished data), grounded in the dialectic between research and practice, in which the integration of transformative knowledge—the reflexive knowledge that makes visible and critiques relations of power operating through social relations and structures, and envisions actions that shift these power relations—leads to transformations in practice. In clinical environments where the language of clinical pathways, best practice guidelines, and care maps predominate, we are exploring how to best incorporate knowledge from this established program of research that has drawn extensively on postcolonial and feminist theories.

The concept of cultural safety, originating in the Maori context of New Zealand, has served as a starting

This knowledge translation study is funded by the Canadian Institutes of Health Research (2005–2008). Principal Investigator: Dr J. Anderson; Coprincipal investigators: Dr M. Judith Lynam, Dr Sheryl Reimer Kirkham, Dr Annette Browne; Coinvestigators: Dr Paddy Rodney, Dr Colleen Varcoe; Dr Sabrina Wong). For more information, see the project Web site at: http://www.cghru.nursing.ubc.ca/.

point for several of our projects.[9,63] Conceptualized by Irihapeti Ramsden and incorporated into New Zealand's Nursing Council guidelines in 1992, *cultural safety* is defined as

> *The effective nursing of a person/family from another culture by a nurse who has undertaken a process of reflection on own cultural identity and recognizes the impact of the nurse's culture on own nursing practice. Unsafe cultural practice is any action which diminishes, demeans, or disempowers the cultural identity and wellbeing of an individual, (cited in Clarke[64(pv)])*

Cultural safety underscores the importance of acknowledging the historical sociopolitical context that shapes people's health and healthcare encounters, and in this way aligns with a postcolonial feminist framework. Yet, even within this framing, the types of knowledge or evidence that may be invoked when the concept of cultural safety is employed are not unproblematic.

Our initial steps to translate this concept into practice highlight the complexities of both the concept itself and some of the challenges of knowledge translation from a postcolonial feminist stance. In our earlier empirical work, we set out to establish what cultural safety looks like in practice.[9,63] However, rather than coming up with a practice guideline (eg, a neat framework of values, attitudes and/or practices characteristic of cultural safety), we concluded that cultural safety can best be understood as an interpretive lens brought to the healthcare encounter by the provider, in which the provider reflects upon his or her own sociocultural positioning with accompanying values and assumptions, and seeks to understand what each patient brings to the healthcare encounter. Clearly, cultural safety then becomes not the *subject* of a clinical pathway but rather a *way* of approaching professional practice. Moreover, "culture" itself is problematized to reveal the widespread tendencies to generalize and/or stereotype on the basis of presumed group affiliations when the nature of culture is itself socially constructed. Indeed, our research has impressed upon us the limitations of the languaging of cultural safety, where the very use of the term "culture" may reinscribe the notion of discrete cultural groups with the all too common accompanying propensities toward stereotyping. To reflect the shifting and contextual nature of how subject identities are enacted and perceived, and the empirical observations that anyone, regardless of social status, ethnic affiliations, gender, and so forth, may face a convergence of events such that they are particularly vulnerable,[9] we have coined the phrase "situated vulnerability" that does not essentialize groups as "vulnerable populations." Rather, we examine the contexts and conditions under which people are made vulnerable. This is not to undermine the suffering of those who have been disadvantaged, but rather, to acknowledge that vulnerability is a social construct, created through the social conditions of people's lives, and not a fixed state of being, or "ethnic trait."

The promotion of reflective practice through the use of transformative knowledge is an important avenue, while less tangible than a clinical pathway, in supporting nurses to provide individualized, client-appropriate care that is attuned to these situated vulnerabilities. Nurses require tools to support not only their objective/technological dimensions of practice but also the relational, contextual, and historical dimensions to assist professional nursing practice. Therefore, while the mechanisms of EBP (ie, clinical pathways, best practice guidelines, care maps) offer one route to clinical decision making applied to a relatively narrow range of clinical phenomena, we advocate for the incorporation of sociological, qualitative, and humanities-based knowledge into the frontline of nursing practice to foster the "critical consciousness"[61] necessary for reflexive thinking and transformative practice.

However, *how* to best translate this type of knowledge into clinical practice poses considerable challenge. We have found that translation of this type of transformative knowledge requires a much more intense relationship between research and practice where researchers embrace a more active role in the process of knowledge translation. In our current knowledge translation efforts, we are exploring more organic ways to facilitate the uptake of a wide range of knowledge, keeping in mind the goal of fostering "understanding, reflection, and action."[62(p23)] Although our initial work with managers and other administrative healthcare decision makers saw a preference for managerial discourses (particularly the language of "numbers") in the communication of research findings, we are now embarking on an exploration of the type of engagement required to facilitate the uptake of transformative knowledge for frontline nurses.

In this more active engagement, our team has been exploring how to translate research-based knowledge from the language of the academy into the language of practice, simultaneously engaging with different discourses in the clinic. We are delving into ways to prepare knowledge in such a way that is accessible to practitioners, resonates with their experiences of the realities of everyday practice, creates a space of openness to the uptake of transformative knowledge, and, ultimately, to transformations in practice. For example, we have taken as starting point practice tools that have been developed for discharge planning (ie, discharge planning guidelines) and used case examples to exemplify how individuals experiencing a vulnerable period in their lives—hospitalization—may not fit within the narrow constructs of the tool. Rather than viewing these individuals as outliers, we then engage practitioners in the process of critical reflection on how this individual's care could have been approached differently, and how guidelines around discharge planning could be written in a way that lead nurses to take up transformative knowledge and translate it into practice within the complex and demanding environments in which they work. Our experiences to date with translation of transformative knowledge has underscored for us the new terrain that this effort represents, particularly as we bring knowledge derived from critical inquiry to the mainstreamed enterprise of knowledge translation and EBP.

 ## Conclusion

Over the past several decades, the discipline of nursing has struggled with the uptake of research-based knowledge at the point of care. EBP has been adapted from medicine and applied to nursing, although not without wide-ranging critique of this approach to knowledge uptake. To these critiques, we have added the perspectives of PCF regarding the shortcomings of EBP, and have recommended an expansion to EBP, in the form of translation of transformative knowledge, as a viable approach to knowledge uptake in clinical settings. This transformative knowledge draws not just on narrow notions of evidence, but seeks inclusive epistemologies that represent the realities of multiple sources of knowledge, including previously marginalized knowledge. The translation of transformative knowledge also guards against discourses of standardization associated with EBP, striving instead to understand the particularities of each situation; and how these particularities are structured by larger historically embedded systems of social classification such as racialization, class, and gender. When employed in this way, knowledge translation has the potential to enhance nursing practice through understanding, reflection, and action.

REFERENCES

1. Dawes M. Evidence-based practice. In: Dawes M, Davies P, Gray A, Mant J, Seers K, Snowball R, eds. *Evidence-Based Practice: A Primer for Health Care Professionals.* London: Churchill Livingstone; 1999:1–8.
2. Meleskie J, Wilson K. Developing regional clinical pathways in rural health. *Can Nurs.* 2003;99(8):25–28.
3. Canadian Nurses Association. *Nursing Now Issues and Trends in Canadian Nursing: Cultural Diversity—Changes and Challenges.* Ottawa, Ontario: Canadian Nurses Association; 2000.

4. Barnes L. The social production of an enterprise clinic: nurses, clinical pathway guidelines and contemporary healthcare practices. *Nurs Inq.* 2000;7(3):200–208.

5. Estabrooks C. Will evidence-based nursing practice make practice perfect? *Can J Nurs Res.* 1998;30(1):15–36.

6. Traynor M. The oil crisis, risk and evidence-based practice. *Nurs Inq.* 2002;9(3):162–169.

7. Walker K. Why evidence-based practice now? A polemic. *Nurs Inq.* 2003;10(3):145–155.

8. Winch S, Greedy D, Chaboyer W Governing nursing conduct: the rise of evidence-based practice. *Nurs Inq.* 2002;9(3): 156–16l.

9. Anderson J, Perry J, Blue C, et al. "Rewriting" cultural safety within the postcolonial and postnational feminist project: toward new epistemologies of healing. *ANS Adv Nurs Sci.* 2003;26(3): 196–214.

10. Reimer Kirkham S. The politics of belonging and intercultural health care provision. *West J Nurs Res.* 2003; 25(7):762–780.

11. Rogers W. Evidence based medicine and justice: a framework for looking at the impact of EBN upon vulnerable or disadvantaged groups. *J Med Ethics.* 2004;30:141–145.

12. Sackett D, Rosengerg W, Gray JAM, Haynes RB, Richardson WS. Evidence-based medicine: what it is and what it isn't. *BMJ.* 1996;312:71–72.

13. DiCensa A, Ciliska D, Guyatt G. Introduction to evidence-based nursing. In: DiCensa A, Guyatt DG, Ciliska D, eds. *Evidence-Based Nursing: A Guide to Clinical Practice.* St. Louis: Mosby Elsevier; 2005:3–19.

14. Fawcett J, Wilson J, Neuman B, Hinton WP, Fitzpatrick JJ. On nursing theories and evidence. *J Nurs Scholarsh.* 2001;33(2):115–119.

15. The Joanna Briggs Institute. *Evidence Based Practice Information Sheets for Health Professionals: Identification and Nursing Management of Dysphasia in Adults With Neurological Impairment.* Adelaide, Australia: Joanna Briggs Institute; 2000.

16. Thorne S, Sawatzky R. Particularizing the general: challenges in teaching the structure of evidence-based nursing practice. In: Drummond J, Standish P, eds. *The Philosophy of Nursing Education.* New York: Palgrave Macmillan. In press.

17. Carper B. Fundamental ways of knowing in nursing. *ANS Adv Nurs Sci.* 1978; 1(1):13–23.

18. McSherry M, Simmons M, Pearce P *Evidence-Informed Nursing: A Guide for Clinical Nursing.* London: Routledge; 2000.

19. Timmermans S, Berg M. *Gold Standard: The Challenge of Evidence-Based Medicine and Standardization in Health Care.* Philadelphia: Temple University Press; 2003.

20. Fanon F. *The Wretched of the Earth.* Harmondsworth, England: Penguin; 1963.

21. Said EW. *Orientalism.* New York: Vintage Books; 1978.

22. Collins PH. *Black Feminist Thought: Knowledge, Consciousness, and the Politics of Empowerment.* New York: Routledge; 1990.

23. Hooks B. *Black Looks: Race and Representation.* New York: Routledge; 1992.

24. Morrison T. *Playing in the Dark: Whiteness and the Literary Imagination.* Cambridge: Harvard University Press; 1992.

25. Brewer R. Theorizing race, class and gender: the new scholarship of black feminist intellectuals and black women's labour. In: James SM, Busia APA, eds. *Theorizing Black Feminisms: The Visionary Pragmatism of Black Women.* London: Routledge; 2006:13–30.

26. Anderson JM. Writing in subjugated knowledges: towards a transformative agenda in nursing research and practice. *Nurs Inq.* 2000;7(3):145.

27. Anderson JM. Toward a post-colonial feminist methodology in nursing research: exploring the convergence of post-colonial and black feminist scholarship. *Nurs Res.* 2002; 9(3):7–27.

28. Anderson JM. Lessons from a postcolonial-feminist perspective: suffering and a path to healing. *Nurs Inq.* 2004; 11(4):238–246.

29. Blackford J. Cultural frameworks of nursing practice: exposing an exclusionary healthcare culture. *Nurs Inq.* 2003; 10(4):236–244.

30. Browne AJ, Smye V, Varcoe C. The relevance of postcolonial theoretical perspectives to research in aboriginal health. *Can J Nurs Res.* 2005; 37(4):16–37.

31. Mohammed S. Moving beyond the "exotic": applying postcolonial theory in health research. *ANS Adv Nurs Sci.* 2006;29(2): 98–109.

32. Racine L. Implementing a postcolonial feminist perspective in nursing research related to non-Western populations. *Nurs Inq.* 2003;10(2):91–102.

33. Reimer Kirkham S, Anderson JM. Postcolonial nursing scholarship: from epistemology to method. *ANS Adv Nurs Sci.* 2002; 25(1):1–17.

34. Street A, Blackford J. Cultural conflict: the impact of western feminism(s) on nurses caring for women of non-English speaking background. *J Clin Nurs.* 2002;11:664–671.

35. Ahmad W. *"Race" and Health in Contemporary Britain.* Buckingham, England: Open University Press; 1994.

36. Allen D, Benner P, Diekelmann N. Three paradigms for nursing research: methodological implications. In: Chinn PL, ed. *Nursing Research Methodology: Issues and Implications.* Rockville, Md: Aspen; 1986:23–38.

37. Barbee E. Racism in US nursing. *Med Anthropol Q.* 1993; 3(4):346–362.

38. Campbell J, Bunting S. Voices and paradigms? Perspectives on critical and feminist theory in nursing. *ANS Adv Nurs Sci.* 1991;13(3):1–15.

39. Webb C. Feminist methodology in nursing research. *J Adv Nurs.* 1984;9:249–256.

40. Allen D. Whiteness and difference in nursing. *Nurs Phil.* 2006;7:65–78.

41. Canales M. Toward an understanding of difference. *ANS Adv Nurs Sci.* 2000;22(4):16–31.

42. Drevdahl D, Phillips D, Taylor J. Uncontested categories: the use of race and ethnicity variables in nursing research. *Nurs Inq.* 2006;13(l):52–63.

43. Kendall J, Hatton D, Beckett A, Leo M. Racism as a source of health disparity in children with attention-deflcit/hyperactivity disorder. *ANS Adv Nurs Sci.* 2002;26(2):114–130.

44. Phillips D, Drevdahl D. "Race" and the difficulties of language. *ANS Adv Nurs Sci.* 2003;26(1):17–29.

45. McConaghy C. *Rethinking Indigenous Education: Culturalism, Colonialism, and the Politics of Knowing.* Brisbane, Australia: Post Pressed; 2000.

46. Meleis A, Im E. Transcending marginalization in knowledge development. *Nurs Inq.* 1999;6:94–102.

47. Horton R. Medical journals: evidence of bias against the diseases of poverty. *Lancet.* 2003;36l:712–713.

48. Whitehead M, Dahlgren G, Gilson L. Developing the policy response to inequities in health: a global perspective. In: Evans T, Whitehead M, Diderichsen F, Bhuiya A, Wirth M, eds. *Challenging Inequities in Health: From Ethics to Action.* New York: Oxford University Press; 2001:308–323.

49. Kemm J. The limitations of "evidence-based" public health. *J Eval Clin Pract.* 2006;12(3):319–324.

50. Estroff S, Henderson G. Social and cultural contributions to health, difference, and inequality. In: Henderson G, Estroff S, Churchill L, King N, Oberlander J, Strauss R, eds. *The Social Medicine Reader: Social and Cultural Contributions to Health, Difference, and Inequality.* Durham, NC: Duke University Press; 2005:4–26.

51. Browne AJ, Smye V. A critical analysis of the relevance of collecting "ethnicity data" in health care contexts. Paper presented at: the Society for Applied Anthropology Conference; April 28, 2006; Vancouver, British Columbia.

52. Bhopal R, Donaldson L. White, European, Western, Caucasian, or what? Inappropriate labeling in research on race, ethnicity, and health. In: Henderson G, Estroff S, Churchill L, King N, Oberlander J, Strauss R, eds. *The Social Medicine Reader: Social and Cultural Contributions to Health, Difference, and Inequality.* Durham, NC: Duke University Press; 2005:252–262.

53. Georges JM, McGuire S. Deconstructing clinical pathways: mapping the landscape of health care. *ANS Adv Nurs Sci.* 2004; 27(1):2–11.

54. Frenkel M, Shenhav Y. From binarism back to hybridity: a postcolonial reading of management and organization studies. *Org Stud.* 2006;27(5):855–876.

55. Acker J. The future of "gender and organizations": connections and boundaries. *Gend Work Organ.* 1998;5(4):195–206.

56. Prasad A, Machel G. *Postcolonial Theory and Organizational Analysis: A Critical Engagement.* New York: Palgrave Macmillan; 2003.

57. Henley E, Peters K. 10 steps for avoiding health disparities in your practice. *J Fam Pract.* 2006;53(3):193–196.

58. Lynam J, Henderson A, Browne A, et al. Healthcare restructuring with a view to equity and efficiency: reflections on unintended consequences. *Can J Nurs Leadersh.* 2003;16(1):112–140.

59. Browne A. Discourses influencing nurses perceptions of First Nations patients. *Can J Nurs Res.* 2005;37(4):62–87.

60. McCall J. *"I Chose to Fight": The Lives and Experiences of Women Who are Living With HIV/AIDS* [unpublished master's thesis]. Vancouver, British Columbia: University of British Columbia; 2006.

61. Anderson JM. Speaking of illness: issues of first generation Canadian women—implications for patient education and counseling. *Patient Educ Couns.* 1998;33:197–207.

62. Lather P. This is your father's paradigm? Government intrusion and the case of qualitative research in education. *Qual Inq.* 2004;10(1):15–34.

63. Reimer Kirkham S, Smye V, Tang S, et al. Rethinking cultural safety while waiting to do fieldwork: methodological implications for nursing research. *Res Nurs Health.* 2002;25:222–232.

64. Clarke M. Preface. In: Wepa D, ed. *Cultural Safety in Aotearoa New Zealand.* Auckland: Pearson Education New Zealand; 2005:v–vii.

THE AUTHORS COMMENT

Knowledge Development and Evidence-Based Practice: Insights and Opportunities from a Postcolonial Feminist Perspective for Transformative Nursing Practice

This article had its genesis in a seminar aimed at discussing the relevance of postcolonial feminist theories for nursing and health-care scholarship, made possible by support from the Elizabeth Kenny McCann (EKM) Professorship held by Dr. Joan Anderson (2001–2005) at the University of British Columbia and the EKM Doctoral Award held by J. Baumbusch. We dedicate this article to the late Professor McCann, whose vision of the connectedness between nursing education and practice inspired the direction of this article. The article signals the challenges facing the profession in regard to how nursing knowledge—particularly that which is framed as "evidence"—is generated and translated in practice and offers insight into how theoretical perspectives in the critical traditions of postcolonial feminist scholarship might be drawn upon in response to these challenges.

SHERYL REIMER-KIRKHAM
JENNIFER L. BAUMBUSCH
ANNETTE S.H. SCHULTZ
JOAN M. ANDERSON

The Use of Postcolonialism in the Nursing Domain
Colonial Patronage, Conversion, and Resistance

DAVE HOLMES, RN, PhD
BERNARD ROY, RN, PhD
AMÉLIE PERRON, RN, BScN

The current context in nursing requires radical political analyses to deconstruct the dominant discourses that map both the discipline and the profession. In response to the strong reaction to articles, which critically examined the evidence-based movement in health sciences, we believe that it is essential to offer a perspective that is capable of resisting the progress of such discourses, which currently prevail in nursing and thus shape our profession. We believe that the biomedical model/ideology is a form of colonial patronage that is becoming more and more influential in nursing. Such colonization takes the forms of powerful discourses (eg, evidence-based medicine) and institutional practices that pervade all spheres of nursing: practice, research, education, and administration. In previous articles, we have criticized this trend; consequently, the objective of this article is not to replicate our previous arguments but rather to demonstrate that to what extent a postcolonial approach to nursing constitutes an efficient tool for disrupting the colonizing effects of the biomedical discourse. **Key words:** biomedicine, critique, epistemology, evidence-based, nursing, postcolonialism, power

The exteriority of the war machine is also attested to be epistemology, which intimates the existence and perpetuation of a nomad or minor science.

Deleuze and Guattari

Be obedient always; the better you obey, the more you will be master, for you will be obeying pure reason.

Deleuze and Guattari

The current context in nursing often requires radical political analyses to deconstruct the dominant discourses/truths that map both the discipline and the profession. In response to the strong reaction to articles which critically examined the evidence-based movement in health sciences,[1,2] we believe that it is essential to offer a perspective that is capable of resisting the progress of the discourses which currently prevail in nursing, and thus shape both our discipline and our profession.

Despite previous attempts to critique the relationship between nursing and medicine,[3] we believe that the biomedical model/ideology is a form of *colonial patronage* that is becoming more and more influential in nursing. Such colonization takes the forms of powerful discourses, such as evidence-based medicine (EBM) and institutional practices (best practice guidelines), that pervade all spheres of nursing: research, education, administration,

and practice. In previous articles, we have criticized this trend.[1,2,4] Consequently, the objective of this article is not to replicate our previous arguments but rather to demonstrate that to what extent a postcolonial approach to nursing constitutes an efficient tool for disrupting the colonizing effects of the biomedical discourse.

We maintain that a postcolonial approach should be used in nursing to look not only at class, race, gender, politics, and language in the fields of aboriginal health and culture-related matters but also at the colonization of nursing itself. Postcolonialism provides a necessary perspective to account for the active colonizing trend in which nursing is now willfully engaged. Using EBM as a starting point, our argument is 2-fold: to describe the colonization of nursing both by the influence of outside forces and from within the nursing apparatus itself. In this way, we wish to demonstrate that nursing is not only far from being (passively) subordinate to colonial patronage but also actively involved in its own colonizing process subsequent to a *conversion* phase.

In French postmodern thought, to critique is not merely an intellectual activity; it is an obligation—hence our extensive use of French philosophers to sustain our argument. To critique means to use politically charged concepts as tools for disrupting the status quo.

ABOUT THE AUTHORS

DAVE HOLMES is a Professor, Vice Dean (Academic), and University Research Chair in Forensic Nursing at the University of Ottawa, Faculty of Health Sciences. After completing his BSc (Ottawa, 1991), MSc (Montreal, 1998), and PhD (Montreal, 2002) in Nursing, Professor Holmes completed a CIHR Post-Doctoral Fellowship in Health Care, Technology and Place at the University of Toronto, Faculty of Social Work (2003). To date, Professor Holmes received funding from the Government of Canada (CIHR and SSHRC), to conduct his research program on risk management in the fields of Public Health and Forensic Nursing. Most of his work, comments, essays, analyses, and research are based on the poststructuralist works of Deleuze & Guattari and Michel Foucault. Professor Holmes has published over 105 articles in peer-reviewed journals and 20 book chapters. He is Editor in Chief for *Aporia—The Nursing Journal* (www.aporiajournal.com). Professor Holmes is Coeditor of *Critical Interventions in the Ethics of Health Care* (Surrey, Ashgate, 2009), *Abjectly Boundless: Boundaries, Bodies and Health Care* (Surrey, Ashgate, 2010), and *(Re)Thinking Violence in Health Care Settings: A Critical Approach* (Surrey, Ashgate, 2011). He has presented at numerous national and international conferences. He was appointed as Honorary Visiting Professor in Australia, the United States, and the United Kingdom.

BERNARD ROY worked for about 10 years with First Nations populations in Northern Quebec. After an MA degree in Applied Social Research (Laurentian University), he obtained his PhD (Anthropology) from Université Laval, Québec. His research program is based on critical perspectives, more specifically postcolonial studies. Dr. Roy's research examines the social, economic, and political dimensions of the Type 2 diabetes epidemic among First Nations. His work explores the way diabetic patients resist normative prescriptions of health professionals. Dr. Roy has been teaching nursing at the Faculté des sciences infirmières, Université Laval since 2004. His teaching focuses mainly on community health, sociocultural dimensions of health, and First Nations health issues. He is also the Editor in Chief of *Infirmières, Communautés et Sociétés*.

AMÉLIE PERRON is an Assistant Professor at the School of Nursing, Faculty of Health Sciences, University of Ottawa. Besides her doctoral research on psychiatric nursing care in a correctional setting, she has worked on many research projects in the fields of psychiatry and forensic psychiatry in Canada, France, and Australia. Her fields of interest include nursing care provided to captive and marginalized populations, psychiatric nursing, forensic psychiatry, power relationships between healthcare professionals and patients, as well as issues of discourse, risk, gender, and ethics. She also writes on issues relating to the state of nursing knowledge and epistemology. Her clinical practice is grounded in community psychiatry and crisis intervention. She is Coeditor of *(Re)Thinking Violence in Health Care Settings: A Critical Approach* (Surrey, Ashgate, 2011) and is the Receiving Editor for *Aporia—The Nursing Journal*.

Defining and Expanding Postcolonialism

For the sake of clarity, this section will provide definitions of the concepts used in our article, and discuss the epistemological underpinnings of postcolonialism. According to Guba and Lincoln,[5] a paradigm is a worldview, a vision of the world and although definitions of a paradigm are numerous, we concur with them that it comprises ontological and epistemological underpinnings as well as methodological orientations. It is our belief that there is no single methodology that is superior to all others and different research questions lend themselves to different methodologies. We do believe, however, that methodology and theoretical, philosophical, and epistemological foundations are inevitably interrelated in any research endeavor, and thus our call for a thorough understanding of paradigmatic influences.

According to Guba and Lincoln,[5] 4 paradigms are said to coexist: positivism, postpositivism, critical theory, and constructivism. Although this coexistence is not always harmonious because of their incommensurable features,[6] we posit that none should prevail, that is, attain a hegemonic position, even if they compete constantly with one another. Boje[7] argues that Guba and

Lincoln's grouping of critical theory, poststructuralism, and postmodernism into 1 paradigm, defined as "critical theory," is problematic because of the significant distinctions among these 3 perspectives. Although we agree with Boje[7] that definite differences do exist, we posit that Guba and Lincoln's definition of the critical theory paradigm is broad enough to include the 3 aforementioned perspectives.

The term *critical theory* originated in the 20th century Frankfurt School, and is now associated with scholars across a vast range of disciplines. While early research in this tradition focused on class oppression, more recent works have focused on the frequent interconnections to be found among class, gender, race, and sexual orientation. According to Guba and Lincoln,[5] critical theory encompasses several perspectives such as feminism, neo-Marxism, queer studies, and (critical) postmodern perspectives, including both poststructuralism and postcolonialism. Research that aims to be critical seeks, as its purpose of inquiry, a confrontation of the injustices in society as well as a questioning of the status quo, while giving a voice to vulnerable persons (including marginalized discourses). Critical researchers believe that the knowledge developed in their research may serve as a first step toward addressing such injustices. As a consequence, the research aims for a transformative outcome, and therefore, is not interested in knowledge for knowledge's sake.[8] In fact, some critical researchers argue that such a "neutral" stance toward research can too easily play into the conservative agendas of those who would rather preserve than challenge the status quo.[9]

Critical theorists require a large measure of autonomy from the phenomena being studied, or, to use anthropological terms, a more "etic" than "emic" position from which to analyze and construct arguments. Moreover, critical researchers defend their attention to the politics of social reality. In fact, Hoy[10] suggests that these researchers are part of a "critical resistance" group. They often encompass and draw upon research from other paradigms, offering an explanation of the workings of power that are often unexamined in logical (post)positivist approaches (with their focus on causal relations between variables) and in humanistic approaches (with their focus on human explanations of actions or meanings).[9]

The postmodern perspective offers an alternative to logical (post)positivist and humanistic approaches. Postmodernism does not promote a particular cause, but rather a "condition," a state of mind and of being. It provides theoretical support for nonlinear thinking and *multivocality*, thus moving away from the concept of a transcendental signified, aesthetic/critical approach to scholarship and toward in-depth and deconstructive readings to provide careful and thoughtful analyses of the political implications of knowledge development. The postcolonial perspective includes

a broad postmodern ethos, which is understood to be detotalizing, deessentializing, local, and rhizomatic.[7] Therefore, a conceptual link can be established between postmodernism and postcolonialism, one that has been described by Anderson as the "commitment to difference and to multiplicity of perspectives and truths."[11 (p240)]

The postcolonial approach has gained momentum in nursing—see Joan Anderson's influential works.[11] Postcolonial nursing studies deal with the effects of colonization on cultures and societies while addressing the issues of culture and race (including racism) within the domain of nursing and health.[12,13] Postcolonialism is used in wide and diverse ways to include the study and analysis of the discursive operations of all types of empires.[14] We argue that a discipline may also act like an empire in that it can enforce specific pathways or programs within which research, practice, education, and administration have to be undertaken.

One of the preferred tools used to conduct postcolonial critiques is *counter-discourse*. Within the postcolonial realm, this has been understood less in terms of historical processes than through the challenges posed to a variety of imperial ideologies including the one promoted/imposed by biomedicine and its preferred research methodologies. This postcolonial intellectual activity promotes the identification/illumination of the unspoken rules controlling which statements can be made and which cannot.[14] Discourses are strongly bound to all areas of knowledge, and convey a system of statements from which the world can be known.[15] For example, "power in academia is reflected in the existence of hierarchies, that is, in the hierarchical organization of the purveyors of knowledge and in a ranking of *knowledges* … other knowledge is considered lower if expressed in different idioms, for example, the writing of journalists but also writing in unconventional academic styles."[16(p122)] As stated by Racine: "the postcolonial approach is directed at uncovering the exclusionary effects of dominant ideologies in 'Othering' other forms of knowledge—the subjugated knowledge."[17(p95)]

The objectives of the critique of discourses from a postcolonial perspective are linked to the following important questions. What are the rules that allow certain statements to be made and not others? Which rules order these statements? Which rules allow the development of a classificatory system (eg, the Cochrane evidences hierarchy)? Which rules allow us to identify certain players as leaders? These questions are vital if one wishes to critique the classification, ordering, and distribution of the forms of knowledge that discourses both enable and exclude. In short, this has to do with the politics of academia.[18] Discourses are very important because they join knowledge to power.[19] Those who have (or think they have) control of what is known and how things should be known act as colonizers in the scientific arena by excluding discourses which are counter to the hegemonic ones (subjugated knowledge) that they support. Such exclusionary practices are strong negative responses to the threat posed by counter-discourses (forms of *savoirs délinquants*) in a specific area of study. The crucial idea in postcolonial study is that the will to truth is linked to the will to power. In the realm of research, truth is a system of statements about science that involve assumptions, prejudices, blindness, and insights, but exclude other potentially valid scientific statements.[19]

A postcolonial reading of the influences of medicine (and the biomedical model) need not be restricted to interrogating a body of work, but may involve far greater attention to the colonial relations between medicine and the allied health sciences, including nursing.[3] The evidence-based movement constitutes a salient example of the colonizing process of medicine in the nursing domain. Nursing takes its lead from institutional medicine, whose authority is rarely challenged or tested probably because it alone controls the terms by which any challenge or test may proceed.[1,2,20] For example, after it had been adopted by medicine, nursing accepted random control testing as the gold standard of evidence-based nursing knowledge.[21] This is a direct contradiction to the fact that nursing is supposed to rely on a variety of ways of knowing (see reference 22). It is deeply questionable whether EBM, as a reflection of stratification (hierarchy of evidences) and segmentation, promotes the multiple ways of knowing deemed important within nursing.[2] Moreover, we must ask whether EBM serves a state or governmental function, where readymade and convenient "goals and targets" can be used to justify cuts to healthcare funding.[23]

Although attempts have been made to distinguish nursing from medicine,[3] the colonizing process of the former by the latter has been going on for some time without any substantive and efficient means for disrupting the process. We maintain that nursing is part of the colonization process when it integrates colonial agendas and principles, makes them its own, and promotes a nursing agenda that resonates with this colonial patronage. The dominance of colonial patronage is exerted by force, but also and foremost, by a more subtle and inclusive power through state apparatuses (following Foucault's notion of *dispositifs*) such as colleges and universities where the colonizers' interests are presented as the common interest, and thus come to be taken for granted.

Furthermore, in our view, nursing is not only colonized by powerful external medical discourses through the deployment of a rigid nursing agenda that conveys dominant biomedical discourses but also controlled from within, when nursing imposes nursing conceptual models or theories to differentiate itself from medicine. While, on the one hand, nursing may try to escape the effects of the colonial (biomedical)

force, on the other hand, it simultaneously creates a "nursing apparatus of capture" by promoting an exclusive "nursing-based" knowledge.[24] As a consequence, nursing faces 2 political threats—one from without and one from within—both trying to colonize/impose a rigid grid on nursing knowledge development.

We believe that resistance (counter-discourse through decolonization) is imperative on 2 fronts. First, in resisting the biomedical hegemonic plan (the deployment of a powerful postpositivistic agenda, eg, EBM, etc) and second, by avoiding the establishment of a rigid road map within nursing (the imposition of nursing conceptual models or theories) in reaction to the colonial patronage of the biomedical model. At the moment, nursing is colonized by both medicine and the nursing *intelligentsia*. Therefore, a "double" decolonizing process is imperative if we wish to escape, even if temporarily, from the violence of these colonization processes. Postcolonial counter-discursive practices constitute an efficient way of resisting an imposed (scientific) agenda.

 ## Playing the Game

The work of Collière[25] eloquently illustrates the various dimensions in which historically colonial endeavors have shaped nursing; as "heirs of the religious world," nurses have always been under the influence (if not the authority) of biomedicine. Can we now assume that nurses have been fully emancipated from their colonial past, or is there room for doubt about this?

While the vigor of the pro-nursing discourse demonstrates a powerful drive for identity, distinction, and affirmation, the dominant discourse seems to betray strong subjection to the biomedical paradigm. However, our goal is not to question the crucial place of biomedical knowledge in nursing but rather to suggest that by strictly adopting such an epistemological stance, nursing plays the role of a vassal to medicine and, as such, turns away from that which makes nursing distinct.

Nursing rhetoric regarding EBM is an example of the subjugation of the nursing discipline and profession to a paradigm that is not and cannot be its own. Surely, a paradigm that makes a marginal space for the voices of patients and for the expertize of professionals should be problematized instead of being accepted uncritically.[26] Unfortunately, both researchers and clinicians are pressured into adopting a discourse that promotes a "ritualistic" process, one that is randomized and statistically significant and in which the concept of the "average" patient predominates. Along with Misonier,[27] we ask, shouldn't the patient's voice and experience be part of the semantic matrix of care?

If, as nurses, we subscribe to the concept of health promotion as defined in the Ottawa Charter for instance, our values cannot escape coming into opposition with those promoted by the usual scientific endeavors, which aim to produce evidence that tends to marginalize, exclude, or even deny the individual.[28] We fully agree with Gori and Del Volgo,[29] who state that care cannot exist without the patient's right to his or her own experience. However, such a right can exist only in a space where the person can speak and where power is exerted by or for them. Unfortunately, as with EBM, evidence-based nursing is authenticated through best practice guidelines, which are best suited to the average patient, and overlook individual experience. In contradistinction, Canguilhem[30] believes that the average patient simply does not exist. Such a perspective in nursing, unconditionally borrowed from the "hard sciences," dismisses the patient by reducing him or her to the appropriate biological (dys)functions. Hatem and Halabi-Nassif[31] eloquently illustrate this position in nursing, a discipline and profession in which the medical postulates elaborated by Sackett and his colleagues are uncritically endorsed: "Health professionals, especially doctors and nurses, are asked to base their clinical decisions on science, research and evidence."[32(p71)] Faced with this quest for answers, we believe that it is preferable by far to remain with questions without answers than with "answers that are never questioned."[33(p70)]

As part of the strategy to assert its specificity, nursing discourse states that its care process is global and holistic. However, the difficulty lies in reconciling this rhetoric with the predominance of the biomedical paradigm. The hierarchy of evidence encourages a reductionist view of nursing, which segments and accessorizes the experiences of both the care provider and the care recipient. Unfortunately, as French mathematician Henri Poincaré aptly pointed out, accumulated facts are no more science than accumulated rocks are a house.

From the EBM perspective, treatment is no more than a rational affair in which reflection dismisses the person and focuses instead on the illness. The person thus becomes a surface needing to be informed of the latest evidence, a surface whose informed consent is fully expected,[34] a consent that will go mainly toward the patient's subjugation to expert knowledge.[35]

knowledge and research methodologies are not only ruling the actual nursing agenda but also (as thinkers and producers of ideas) they determine how research should be conducted to obtain what they consider to be "best evidence." The hegemonic discourse of EBM and its correlates is unquestionably ideological from an Althusserian perspective.[36] EBM ideology constructs subjectivities—good/bad researchers and good/bad scholars—and is perpetuated/supported by ideological state apparatuses such as universities, especially in Australia, North America, and the United Kingdom. The promotion of a single truth (EBM) by departments, schools, faculties, and universities is reminiscent of the "total" or "global" program imposed on groups in total institutions (see reference 37) such as asylums, army barracks, and so forth, where everybody has to obey a specific set of rules to foster a sense of community and harmony.

The panoptic gaze of EBM disciples, such as the Cochrane Collaboration Group, provides the necessary disciplinary technology to sustain such an ideology in that it observes (hierarchical observation), includes/excludes (normalizing judgment), and judges (examination) that which forms of knowledge are closest to the gold standard and which are not, regardless of the epistemological biases that steer this inclusion-exclusion process. The effects of the panoptic (academic) machinery, which is far from the intellectual ethos as proposed by Bourdieu,[18] are legion. One important consequence of this quality-control surveillance is termed *conversion*.

Conversion could be defined as the process whereby the colonized appear to internalize the colonizers' discourse, and make it their own.[37] Although conversion is not always imposed by force in the academic sphere, power over any group of people can be exerted in multiple ways, for example, by rewards and punishments. As a result of conversion, the colonized accept the colonizers' views and, in turn, impose these views on their peers.[37] This is exactly what is happening in the nursing domain at this time, as nursing is colonized by powerful external and internal discourses. Therefore, ongoing resistance is imperative.

The Singing of the Biomedical Mermaid and the Conversion of Nursing

Escaping the Game: Resistance to Colonial Patronage

The authoritative discourse of biomedicine (the biomedical model) regarding what counts as "best evidence" in the field of medicine and health sciences represents, metaphorically, a ruling class. In the scientific domain, the proponents of evidence-based medicine promoting the *hierarchization* of scientific

Patronage is a term referring to a socioeconomic power that allows institutions and agencies to come into existence and to be valued and promoted (imposed). As with social ones, scientific patronages are powerful discourses known for endorsing and promoting certain ways of knowing (and paradigms) while discrediting other marginal (minor) forms of scientific endeavors.[19] The dominance of the postpositivistic paradigm in biomedical science is a good example of a dominant discourse, which pervades all levels of nursing, and is often praised uncritically as the favorable path for knowledge development. In addition, trends such as EBM, and the best practice guidelines that arise from these evidences are prominent examples of biomedical patronage. A postcolonial posture permits us to examine this scientific patronage and unmask the power of the colonial institutions, ideologies, and governing systems that confirm some forms of knowledge while denying the importance/validity of others.

To address this challenge, the work of Deleuze and Guattari[38] provides a useful way of decolonizing nursing through the principles of *nomadology* (see also Holmes and Gastaldo[4]), which could be defined as a treaty on resistance, an ethos that engages the self in the political arena. Since research and knowledge development are political enterprises, we should not recoil from this reality, even if the exercise is perceived as threatening and risky. The use of politically charged concepts to deconstruct dominant discourses in nursing is imperative if we wish to engage in the decolonization of our profession.

According to Deleuze and Guattari,[39] 2 forms of science exist: *royal* (dominant) and *minor* (nomad). *Royal* (sovereign) or *State Science* is the science of the governors, the patrons, and the colonial force. This form of science tolerates and legitimizes only knowledge that reinforces the primacy of the fixed model of form, mathematical figures, and measurement. One of the major objectives of *royal science* is to "striate" (control/refuse access/survey/map) the space it occupies and over which it reigns. The political power of *royal science* is a form of policing that designates and regulates what is good or bad science. Like gated communities, it filters what is coming in, and attempts to block or exclude those who do not represent the pre-designated norm.[40]

Nomad Science, on the other hand, creates forms of knowledge, which disrupt the dominant configuration of (royal) science. *Nomad science* is fractured, discontinuous, and pluralistic; it is viewed as barbaric from the *royal* scientists' perspective. Rooted in a highly political mindset, *nomad science* seeks to seize singularities instead of working toward the reinforcement of a single truth/form of domination (eg, the idea of the "average" patient). There have been calls by some thinkers[41,42] to use education as a fertile terrain to defy any prevailing consensus or truth. Critical pedagogy, in particular, aims to challenge the pressures brought on by the commodification of knowledge. However to become a minor-scientist is not without risks, as the apparatus of *royal science* will do whatever it can to stop the *nomad* scientists from progressing.

The intense reactions to a recent article[1] published in an evidence-based journal constitutes a clear example of the violent and defensive position adopted by some *royal* scientists (see Jefferson's comment following our critique of the Cochrane taxonomy). The *royal science* establishment finds it necessary to repress and discredit *nomads* because they threaten the "total/global" order of the hegemonic research paradigm. According to Deleuze and Guattari, "royal science is inseparable from a *holomorphic* model implying both a form that organizes matter, and a matter prepared for the form; it has been shown that this schema derives less from technology or life than from a society divided into governors and governed."[39(p31)]

The *royal* scientists (outside and within nursing) are represented by individuals, who impose an authoritarian nursing knowledge development pathway, and demand/command obedience, domestication, and subjugation on the part of nursing researchers, clinicians, and educators. This assertion may sound controversial, even subversive, but many other nursing critics of the biomedical model and its correlates[3,21,23,43] are also making this same point quite clearly; although some of us may wish to discredit/disqualify this assertion, labeling it as polemical as opposed to nuanced (read scientific) and as if it is unthinkable to be political, controversial, and scientific at the same time. We believe that political correctness is often a means of domesticating the masses and forcing authors/thinkers to use words while saying nothing.[16] Unfortunately, the current issues regarding the evidence-based movement fall short of leading nursing scholars/researchers toward an epistemological debate, which should constitute the core of the discussion.

Final Remarks

The production of knowledge and its use are a form of social practice[16] saturated with political struggles. In this article, we have used a postcolonial stance to discuss the way in which nursing is doubly colonized from both outside and within. EBM, with its associated *hierarchization* of knowledge, has been employed as a salient example of the dominant biomedical discourse currently in vogue in nursing. We have also introduced the politically charged concept of *nomadology* to give form to this resistance. We contend that decolonizing nursing is an ongoing process already addressed by other authors. However, the actual momentum with EBM/best practice guidelines pervading the nursing domain requires a tougher response.

Universities are panoptic apparatuses, which often supervise "with the view of repressing, mastering, and domesticating (cultivating) the errant impulses that threaten to disrupt the authority and hegemony of the privileged majority discourse."[44(p183)] To paraphrase Deleuze and Guattari, the monolithic discourse that pervades nursing in Australia, North America, and the United Kingdom is clearly aligned with *royal science*. Furthermore, we contend that the emancipation of nursing cannot be assured only through a biomedical discourse. As stated before, multiple paradigms in research must coexist in the nursing domain, if we wish to grasp the complexity of this practice.

It is essential that different types of knowledge should be made accessible to both care providers and recipients in order to break free from nursing's colonial past, which is still grounded in postpositivism. Nursing should never rest on a single research paradigm or on nursing theories alone; it should draw from different types of knowledge and learn to recognize (from specific situations) the multiple forms that nursing can take. This, in turn, should mobilize both care providers and patients.[25] The type of withdrawal that is encouraged by nursing fundamentalism in reaction to EBM condemns nursing to dangerously restrict future perspectives. Consequently, decolonization must include the following items: first, a critical challenge to the dominant paradigm and second, emancipation from the idea that in order to resist the dominant paradigm, it is imperative to resort to nursing conceptual models exclusively.

Nursing practice falls within the social domain, and thus underlines the commitment of those who provide care. Nursing care helps manage life and, therefore, influences all social projects[45]; as such, political reflection should be encouraged. We agree with Latour,[46] who believes that science is a continuation of politics through a different means. In fact, many researchers have allowed an appreciation of the political influence of science, especially, the health sciences. We believe that, rather than being strictly "objective" or "scientific," EBM is above all a political statement, one that subjugates nursing and extends this subjugation to the person in need of care. This power position falls within Foucault's conception of the *government* of bodies and the standardization of existence, brought on by postpositivistic epistemology. This approach bears some resemblance to a regime that does not *prohibit* one to speak, but *forces* one to speak in a specific way.[47]

Clinical nurses as well as researchers should not refrain from being political; the (de)colonization of nursing is a highly political process. We acknowledge that engagement in the nursing critique (decolonization) of EBM is a risky endeavor—an intellectual edgework—but we assert, along with Lyng,[48] that it is institutionalized dissent rather than consensus formation that is a cornerstone of a robust democratic order in all societies as well as within universities. This article is thus a direct call for the *politicization* of nursing affairs.

REFERENCES

1. Holmes D, Murray SJ, Perron A, Rail G. Deconstructing the evidence-based discourse in health sciences: truth, power, and fascism. *Int J Evid Based Healthc.* 2006;4:180–186.
2. Holmes D, Perron A, O'Byrne P. Evidence, virulence, and the disappearance of nursing knowledge: a critique of the evidence-based dogma. *Worldviews Evid Based Nurs.* 2006;3(3):95–102.
3. Freshwater D, Rolfe G. *Deconstructing Evidence-Based Practice.* London: Routledge; 2004.
4. Holmes D, Gastaldo D. Rhizomatic thought in nursing: an alternative path for the development of the discipline. *Nurs Philos.* 2004;5:258–267.
5. Guba EG, Lincoln YS. Competing paradigms in qualitative research. In: Denzin NK, Lincoln YS, eds. *The Landscape of Qualitative Research: Theories and Issues.* Thousand Oaks, CA: Sage; 1998:195–220.
6. Kuhn T. *La structure des révolutions scientifiques.* Paris: Flammarion; 1970.
7. Boje DM. Alternative postmodern spectacles: the skeptical and affirmative postmodernist (organization) theory debates. 1999. http://business.nmsu. edu/~dboje/canary.html. Accessed September 20, 2006.
8. Clark L. Critical theory and constructivism: theory and methods for the teens and the new media. 2006. http:// www.colorado.edu/journalism/mcm/ qmr-crit-theory.htm. Accessed September 14, 2006.
9. Ferguson M, Golding P. *Cultural Studies in Question.* London: Sage; 1997.
10. Hoy DC. *Critical Resistance: From Poststructuralism to Post-Critique.* Boston: MIT; 2004.
11. Anderson JM. Lessons from a postcolonial-feminist perspective: suffering and a path to healing. *Nurs Inq.* 2004;11(4):238–246.
12. Browne AJ, Smye V Varcoe C. The relevance of postcolonial theoretical perspectives to research in aboriginal health. *Can J Nurs Res.* 2005;37(4):17–37.
13. Kirkham SR, Anderson JM. Postcolonial nursing scholarship: from epistemology to method. *Adv Nurs Sci.* 2002;25(1):1–17.
14. Ashcroft B, Griffiths G, Tiffin H. *Key Concepts in Post-Colonial Studies.* New York: Routledge; 1998.
15. Foucault M. *L'ordre du discours.* Paris: Gallimard; 1971.
16. Sibley D. *Geographies of Exclusion.* New York: Routledge; 1995.
17. Racine L. Implementing a postcolonial feminist perspective in nursing research related to non-Western populations. *Nurs Inq.* 2003;10(2):91–102.
18. Bourdieu P. *Homo Academicus.* Paris: Éditions de Minuit; 1984.
19. Foucault M. *Power/Knowledge and Selected Interviews and Other Writings, 1972–1977.* New York: Pantheon Books; 1980.
20. Miles A, Loughlin M. Continuing the evidence-based health care debate in 2006. The progress and price of EBM. *J Eval Clin Pract.* 2006;12(4):385–398.
21. Walker K. Why evidence-based practice now? A polemic. *Nurs Inq.* 2003;10(3):145–155.
22. Carper BA. Fundamental patterns of knowing in nursing. *Adv Nurs Sci.* 1978;1(1):13–23.
23. Traynor M. The oil crisis, risk and evidence-based practice. *Nurs Inq.* 2002;9(3):162–169.

24. Parse RR. Building the realm of nursing knowledge. Nurs Sci Q. 1995;8:51.

25. Collière MF. *Promouvoir la vie.* Paris: InterEditions; 1982.

26. De Simone J. Reductionist inference-based medicine, *i.e. EBM. J Eval Clin Pract.* 2006;12(4):445–449.

27. Misonier S. Prolégomènes à un consentement mutuellement éeclaireé. In: Caverni JP, Gori R, eds. *Le consentement. Droit nouveau du patient ou imposture.* Paris: In Press Editions; 2005:171–186.

28. O'Neil M. Données probantes et promotion de la santé: les principaux enjeux. In: Morin D, ed. La pratique professionnelle en santé. Données, résultats et savoirs probants. Montréal, Quebec, Canada: ACFAS; 2005:35–47.

29. Gori R, Del Volgo MJ. *La santé totalitaire.* Paris: Denoël; 2005.

30. Canguilhem G. *Le normal et le pathologique.* Paris: PUF; 1957.

31. Hatem M, Halabi-Nassif H. L'infirmière et les résultats probants. In: Morin D, ed. *La pratique professionnelle en santé. Données, résultats et savoirs probants.* Montréal, Quebec, Canada: Cahiers de l'ACFAS; 2005:49–65.

32. Sackett D, Rosemberg W Gray J, Haynes R, Richardson W. Evidence-based medicine: what it is and what it isn't? *BMJ. 1996;312:71–72.*

33. Paquet M. *Vivre une expérience de soins à domicile.* Québec, Canada: Presses de l'Université Laval; 2003.

34. Couturier Y Carrier S. Scientificité et logiques de preuve en contexte de pratiques fondées sur les données probantes (evidence-based practice). In: Morin D, ed. Les pratiques professionnelles fondées sur les réesultats probants: questionnons à nouveau ce paradigme. Montréal, Quebec, Canada: Cahiers de l'ACFAS; 2005:9–25.

35. Caverni JP, Gori R, eds. *Le consentement. Droit nouveau du patient ou imposture.* Paris: In Press Editions; 2005.

36. Althusser L. *Essays on Ideology.* London: Verso; 1984.

37. Goffman E. *Asiles: études sur la condition sociale des malades mentaux.* Paris: Éditions de Minuit; 1968.

38. Deleuze G, Guattari F. *Nomadology.* New York: Semiotext; 2002.

39. Deleuze G, Guattari F. *Anti-Oedipus: Capitalism and Schizophrenia.* Minneapolis: University of Minnesota Press; 1998.

40. Virilio P. *City of Panic.* London: Berg; 2004.

41. Bauman Z. *Liquid Life.* Cambridge, UK: Polity Press; 2005.

42. Giroux HA, Giroux SS. *Take Back Higher Education: Race, Youth, and the Crisis of Democracy in the Post-Civil Rights Era.* New York: Palgrave MacMillan; 2004.

43. Winch S, Creedy D, Chaboyer W. Governing nursing conduct: the rise of evidence-based practice. *Nurs Inq.* 2002;9(3):156–161.

44. Spanos WV. *The End of Education: Toward Posthumanism.* Minneapolis: University of Minnesota Press; 1993.

45. Cognet M, Bourgon A, Bouvier L, Dufour L. Citoyenneté et soins de santé aux immigrants: les infirmières jouent-elles un rôle dans la construction de la citoyenneté des immigrants au Québec? *Cahier METISS.* 2006;1(1): 25–36.

46. Latour B. *Le métier de chercheur: regard d'un anthropologue.* Paris: INRA Éditions; 1995.

47. Barthes R. *Barthes: Selected Writings.* Oxford, UK: Fontana; 1982.

48. Lyng S. *Edgework: A Sociology of Risk Taking.* New York: Routledge; 2005.

THE AUTHORS COMMENT | The Use of Postcolonialism in the Nursing Domain: Colonial Patronage, Conversion, and Resistance

The purpose of this article is to engage in a radical critique of the ongoing yet subtle incursion of biomedical thought and practice in all nursing domains. To achieve this, the concept of colonization is used to examine the way powerful discourses such as the evidence-based movement currently shape nursing.

A postcolonial perspective is used as an innovative approach to deconstruct this trend and offer a counter-discourse.

DAVE HOLMES
BERNARD ROY
AMÉLIE PERRON

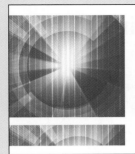

Tools for Theory Development

Just as *research* has its tools and methods for knowledge development and testing, *theory* has its tools and methods for building and evaluating knowledge. This unit highlights various tools for theory development. The chapters do not exhaust the topic but present a sampling of tools that are used across different phases of knowledge development—tools that might not be included in a standard course on theory development strategies.

The tools that are discussed include concept development and a critique of concept analysis, a framework for thinking about theories in terms of levels of abstractions from micro to macro, an extension of the usual typology of theories to include situation-specific theories that privilege the context of practice, and new strategies involving research and practice to develop midrange theories. The chapters also reveal the natural synergy between nursing theories, practice, and research in producing nursing knowledge. Readers may be impressed with the repertoire of tools available to them for knowledge development.

QUESTIONS FOR DISCUSSION

- How might nurses' contexts (for example, the contexts of practice or academia) influence their comfort with or selection of approaches in theory development?

- Are certain tools or strategies of theory development more effectively used by nurses with the *practice doctorate*? By nurses with the *research doctorate*?

- What other strategies, beyond the traditional inductive and deductive approaches, might be invented or identified to develop theoretical ideas?

- Is development of situation-specific theories restricted to practice situations or might they be applied to research and data collection as other *situations* for generating theory?

- Is development of midrange theories best done through standard research or might other forms of inquiry be used?

Concept Analysis: Examining the State of the Science

JUDITH E. HUPCEY, RN, EdD, CRNP

JANICE PENROD, RN, PhD

*A*s methods for analyzing concepts have proliferated in nursing, a critical methodological issue has arisen. Analytic techniques for examining conceptual meaning have incorporated varied strategies for advancing the concept under the rubric of concept analysis, concept development, and theory building. The authors argue that this evolution has created methodological confusion. Following a discussion of a conceptualization of concepts and concept-theory-truth linkages, methods of concept analysis are critiqued in terms of the purpose and the nature of the findings produced by analyses using both traditional and emergent methods. The authors argue that concept analysis is a process of strategic examination of the scientific literature that results in an integrated perspective of the state of the science, or what is known about the concept. In contrast, concept advancement refers to techniques that emphasize the synthesis of new or deeper knowledge that is relevant to the discipline. The authors conclude that disentangling concept analysis from techniques for concept advancement is critical to enhancing the utility of concept-based research in nursing.

Over the past several decades, multiple methods of concept analysis have been developed and applied in nursing. These techniques have provided nursing researchers with much needed analytic processes to examine the conceptual understanding of phenomena of interest to nursing science. Such conceptual understanding guides translational research that in turn directs the development of evidence-based practice. Thus, phenomena-concepts-practice are inherently linked in the science of nursing.

The proliferation of methods of concept analysis has resulted in a critical methodological issue: Is concept analysis synonymous with concept advancement? In this article we review the commonly employed techniques of concept analysis and the products of such analyses to set the scene for a deeper discussion of concept advancement techniques. We conclude that concept analysis is ideally employed to determine the state of the science; the point from which the concept may be strategically advanced toward a higher level of scientific utility.

Types of Concepts

What are concepts? Before launching a discussion of analytic techniques, it is useful to describe a conceptualization of concepts. Concepts are mental abstractions or units of meaning derived to represent some aspect or element of the human experience (Chinn & Kramer, 1995; King, 1988). It is important to keep in mind that concepts are manifested in phenomena but that they never assume a concrete form; a concept is a *mental image,* not the thing or behavior itself (Walker & Avant, 1995). For example, the classic exercise of asking students to play word games involving a thing (e.g., What is a table?) attempts to draw their thinking into abstraction to demonstrate how the concept is a unit of meaning rather than a material entity that appears before them.

Concepts are second order expressions; they package complex sensible or precognitive meaning with cognitive processing into some form of categorical meaning (Merleau-Ponty, 1998). Concepts are brought forth through language; they are embedded in discourse (see Merleau-Ponty, 1998; Rodgers, 2000a; or Walker & Avant, 1995). Concepts are not purely a scientific endeavor; rather concept formation is a natural human process that occurs through being in the world with others.

But there is an important differentiation of concepts that is critical to this discussion. Ordinary or everyday concepts are not the same as scientific concepts (for this discussion, see Mitcham, 1999; Morse, 2000; Rodgers, 2000a). Ordinary concepts are those used by

ABOUT THE AUTHORS

JUDITH E. HUPCEY was raised in New York and attended college and worked in New York City. She received her BS and MS in nursing from Columbia University and a Master's and Doctoral degree in nursing education from Teachers College, Columbia University. Dr. Hupcey held numerous clinical positions at St. Luke's-Roosevelt Hospital Center including working as an Adult Nurse Practitioner in a medical clinic that specialized in the care of underserved adolescents and adults. After joining the faculty at the Penn State School of Nursing, Dr. Hupcey was awarded a National Research Service Award (NRSA) postdoctoral fellowship focusing on qualitative method and concept development. She is an Associate Professor of Nursing, Associate Professor of Medicine, and serves as Professor-in-Charge of Graduate Programs in Nursing. Her research interests include family caregiving, in particular spousal caregivers, palliative care, and heart failure. She spends her summers with her husband, three children, and dogs in New Hampshire, where she enjoys racing sailboats and trailoring kids' boats to sailing regattas throughout New England.

JANICE PENROD was born and raised in central Pennsylvania. She studied nursing at the University of Pittsburgh (BSN 1976) and then continued her graduate education at the Pennsylvania State University (MS 1996; PhD 2001). Dr. Penrod held varied positions in nursing education and practice before joining the faculty at the Penn State School of Nursing, where she is an Associate Professor of Nursing. The foci of her scholarship are family caregiving, end-of-life care, and geriatric nursing. She unwinds by spending time with her family and simply enjoying life at her rural home along a river.

people in everyday life. They have a common meaning, which may be implicit but is understandable within that cultural unit. Ordinary definitions of concepts are found in the dictionary. They change over time to reflect common usage, for example, "soccer mom" or "globalization" now carry conceptual meanings that have evolved through usage. Twenty or 30 years ago, these concepts would have been meaningless.

Scientific concepts are a different entity in that a degree of precision is required in order for the conceptual label to encompass a unit of meaning that is used consistently within a scientific discipline. These concepts require a more specific or narrow definition so that those using the conceptual unit in scientific endeavors are clearly using it in the same way, with the same meaning, so that findings are meaningfully understood (Morse, 2000). The concern of science with specification of concept usage is reflected in the issues of construct validity. Conceptual clarity is necessary for solid theoretical integration (Knafl & Deatrick, 2000). Therefore, scientific concepts are more precise meaning units that when linked together propositionally form a theoretical representation of reality.

This difference in types of concepts (ordinary vs. scientific) is important to concept analysis techniques. Scientific endeavors rely on more precisely defined concepts (Mitcham, 1999; Morse, 2000). When ordinary or implied meanings of concepts are used to build theory in scientific enterprises, the waters are muddied (e.g., see Hupcey, Penrod, Morse, & Mitcham, 2001). For example, when considering trust in nurse-patient relationships, is *my* conceptualization of trust the same as the next reader's? Is trust different from *reliance*? If so, how? It is important for conceptual units of scientific theory to be explicit in their representation of a precise meaning of an element of human experience. In this article, we assert that the *scientific* understanding of a concept is the concern of concept analysis, not ordinary conceptual meaning. This is not to say that ordinary meaning has no merit in scientific work, rather this form of data is relevant to concept advancement techniques, not concept analysis.

 ## Concepts-Theory Linkages

Often, as scientific units of meaning, concepts are described as building blocks of theory (Fawcett, 1978), triggering images of a brick and mortar wall. Using this analogy, theory is built block by block as a process of stacking and securing concepts together. This view is problematic in that the linkages between concepts are presented as linear, a rather simplistic approach. For example, a "block" (concept) on the first course of the "wall" (theory) may be integrally linked with a "block" on the third course—yet the two don't touch or link in any way except to support the "wall" (theory). Thus, this representation is inadequate in illustrating the complex integration of concepts important to nursing and other sciences concerned with human experiences or behaviors.

Hempel (1966) offers a different concept-theory analogy in his work in natural science, describing concepts as the "knots in a network of systematic interrelationships" (p. 94). Extending this analogy, theory could be represented as a tapestry of interwoven, knotted conceptual threads (Penrod & Hupcey, 2005). Thus, no single strand (i.e., concept) in the tapestry (i.e., theory) stands apart from the others in a meaningful way. To pull one conceptual thread from the tapestry produces a piece of string or thread (i.e., the concept) that no longer reveals its accent or color within the larger pattern (i.e., conceptual meaning).

The tapestry analogy is useful to emphasize the importance of strong, well-integrated concepts for supporting theory. However, there is a deeper implication in this analogy that warrants some consideration: concepts are assigned meaning through placement within the context of theory. If we were to examine only red threads pulled from different tapestries, we could analyze the characteristics of threads themselves; however, the contribution of these threads to each tapestry lies in the contrast and intricacies developed when the red thread is knotted and woven with other strands in the larger work. That is, concepts cannot be analyzed irrespective of their theoretical frame. Paley (1996) has argued that concepts must be examined within the niches created in specific theories integrating those concepts. He asserts that the most meaningful way to clarify concepts is to examine the theories in which the concepts are embedded. We agree with Paley and have further asserted that the power of concept analysis (and subsequently, methods of advancing the concept) is to identify the existing theoretical strands and, ultimately, to tie and retie the conceptual knots to form a stronger, more coherent tapestry of nursing theory (Penrod & Hupcey, 2005).

Concepts that are of concern to the caring sciences, including nursing, are embedded in complex tapestries of behavioral, cognitive and emotive meaning (e.g., theories). It is difficult, if not impossible, to untangle the discrete thread of a concept from this tapestry of meaning. Therefore, attempts to isolate a concept in the process of analysis become an artificial endeavor. We cannot isolate concepts that are inherently linked in abstract meaning without in some way limiting the utility of analysis for understanding complex human experiences. From a practical perspective, this means that the scientific literature that precisely orders or interprets ordinary conceptual meaning, must be analyzed for explicit and implicit meaning during the analytic process. Implicit meaning may be derived through an analysis of the positioning of concepts in a theoretical frame or by linguistic cues. We assert that scientific concepts cannot be critically analyzed if pulled from or isolated from the broader theoretical landscape without seriously compromising the value of the analytic product. In other words, processes

of concept analysis must examine multiple theoretical frames to derive insights regarding conceptual meaning that transcend specific theoretical bounds and ring true to the human construction of meaning with the degree of precision required in scientific endeavors.

Far too often, manuscripts related to concept analyses describe the literature surrounding a word label without ever addressing the scientific meaning of the concept in any depth. In these papers, there is an obvious lack of conceptual thinking as the author processes mounds of literature from a narrow and restricted perspective. Available methods of concept analysis may be easily misconstrued to permit such superficial analysis, especially those that prescribe the concoction of contrived cases to support the analysis. Often, these model cases suffer an obvious lack of depth and the derived conceptualization is unable to capture the meanings inherent to complex human experiences (for further discussion, see Hupcey, Morse, Lenz, & Tasón, 1996). Such endeavors fall short of truly determining scientific meaning in a way that permits an understanding of the state of the science surrounding the concept.

Concept-Truth Linkages

We believe that the power of concept analysis lies in identifying how a concept works within existing theories in order to derive a theoretical definition of the meaning ascribed to that concept. This definition of meaning derived from the contextual basis of the science (that is, theories) represents the "state of the science." This assertion is rooted in our metaphysical perspectives of truth or reality, primarily ontology. On one hand, truth could be conceived as an absolute value that can be discovered through precise scientific endeavors. On the other hand, truth can be conceived as a construction of those who experience a given phenomenon at a given point in time. Somewhere between these two endpoints of a continuum, there is a middle ground—a stance that accepts the power of the human experience in formulating conceptual meaning that is subsequently clarified through language expounding that meaning within a specific theoretical context for scientific use.

Kikuchi's (2003) interpretation of moderate realism embraces a quest for understanding reality focusing on *probable* truth rather than *absolute* truth. Concepts are abstracted through a cognitive process that is based on percepts (formed through perceptions along with memory and imagination). Concepts are, therefore, "grounded in reality or empirically derived" (p. 12). Context becomes critical as the individual is situated in a set of circumstances that influences percepts and the abstraction of concepts. Yet the convergence of what is known through a rigorous examination of these multiple contextually based conceptions reveals the *probable* truth that is embraced by moderate realists. Moderate realism asserts, "reality exists independent of the human mind" (p. 12), supporting a notion that probable truth transcends individual experience.

Using the tapestry analogy, concept analysis centers on following and pulling selected conceptual threads in multiple tapestries of meaning. The insights gleaned through each examination (now new threads of meaning) are then rewoven or reknotted and tie into a new tapestry of meaning for that concept. The theoretical tapestry represents the probable truth revealed through an examination of multiple, and often, divergent contextual conceptualizations of concepts grounded in empirical, human experiences.

This is the position that we adopt in this series of papers. Through techniques of concept analysis, conceptual insights are isolated and examined. These insights are then integrated into a summative view of the state of the science surrounding the concept of interest. Since concepts are the backbone of theory *in practice* (that is, concepts help nurses to organize meaning to understand complex human experiences and behaviors in ways that influence the practice of nursing) such work is a critically important scientific endeavor.

Given this perspective, we propose that it is time to clarify methodological approaches to concept analysis and concept advancement. Concept analysis is a means for identifying scholars' best efforts at establishing the probable truth as reflected in the scientific literature. In this case, the label "scientific literature" refers to scholarly works pertaining to the concept of interest, including empirical, theoretical, and philosophical writings. The goal of concept analysis is to establish the state of the science. As such, concept analysis has the potential to serve as an essential method of inquiry in a progressive nursing science, not merely as an academic exercise. We believe that the findings of a critical concept analysis provide evidence for determining the most appropriate means for subsequently advancing the concept. In essence, concept advancement techniques progressively build the concept by explicating implicit meaning into more abstract theoretical formulations that transcend contextual conceptions. Such a clarification of methods supports an evolutionary turn toward praxis by uniting nursing research, theory, and practice in a way that, we believe, could advance the science of nursing significantly.

Traditional Approaches to Concept Analysis

A number of approaches are used to guide the process of "concept analysis" in nursing. It is important to note, however, that the terms describing the overarching analytic processes, purposes for using such techniques, and the nature of the findings produced by each method differ. Ultimately these factors affect the critical examination of the concept, and may result in analytic findings that do not truly reflect the state of the science. Others have critiqued common techniques of concept analysis (for example, see Hupcey, Morse, Lenz, & Tasón, 1996). For clarity, we provide a brief overview of the approaches described by: Wilson (1963), Walker and Avant (1995), Chinn and Kramer (1995), Rodgers (2000b), and Schwartz-Barcott and Kim (2000) (further delineated by Schwartz-Barcott, Patterson, Lusardi, & Farmer, 2002). Our focus in this review centers on the purpose, process, and products of these methods.

Wilson (1963) introduced a method of examining concepts that involved discussion of 11 considerations: questions of concept; 'right answers'; model cases; contrary cases; related cases; borderline cases; invented cases; social context; underlying anxiety (of the researcher); practical results; and results in language. This ambitious discourse endures as a classic reference in concept analysis literature. While Wilson's intent was not to delineate a method of concept analysis, this analytic process serves as the basis for many methods of concept analysis in nursing.

Although Wilson (1963) described the purpose of his work as, "set[ting] forth a framework through which one can build understanding of the essential meaning of a concept in varied contexts" (p. 93), he also stated that "the analysis of concepts is essentially an imaginative process; certainly it is more of an art than a science" (p. 33). This emphasis on process or the art of exploring concepts overshadows the notion of a product. A Wilsonian analysis enhances critical thinking processes, but does not necessarily produce documentation of a scientific examination of a concept (i.e., a product). Herein arises the difficulty in applying this method to scientific endeavors; while the art of the imagination contributes to the derivation of the scientific conceptualization, the influence of imaginative processes often precludes the "evidence" found in the literature that reflects the essential meaning of the concept within a scientific context (especially complex behavioral concepts, like trust or uncertainty). The difficulty with Wilson's text is that, while insightful and very comprehensive, it fails to prepare one to embark on a methodological analysis of the state of the concept in the science (reflected soundly in the literature).

Walker and Avant (1983, 1988, 1995) describe concept analysis as a technique of concept development that is used when the concept is unclear, outmoded, or unhelpful. This method adapts Wilson's work into an eight-step process: select a concept; determine aims or purposes of analysis; identify uses; determine defining attributes; construct a model case; construct borderline/related/contrary/invented/and illegitimate cases; identify antecedents and consequences; and define empirical referents. Both qualitative and quantitative techniques are prescribed within this process. The purpose of this technique is described as theory development. The products of the process include clear and precise theoretical and operational definitions for use in research (1995, p. 46), thus supporting the achievement of the purpose. Concepts are defined as evolving ("change over time," 1995, p. 37) within a constructivist perspective. "The best one can hope for from a concept analysis is to capture the critical elements of it at the current moment in time" (1995, p. 37). While this approach to concept analysis is perhaps, in our experience, the most commonly used in nursing, this method often fails to produce an analysis of the concept that reaches the degree of insight implied by the authors. Of primary concern, how does the researcher come to know that the concept is unclear, outmoded, or unhelpful without a full analytic review of the state of the science?

Chinn and Kramer's (1991, 1995; Chinn & Jacobs, 1983, 1987) approach to concept analysis is an adaptation of the work of Wilson and Walker and Avant. They assert that the primary purpose of concept analysis is the development of theory. Their technique focuses on five steps: select a concept; clarify the purpose; identify data sources; explore context and values; and formulate criteria. It is interesting to note their emphasis on constructed exemplary cases and the inclusion of diverse data sources including popular literature, visual images, and people. The purpose of the analytic process described by these scholars is to identify, clarify, and examine the word label, the phenomenon represented by the label, and the values, feelings, and attitudes that are associated with both the symbol and the phenomenon. The product of this process is considered to be tentative in nature and subject to alteration and change as new evidence becomes available. This method extends analysis beyond the state of the science into the personal and societal realms. While we agree that such conceptualizations (the personal and the societal) are critical to advancing a concept to capture the empirical essence of the human experience, we do not believe that these realms of meaning are appropriate to discerning the probable truth exposed in the scientific literature.

Rodgers (1993, 2000b) described an 'Evolutionary View' of concept analysis that is embedded in the cycle of concept development. The purpose of concept analysis is "clarification of the concept and its current use, and uncovering the attributes of the concept as a basis for further development" (2000b, p. 83). In this method, Rodgers attempted to move beyond the essential features of a concept to capture "the dynamic nature of concepts, changing with both time and context" (2000b, p. 99). The process in this form of concept analysis was designed around the dynamic (not static) perspective of a concept: identifying the

concept; choosing the setting and sample (literature); collecting and managing the data; analyzing the data; identifying a model case; interpreting the results; and identifying implications. The product of analysis (or results) is described as a heuristic device to provide "the clarity necessary to create a foundation for further inquiry and development" (2000b, p. 84). Emphasizing the cyclic nature of concept development even further, Rodgers (1993) said,

> I do not consider the attributes of a concept to be a fixed set of necessary and sufficient conditions, or an **essence**. Consequently, … this cluster of attributes may change, by convention or by purposeful redefinition, over time to maintain a useful, applicable, and effective concept. (p. 75)

The evolutionary approach challenges an essentialist position on concepts. This method of concept analysis is based in a complex, intellectually rigorous integration of more contemporary philosophical positions. Such complexity makes it difficult to disentangle the process of concept analysis as separate and discrete from concept development. Application of this method has been more limited than more traditional forms of concept analysis (e.g., Walker & Avant), perhaps because it challenges our philosophical interpretation of concepts or perhaps because it depicts concepts as such dynamic entities that are difficult to grasp for scientific examination and use.

Schwartz-Barcott and Kim (1986, 1993, 2000) described their "Hybrid Model," which was originally developed in a doctoral course to merge philosophy of science, sociology, and field research into a three-phase approach to concept analysis: theoretical work (based in the literature); field work (based on empirical data); and analytical work (integrating the final product). Schwartz-Barcott and Kim (2000) described this process in terms of concept development and analysis with the implicit purpose of fortifying the "building blocks of a theory" (2000, p. 130) for ultimate integration. This method moves concept analysis from an academic mental exercise into the realm of clinically based fieldwork, thus making an important contribution methodologically. However, the basis of the fieldwork (i.e., the theoretical work) remains underdeveloped. The method does not formulate a strong analysis of the state of the science from which to launch appropriate and well-focused fieldwork. Recently, Schwartz-Barcott and colleagues (2002) clarified their fieldwork strategies into three distinct pathways for clarifying and establishing theoretical congruence between a concept and clinical settings: theoretical selectivity; theoretical integration; and theory creation. The resultant products of the procedural application of the refined pathways are yet to be seen.

Emergent Perspectives on Concept Analysis

Despite the fact that the aforementioned methods of concept analysis were available and used in nursing, their application to phenomena of concern to nursing had varying degrees of success (Morse, Hupcey, Mitcham, & Lenz, 1996). In critical response to these methods, a series of papers on concept analysis published by Morse and colleagues (Hupcey et al., 1996; Morse, 1995; Morse, Hupcey, et al., 1996; Morse, Mitcham, Hupcey, & Tasón, 1996) presented new perspectives on concept analysis. One of the insightful notions regarding concept analysis was the need to establish "criteria for the evaluation of the level of maturity of concepts" (Morse, Mitcham, et al., p. 387). Maturity was defined as a concept which "is well-defined, has clearly described characteristics, delineated boundaries, and documented preconditions and outcomes" (Morse, Mitcham, et al., 1996, p. 387). The evaluation of conceptual maturity was based on four broad philosophical principles, epistemological, pragmatic, linguistic, and logical (Morse, Hupcey, et al., 1996). The epistemological principle sets criteria for conceptual definitions and differentiation. The pragmatic principle addresses criteria surrounding utility and fit of conceptualizations. The linguistic principle centers on consistency and appropriateness of use. And finally, the logical principle develops criteria for examination of theoretical integration with other concepts. Thus, this series of papers provides an analytic lens through which the truth-value of current conceptualizations may be examined.

We believe that the principles described by Morse and colleagues (Hupcey et al., 1996; Morse, 1995; Morse, Hupcey, et al., 1996; Morse, Mitcham, et al., 1996) reveals the best estimate of probable truth evident in the scientific literature. The application of these analytic criteria has the potential to produce a principle-based examination of the concept as it appears in the scientific literature; however, use to date has been limited. From our experience, we have come to discover that the entanglement of analysis and advancement techniques muddles analytic processes, resulting in novice analysts wallowing in data and wondering when, or if, they will ever be finished with the project. Further, in order to address operational difficulties, we have clarified strategies for applying these principles in a concept analysis (Penrod & Hupcey, 2005). Yet, one thing is clear: principle-based concept analysis is a complex method and demands that the researcher *analyzes* scientific meaning (not everyday notions) and *thinks critically* (not imaginatively).

 ## Discussion

Given these diverse approaches to concept analysis, it is not surprising that the potential contribution of concept analyses on the evolution of nursing science has been constrained. We believe that some of the limitations in the utility of the product of concept analyses are related to how nurse researchers and educators *think* about concept analysis. For example, while all of the approaches discussed above are somehow related (and taught) under the rubric of *concept analysis,* analytic terms are confused and entangled within broader concept-based research techniques, including concept development, creating conceptual meaning, and theory building. Data collection/field work appears to be premature in some approaches: how can the researcher proceed with fieldwork strategically until a thorough understanding of the state of the science is fully established? Therefore, clarifying the principles underlying concept analysis is a logical first step in addressing these methodological limitations.

First, we assert that the purpose of concept analysis is to determine the state of the science (or best estimate of probable truth) surrounding a concept of interest. Thus, concept analyses are concerned with scientific literature, not creative imagination, art forms, fiction, interview data, or any other form of representation. Second, the process of concept analysis is primarily at the level of integration, not synthesis. The researcher must engage in a thorough and thoughtful analysis of what is known by examining the implicit and explicit assumptions cited in the scientific literature (i.e., scholarly works pertaining to the concept of interest, including empirical, theoretical, and philosophical writings). Concept analysis is more than an organization of findings; the integrated perspective produces a higher level understanding of the concept of interest. In other words, when theoretical frameworks are examined for meaning and contextual boundaries are transcended, the evidence of probable truth is revealed. Therefore, the product of concept analysis is some form of a summary of the state of the science that reveals the scientific community's best estimate of probable truth, given the evidence portrayed in the extant literature. While this product certainly contributes to the science of nursing, it is not a form of concept advancement; it is an analysis of what is known.

In our view, principle-based concept analysis (Penrod & Hupcey, 2005) provides a useful and meaningful framework for determining the global state of the science (or probable truth) surrounding a concept. However, the real value of this emergent method lies in the evidence culled to support the summative conclusions (truth-value) related to each principle rather than on an assigned word label that denotes the degree of maturity (e.g., immature vs. partially mature). The notion of conceptual maturity is a significant contribution to understanding concepts, but the label that connotes level of maturity is insufficient for determining the most appropriate techniques for concept advancement.

This is an important methodological distinction. Concept analysis is an integration of what is known, not an evaluation of quality or maturity of the concept. Concept advancement is not driven by the label denoting level of maturity; rather, gaps in understanding identified through comprehensive principle-based concept analysis are the most significant findings that direct subsequent concept-based inquiries.

Principle-based concept analysis requires the researcher to focus on evidence found in the scientific literature, not constructed cases, imaginative exploration, or hypothetical exemplars. Through the integration of insights derived from a principle-based examination of the scientific literature, the researcher should be able to derive a summative paragraph (or theoretical definition) on what is known in order to expose gaps or inconsistencies in current thinking. This enables the researcher to strategically progress toward a deeper examination of divergent views to advance a better explication of probable truth.

Principle-based concept analysis appears to provide the most comprehensive examination of the concept within theoretical frames of reference documented in the scientific literature. By applying the overarching principles based in the philosophy of science, the analyst is forced to take a much broader stance in an examination of theory, research, and philosophy papers; but most importantly, the analysis is based in the scientific literature (not lay literature or other forms of representation). This analysis reveals the state of the science, and must be based in the literature of the selected disciplines.

Yet, even the application of such a comprehensive analytic technique will only provide us with a perspective of the state of the science, that is, the baseline understanding that enables the researcher to determine how to strategically advance the concept of interest by addressing identified gaps or inconsistencies. Concept analysis is the initial step in concept advancement; analysis must precede efforts at advancement. Analysis of a concept clarifies what is known of the concept at that time. As such, concept analysis can be used to estimate the probable truth revealed in the scientific literature as a first step in enhancing the knowledge base of the discipline. Such delimitation of analytic processes focuses the researcher on scientific perspectives of reality that can then be further developed through processes of concept advancement.

REFERENCES

Chinn, P. L., & Jacobs, M. K. (1983). *Theory and nursing: A systematic approach.* St. Louis: Mosby.

Chinn, P. L., & Jacobs, M. K. (1987). *Theory and nursing: A systematic approach* (2nd ed.). St. Louis: Mosby.

Chinn, P. L., & Kramer, M. K. (1991). *Theory and nursing: A systematic approach* (3rd ed). St. Louis: Mosby.

Chinn, P. L, & Kramer, M. K. (1995). *Theory and nursing: A systematic approach* (4th ed.). St. Louis: Mosby.

Fawcett, J. (1978). The relationship between theory and research: A double helix. *Advances in Nursing Science, 1*(1), 49–62.

Hempel, C. G. (1966). *Philosophy of natural science.* Englewood Cliffs, NJ: Prentice-Hall.

Hupcey, J. E., Morse, J. M., Lenz, E., & Tasón, M. C. (1996). Wilsonian methods of concept analysis: A critique. *Scholarly Inquiry for Nursing Practice, 10,* 185–210.

Hupcey, J. E., Penrod, J., Morse, J. M., & Mitcham, C. (2001). An exploration and advancement of the concept of trust. *Journal of Advanced Nursing, 36,* 282–293.

Kikuchi, J. (2003). Nursing knowledge and the problem of worldviews. *Research and Theory for Nursing Practice: An International Journal, 17*(1), 7–17.

King, I. M. (1988). Concepts: Essential elements of theories. *Nursing Science Quarterly, 7*(1), 22–25.

Knafl, K. A., & Deatrick, J. A. (2000). Knowledge synthesis and concept development in nursing. In B. L. Rodgers & K. A. Knafl (Eds.), *Concept development in nursing: Foundations, techniques, and applications* (2nd ed., pp. 39–54). Philadelphia: W. B. Saunders.

Merleau-Ponty, M. (1998). *Phenomenology of perception* (C. Smith, Trans.). New York: Routledge. (Original work published 1962).

Mitcham, C. (1999, February). Concepts of concepts: Philosophical perspectives. In J. M. Morse (Chair), *Issues in concept and theory development.* Symposium conducted at the Advances in Qualitative Methodology Conference, Edmonton, Canada.

Morse, J. M. (1995). Exploring the theoretical basis of nursing using advanced techniques of concept analysis. *Advances in Nursing Science, 17*(3), 31–46.

Morse, J. M. (2000). Exploring pragmatic utility: Concept analysis by critically appraising the literature. In B. L. Rodgers & K. A. Knafl (Eds.), *Concept development in nursing: Foundations, techniques, and applications* (2nd ed., pp. 333–352). Philadelphia: W. B. Saunders.

Morse, J. M., Hupcey, J., Mitcham, C., & Lenz, E. (1996). Concept analysis in nursing research: A critical appraisal. *Scholarly Inquiry for Nursing Practice, 10,* 257–281.

Morse, J. M., Mitcham, C., Hupcey, J. E., & Tasón, M. C. (1996). Criteria for concept evaluation. *Journal of Advanced Nursing, 24,* 385–390.

Paley, J. (1996). How not to clarify concepts in nursing. *Journal of Advanced Nursing, 24,* 572–577.

Penrod, J., & Hupcey, J. E. (2005). Enhancing methodological clarity: Principle-based concept analysis. *Journal of Advanced Nursing, 50*(4), 403–409.

Rodgers, B. L. (1993). Concept analysis: An evolutionary view. In B. L. Rodgers & K. A. Knafl (Eds.), *Concept development in nursing: Foundations, techniques, and applications* (2nd ed., pp. 73–92). Philadelphia: W. B. Saunders.

Rodgers, B. L. (2000a). Philosophical foundations of concept development. In B. L. Rodgers & K. A. Knafl (Eds.), *Concept development in nursing: Foundations, techniques, and applications* (2nd ed., pp. 7–38). Philadelphia: W. B. Saunders.

Rodgers, B. L. (2000b). Concept analysis: An evolutionary view. In B. L. Rodgers & K. A. Knafl (Eds.), *Concept development in nursing: Foundations, techniques, and applications* (2nd ed., pp. 77–102). Philadelphia: W. B. Saunders.

Schwartz-Barcott, D., & Kim, H. S. (1986). A hybrid model for concept development. In P. L. Chinn (Ed.), *Nursing research methodology: Issues and implementation* (2nd ed., pp. 91–101). Rockville, MD: Aspen.

Schwartz-Barcott, D., & Kim, H. S. (1993). An expansion and elaboration of the hybrid model of concept development. In B. L. Rodgers & K. A. Knafl (Eds.), *Concept development in nursing: Foundations, techniques, and applications* (pp. 107–133). Philadelphia: W. B. Saunders.

Schwartz-Barcott, D., & Kim, H. S. (2000). An expansion and elaboration of the hybrid model of concept development. In B. L. Rodgers & K. A. Knafl (Eds.), *Concept development in nursing: Foundations, techniques, and applications* (2nd ed., pp. 129–160). Philadelphia: W. B. Saunders.

Schwartz-Barcott, D., Patterson, B. J., Lusardi, P., & Farmer, B. C. (2002). From practice to theory: Tightening the link via three fieldwork strategies. *Journal of Advanced Nursing, 39,* 281–289.

Walker, L. O., & Avant, K. C. (1983). *Strategies for theory construction in nursing.* Norwalk, CT: Appleton Century-Crofts.

Walker, L. O., & Avant, K. C. (1988). *Strategies for theory construction in nursing* (2nd ed.). Norwalk, CT: Appleton & Lange.

Walker, L. O., & Avant, K. C. (1995). *Strategies for theory construction in nursing* (3rd ed.). Norwalk, CT: Appleton & Lange.

Wilson, J. (1963). *Thinking with concepts.* Cambridge, England: Cambridge University Press.

THE AUTHORS COMMENT

Concept Analysis: Examining the State of the Science

Immersed in our work involving concept analysis, qualitative methodology, and theory building, we found the earlier writings on methods and the products of concept-driven work to be confusing or poorly integrated. Despite the potential power of this endeavor, it appeared that concept analyses were drifting toward becoming academic exercises, partly because the methods were not fully explicated. We launched this work in an effort to refocus thinking by stimulating discussion of a new interpretive framework. This and the accompanying article on concept advancement are benchmarks in the evolution in our thinking as we tried to assemble a coherent and meaningful framework for concept advancement that was useful to nurse scientists. We are indebted to our colleagues, especially the expert reviewers at *Research and Theory for Nursing Practice* who guided revisions with both enthusiastic encouragement and sharp critique.

JUDITH E. HUPCEY
JANICE PENROD

Rethinking Concept Analysis

MARK RISJORD, PhD

Aim: This study reports ways to strengthen the epistemological foundation of concept analysis and to clarify its ontology. **Background:** Nursing methods of concept analysis were derived from philosophy. In applying the philosophical ideas to nursing, changes were made that weakened the method. As a result, concept analyses often do not produce meaningful results. **Data sources:** Essays in nursing journals that critique or develop methods of concept analysis and philosophical writing about language. **Findings:** Many methods of concept analysis presuppose that the meaning of a concept depends on context. This 'contextualism' has epistemological and ontological consequences. Epistemologically, justifying a proposed set of defining attributes requires showing that the attributes explain the contextual pattern of use. Ontologically, concepts change their meaning as the theoretical contexts change. This means that concepts can only be developed as part of larger theories. Theory development requires a commitment to moderate realism and so, concept development also presupposes moderate realism. **Conclusion:** There are two forms of concept analysis: theoretical and colloquial. Each has its own purpose and evidence. The two forms can be used together and some theoretical developments will require both. Concept analysis must be based either on scientific literature or on colloquial usage. Concept analysis is not prior to theory development, but it must be part of theory development. It makes the meaning of a concept explicit, so that it can be part of testable and practical nursing theories. **Key words:** *concept analysis, epistemology, nursing theory, philosophy.*

Introduction

Concept analysis has a mixed reputation in nursing scholarship. As Walker and Avant (2005) introduced it in *Strategies for Theory Construction in Nursing* (first edition 1983), textbook authors have stated that concept analysis is necessary for theory development. However, many commentators have found concept analysis troublesome. Rodgers (1989, p. 331) remarked that it is 'not clear' how Walker and Avant's method 'actually contributes to further intellectual progression'. After discussing Walker and Avant's method and Rodgers' evolutionary method, Morse (1995, p. 32) concluded that such methods 'fail to produce a useful theoretical base'. Paley (1996, p. 578) concurred that concept analysis is 'an arbitrary and vacuous exercise'. Ten years later, after reviewing techniques for concept analysis, Hupcey and Penrod (2005, p. 205) concluded that 'the potential contribution of concept analysis on the evolution of nursing science has been constrained'. If these critics are right, then something is wrong with concept analysis in nursing.

Background

The character of concepts is a longstanding issue, both in philosophy and in nursing (Rodgers 2000b). One of the outstanding questions is how concepts relate to theories. Concepts are sometimes called 'the building blocks of theory' (Walker & Avant 2005, p. 26) and published concept analyses often include the suggestion that concepts can be fruitfully developed prior to any significant theorizing. This idea has been criticized in nursing (Rodgers 1989, 2000b, Paley 1996) as well as in philosophy (Quine 1953, Wittgenstein 1953). According to these critics, concepts are 'theory-formed' rather than 'theory-forming' (*cf.* Morse 1995, p. 42). This idea of 'contextualism' is often expressed with Carl Hempel's image of concepts as knots in the net of scientific theory (Hempel 1966, p. 94). As knots cannot exist without the cord, concepts cannot exist without the context. Paley (1996, p. 577) opts for the related image of concepts as 'niches' within theory. Whatever the metaphor, the underlying idea is that concepts

ABOUT THE AUTHOR

MARK RISJORD was raised in Madison, Wisconsin. He earned a BA in philosophy and a BA in anthropology at the University of Wisconsin, and a PhD in philosophy from the University of North Carolina at Chapel Hill. In 1993, he joined the Philosophy Department at Emory University. Since 1999, he has had an adjunct appointment with the Nell Hodgson Woodruff School of Nursing. His research focuses on philosophical issues that arise in the social and health sciences. In his spare time, he plays jazz bass and enjoys the outdoors with his wife and two daughters.

get their content from context. Contextualism played an important role in the development of concept analysis in nursing. Wilson's method (Wilson 1963) was the first method used by nurses and it presupposed that context determined word meaning. When it was adopted by nurse theorists, the method was transformed and the commitment to contextualism was elided. Contemporary concept analysis thus sits uneasily between the idea that concepts are theory-formed (contextualism) and the idea that they are theory-forming (building blocks).

The philosophical questions about concept analysis are both epistemological and ontological. According to some commentators, (Paley 1996, Hupcey & Penrod 2005), the fundamental problem with published concept analyses is that there is a very weak relationship between the evidence and the result. This raises epistemological questions: what *is* the evidence for a concept analysis and how should concept analyses be justified? In this study, I will argue that these questions can best be answered by reaffirming the idea that concepts must be related to contexts, such as theories, discourses or speech communities. The ontological consequences of this form of contextualism have been the subject of a recent dispute. Hupcey and Penrod (2005) have argued that contextualism entails a moderate realist ontological framework. In response, Duncan *et al.* (2007) have argued that contextualism requires a relativist, context-bound ontology. Once the relationship of contextualism to the epistemology of concept analysis has been made clear, this ontological dispute can be resolved.

Many discussions of concepts and concept analysis have been committed to the idea that concepts are contextual (Rodgers 1989, 2000b, Paley 1996, Hupcey & Penrod 2005, Duncan *et al.* 2007). Others have either been committed to a view of concepts as prior to theories or have been ambivalent about the possibilities (Morse 1995, Walker & Avant 2005). In this study, I will recommend a renewed commitment to contextualism by arguing that if it is adopted, then concept analysis and development can be put on a more robust epistemological and ontological footing.

Data Sources

In this study, I use historical and philosophical methods to critique arguments found in the nursing literature. The project began with an analysis of the arguments in widely-cited books and essays about concept analysis. Historical influences on these key essays were traced through their bibliographies. Google Scholar was used to identify subsequent publications by authors responding to the key essays. Finally, arguments concerning the epistemology or ontology of concept analysis were evaluated in the light of philosophical literature on concepts and word meaning.

Findings

Wilson's Method

In *Thinking with Concepts*, Wilson (1963) intended to popularize a method that was common among the so-called 'ordinary language philosophers'. Thinkers in this mid-twentieth century school held that philosophical problems were often the result of linguistic muddles. Therefore, prior to answering the deep questions about, say, freedom or moral responsibility, philosophers should be clear about the meaning of words such as 'free' and 'responsible'. To do this, ordinary language philosophers emphasized the need for careful analysis of how words were commonly used. In their work, they made two presuppositions. First, conceptual content is closely related to (if not identical to) word meaning. Second, ordinary language philosophers generally held that 'the meaning of a word is its use in the language' (Wittgenstein 1953, p. 20). It follows from these two assumptions that clarity about concepts required attending closely to the use of words. By 'use', ordinary language philosophers meant the utterance of a word as part of a sentence in a particular context or situation. Situations where a word was naturally used must exhibit attributes of the word's meaning. If speakers refrained from using a word in a situation, preferring a contrasting word, then the situation must lack some attribute necessary to the word's meaning. Ziff (1960) framed the idea in terms of such contrast: the meaning of a word is the difference it makes to the use of a sentence. To state the meaning of a word, then, is to articulate the difference between those situations where we are inclined to use the word and those where we are inclined to refrain from doing so.

Wilson's method of concept analysis relied on the ideas of the ordinary language philosophers. He recommended developing examples (cases) designed to highlight the difference a word makes to the use of a sentence. In nursing, Wilson's cases are sometimes treated as if an analyst could chose to use some kinds of cases without others. This is a misunderstanding of Wilson and the philosophical background of ordinary language philosophy shows why. The model case is an example where the word is naturally and commonly used. For example, an analysis of the concept of 'ache' might begin with the model case of Sally, who has had a dull, throbbing pain in her wrist for a half hour. It would be natural to say, 'Sally has an ache in her wrist'. The problem is that every feature of the model case is a possible defining attribute, including Sally's gender, or the fact that the pain is in her wrist. The problem is to narrow down the list and this can only be done by finding more examples. Additional model cases are a first step. Gender and location can be eliminated as possible features by finding other model cases where the protagonist is male and has a pain in his tooth. Model cases alone, however, cannot be used to identify the *difference* that the word makes to the use of the sentence. Identifying difference requires examples where the word would not be used. A contrary case for 'ache' would be one where Sally is free from pain. This shows that being painful is a necessary attribute of the concept of an ache. Related cases show that the pain must have a certain character. If Sally had only a quick flash of pain, it might be a 'twinge' or 'prick', but not an 'ache'. Contrary and related cases thus work to identify difference, and must therefore work along with the model case to isolate a set of candidates for attributes.

Epistemically, the cases form the evidence for a concept analysis. The function of evidence is to justify a belief or theory. In a Wilsonian concept analysis, the object is to create something like a dictionary definition. Dictionaries show that words typically have many different uses. Sometimes, the differences are small and we speak of different senses of a single word (*eg*, the physical and emotional senses of 'comfort'). Sometimes, the differences are large and the dictionary says that there is not one word, but a set of homonyms (*eg*, at least three different words are spelled 'bank'). A good Wilsonian concept analysis will identify the different uses, sort these into senses of the

word and articulate a definition. The definition will be justified insofar as it accounts for the whole range of examples. A good concept analysis should explain why the model and contrary cases are clear as well as why we hesitate in the borderline cases.

Walker and Avant's Transformation of Wilson's Method

The intention behind Wilson's method was to help clarify concepts that were used in common, colloquial speech. Walker and Avant wanted to use concept analysis in their strategies for theory construction and this motivated one important change in method. Scientific literature had to be made relevant. They thus recommended a broad review of sources: 'dictionaries, thesauruses, colleagues and available literature' (Walker & Avant 2005, p. 67). Scientific literature is important, they said, but the literature review should not be restricted to 'just nursing and medical literature'. By itself, this modification of Wilson's method is salutary. The latter put the speaker in a privileged position, as if they were the ultimate authority on a word's meaning. But speakers may be idiosyncratic and words may have well-established uses of which the speaker is unaware. Therefore, to undertake a comprehensive review of literature is good advice. A problem arose when Walker and Avant (2005) presented concept analysis as a process of eight steps, beginning with a literature review, determining the attributes and only then working through Wilson's cases. Readers took this to be a linear process (in spite of Walker and Avant's advice to the contrary). In many published concept analyses, the defining attributes are identified before the discussion of cases. Wilson's cases are thereby transformed from evidence into illustrations. Treated as illustrations, they add little or no substance to the analysis. As a result, the most common modification of Walker and Avant's method is to reduce the number of cases or eliminate them entirely (Chinn & Kramer 1999, Morse 1995, Rodgers 1989, 2000a, Schwartz-Barcott & Kim 2000).

The practice of concept analysis in nursing, then, turns Wilson's method upside down. The cases were supposed to be evidence that justified the choice of defining attributes. The literature review replaced the cases, but there was no account of how the literature was supposed to support the particular attributes. By turning Wilson's cases into illustrative examples (or worse, eliminating them entirely), nursing methods of concept analysis created a gap between evidence and result. Paley (1996) and Hupcey and Penrod (2005) have pointed out that one of the chief weaknesses of published concept analyses is that the author never justifies the choice of defining attributes.

The reader is left wondering why the concept has these attributes and not others. The transformation of Wilson's method explains why published concept analyses are so weakly supported by the evidence. The source of the problem is that, after Walker and Avant, the methods provide no guidance for how the attributes are to be justified. It is no wonder that concept analysis seems an arbitrary and vacuous exercise.

Epistemological Foundation of Concept Analysis

The central idea of Wilson's method is that a concept analysis is justified by a pattern of usage in a particular context. The gap between evidence and result was created when the commitment to contextualism was lost and this happened when Walker and Avant applied the method to scientific literature. One tradition, starting with Rodgers (1989), continuing through Paley (1996) and re-expressed by Hupcey and Penrod (2005), held that scientific concepts are contextual in just the same way as ordinary language concepts. For a scientific concept, the context of use is a theory or related group of theories. To articulate the meaning of a scientific term, then, one needs to look on the difference it makes to the theory: the pattern of inferences, observations and practical interventions that the term enables. The justification for a concept analysis in a scientific context is, therefore, largely the same as the justification for the analysis of a colloquial term. In both cases, the evidential basis for a concept analysis is a pattern of use and a particular analysis is justified if it accounts for that pattern. The specific difference is that scientific concept analyses need to attend to the scientific usage of a word, while colloquial analyses may rely on a broader range of uses.

If the content of a concept depends on the context of use, as contextualism holds, then when the context of use changes, the meaning must change too. This idea is a cornerstone of Rodgers (1989, 2000a) 'evolutionary method'. While she emphasizes the way in which concepts and theories change together over time, this point also applies to different contexts at the same time point. For example, the word 'depression' is used in the psychology, weather forecasting, economics and common speech. These contexts are independent insofar as the use of 'depression' in one domain may change without corresponding changes in the others. Moreover, as Hupcey and Penrod (2005) point out, when a term is part of a scientific theory, it is often explicitly defined and its implications are restricted. Scientific concepts are thus more precise than their colloquial counterparts and when similar terms appear in different theories they may have different meanings. As psychology and meteorology are very different contexts, they support different concepts

of 'depression', even though they use the same word. It is therefore a mistake to indiscriminately mix literary, colloquial and scientific sources. By failing to attend to contextual differences, authors dilute their evidence base to the point that it is impossible to justify any selection of attributes. A 'tropical depression', a psychological 'depression', the 'Great Depression' and a 'depression in the grass' have no more in common than a vague sense of going down. A concept analysis that does not carefully attend to a specific context of use is robbed of its power to justify a nuanced analysis.

Ontological Consequences of Contextualism

Contextualism has some ontological consequences that have recently been dispute in the nursing literature. Duncan et al. 2007, p. 297 argued that the contextual character of concepts implies a 'relativist ontological perspective'. They explicitly contrast this relativism with the 'moderate realism' adopted by Hupcey and Penrod (2005, p. 201) in their work on concept analysis. Both sides of this debate agree on the fundamental premise that 'concepts are assigned meaning through placement within the context of theory' (cf. Hupcey & Penrod 2005, p. 199, Duncan et al. 2007, p. 296). Their dispute is about what this premise entails.

Hupcey and Penrod (2005, p. 201) describe their 'moderate realism' as a commitment to the 'probable truth' of scientific theories. The notion of 'truth' they deploy makes their view a form of realism in which the statements of a theory can be true or false only if the concepts represent some mind-independent objects. A strong or absolute form of realism would hold that the truth or falsity of theoretical statements is determined solely by the way things are and that an objective scientific method will guarantee truth. The antirealist view holds that truth is 'a construction of those who experience a given phenomenon at a given point in time' (Hupcey & Penrod 2005, p. 200). Hupcey and Penrod's moderate realism occupies a middle ground between these extremes and it does so in two ways. First, they invoke the 'probable' truth of scientific theory. To say that the truth of theories is 'probable' rather than 'absolute' is to admit that scientific inquiry is fallible. At any given time, we judge our theories to be true, but recognize that they may be overturned by future evidence. Second, Hupcey and Penrod affirm the importance of context for conceptual meaning. This means that when theories are changed, the concepts take on new meaning. Scientists decide how to construct theories and thus determine the meaning of the concepts, but they do not thereby determine the truth of a theory. On a moderate realist view, 'probable truth transcends individual experience' (Hupcey & Penrod 2005, p. 201).

Duncan *et al.* (2007) argue that Hupcey and Penrod are part of a realist tradition of concept analysis that is at odds with contextualism. They argue that the realist tradition of concept analysis arose because Walker & Avant (2005) attempted to 'transcend context and thereby accommodate the requirement of a product useful for empirical work' (Duncan *et al.* 2007, p. 297). After Walker and Avant, they argue, methods of concept analysis stripped concepts from their context and attempted to provide definitions that are free from entanglement with any theory: 'The outcome of Walker and Avant's analysis is fixed truth; concepts as measurable variables that ideally are knowable outside of context and function in a realist research world' (Duncan *et al.* 2007, p. 297). Realism, Duncan *et al.* argue, requires concepts that are not contextual. Only then can scientific methods demonstrate that a theory is true or false in a realist sense of 'truth'.

The key to Duncan *et al.*'s argument is their claim that realism and contextualism are inconsistent. Realism holds that theories are true when they correctly represent a mind-independent reality. Realism therefore requires a distinction between representations (words, concepts, propositions or theories) and the things represented. Contextualism means that concepts get their content from a context, which may be a theory or colloquial use. Contextualism tells us something about representations, not the things represented. It is therefore consistent to hold that the content of a concept is fixed by the theoretical context, but that, once fixed, it represents something. It follows that as the theory changes, what gets represented changes. This is part of what Hupcey and Penrod are expressing in their 'moderate realism'. When new evidence undermines a theory, it is taken to be an inaccurate representation of a mind-independent reality (*ie*, false). When the theory is modified and its concepts change, something new is thereby represented. If the new theory is supported, it is provisionally taken as an accurate representation (*ie*, probably true). Contrary to Duncan *et al.*, realism and contextualism are fully consistent. Therefore, contextualism does not entail relativism.

Once we have understood why realism and contextualism are consistent, a stronger link between them appears. If concepts are 'knots' or 'niches' within larger contexts, then the only way to change concepts is to change the context. Where the concepts are scientific, the larger context is a theory. Theories change when they are tested. Even abstract theories or conceptual models are indirectly supported by evidence and should be developed in the light of empirical investigation. Contextualism about meaning thus entails that the only way to develop scientific concepts is to test theories. A theory can be supported (or undermined) by evidence only if its propositions are taken to be true or false and this in turn requires that the concepts represent something real. Therefore, if nursing is to develop its concepts, a commitment to contextualism *requires* a commitment to moderate realism.

 ## Discussion

A concept analysis makes a pattern of usage explicit. Because nursing concept analyses are intended to contribute to theory development, the scientific pattern of use is important. As we have seen, there are significant differences between the scientific context and the context of colloquial speech. This difference leads Hupcey and Penrod (2005) to conclude that the concept analysis should be restricted to scientific literature:

> *We assert that the purpose of concept analysis is to determine the state of the science (or best estimate of probable truth) surrounding the concept of interest. Thus, concept analyses are concerned with scientific literature, not creative imagination, art forms, fiction, interview data or any other form of representation. (p. 205)*

This conclusion will be troublesome to nurse scholars who pursue qualitative research. Interviews are the backbone of qualitative methods. When a researcher conducts interviews, the goal is to understand how the participants experience or conceptualize some domain. Attributing a world of meaning (which always includes concepts) to a person or community on the basis of patterns found in interviews is part of any interview-based method. Where the researcher is trying to discover the participants' conceptions, the researcher is doing a form of concept analysis. Therefore, excluding interview data and similar sources from the evidence for concept analysis would make qualitative research impossible.

Hupcey and Penrod probably did not mean to exclude qualitative research. The apparent exclusion arises because they focused on scientific concepts. To resolve the problem, we need only to remind ourselves of the importance of context. The context for a scientific concept is a theory or group of theories. When an interviewer explores the concepts of a community, on the other hand, the context is their everyday speech. This difference in context suggests that we should recognize two forms of concept analysis. Each has its own purposes and kinds of evidence. In the first, 'theoretical concept analysis,' the aim is to represent concepts as they appear in particular scientific literatures and the relevant evidence must be restricted to scientific literature. In the second, 'colloquial concept analysis,' the aim is to represent the concepts of a particular group of people. Evidence of what people say and do, including formal interviews, participant observation, casual speech and imaginative literature, is relevant to these analyses. Notice that these are forms of analysis, not methods. Choice of methods (eg, semistructured interviews or focus groups) is determined by the needs of the particular study.

Theoretical Concept Analysis

To make the meaning of a scientific concept clear, a theoretical concept analysis must make explicit both the theoretical role of the concept and its relationship to observation or practice. Again, the meaning of a term or concept is the difference it makes in the context. For a scientific concept, this means answering questions such as: how is the term defined in the theory? Is it used to define other terms? What predictions or explanations does the concept make possible that would be impossible otherwise? In what causal generalizations or descriptions of patterns does the concept appear? If the theory has immediate practical application, how does the use of the term make a difference to what is done? An explicit formulation of the meaning of the term will make its theoretical contribution and application to observation and practice clear. In so doing, the analyst will, as Hupcey and Penrod (2005) say, determine the state of the science surrounding the concept.

One of the challenges of theoretical concept analysis is the choice of an appropriate domain of discourse. To avoid ambiguities, the analyst should choose a domain that promises to be coherent and yield an informative set of attributes. If the concept is widely used, the data for the analysis may include a broad range of theories from different disciplines. However, the analyst must remain alert for differences among the scientific uses of the concept. Even within one discipline, theories might use a term in different ways. In nursing, for example, the concept of coping has been treated slightly differently in different theories. A good theoretical analysis of 'coping' would isolate these differences and determine whether there is one concept or many concepts of coping in nursing theories. Identification of such differences is an important kind of theoretical progress. Making the differences explicit allows the theories to be more rigorously compared and evaluated. Left unrecognized, such ambiguities make studies incommensurable and applications impractical.

Theoretical concept analysis is primarily useful for making the content of an existing theoretical concept explicit. When its content is clear, researchers will be able to judge whether the theory is applicable to nursing phenomena and whether it is consistent with other theories. Ultimately, however, the goal of nursing researchers is to develop solutions to nursing problems. This means that the theories will have to be modified and changing the concepts is a part of theoretical change. Theoretical concept analysis contributes to theory development by clarifying conceptual materials that nurse theorists will rework for their own ends.

Colloquial Concept Analysis

The objective of colloquial concept analysis is to characterize the concepts prevalent in a particular community, typically a community of nurses or nursing clients. Colloquial concept analysis thus focuses on people, while theoretical concept analysis focuses on literature. To capture the appropriate context, the colloquial analyst needs to delimit a target population. If the analyst is concerned to understand, say, adolescents' concept of 'depression,' it will not be helpful to ask healthcare professionals; teenagers must be interviewed. Focus groups and interviews are appropriate methods for colloquial analysis. Wilson's method was intended as a way of identifying concepts in the context of common speech. The addition of focus groups or interviews expands the data available for analysis, as does the exploration of literature and imagery that is read or produced by the target group. While the range of examples is broader and the details of the method different, the underlying philosophical principles are the same as Wilson's.

Colloquial concept analysis faces several unique challenges. First, colloquial concepts are unlikely to have the clear definitions found in scientific theories. Everyday concepts can be fluid and vague. Indeed, cognitive psychologists have found evidence that human concepts are not structured by necessary and sufficient conditions. Rather, humans tend to think in terms of paradigms, exemplars or family resemblances (for a discussion of this literature as it relates to concept analysis, see Paley 1996 and Rodgers 2000b). The colloquial analyst thus needs to take care not to force the analysis into an artificial form. Second, while words are shared, their meanings may differ among communities. The analyst thus needs to consider whether there are subgroups within the study population that might have different ways of thinking about the phenomenon. There is no reason, for example, to suppose in advance that all nurses think about 'caring' in the same way. Pediatric nurses in urban hospitals may have one concept, while nurse practitioners in rural clinics have another. In any concept analysis, the existence of conceptual similarities and differences is something to be discovered, not presupposed. Finally, the colloquial analyst has to be alert for contested concepts, where subgroups have a stake in the way something is represented.

What is already known about this topic

- Methods of concept analysis in nursing are an important part of theory development.
- Nursing theorists have adopted methods of concept analysis from philosophy.
- Conceptual meaning depends on the context of use.

What this paper adds

- There are two forms of concept analysis: theoretical and colloquial.
- Theoretical concept analysis and colloquial concept analysis have different purposes and evidence bases.
- Concept development requires a commitment to moderate realism.

Implications for practice and/or policy

- When using a concept analysis, researchers should attend carefully to the evidence base of the analysis.
- Concepts are developed by testing and modifying the theories of which they are a part.

Once we identify the purpose, methods and evidence for colloquial concept analysis, it becomes clear that it is not much different from some of the best qualitative research in nursing. The aim in ethnography, phenomenology and grounded theory is often to uncover how some nurses or nursing clients conceptualize their environment. The usefulness of colloquial concept analysis is thus very similar to the value of descriptive, qualitative research. In addition, colloquial concept analysis can be a first step toward extracting the knowledge embedded in nursing practice. We are often unaware of the full extent of the patterns in our speech and behavior (Wittgenstein 1953, Ziff 1960) and nurses successfully respond to situations in ways they cannot fully express (Benner 1984). A colloquial concept analysis makes explicit such implicit regularities, thereby uncovering new concepts for theory development.

Mixed Analyses

Theoretical and colloquial concept analyses have distinct goals and evidence. They are, nonetheless, compatible and some of the more sophisticated forms of nursing research require both. Many nursing phenomena are patient-centered in the sense that how the patient feels, thinks or responds is a central part of what is being theorized. In symptom management, for example, the patient's way of conceptualizing a symptom will be important for its expression, evaluation and mitigation. To understand the phenomenon, the theorist will need to know how patients are thinking about it and responding to it. Clearly, this phase of

the research will require colloquial concept analyses. At the same time, concepts like 'depression' or 'pain' have been developed within scientific theories that do not begin from the patient's point of view. Many nursing phenomena have a biological, psychological or social dimension. A theoretical concept analysis is likely to show that the meaning of, say, pain in a neurological theory is much different from the meaning of pain to a patient. Nursing theories of pain cannot afford to ignore either the neurological or the patient-centered concepts of pain. Nurse scholars thus face the profound challenge of developing theories that encompass both the subjective and physical character of phenomena like pain. Using both theoretical and colloquial concept analyses, nurse theorists can begin to forge new concepts (in new theories) that do justice to the whole phenomenon.

 ## Conclusion

Concept analysis, whether theoretical or colloquial, articulates concepts that already have a home in some domain: in scientific theories, among people in a community or both. Concept analysis is thus merely a phase of the concept development process. It makes existing concepts explicit objects of reflection and this is especially important where theories are being borrowed and modified. Nurses have also found that where theory does not yet exist, it is useful to start with the knowledge embedded in nursing practice. Colloquial concept analysis (often as part of a qualitative research project) is one way to make this knowledge explicit. Whether colloquial or theoretical, concept analysis is never an end in itself; it is a means toward theoretical development. Contextualism entails that if concepts are to be developed, they must be embedded within theories and these theories must be tested. The evidence for concept development is therefore nothing more (or less) than the evidence for theory development. We keep those concepts that are parts of well-confirmed and useful theories and when theories are changed, the concepts change. Therefore, neither concept analysis nor concept development is an independent form of research. Both are adjuncts to theory development. If nursing is to develop mature concepts, the emphasis must be on the testing and subsequent modification of theories.

 ## Funding

This research received no specific grant from any funding agency in the public, commercial, or not-for-profit sectors.

REFERENCES

Benner P. (1984) *From Novice to Expert*. Addison-Wesley, Menlo Park CA.

Chinn P.L. & Kramer M.K. (1999) *Theory and Nursing: Integrated Knowledge Development*, 5th edn. Mosby, St. Louis.

Duncan C., Cloutier J.D. & Bailey P.H. (2007) Concept analysis: the importance of differentiating the ontological focus. *Journal of Advanced Nursing* **58**, 293–300.

Hempel C. (1966) *Philosophy of Natural Science*. Prentice Hall, Englewood Cliffs, NJ.

Hupcey J.E. & Penrod J. (2005) Concept analysis: examining the state of the science. *Research and Theory for Nursing Practice: An International Journal* **19**, 197–208.

Morse J.M. (1995) Exploring the theoretical basis of nursing knowledge using advanced techniques of concept analysis. *Advances in Nursing Science* **17**, 31–46.

Paley J. (1996) How not to clarify concepts in nursing. *Journal of Advanced Nursing* **24**, 572–578.

Quine W.V.O. (1953) *From a Logical Point of View*. Harper and Row, New York.

Rodgers B.L. (1989) Concepts, analysis, and the development of nursing knowledge: the evolutionary cycle. *Journal of Advanced Nursing* **14**, 330–335.

Rodgers B.L. (2000a) Concept analysis: an evolutionary view. In *Concept Development in Nursing: Foundations, Techniques, and Applications* (Rodgers B.L. & Knafl K.A., eds), W. B. Saunders Company, Philadelphia, pp. 77–102.

Rodgers B.L. (2000b) Philosophical foundations of concept development. In *Concept Development in Nursing: Foundations, Techniques, and Applications* (Rodgers B.L. & Knafl K.A., eds), W. B. Saunders Company, Philadelphia, pp. 7–38.

Schwartz-Barcott D. & Kim H.S. (2000) An expansion and elaboration of the hybrid model of concept development. In *Concept Development in Nursing: Foundations, Techniques, and Applications* (Rogers B.L. & Knafl K., eds), W. B. Saunders Company, Philadelphia, pp. 129–159.

Walker L.O. & Avant K.C. (2005) *Strategies for Theory Construction in Nursing*, 4th edn. Pearson Prentice Hall, Upper Saddle River, NJ. Wilson J. (1963) *Thinking with Concepts*. Cambridge. University Press, Cambridge.

Wittgenstein L. (1953) *Philosophical Investigations* (G. E. M. Anscombe, Trans.). Macmillan Publishing Company, New York.

Ziff P. (1960) *Semantic Analysis*. Cornell University Press, Ithaca.

THE AUTHOR COMMENTS │ Rethinking Concept Analysis

When I first encountered concept analysis in nursing, I was struck by the way it reproduced philosophical ideas that had been subject to severe criticism in philosophy. I was also concerned that many published concept analyses were uninformative. This essay criticizes some philosophical presuppositions about concept analysis that I think are responsible for the problems with concept analysis as currently practiced. Properly understood, clarifying concepts is an essential part of developing nursing theories, and this essay tries to rest concept analysis on a more secure epistemological foundation.

MARK RISJORD

Levels of Theoretical Thinking in Nursing

PATRICIA A. HIGGINS, RN, PhD

SHIRLEY M. MOORE, RN, PhD, FAAN

*D*evelopment of a knowledge base is an iterative and ongoing process that requires periodic analysis and synthesis of an entire body of work. This article examines 4 related levels of theoretical thinking that are currently used in developing knowledge for nursing practice, education, and science: metatheory, grand theory, middle-range theory, and micro-range theory. Each level of theory is discussed according to typology, scope, and generalizability, level of abstraction, and role. Suggestions are made for clarification of terminology, and examples are provided for each level of theoretical thinking. Evidence associated with the 4 levels of theoretical thinking is discussed, and applications for use of the levels of theoretical thinking to meet future challenges in nursing's knowledge development are offered.*

In an effort to build a knowledge base for the clinical, educational, and scientific endeavors of the discipline, nursing theory has undergone several phases of development. In the earliest period, scholars focused their attention on building grand theory and debating the structure and methods for developing nursing theory. More recently, there has been a call for the development of middle-range theory. Thus theory in nursing has been conceptualized as existing on several levels although there are wide differences in the definitions and terminology associated with the levels of theoretical thinking and the classification of theoretical products. This lack of clarity impedes our use of theoretical thinking to extend and communicate our nursing knowledge. Therefore, the purpose of this article is to present an examination of levels of theoretical thinking in nursing and provide examples of how several existing nursing theories can be classified within the theoretical levels. Applications of levels of theoretical thinking to meet challenges in knowledge development in nursing are suggested.

A theory in its simplest view is the creation of relationships among two or more concepts to form a specific view of a phenomenon. As constructions of our mind, theories provide explanations about our experiences of phenomena in the world.[1] The understanding provided by theories is of two types: explanatory (describing concepts and understanding interactions among concepts) or predictive (anticipating a particular set of outcomes).[2] Theories consist of the following components: (1) concepts that are identified and defined, (2) assumptions that clarify the basic underlying truths from which and within which theoretical reasoning proceeds, (3) context within which the theory is placed, and (4) identified relationships between and among the concepts.[3]

The terms theory, theoretical (or conceptual) model, theoretical framework, and theoretical system are often used to distinguish different types of theory. This practice has created confusion among scholars and practitioners, and we believe a more useful approach to understanding theory is to consider all of the aforementioned terms as parallel synonyms. Each can be used interchangeably, but each term also requires further specification through an adjective modifier, such as "grand" or "middle range," that describes its fit with other theoretical work. Thus the notion of different levels of theoretical thinking can be a more useful way to develop, disseminate, and use knowledge in nursing. We use the word "level" to imply a relative degree of relationship rather than a ranking or a distinct advantage. Each level of theoretical thinking has defining characteristics and purposes that are specific to that level. The scope or breadth of the concepts and goals of a theoretical system determine its use for research and practice. Therefore, theoretical thinking in nursing uses concepts and their relationships to organize and critique existing knowledge and guide new discoveries to advance practice.

Reprinted from Nursing Outlook, 48(4), P. A. Higgins & S. M. Moore, Levels of theoretical thinking, 179–183.
Copyright © 2000 with permission from Elsevier Science.

ABOUT THE AUTHORS

PATRICIA HIGGINS is Associate Professor of Nursing, Case Western Reserve University (CWRU). Her first nursing diploma was from Henry Ford Hospital (1970) and her second from Akron University (BSN, 1986). These were followed by graduate degrees from CWRU (MSN, 1989; PhD, 1996). Her teaching concentrates on theory and philosophy of science, and her program of research focuses on understanding and improving the health of adults who live with chronic conditions. In her time off, Dr. Higgins enjoys her family, gardening, and reading.

SHIRLEY MOORE is the Edward J. & Louise Mellen Professor of Nursing and Associate Dean for Research at Case Western Reserve University (CWRU) Frances Payne Bolton School of Nursing, Cleveland, OH. Born at the beginning of the baby boom, she began her nursing career during a shift in nursing education from hospital training programs to more academic-focused programs, and she considers herself a product of both. Dr. Moore received her diploma of nursing from the Youngstown Hospital Association School of Nursing (1969) and her bachelor's degree in nursing from Kent State University (1974). At CWRU, she earned a master's degree in nursing-psychiatric mental health nursing (1990) and a PhD in nursing science (1993). Dr. Moore has taught nursing theory and nursing science to all levels of nursing students and has a program of research and theory development that addresses recovery after acute cardiac events. Her hobbies include traveling with her family, reading, and music.

Its development and use is not limited to particular venues, time frames, or formats, and although *all* nurses may not use theoretical thinking *at all times,* its actual use is more frequent than some nurses may acknowledge. For instance, theoretical thinking regarding a family's psychologic well being can be briefly and automatically accessed as part of the gestalt of clinical practice or formally developed into a more permanent, written framework. Both types of theoretical thinking are crucial for practice, and either may be critiqued, modified, and tested.

Linkages between the theoretical world and the empirical world to which it applies are made through the formulation and testing of hypotheses. Both scientists and practitioners use this process to make the empirical world and the theoretical world as congruent as possible. It is important to distinguish an empirical system from a theoretical system. An empirical system is what we apprehend, through senses, in the environment. A theoretical system is what we construct in our mind's eye to model the empirical system.[1] Nurse scientists and practitioners focus on understanding the variables of a particular practice situation. To better understand a specific event, they formulate working definitions and associations among variables (hypotheses) and either develop a new theoretical system or link them to existing organizing frameworks. The theoretical system then serves as guidance about how to proceed, and as long as the abstraction of a theory can be represented with empiric indicators, hypotheses can be generated and empirically tested.[2]

Levels of Theoretical Thinking

Theory in the human sciences has been used to delineate and legitimate the emerging disciplines and substantiate knowledge development.[4] There are 4 levels of theoretical thinking in nursing: metatheory, grand theory, middle-range theory, and micro-range theory.[5] Each level of theory will be discussed according to level of abstraction and scope, generalizability, typology, and role. Figure 33-1 describes the relationships among the 4 levels and provides examples of theoretical thinking for each level.

Meta-theory

Meta-theory, the most abstract and universal of the 4 levels of theoretical thinking, addresses issues related to the conduct of inquiry. Therefore, it is the theory of inquiry. Meta-theory or philosophic inquiry uses logic and analytic reasoning to examine the direction, methods, and standards of inquiry and thus it differs from the other levels of theory as its product is primarily knowledge-about-knowledge (second-order knowledge), rather than specific theoretical frameworks that explain the empirical world (first-order knowledge). Metatheoretical inquiry related to scientific issues is known as philosophy of science, and it focuses on a critical examination of science, its processes, and products. Used by both scientists and practitioners, metatheoretical inquiry also addresses questions that science cannot answer. For example, in the study of death and dying, scientific inquiry seeks

Figure 33-1 *Levels of theoretical thinking.*

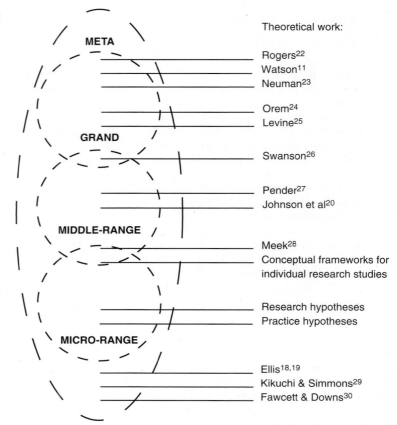

Theoretical work:

Rogers[22]
Watson[11]
Neuman[23]

Orem[24]
Levine[25]

Swanson[26]

Pender[27]
Johnson et al[20]

Meek[28]
Conceptual frameworks for individual research studies

Research hypotheses
Practice hypotheses

Ellis[18,19]
Kikuchi & Simmons[29]
Fawcett & Downs[30]

to answer questions about the physiologic changes leading to death. However, philosophic inquiry is needed to address the question, "Is death best understood as a process or a product?" Therefore, an understanding of metatheoretical thinking is central to both the research and practice of nursing.

As the most well established of the 4 levels, the significance and role of metatheoretical knowledge in nursing is revealed through a partial list of issues addressed through this mode of inquiry: (1) clarification of the relationship between nursing science and practice, (2) definition, development, and testing of nursing theory, (3) establishment of the academic discipline of nursing, and (4) examination and interpretation of fundamental philosophic perspectives and their connection to nursing science. The long list of exemplary scholarship that represents these 4 categories of philosophic inquiry in nursing is well represented in anthologies such as the one by Nicoll,[6] but one example also illustrates the value of the discipline's metatheoretical thinking. In 1978 when Carper[7] published her influential article on the fundamental patterns of knowing in nursing, she initiated a spirited dialogue that continues to this day—in print, classrooms, and practice arenas throughout the world.

Grand Theory

Nursing grand theories are the global paradigms of nursing science.[8] They are formal, highly abstract theoretical systems that frame our disciplinary knowledge within the principles of nursing, and their concepts and propositions transcend specific events and patient populations. The substantial body of analytic and philosophic reasoning that has emerged from grand theory provides evidence of scholarship that distinguishes nursing from other closely related disciplines and legitimizes its existence among academic disciplines.[9] Thus grand theory's most significant contribution to nursing is the establishment and substantiation of the discipline's identity and boundaries.

Given their abstract nature, grand theories provide universal explanations and an understanding of nursing, but not the particulars that are necessary for empirical testing. As a result, they have little predictive capability. Some grand theories also use language that is difficult for the beginning student and unfamiliar to many potential users. Nevertheless, they have significantly influenced knowledge development within the discipline and there are numerous examples of their use in guiding nursing research, practice, and education. Grand theories also contribute to the historical perspective of nursing, reflecting the time and context in which the authors developed their theories, as well as their philosophic underpinnings and their educational and practice perspectives. In charting the growth of the discipline, Nightingale[10] can be considered the first grand theorist and *Notes on Nursing,* the original paradigm of contemporary nursing.

There is debate about what constitutes a grand theory and thus, which nursing scholars' work should be classified as grand theory. For example, is Jean Watson's[11] *Philosophy and Science of Caring* more accurately categorized as a "philosophy" or "grand theory" of nursing? Further, should Madeleine Leininger's[12] conceptual model, *Culture Care: Diversity and Universality Theory,* be classified as a grand or middle-range theory? Our view is that this type of debate reflects the growth of nursing's disciplinary knowledge. Although we may never have a consensus of answers for such questions, it also indicates that we have sufficiently established our external boundaries, and we can now redirect our energy to further distinguish the internal substance and structure of our knowledge through the construction of middle-range theories.

Middle-Range Theory

In terms of historical development, middle-range theory is the relative newcomer to nursing science. Similar to grand theory, middle-range theory explains the empirical world of nursing, but it is more specific and less formal. For example, the philosophic underpinnings and assumptions of the middle-range theorist may be more implicit than explicit. As indicated by its name, any explanation of middle-range theory requires discussing "what it is" and "what comes before and after in its range." Suppe[4] was one of the first to clarify and define middle-range theory for nursing science. By using Merton's examination of sociologic theory,[13] Suppe[4] provided 3 criteria for delimiting middle-range theory from grand theory and the next lower level, micro-range theory. These 3 criteria, scope, level of abstraction, and testability are widely accepted.[14,15]

In terms of scope and level of abstraction, Lenz et al[15] stated that "middle-range theories (are those) that are sufficiently specific to guide research and practice, yet sufficiently general to cross multiple clinical populations and to encompass similar phenomena." In the quote from Lenz et al,[15] the guidance for research and practice is much more direct than is that offered by grand theory; therefore, middle-range theory can be tested in the empirical world. The concepts or phenomena of interest can be coded objectively (by using either qualitative or quantitative methods) and it has the potential to postulate measurable

relationships between the phenomena; thus it has a "time-relativistic distinction."[4] The generalizability of middle-range theory is further defined by boundaries that limit measurement of the person-environment interaction. Although testable across several different patient populations and environments, a particular middle-range theory does *not* address *all* patients in *all* environments. For example, Good and Moore's[14] theory on pain management applies only to adults who experience acute surgical pain and is appropriately tested only during the immediate postoperative period. Because of the aforementioned characteristics, middle-range theory is not as limited as grand theory in its typology and can be classified as either explanatory or predictive. A major role of middle-range theory is to define or refine the substantive content of nursing science and practice, and it should be an important focus of both nurse scholars and practitioners as we continue to build knowledge for the discipline.

Micro-range Theory

Micro-range theory is the least formal and most tentative of the theoretical levels discussed in this article. It also is the most restrictive in terms of time and scope or application. However, its particularistic approach is invaluable for scientists and practitioners as they work to describe, organize, and test their ideas. We propose 2 levels of micro-range theory. At the higher level, micro-range theory is closely related to middle-range theory but is comprised of 1 or 2 major concepts, and its application frequently is limited to a particular event; for example, theories related to decubitus or catheter care.[16]

At the lower level, micro-range theory is defined as a set of working hypotheses or propositions.[17] Scientists and practitioners use these working propositions to tentatively categorize, explain, or test health-related person-environment interactions. As such, they are not coded and entered into a formal theoretical system, but two examples serve to illustrate their invaluable contribution to science and practice. In the first example, scientists interested in developing and testing larger theoretical frameworks isolate and organize proposed conceptual relationships into propositions. The scientific literature is then used to investigate the relationships of the propositions and, if there is evidence for the truth of the relationships, to determine conceptual-empirical correspondence. In the second example, the clinician also uses propositions to identify, describe, and organize the working conceptual relationships in practice. The investigation, although identical in process to the scientist's, differs in terms of its scope and its generalizability; that is, the practitioner investigates more particular and immediate relationships in a smaller group of persons; or frequently, a single person. For instance, a nurse working on a general medical unit is assigned to admit an elderly patient with the medical diagnosis of chronic obstructive pulmonary disease. Before meeting the patient, and in attempt to organize knowledge, the nurse hypothesizes several possible conceptual relationships; for example, the patient's age and medical diagnosis limit the patient's functional status. The nurse then tests the working hypothesis through assessment and works to directly change the concepts' relationships through manipulation of the person-environment interaction.

Any discussion of micro-range theory must consider the term "practice theory." We jump into the debate on what constitutes practice theory with the realization that numerous definitions exist and many authors consider micro-theory, as the most concrete and applicable of all theoretical levels, to be an equivalent term for practice theory.[5,16] We believe this categorization limits the understanding of theoretical thinking in nursing and a broader definition of practice theory is more useful. Based on Ellis,[18,19] who stated that *all* nursing knowledge ultimately is developed for practice, we maintain that all nursing theory, regardless of level, is practice theory.

Evidence and Levels of Theoretical Thinking

Regardless of the method used to create the theory or whether the theory is explanatory or predictive, the amount of evidence accrued to support it promotes confidence in its use by practitioners and scientists. In addition to the previously cited examples, varying degrees of evidence exist among the different types and levels of theoretical thinking.

On the metatheoretical level, the accrual of bodies of research findings (evidence) demonstrates our ability to produce and critique our knowledge. Our progress is measured by the usefulness of the knowledge that is accrued, the explanatory and predictive theories that are created and tested, and the articulation of philosophic perspectives that are connected to nursing science and practice.

At the grand theory level, evidence is represented by practitioners' and scientists' use of the philosophic approaches presented in the theories. As we have sought to build an academic discipline, grand theories have assisted in legitimizing the emerging discipline by providing broad guidelines about the focus of the discipline. There are varying degrees of evidence about the usefulness of existing nursing grand theories. Their frequent use by schools of nursing, care institutions, and practitioners, and their use in guiding research initiatives are examples of their value.

Middle-range theories often have evidence that is acquired by using many repetitions under controlled conditions (scientific method). An example is Johnson's[20,21] self-regulation theory that addresses the use of preparatory information to assist persons in coping with threatening illness situations. Middle-range theoretical frameworks provide some evidence to support the relationships posed. However, to date no nursing theories have sufficient evidence to be considered "laws," which is not unexpected, given that nursing is a newly established discipline and our phenomena of interest are highly complex.

In micro-range theory, relationships exist among a limited number of concepts that characterize a specific situation. The working hypothesis (of either the practitioner or the scientist) has the least amount of evidence behind it. The evidence behind this kind of theoretical thinking is not usually accrued by planned repetitions under controlled situations, but instead it is built from a limited number of repetitions and observations. For example, the best way to approach first-time ambulation for surgical patients may be hypothesized by a nurse as the result of providing postoperative care to a series of patients. The theoretical-empirical congruence of this hypothesis is then tested in subsequent surgical patients.

Use of Levels of Theoretical Thinking to Enhance Knowledge Development in Nursing

Several challenges prevail in the development of nursing knowledge. Conceptualizing theory at different levels of theory may assist us to address some of these challenges. For example, one challenge is to determine how different levels of theory relate to each other. How can one level of theory be used to develop related theories at another level? As we analyze and generate theory, we often use traditional methods of theory construction and substruction. The appropriate use of inductive and deductive approaches to develop nursing knowledge may be improved by the consideration of the relationships among levels of theories. Conceptualizing levels of theories also provides a beginning tool to assess whether the philosophic roots of our grand theories are reflected in our middle-range and micro-range theories. Such analyses can potentially enhance the consistency and logic in our decision making about care issues and the theoretical design of future research.

As a discipline, we also are looking for ways to integrate related theories that have arisen from the multiple ways of building knowledge. For instance, how does the theory about stages of behavior change, developed from grounded theory methods, relate to theories of self-efficacy for health behaviors that were developed by using hypothesis-testing methods? Similarly, we are searching for ways to integrate related theories from different disciplines. For example, how do middle-range theories of health promotion in psychology relate to those in sociology and nursing? The analysis and integration of related theories may be facilitated by comparison of related theories at the same theoretical level across disciplines and arising from multiple methodologic approaches.

Another challenge in the discipline's knowledge development is understanding the mechanisms needed to enhance articulation of the knowledge produced by practitioners and researchers. Regardless of whether the methods used to develop theory are inductive or deductive, and originate from a philosophic, practice, or research perspective, multiple levels of theoretical thinking exist. Although practitioners and researchers may use divergent methods, each uses theoretical thinking for the generation of knowledge. Recognition and discussion about the levels of theoretical thinking can serve as a vehicle for increased communication between practitioners and scientists about the knowledge each is developing.

Conclusion

Knowledge development in any discipline is a dynamic process that pursues probable truths about reality. It begins with creative approaches from multiple perspectives and continues by testing the knowledge according to appropriate truth criteria. In nursing, our "reality" is clinical practice, and we construct theories about probable truths related to the experience of health in the person-environment interaction. Development of a knowledge base is an iterative and ongoing process that requires periodic analysis and synthesis of an entire body of work. In an attempt to further the understanding of the current status of nursing theory, we provided an examination of the different levels of theory currently being used to develop nursing knowledge. This metatheoretical discussion of theory is not meant to create artificial domains; rather, it is an attempt to understand the current status of nursing theory through clarification of the terminology and a discussion of the related categories of theoretical thinking. Perhaps more important, the final purpose of this article is to recognize the strength of our disciplinary knowledge base and generate public discussion about the future of theory development and testing.

REFERENCES

1. Stevens BJ. Nursing theory, analysis, application, evaluation. 2nd ed. Boston: Little Brown & Co Inc; 1984.
2. Dubin R. Theory building. 2nd ed. New York: Free Press; 1978.
3. Chinn PL, Kramer MK. Theory and nursing. 5th ed. St. Louis: Mosby; 1999.
4. Suppe F. Middle range theories: what they are and why nursing science needs them. Proceedings of the ANA/Council of Nurse Researchers Symposium; 1993 Nov 15.
5. Walker LO, Avant KC. Strategies for theory construction in nursing. 3rd ed. Norwalk (CT): Appleton & Lange; 1995.
6. Nicoll LH. Perspectives on nursing theory. 3rd ed. Philadelphia (PA): Lippincott-Raven; 1997.
7. Carper BA. Fundamental patterns of knowing in nursing. Adv Nurs Sci 1978;1:13–23.
8. Whall AL. Current debates and issues critical to the discipline of nursing. In: Fitzpatrick JJ, Whall AL. Conceptual modes of nursing. 3rd ed. Stamford (CT): Appleton & Lange; 1996. p. 1–12.
9. Fawcett J. Analysis and evaluation of conceptual models of nursing. 3rd ed. Philadelphia (PA): FA Davis Co; 1995.
10. Nightingale F. Notes on nursing. New York: Churchill Livingstone; 1859.
11. Watson J. Nursing: the philosophy and science of caring. Boston: Little Brown & Co Inc; 1979.
12. Leininger M. Transcultural nursing: concepts, theories, and practices. New York: Wiley; 1978.
13. Merton RK. On sociological theories of the middle range. In: Merton RK. Social theory and social structure. New York: Free Press; 1968. p. 39–72.
14. Good M, Moore SM. Clinical Practice guidelines as a new source of middle-range theory: focus on acute pain. Nurs Outlook 1996;44:74–9.
15. Lenz ER, Suppe F, Gift AG, Pugh LC, Milligan RA. Collaborative development of middle-range nursing theories: toward a theory of unpleasant symptoms. Adv Nurs Sci 1995;17(3): 1–13.
16. Whall AL. The structure of nursing knowledge: analysis and evaluation of practice, middle-range, and grand theory. In: Fitzpatrick JJ, Whall AL. Conceptual modes of nursing. 3rd ed. Stamford (CT): Appleton & Lange; 1996. p. 13–25.
17. Kim HS. The nature of theoretical thinking in nursing. East Norwalk (CT): Appleton-Century-Crofts; 1983.
18. Ellis R. The practitioner as theorist. Am J Nurs 1969;69: 428–35.
19. Ellis R. Values and vicissitudes of the scientist nurse. Nurs Res 1970;19:440–5.
20. Johnson JE, Fieler VK, Jones LS, Wlasowicz GS, Mitchell ML. Self-regulation theory: applying theory to your practice. Pittsburgh (PA): Oncology Nursing Press; 1997.
21. Leventhal H, Johnson JE. Laboratory and field experimentation: development of a theory of self-regulation. In: Wooldridge PJ, Schmitt MH, Skipper JK, Leonard RC, editors. Behavioral science and nursing theory. St Louis: Mosby; 1983, p. 189–262.
22. Rogers ME. An introduction to the theoretical basis of nursing. Philadelphia (PA): F. A. Davis Company; 1970.
23. Neuman B. The Neuman systems model: application to nursing education and practice. New York: Appleton-Century-Crofts; 1982.

24. Orem DE. Nursing: concepts of practice. New York: McGraw Hill; 1971.

25. Levine ME. The four conservation principles of nursing. Nurs Forum 1967;6:45–59.

26. Swanson KM. Empirical development of a middle range theory of caring. Nurs Res 1991;40(3): 161–6.

27. Pender NJ. Health Promotion in nursing practice. New York: Appleton-Century-Crofts; 1982.

28. Meek SS. Effects of slow stroke back massage on relaxation in hospice clients. IMAGE J Nurs Sch 1993;25:17–20.

29. Kikuchi JF, Simmons H, editors. Philosophic inquiry in nursing. Newbury Park (CA): Sage Publications; 1992.

30. Fawcett J, Downs FS. The relationship of theory and research. 2nd ed. Philadelphia (PA): FA Davis Co; 1992.

THE AUTHORS COMMENT | Levels of Theoretical Thinking in Nursing

We wrote this article in response to our need to understand and explain middle-range theory to our students. As the discipline's understanding of theoretic thinking evolved, we were asked for detailed definitions of theory and how to distinguish the meaning and application of the different types. Because we both also have programs of research, we're pragmatists when it comes to theoretic thinking. Therefore, using "levels" of theory was a natural approach for categorizing and explaining the range of theoretic thinking used by all nurse theorists, from practitioners to scientists to philosophers. The article is dedicated to all our students. Thank you for your questions, skepticism, and willingness to take on the adventure of understanding human health and illness.

PATRICIA A. HIGGINS
SHIRLEY M. MOORE

34

Development of Situation-Specific Theories
An Integrative Approach

E U N - O K   I M ,   R N ,   P h D ,   M P H ,   C N S ,   F A A N

One type of "ready-to-wear" theories that can bring about better nursing care outcomes regardless of their philosophical bases is situation-specific theories proposed by Im and Meleis in 1999. In this paper, some propositions for an integrative approach to the development of situation-specific theories are made. First, situation-specific theories are described as practice theories while they are compared with middle-range theories. Then the integrative approach is detailed, which includes (a) checking assumptions for theory development; (b) exploring through multiple sources; (c) theorizing; and (d) reporting, sharing, and validating. Finally, the paper concludes with suggestions for further development of the integrative approach.

ACROSS disciplines, scholars can now sympathize with the epistemic pluralism that is the practical philosophy of most working scientists in general.[1] Until recently, scholars believed in the unity of scientific knowledge, and they accepted its fragmentation only as a pragmatic necessity. However, these days, scholars are quite happy to go along with philosophical plurality across many disciplines.[2]

Nursing history also shows the same changes toward epistemic pluralism in theoretical and philosophical thinking. In the 1950s, under the tremendous influences of logical positivism, grand theories were developed and used to answer questions on the nature, mission, and goals of nursing, and nursing scholars and theorists believed in the unity of nursing knowledge. In the 1960s–1980s, metatheoretical questions on the types and contents of theories were asked and argued, yet their philosophical basis was still empiricism.[3–6] From the middle of the 1980s onward, tremendous efforts in concept development were made with the introduction of qualitative philosophical thinking.[7–11] From the beginning of the 1990s, numerous middle-range theories were developed and published,[14–17] and philosophical pluralism in theoretical nursing became more prominent.[12–14] Through these historical changes, now, nursing scholars even envision and sympathize with epistemic pluralism, and seek ready-to-wear theories in nursing practice that may bring about better nursing care outcomes regardless of their philosophical bases.[15]

Nursing has struggled to develop "ready-to-wear" theories. "Ready to wear" refers to easy applicability to research and practice. One type of "ready-to-wear" theories is situation-specific theories, proposed by Im and Meleis in 1999.[16] *Situation-specific theories* are defined as theories that focus on specific nursing phenomena, that reflect clinical practice, and that are limited to specific populations or to particular fields of practice.[16,17] Situation-specific theories belong to a different level than grand theories and middle-range theories, which can incorporate diversities and complexities in nursing phenomenon, consider sociopolitical, cultural, and historical contexts of nursing encounters, and be easily applicable to nursing practice.[17] In this paper, *middle-range theories* mean theories that have more limited scope and less abstraction than grand theories, address specific phenomena or concepts, reflect practice, and aim to be easily testable[18]; *grand theories* are systematic constructions of the nature of nursing, the mission of nursing, and the goals of nursing care.[17] Situation-specific theories are also intended not to be universal theories that can be applicable to any time, any socially constraining structures, or any politically limiting situations. Rather, they are intended to be more clinically specific, reflect a particular context, and include blueprints for action.[16,17] Philosophically, this new type of theory has roots in postempiricism, critical social theory, feminism, and hermeneutics,[16] all of which agree with current epistemic pluralism in nursing.

When situation-specific theories were proposed, an integrative approach was also proposed as a strategy for developing them. *The integrative approach* was originally proposed by Meleis[17] and has been

ABOUT THE AUTHOR

EUN-OK IM was born in South Korea and moved to the United States in her 20s. She received a PhD in nursing from the University of California, San Francisco, where she also held a postdoctoral position. She is currently a Professor at The University of Pennsylvania School of Nursing. Professor Im has gained national and international recognition as a methodologist and theorist in international cross-cultural Internet research through more than 90 peer-reviewed publications and over 150 professional presentations. Her published articles on situation-specific theories, feminist critique, and Internet research methodologies are cited by many researchers around the world. Her hobbies include reading novels, knitting, and watching movies.

extended through later work by Im and Meleis.[16] The integrative approach has some essential components, such as the clinical grounding that drives the basic or clinical questions as well as the questions themselves. Also essential are opportunities for clinical involvement and for conceptually thinking about the health/illness responses, the situations, and the environment.[17] However, the propositions of the integrative approach tended to be too abstract for novice theorists to utilize in actual theory development. Further development/refinement of the integrative approach is essential for the future development and practical use of situation-specific theories, which may ultimately result in a stronger link between theory and practice and subsequently produce better nursing care outcomes than other types of theories. In this paper, some propositions for the integrative approach to the development of situation-specific theories are made. First, situation-specific theories are described as practice theories while they are compared with other types of theories. Then the integrative approach is detailed. Finally, the paper concludes with suggestions for further development of the integrative approach.

Situation-Specific Theories, Practice Theories, and Middle-Range Theories

Figure 34-1 shows the relationships among practice theories, situation-specific theories, middle-range theories, and grand theories reported in the literature. In recent literature, situation-specific theories are sometimes labeled as *micro-theories* or *practice theories* (a term that is interchangeable with *micro-theories),* or even as middle-range theories.[11,13,18] In a sense, situation-specific theories can be categorized as practice theories because situation-specific theories certainly aim at functioning as practice theories. Jacox[6] proposed that *practice theories* be considered those

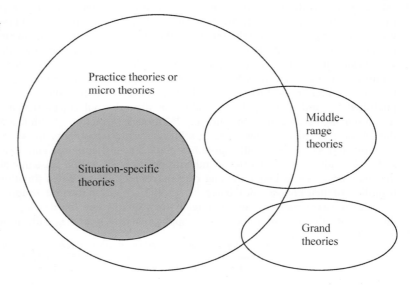

Figure 34-1 *Relationships among practice theories, middle-range theories, grand theories, and situation-specific theories.*

theories that outline the actions that nurses must take to meet a nursing goal (producing some desired change or effect in the patient's condition). In these terms, situation-specific theories can be considered practice theories because one of the goals of situation-specific theories is to provide a blueprint for nursing practice.[16] Peterson[18] even categorized situation-specific theories and practice theories in the same category, noting that the literature included a confusing variety of terms to refer to the level of theory that is considered less abstract, more specific, and narrower in scope than middle-range theories.

Although practice theories have been welcome in nursing because nursing is inherently a practice-oriented discipline, they have often been criticized as well. The major criticism is that they are procedural and not based on a well-developed body of nursing science.[18] For this reason, some theorists have worked to blend middle-range theories with practice theories, and their hybrid efforts have been highly evaluated because they elevate the resulting practice above simple dictates or imperatives.[11] Since situation-specific theories, in nature, are practice theories, those blending efforts are unnecessary for situation-specific theories. In addition, situation-specific theories can provide a basis for the development of the knowledge base for nursing practices through research and practice efforts in specific nursing situations because they are more than just guidelines or standardized procedures for nursing practice.[16]

Situation-specific theories, however, are different from middle-range theories because the former can be applicable only to specific nursing phenomenon or particular nursing clients while the latter can be applicable across nursing practice fields.[16,18] For example, the middle-range theory of transition proposed by Meleis and her colleagues[19] was developed based on several studies of ethnically diverse samples undergoing a wide range of transitions, including menopausal, maternal, and caregiving transition; subsequently, they aimed to cover all types of transitions in nursing situations. However, the situation-specific theory of the menopausal transition of Korean immigrant women by Im and Meleis[20] aimed at only the specific population of menopausal low-income Korean immigrant women in the United States.

Situation-specific theories are also different from middle-range theories in terms of their testability. Middle-range theories contain a limited number of variables and testable relationships.[21] In other words, middle-range theories are based on logical positivistic and/or postpositivistic ideas that assume the testability of a theory.[18] Grand theories are criticized as too abstract to be tested empirically. The basic assumption here is that the testability of theories is based on a logical positivistic idea.

Situation-specific theories do not always assume their testability.[16] Some situation-specific theories will certainly aim at the operationalization of central concepts for hypotheses testing in real settings. However, other situation-specific theories are not supposed to be testable because they are developed on philosophical foundations (e.g., hermeneutics, phenomenology, critical theory, postmodernism) in which positivistic apparatuses such as hypotheses do not have a place.[16] Rather, the situation-specific theories aim at helping researchers understand central concepts through qualitative fieldwork and/or participant observation. If a situation-specific theory was developed based on postempiricism, it can aim at operationalization, measurements, and hypothesis testing. On the contrary, if a situation-specific theory originated with a phenomenological perspective, the theory may not be used to operationalize, measure, and/or test a hypothesis. Rather, the theory may aim at explaining and understanding the lived experience of human beings in the middle of the phenomenon.

In the discipline of nursing, many strategies for concept development and theory development have been proposed. The concept development strategies proposed and used in nursing include the Wilsonian method,[21,22] the Walker and Avant approach,[10,11] Rogers' evolutionary concept analysis method,[23] the Hybrid method,[9] and the simultaneous analysis method.[7,8] Many strategies for developing a theory have been also proposed, and used as well.[10,11,17,23,24] Rodgers and Knafl[23] asserted that these currently existing concept and theory development strategies for grand theories and middle-range theories do not adequately consider that the theory development process, specifically the concept development process, is evolutionary, and that there is no step-by-step recipe for developing a theory.

The view of Rodgers and Knafl assumes that concepts are formed by the identification of characteristics common to a class of objects or phenomena and the abstraction and clustering of these characteristics, which is influenced heavily by socialization and public interaction.[23,25] This view assumes that, because these contextual factors vary, there will be variations in concepts over time or across situations. Currently, most nursing theorists and scholars agree that the theory development process is a continuous, dynamic, and evolutionary process influenced by contexts surrounding the theory development process.[11,23] This is somewhat problematic in practical applications to nursing practice and research, however. It is easy to understand in an abstract way, but in reality, the assumption that theory development is evolutionary, not algorithmic and linear, poses a potential contradiction because a theory might evolve away from the specific time, place, and population for which it was originally conceived. Since situation-specific theories are limited to a specific population and a particular nursing phenomenon/situation, which, in turn, limits the contexts (eg, time, place, situation) for theory applications, the theory development process becomes more feasible and easily applicable to nursing practice and research even in light of the evolutionary nature of theory development.[16] Consequently, with the specificity and easy applicability of situation-specific theories, nurses may produce better nursing care outcomes than with other types of theories that do not limit the time, nursing situations, or nursing clients.

The Integrative Approach

In the integrative approach, the conceptualization and theorizing processes can happen all at once, or they might take years and never quite evolve into a useful integrated view of reality.[17] Yet, to provide a convenient guideline, in this section, the process of the integrative approach to the development of situation-specific

theories is proposed step by step. This process may not happen subsequently or in a continuous way. Rather, some steps of the process would be skipped, while others could happen repetitively. The steps suggested in this paper are actually what nursing researchers and practitioners have frequently used in their research projects and practice without recognition. Based on an in-depth review of the literature published within the past 5 years, the steps used in the development of situation-specific theories in the literature are summarized and proposed as follows. The process of the integrative approach is also summarized in Figure 34-2.

Checking Assumptions for Theory Development

A theorist who wants to develop a situation-specific theory needs to check her or his assumptions for theory development first. The assumptions for the development of situation-specific theories include (a) multiple truths; (b) evolutionary nature of theory development; (c) sociopolitical contextuality; and

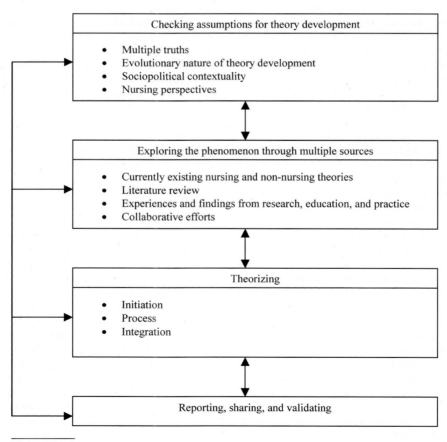

Figure 34-2 *An integrative approach to situation-specific theories.*

(*d*) nursing perspectives. These assumptions are the basis for the whole theory development process of situation-specific theories. If a theorist does not agree with these assumptions, she or he may need to reconsider if she or he really wants to develop a situation-specific theory. For example, if her or his assumption for theory development is based on the universality of health/illness experience, she or he might not aim at the development of a situation-specific theory because a situation-specific theory assumes multiple truths, which negates the universality of health/illness experience. Rather, she or he needs to aim at developing a grand theory or a middle-range theory.

Multiple Truths

Under the influences of positivism and scientism, nursing phenomena have been considered to be universal phenomena which can occur to any racial, cultural, and gender groups in the same way.[29,30] Thus, most nursing theories have also assumed that nursing phenomena are universal and homogeneous, and traditional approaches to knowledge development depend on the assumptions of universality, homogeneity, and normality.[29] Yet nursing phenomenon are becoming more complex and are complicated by multiple factors, including the increasing diversity of nursing clients.[30] A consensus has developed among nurse scholars recently in which theoretical development must take into consideration the diversity and complexity of nursing phenomena.[30,31] Without doing so, the theoretical foundation of the nursing discipline cannot achieve the connections for which nursing has been striving.

As posited in the paper by Im and Meleis,[16] the development of situation-specific theories assumes philosophical, theoretical, and methodological plurality, which is more congruent with the nature and goals of nursing and which can incorporate the diversity and complexity of nursing phenomenon. The philosophical bases of the substance and syntax of nursing knowledge have been debated by many nursing scholars.[26-28] Meleis[17] divided the philosophical positions of nursing scholars into three: (*a*) the purist position; (*b*) the radical separationist position; and (*c*) the nonpurist position. The bona fide purist position claims that a philosophical viewpoint should guide and direct theory development, research strategy, and clinical practice.[17] The radical separationist position asserts that a discipline's theory and research are distinct entities and do not necessarily have to be congruent philosophically and methodologically.[17] The nonpurist position takes a philosophical, theoretical, and methodological pluralistic position.[17] The project to develop situation-specific theories assumes this nonpurist philosophical position as well as the existence of multiple truths, not one universal scientific truth.

Evolutionary Nature of Theory Development

Another assumption for the development of situation-specific theories is that the theory development process is cyclic and evolutionary. As discussed above, a concept which is currently regarded as a norm or a standard may not be a norm or a standard in the future.[23] In other words, the integrity or stability of that norm through time cannot be predicted or ensured. Concepts are formed by the identification of characteristics common to a class of objects or phenomena and the abstraction and clustering of these characteristics.[25] Therefore, as characteristics of nursing phenomena change, concepts also change. A concept which is not considered as important now can evolve into an important concept in future nursing. Consequently, a situation-specific theory which is developed for a particular population in a specific situation will not be appropriate for the same population in a different time or a different sociopolitical context. Thus, the situation-specific theory for the same population in the same situation also needs to be changed with changes in time and sociopolitical contexts.

Sociopolitical Contextuality

A third assumption for the development of situation-specific theories is the sociopolitical contextuality of nursing phenomena. The current theory development process involved in the development of grand theories and middle-range theories rarely considers the sociopolitical, cultural, and/or historic contexts inherent to each client-nurse encounter.[32] Rather than accounting for the contextuality of nursing phenomenon, they usually try to reduce the phenomenon into several central concepts; operationalize and measure the concepts; explore/test the concepts and constructs through quantitative and qualitative data collections; and refine the theories.[11,18] Consequently, they frequently aim at theories that can be applicable to all nursing fields and explain central concepts across the fields. Since situation-specific theories are limited to a specific population and/or a particular area of interest, the theories can easily incorporate the contextuality of the phenomenon.[16] Indeed, the development of situation-specific theories assumes that nursing phenomena or client-nurse encounters happen in sociopolitical contexts, that sociopolitical contexts need to be incorporated in the theory development process, and that the theories cannot be always applicable to any historical moment, any social structure, or any political situation.

Nursing Perspectives

An essential assumption for the development of situation-specific theories is that they are based on nursing perspectives. Nursing perspectives give a unique view on a phenomenon. When we view a same phenomenon with two different perspectives, the phenomenon described by each of the two different perspectives may be different from each other. For example, when we view Asian American cancer patients' lack of pain reporting using a biological perspective, we may focus on the physiological characteristics of Asian Americans without considering their whole beings in the contexts of their daily lives. Consequently, we may assume that Asian Americans' lack of pain reporting is a simple biological difference from other ethnic groups, which may lead us to look for basic biological difference between the ethnic groups. When we view the same phenomenon (lack of pain reporting) from a nursing perspective, we may view the patients' bio-psycho-socio-cultural beings within the contexts of their daily lives. Rather than focusing on interethnic biological differences, we may focus on how their psycho-socio-cultural contexts circumscribe their pain experience and how we could provide adequate pain management while considering their unique pain experience.

In the development of situation-specific theories, a nursing perspective is mandatory.[16] The theories developed without a nursing perspective might distort the descriptions of nursing phenomenon and mislead nursing research and/or practice. Yet more than one nursing perspective exists.[17] A nursing perspective may be based on biomedical models; it may also be based on feminist perspectives emphasizing sociopolitical environments and reflecting oppressed groups' interests (mostly women's). In either case, it should also reflect nurses' concerns, views, values, and attitudes.

Exploring Through Multiple Sources

After checking assumptions for her or his theory development, a theorist needs to explore her or his phenomenon of interest through multiple sources. The multiple sources may include: (*a*) currently existing nursing and nonnursing theories related to the phenomenon of interest; (*b*) literature reviews; (*c*) findings and experiences from research, education, and practice; and (*d*) collaborative efforts. Theorists usually use more than one of these sources for theory development at the same time. Each source is discussed in detail as follows.

Currently Existing Nursing and Nonnursing Theories

Nursing and nonnursing conceptual models, grand theories, and middle-range theories can serve as the foundation for the development of situation-specific

theories. From the early days of nursing theory development, theory derivation has been prevalent in nursing.[11] Usually, theory derivation in nursing has been done by using analogy to obtain explanations or predictions about a phenomenon in nursing from the explanations or predictions in another field including medicine, psychology, sociology, and public health.[13] Recently, theories from nursing have been combined with those from other disciplines to create middle-range theories.[11,18] In the development of situation-specific theories, both nursing and/or nonnursing theories may provide the basis for analogy for explanations, understandings, or predictions of a particular situation of a specific population of interest as well.

An example is the above mentioned theory of menopausal transition of Korean immigrant women,[20] which was developed based on a middle-range theory of transition.[33] In the development of the situation-specific theory, major research questions were set based on the middle-range theory of transition. Then, each concept was explored through both quantitative and qualitative findings from a study on menopausal transition of Korean immigrant women. Based on the findings related to the concepts, the theory of transition was modified, and further developed as a situation-specific theory for menopausal transition of Korean immigrant women. Compared with the middle-range theory of transition, the situation-specific theory of menopausal transition of Korean immigrant women has increased specificity of the conceptualization and is easily applicable to the situation through the modifications based on actual study findings.

Literature Reviews

An extensive review of literature can provide a systematic analysis of currently existing knowledge about a nursing phenomenon and frequently provide an excellent source for theory development.[10,11] In this paper, the literature review means a review of previous research findings, theoretical work, and statistical governmental reports. Indeed, the literature review has been an essential basis for concept development and theory development. Walker and Avant[11] included literature synthesis as a method of concept synthesis and suggested that theory synthesis incorporate published research literature, direct statistical information, and qualitative research as the second step of three phases of theory development.

Many examples of theory development through literature review can be easily found in the nursing literature. An example would be the transition theory by Schumacher and Meleis[33] who conducted an extensive literature review on all types of transitions in nursing and proposed a theoretical framework of transitions. Based on the analysis of the literature, they proposed a set of major concepts related to transitions, which include types of transitions, properties of transitions, transition conditions, and nursing therapeutics. Although this example of the transition theory aims to be a middle-range theory, the review of the literature as a source of theory development can be easily incorporated into the integrative approach. In addition, a literature review frequently provides a starting point for theory development by giving us a picture of the state of the science in the area and initiating our theoretical thinking on the major and/or central concept(s) in the nursing phenomenon in question.[11] Hulme[34] provided an excellent example of an integrative literature review on currently existing grand, middle-range, and situation-specific theories related to health problems of adults who experienced childhood sexual abuse.

Findings and Experiences from Research, Education, and Practice

Findings and experiences from research projects, educational programs, and/or clinical practice in hospital and/or community settings can provide a source for theoretical development. Most nursing theories tend to be initiated by the theorists' experiences from their long clinical, academic, or research experience in nursing.[17] Theorists can easily raise theoretical questions from their own experience. Kirkevold[35] posited that integrative nursing research experience has great potential for clarifying the theoretical perspective and substance of the nursing discipline, as well as making research-based knowledge more accessible to clinical nurses. Lyons[36] argued that nursing can generate a knowledge base through reflecting on nurses' own experience. Reed[37] mentioned that her theory of self-transcendence was developed using clinical experience and empirical investigations.

Collaborative Efforts

International and interdisciplinary collaborative efforts may provide sources for the development of situation-specific theories as well. To be specific to a situation and/or a population, such a theory sometimes needs to incorporate a more detailed and exact source for theory development. Collaborative efforts allow comparisons of ideas, scholarly dialogues, and an integration of different and/or disperse opinions and findings.[38] Experts in different areas of nursing who are working on the same nursing phenomenon will give different and new views/visions on nursing phenomena which cannot be easily obtained by independent work by one person. For example, when a collaborative team is working together on midlife women's menopausal experience, a nurse whose expertise is physiology can provide a different view on

menopausal experience from a nurse anthropologist or a nurse feminist. In terms of theoretical development, the theory will be a nursing theory, but it will be based on diverse views on menopause.

Collaborations between academics and clinicians can also provide a source for theory development, which will provide a strong link between theory and practice. Gassner et al.[39] proposed a model devised by the project team, including four academics and six clinicians, and concluded that the model was effective in facilitating the collaborative relationships necessary for successful development and implementation of reality-based learning for nursing students. Collaboration with research participants can also provide an excellent source of theory development.[40] Taking the lead in identifying areas of practice for action research is a natural extension of nurses' role as advocates for nursing clients, and it may provide a new view of the research participants.[40]

International collaborative efforts also can provide an excellent source for theory development, especially for situation-specific theories, because such theories need to provide blueprints for nursing practice with a specific population that can be usually categorized along ethnic/cultural lines. Walker and Avant[11] even envision that international efforts of nursing theory development will strengthen nursing knowledge and theory development by incorporating different perspectives/views from different cultural backgrounds. International collaboration can give a new view on everything from the philosophy of life, accepted behaviors, and human relations to the way in which people live.[41–42] Recent advances in computer and communication technologies may facilitate international collaboration through electronic networks more easily than in the past, and we will see more and more international collaborative works in theoretical nursing.[43]

Theorizing
Initiation

While exploring the phenomenon of interest through multiple sources, a theorist may initiate her or his theory development with a simple literature review on a specific nursing phenomenon of her or his interests, from her or his own research, and/or from her or his practice experiences even before the review of the literature. Theory development can start from a mother theory and result in a modified form of the theory, which is more specific to the population of her or his interest or to the nursing situation. Theory development can be initiated by a single person or a group of colleagues who have been involved in the same area of interests. Recently, some theories have been even developed through international or interdisciplinary

Figure 34-3 *The process involved in the development of the theoretical work by Falk-Rafael.*

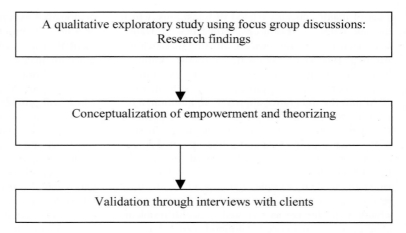

collaboration.[11,41–42] Theory development in the integrative approach may be initiated from one source or multiple sources at a time or at separate time points.

Process

Developing a situation-specific theory can take place through a theorizing process in several different ways. Although few nursing theorists claim to have developed situation-specific theories, many theories in nursing meet the definition of situation-specific theories. The following examples show that the process involved in the development of situation-specific theories can be diverse. These examples were searched using the PUBMED database. For the PUBMED search, key words including *nursing, theory,* and *theory development* were used, and only the articles published in English during the past 5 years were searched in order to capture the current trends in nursing theory development. From the 215 articles retrieved through the search, tutorials, editorials, and literature review articles were excluded. Then, all the articles were reviewed in order to identify the process used in theory development. Among them, only the articles presenting situation-specific theories were selected for this paper.

One of the examples is the theoretical work by Falk-Rafael[44] (see Fig. 34-3). Her theoretical work shows a unique type of process for theory development. She initiated her theoretical work through a qualitative exploratory study. She began the study by using a nominal group technique in a series of focus groups with public health nurses to identify their conceptualization of empowerment, the strategies they identified as empowering, and the outcomes of empowering strategies they observed in their practice. Based on the qualitative study, she then initiated the theorizing process and developed a model that conceptualized empowerment as a process of evolving consciousness in which increasing awareness, knowledge, and skills interacted with the clients' active participation to move toward actualizing potential. Finally, the developed model was shared and validated through interviews with clients whom nurses identified as having been empowered through their practice.

Recent nursing literature notes a type of theory development that integrates theory, research and practice. For example, LaCoursiere's theory of online social support (see Fig. 34-4) was developed with an integrated framework that incorporates knowledge from multiple sources including (*a*) a conceptual literature review of existing frameworks and research findings

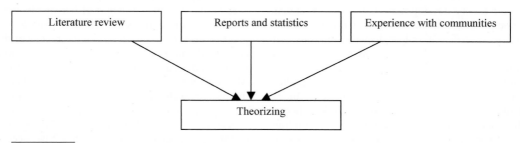

Figure 34-4 *The process involved in the development of the theoretical work by LaCoursiere.*

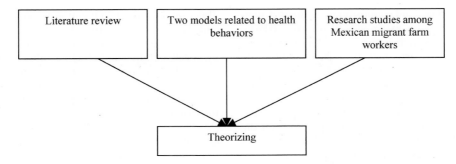

Figure 34-5 *The process involved in the development of the theoretical work by Poss.*

related to social support, online communications, and the effect of the Internet or the Web; (*b*) reports and statistics from agencies and organizations focusing on the online health care experience; and (*c*) the author's experiences with online social support communities over a number of years. This type of theorizing can be easily found in nursing.

Another example of this type of theorizing is Poss's model for cross-cultural research among Mexican migrant workers in tuberculosis screening tests (see Fig. 34-5).[46] In the theoretical work, the model was developed based on a literature review, two models that are often used to study health behaviors (the Health Belief Model and the Theory of Reasoned Action), and previous research studies among Mexican migrant farm workers participating in a tuberculosis screening program.

The theory development process of situation-specific theories can also be found in the development of the integrative model for environmental health research by Dixon and Dixon (see Fig. 34-6).[47] The theorists developed the theory based on their experiences

in both academic and activist communities relative to environmental health and a review of the research literature. Then, a working hypothesis that may be useful in guiding investigations or suggesting needed policies was extracted and used in their research on the engagement in environmental health issues at the individual and community levels.

Integration

While initiating and proceeding theorizing process based on explorations of nursing phenomenon through multiple sources, a theorist can integrate her or his analysis, discovery, formulation, and evaluation through conceptual schemes, reflexivity, and documentation.

The integration process that a theorist can adopt includes several different components. From existing nursing and nonnursing theories, a theorist may start with broad established facts, principles, laws, or theories that are known and generally accepted as true and use them to address narrower yet related phenomena,

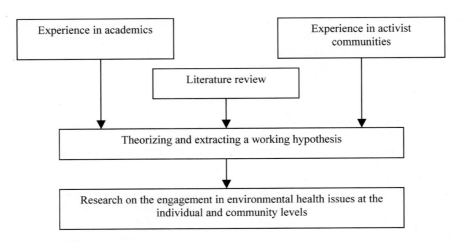

Figure 34-6 *The process involved in the development of the theoretical work by Dixon and Dixon.*

concepts/variables, and propositions. A theorist may start from her or his experience in research, education, practice, research findings, or literature review with smaller, narrower concepts/variables and formulates new propositions that may ultimately lead to the development of new facts, principles, laws, and theories. A theorist may also formulate potential propositions based on personal and nursing knowledge, skills, values, meanings, and experience and not on empirically-based evidence or facts. Although distinctively different, these ways of integration may combine. Furthermore, these integration processes can happen for a long period of time, and a theorist might go through several waves of integration through her or his research projects and practice in clinical settings.

In these integration efforts, conceptual schemes with beginning hunches can be instrumental.[16] Conceptual schemes can be initiated, developed, and refined throughout the theory development process. The most important part of the conceptual schemes is internal and external dialogues.[16,17] Through conceptual thinking, memo writing, and journal writing, a theorist can initiate and maintain her or his internal dialogues so that her or his theorizing process can be further organized, refined, and integrated.[17] In addition, a theorist may initiate and maintain an external dialogue through discussions with colleagues, research members, students, and research participants and through participation in seminars, conferences, and/or panel discussions. In both ways, the theorist can develop and refine her or his conceptual schemes that are related to the nursing phenomenon of her or his interests and can integrate various theorizing processes.

Reflectivity is also instrumental in the process of integration. Situation-specific theories consider social, cultural, and historical contexts, but their scope and the questions are limited to specific situations and/or specific populations.[17,30] Therefore, in the development of situation-specific theories, considerations of social, cultural, and historical contexts should be incorporated from the beginning stage of the theory development process, which requires reflectivity of the theorists. Sufficient reflectivity to uncover what may be deep-seated but poorly recognized views on the specific situations and/or the specific populations central to the theory development and a full account of the theorists' views, thinking, and conduct can help the theorist's integration of her or his theorizing processes.[17]

The theorists also need to be reflective about their own values and meanings related to specific situations and/or specific populations. Values are enduring beliefs, attributes, or ideals that establish moral and ethical boundaries of what is right and wrong in thought, judgment, character, attitude, and behavior.[48]

Thus, values form a foundation for correct thinking and decision making throughout the theorist's life; values develop over time and reflect individual, family, social, cultural, and religious influences as well as personal choice.[48] Thus, during the integration process, a theorist needs to be reflective on their own meanings attached to the specific situations and/or the specific populations.

Documentation of all stages involved in the theory development process can be instrumental in integration efforts. As situation-specific theories emphasize contextuality and reflectivity in the process of theory development, the theoretical and analytic decision trails created by the theorists during the development process need to be ascertained as well.[16] Theorists may continually question their conceptualization and theorizing, critiquing each step of the development process and the impact of the theories within their social and political environment. This process needs to be well documented through theoretical diaries and/or memos, so that the documentation supports the integration of the theory development process.[17] Systematically documenting the rationale, outcome, and evaluation of all actions related to theory development is an important component of the development of the situation-specific theories.[17] This documentation will result in well-grounded, cogent, justifiable, relevant, and meaningful theory development processes and outcomes.

Reporting, Sharing, and Validating

When the documenting of theorizing and integration takes the form of a manuscript, a model, or a research report, these need to be reported and shared with nursing communities. Nurse theorists have emphasized reporting and sharing of their work.[29] The criteria for theory evaluation that have been proposed and used in nursing usually include social utility and/or contagiousness as an important criterion.[17,50] Through reporting and sharing, theory development may be constructively critiqued by peers, and theoretical products can be further developed.

The validation of theories by nursing clients can also enhance the efforts to develop a theory. The relevance of an approach needs to be reflected from the very beginning of the process. Here, relevance means that a nursing theory can serve nursing clients' own issues and interests in improving their lives.[32] To ensure relevance, situation-specific theories may be checked with nursing clients in the specific situation and/or with the particular population through a member validation process, and theorists always need to be reflective about nursing clients' own views, needs, and interests throughout the theory development process. When nursing clients perceive a theory to be representative of their real experience, the theorized model is more easily applicable to the nursing phenomenon that the clients are experiencing, which subsequently improves understanding and nursing care outcomes.

Conclusions

In this article, an integrative approach to the development of situation-specific theories is proposed. This proposition is an extension of a suggested outline of the integrative approach previously drawn by Im and Meleis.[16] The proposed integrative approach describes the development process of situation-specific theories that aim to produce ready-to-wear theories and that ultimately aim to link better nursing care outcomes through their specificity and diversity. None of the steps/stages in the proposed approach is entirely new to nurses, whether they are clinicians, theorists, or researchers.[17] Nurses may be involved in the theory development process in many ways, and we can see the growing acceptance of theory development as a significant aspect of knowledge development in nursing.

Theory development cannot grow in isolation.[17] The integrative approach proposed in this paper needs more discussion, constructive criticism, and feedback from researchers, practitioners, and theorists alike. The integrative approach should not be limited only to the proposed process. As knowledge and technology in nursing advance, we may see different types and processes of theory development in nursing in the near future.[11] As we keep in mind that theory development process is dynamic, cyclic, and changing over time, we need to continue to welcome the changes and remain open to the potential growth of theoretical nursing for better nursing care outcomes.

REFERENCES

1. Ziman J, Midgley M. Pluralism in science: a statement. *Interdisc Sci Rev.* 2001;26:153.
2. Ziman J. Emerging out of nature into history: the plurality of the sciences. *Phil Trans R Soc Lond.* 2003:361:1617–1633.
3. Chinn PL. Response: revision and passion. *Sch Inq Nurs Pract.* 1987;l:21–24.
4. Ellis R. Characteristics of significant theories. *Nurs Res.* 1968; 17:217–222.
5. Hardy ME. The nature of theories. In: Hardy ME, ed. *Theoretical Foundations for Nursing.* New York: MSS Information Corp; 1974.
6. Jacox A. Theory construction in nursing: an overview. *Nurs Res.* 1974;23:4–13.
7. Haase JE, Britt T, Coward DD, Leidy NK, Penn PE. Simultaneous concept analysis of spiritual perspective, hope, acceptance, and self transcendence. *Image J Nurs Sch.* 1992; 24:l4l–147.
8. Haase JE, Leidy NK, Coward DD, Britt T, Penn PE. Simultaneous concept analysis: a strategy for developing multiple interrelated concepts. In: Rodgers B, Knafl K, eds. *Concept Development in Nursing.* Philadelphia: WB Saunders Co; 1993: 175–192.
9. Schwartz-Barcott D, Kim HS. An expansion and elaboration of the hybrid model of concept development. In: Rodgers BL, Knafl KA, eds. *Concept Development in Nursing: Foundations, Techniques, and Applications.* Philadelphia, PA: WB Saunders Co; 2000:129–160.
10. Walker LO, Avant KC. *Strategies for Theory Construction in Nursing.* 3rd ed.. Norwalk, CT: Appleton & Lange; 1995.
11. Walker LO, Avant KC. *Strategies for Theory Construction in Nursing.* 4th ed.. Norwalk, CT: Appleton & Lange; 2005.
12. Chinn PL. Why middle-range theory? *Adv Nurs Sci.* 1997; 19(3): viii.
13. Peterson SJ, Bredow TS. *Middle Range Theories: Application to Nursing Research.* Philadelphia, PA: Lippincott Williams & Wilkins; 2004.
14. Smith MJ, Liehr PR. *Middle Range Theory for Nursing.* New York: Springer Publishing Co; 2003.
15. Gortner SR. The history and philosophy of nursing science and research. In: Reed PG, Shearer NC, Nicoll LH, eds. *Perspectives on Nursing Theory.* Philadelphia: JB Lippincott; 2003: 105–112.
16. Im EO, Meleis AI. Situation-specific theories: philosophical roots, properties, and approach. *Adv Nurs Sci.* 1999;22(2): 11–24.
17. Meleis AI. *Theoretical Nursing: Development and Progress.* 3rd ed. Philadelphia: Lippincott; 1997.
18. Peterson SJ. Introduction to the nature of nursing knowledge. In: Peterson SJ, Bredow TS, eds. *Middle Range Theories: Application to Nursing Research.* Philadelphia, PA: Lippincott Williams & Wilkins; 2004:3–41.
19. Meleis AI, Sawyer LM, Im EO, Messias DK, Schumacher K. Experiencing transitions: an emerging middle-range theory. *Adv Nurs Sci.* 2000;23(1):12–28.
20. Im EO, Meleis AI. A situation-specific theory of Korean immigrant women's menopausal transition. *Image.* 1999;31: 333–338.
21. Whittemore R, Roy SC. Adapting to diabetes mellitus: a theory synthesis. *Nurs Sci Q.* 2002;15(4):311–317.
22. Hupcey JE, Morse JM, Lenz ER, Tason MC. Wilsonian methods of concept analysis: a critique. *Sch Inq Nurs Pract.* 1996;10:253–277.
23. Rodgers BL, Knafl KA. *Concept Development in Nursing: Foundations, Techniques, and Applications.* Philadelphia, PA: WB Saunders Co; 2000.
24. Chinn PL, Kramer MK. *Theory and Nursing: Integrated Knowledge Development.* St Louise: CV Mosby; 1999.
25. Rodgers BL. Philosophical foundations of concept development. In: Rodgers BL, Knafl KA, eds. *Concept Development in Nursing: Foundations, Techniques, and Applications.* Philadelphia, PA: WB Saunders Co; 2000:7–37.
26. Kim HS. Putting theory into practice: problems and prospects. *J Adv Nurs.* 1993;18(1):1632–1639.
27. Moccia PA. A critique of compromise: Beyond the methods debate. *Adv Nurs Sci.* 1988; 10:1–9.
28. Thompson JL. Practical discourse on nursing: going beyond empiricism and historicism. *Adv Nurs Sci.* 1985;7:59–71.
29. Hall JM, Stevens PE. Rigor in feminist research. *Adv Nurs Sci.* 1991;13:l6–29.

30. Meleis AI. A passion for making a difference: Revisions for empowerment. *Sch Inq Nurs Pract*. 1998;12:87–94.
31. Baker C. Cultural relativism and cultural diversity: implications for nursing practice. *Nurs Sci*. 1997;20:3–11.
32. Hall JM, Stevens PE, Meleis AI. Marginalization: a guiding concept or valuing diversity in nursing knowledge development. *Adv Nurs Sci*. 1994; 16(4):23–41.
33. Schumacher KL, Meleis AI. Transitions: a central concept in nursing. *Image*. 1994;26:119–127.
34. Hulme PA. Theoretical perspectives on the health problems of adults who experienced childhood sexual abuse. *Issues Mental Health Nurs*. 2004;25:339–361.
35. Kirkevold M. Integrative nursing research—an important strategy to further the development of nursing science and nursing practice. *J Adv Nurs*. 1997;25(5):977–984.
36. Lyons J. Reflective education for professional practice: discovering knowledge from experience. *Nurse Educ Today*. 1999; 19(l):29–34.
37. Reed PG. Toward a nursing theory of self-transcendence: deductive reformulation using developmental theories. *Adv Nurs Sci*. 1991;13(4):64–77.
38. Norbeck JS, Tilden VP International nursing research in social support: theoretical and methodological issues. *J Adv Nurs*. 1988; 13(2): 173–178.
39. Gassner LA, Wotton K, Clare J, Hofmeyer A, Buckman J. Evaluation of a model of collaboration: academic and clinician partnership in the development and implementation of undergraduate teaching. *Collegian*. 1999;6(3): 14–21.
40. Neill SJ. Developing children's nursing through action research. *J Child Health Care*. 1998;2:11–15.
41. Gennaro S. International nursing: the past 25 years and beyond. *MCN Am J Matern Child Nurs*. 2000;25(6):296–299.
42. Beunza I, Boulton N, Ferguson C, Serrano R. Diversity and commonality in international nursing. *Int Nurs Rev*. 1994; 41(2):47–52.
43. Sparks SM. Electronic networking for nurses. *Image*. 1993; 25(3):245–248.
44. Falk-Rafael AR. Empowerment as a process of evolving consciousness: a model of empowered caring. *Adv Nurs Sci*. 2001; 24(1):1–16.
45. LaCoursiere SE A theory of online social support. *Adv Nurs Sci*. 2001;24(l):60–77.
46. Poss JE. Developing a new model for cross-cultural research: synthesizing the health belief model and the theory of reasoned action. *Adv Nurs Sci*. 2001;23(4): 1–15.
47. Dixon JK, Dixon JE An integrative model for environmental health research. *Adv Nurs Sci*. 2002;24(3):43–57.
48. Johnson BM, Webber EB. *An Introduction to Theory and Reasoning in Nursing*. Philadelphia, PA: Lippincott Williams & Wilkins; 2004.
49. Benner P, Tanner CA, Chesla CA. *Expertise in Nursing Practice: Caring, Clinical Judgment, and Ethics*. New York: Springer Publishing Co; 1996.
50. Fawcett J. Framework for analysis and evaluation of conceptual models of nursing. In: Reed PG, Shearer NB, Nicoll LH, eds. *Perspectives on Nursing Theory*. 4th ed. Philadelphia: Lippincott Williams & Wilkins; 2004:87–94.

THE AUTHOR COMMENTS

Development of Situation-Specific Theories: An Integrative Approach

When I taught doctoral theory classes, many students wanted clear directions for theory development, especially for development of situation-specific theories. Despite some philosophical conflicts and disagreement about the level of abstraction, I think that situation-specific theories are an innovative direction for nursing theory that could be easily linked to nursing research and practice, and that could incorporate diversities and complexities of nursing phenomena in our ever-changing 21st century.

EUN-OK IM

Middle Range Theory: Spinning Research and Practice to Create Knowledge for the New Millennium

PATRICIA LIEHR, RN, PhD

MARY JANE SMITH, RN, PhD

*T*he foundation of middle range theory reported during the past decade was described and analyzed. A CINAHL search revealed 22 middle range theories that met selected criteria. This foundation is a firm base for new millennium theorizing. Recommendations for future theorizing include: clear articulation of theory names and approaches for generating theories; clarification of concept linkages with inclusion of diagrammed models; deliberate attention to research-practice connections of theories; creation of theories in concert with the disciplinary perspective; and, movement of middle range theories to the front lines of nursing research and practice for further analysis, critique, and development.

A spinner prepares wool by combing, to discard debris and align the strands of a matted mass in much the same way as content is sifted to tease central ideas out of extraneous ones. Just as the spinner twirls strands to compose a single thread; the nurse theorist spins central ideas into a synthesized thread for research and practice. Twisting single threads with each other enhances the strength of the product; as does the crafting of research-practice links in the creation of strong middle range theory. The beauty of any woven article is dependent on its warp and weft; likewise, the esthetics of the discipline is dependent on its theories. Spinning, like theorizing, is rigorous work aimed at creating esthetic, useful products. This article describes and analyzes a decade of middle range theory products that establish a foundation for the new millennium. This foundation highlights the current structure of middle range theory and offers direction for 21st century spinning.

The Historical Context of Middle Range Theory

Modernism, postmodernism, and neomodernism are historical descriptors that represent change in the course of a developing discipline by influencing thinking and scholarship. Modernism espouses beliefs about human beings that affirm a unidimensional and stable existence, while post modernism adheres to views that affirm multidimensional, ever-changing, and complex human unfolding existence.[1] Watson[2] identified the postmodern for nursing as reconnecting

with "the truths of unfoldment, an expansion and fusing of horizons of meaning, an attending to the authenticity, ethos, and ethic of caring relations, context, continuity, connections, aesthetics, interpretation and construction."[2(p63)] She concludes that these postmodern dimensions tie directly to developing the art and science of nursing as a caring-healing transformative praxis paradigm. Reed[3] moves beyond postmodernism to neomodernism and calls for a synthesis of modernism and postmodernism. She describes the synthesis as a metanarrative reflecting the human developmental potential, transformation, and self-transcendent capacity for health and healing, including a recognition of the developmental histories of persons and their contexts.[3] It is expected that theories that offer direction for the new millennium will emerge from the historical context that defines the time. The current context urges a focus on the human developmental potential of health and healing and supports a nursing knowledge base that synthesizes art and science; practice and research. Theories at the middle range level of discourse are in keeping with the historical context launching the new millennium.

> Merton describes theories of the middle range as those *that lie between the minor but necessary working hypotheses that evolve in abundance during day-to-day research and the all-inclusive systematic efforts to develop unified theory that will explain all the observed uniformities of social behavior, social organization and social change.*[4(p39)]

ABOUT THE AUTHORS

PATRICIA LIEHR was born in Pittsburgh, PA, and received her first nursing education at Ohio Valley General Hospital, School of Nursing in Pittsburgh; her baccalaureate education at Villa Maria College in Erie, PA; and her master's in education at Duquesne University in Pittsburgh. Her doctorate in nursing was completed at the University of Maryland, and she did postdoctoral study as a Robert Wood Johnson Scholar at the University of Pennsylvania. She is now a Professor and Associate Dean for Research & Scholarship at the Christine E. Lynn College of Nursing, Florida Atlantic University in Boca Raton, FL. Over time, in her scholarly work, she has woven the threads of theory, practice, and research together to enhance her understanding of each. Interestingly, she is a weaver with little time for warp and weft these days … but still a weaver in her heart.

Her scholarly endeavors focus on human language, including and extending beyond words, and on the scientific structures, which guide nurse-person dialogue.

MARY JANE SMITH was born in Johnstown, PA, and earned a BSN and an MNEd from the University of Pittsburgh and a PhD from New York University. She has taught nursing theory to master's-level students for 25 years and, more recently, to doctoral students. She has been on the faculty at West Virginia University since 1981, during the past several years as a Professor and Associate Dean for Graduate Academic Affairs. The focus of her scholarly work is gathering and analyzing the stories of becoming pregnant for teenaged high school students, time-pressured busyness for graduate students, and intervening in drinking/driving situations for rural youth. She likes to cook, garden, and dance.

He goes on to describe the principal ideas of middle range theory as relatively simple. Simple, in this sense, means rudimentary straightforward ideas that stem from the perspective of the discipline. An example of such an idea is that when individuals tell their story to one who truly listens, a change takes place. This idea is central to the middle range theory of attentively embracing story.[5] The ideas of middle range theory are simple yet general and are more than mere empirical generalizations.

In keeping with the views of Merton,[4] the following descriptions of middle range theory are found in the nursing literature: testable and intermediate in scope,[6] adequate in empirical foundations,[7] neither too broad nor too narrow,[8] circumscribed and substantively specific,[9] and more circumscribed than grand theory but not as concrete as practice theory.[10] In 1974, Jacox[11] described middle range theories as those including a limited number of variables and focused on a limited aspect of reality. Each of these descriptions highlights a scope somewhere in the middle, allowing for broad definitions. Lenz[12] addresses the issue of definitional clarity and believes that although the definitions of middle range theory are consistent, theories of varying scope have been labeled middle range and the discipline may be well served by recognizing levels of theory within the middle range. She states the challenge for the discipline will be to not generate a plethora of middle range theories, but to develop a few that are empirically sound, coherent, meaningful, useful, and illuminating.[12] To meet the challenge set by Lenz in the next century, it is essential that middle range theories emerge from the twisting of research and practice threads by nurse scholars who are building on the work of others and creating the future direction of the discipline. The spinning of middle range theory in the next century will be guided by the existing middle range theory foundation.

The Existing Middle Range Theory Foundation

To assess the current foundation of middle range theory, a CINAHL search of the past 10 years of nursing literature was done entering middle range theory, midrange theory, and nursing as search terms. The search was conducted independently in two institutions. All papers written in English that surfaced from the combined search were evaluated for inclusion in the foundation list of middle range theories (Table 35-1). Criteria for inclusion were

1. The theory was identified as middle range by its author;
2. The theory name was accessible in the paper;
3. Concepts of the theory were explicitly identified or implicitly identified in propositions; and
4. The development of the theory was the major focus of the paper.

TABLE 35-1	Middle Range Theories Over the Decade: 1988–1998				
			Inclusion of Model		
Year Published	**Author(s), Journal**	**Name of Theory**	**Yes**	**No**	**Theory Generating Approach**
1988	Mishel *Image*	Uncertainty in Illness	X		Empirical research, literature synthesis from nursing and other disciplines
1989	Thompson, et al. *Journal of Nurse Midwifery*	Nurse Midwifery Care		X	Philosophy of nurse-midwifery profession, survey data, patient-nurse practice videotapes, empirical research
1990	Kinney *Issues in Mental Health Nursing*	Facilitating Growth and Development		X	Middle range model from Erickson's Modeling and Role Modeling theory, practice
1991	Reed *ANS*	Self-Transcendence		X	Literature reviews, clinical experience, empirical research, deductive reformulation of life span theories from developmental psychology with Rogers Conceptual System
1991	Burke, Kauffmann, Costello, Dillon *Image*	Hazardous Secrets and Reluctantly Taking Charge	X		Grounded theory
1991	Thomas *Issues in Mental Health Nursing*	Women's Anger	X		Existential and cognitive-behavioral theories, literature review, clinical knowledge, intuition, logic
1991	Swanson *Nursing Research*	Caring		X	Phenomenological studies
1994	Powell-Cope *Nursing Research*	Negotiating Partnership		X	Extending Swanson's Caring theory using grounded theory
1995, 1997	Lenz, et al. *ANS*	Unpleasant Symptoms	X		Empirical research, clinical observation, concept analysis, collaboration
1995	Jezewski *ANS*	Cultural Brokering	X		Concept analysis, ethnography, grounded theory, practice experience, literature synthesis
1995	Tollett, Thomas *ANS*	Homelessness-Hopelessness	X		Testing Miller's Patient Power Resources Model using a quasi-experimental study

(Continued)

TABLE 35-1 Middle Range Theories Over the Decade: 1988–1998 (Continued)

Year Published	Author(s), Journal	Name of Theory	Inclusion of Model		Theory Generating Approach
			Yes	No	
1996, 1998	Good, Moore, Good Nursing Outlook	Balance between Analgesia and Side Effects	X		Clinical practice guidelines; empirical research
1997	Auvil-Novak Nursing Research	Chronotherapeutic Intervention for Postsurgical Pain	X		Chronobiologic theory, literature synthesis, empirical research
1997	Olson, Hanchett Image	Nurse-Expressed Empathy and Patient Distress	X		Orlando's nursing model, empirical research
1997	Brooks, Thomas ANS	Interpersonal Perceptual Awareness	X		Concept analysis to extend King's Interacting System framework
1997	Polk ANS	Resilience	X		Concept synthesis using literature from other disciplines, Roger's Science of Unitary Beings
1997	Gerdner Journal of American Psychiatric Nurses' Association	Individualized Music Intervention for Agitation	X		Clinical practice, literature review, pilot study
1997	Acton Journal of Holistic Nursing	Affiliated Individuation as a Mediator of Stress	X		Middle range model from Erickson's Modeling and Role Modeling theory, Empirical research
1998	Eakes, Burke, Hainsworth Image	Chronic Sorrow	X		Concept analysis, literature review, qualitative research
1998	Huth, Moore Journal of the Society of Pediatric Nurses	Acute Pain Management	X		Clinical practice guidelines
1998	Levesque, et al. Nursing Science Quarterly	Psychological Adaptation	X		Middle range theories from other disciplines, empirical research, collaboration, Roy's Adaptation Model
1998	Ruland, Moore Nursing Outlook	Peaceful End of Life	X		Standards of care

These criteria represent an intent to be inclusive, providing the broadest view of available middle range nursing theory. However, some papers excluded were primarily methodological in focus.[13,14] These were identified in the literature search but did not meet the criteria. Table 35-1 describes the middle range theory foundation that has emerged during the past decade. Along with including identifying and locating information about the theory, it notes the inclusion of a diagrammed model and the approaches for theory generation identified by the author.

Analysis of the Middle Range Theory Foundation

The Middle Range Theories

There are 22 middle range theories proposed as the current foundation. Two theories, Unpleasant Symptoms[7,15] and Balance between Analgesia and Side Effects,[16,17] are accompanied by two citations. Unpleasant Symptoms is the only theory to have documented ongoing development in the past decade. The second citation for Balance between Analgesia and Side Effects provides examples of use of the theory for research but does not alter its original structure. Powell-Cope,[18] using Swanson's[19] theory of Caring—with the intent of extending it—derived yet another theory, Negotiating Partnerships. This was the only instance of one middle range nursing theory generating another. However, Levesque et al.[20] report that a foundation of middle range theories from other disciplines was the basis of their work.

Several theories that have been labeled middle range by persons who are not the primary author of the theory do not appear in the middle range foundation list. For instance, Fawcett[9] labels Orlando's Deliberative Nursing, Peplau's Interpersonal Relations, and Watson's Human Caring theory as middle range; however, none of these came up in the literature search for middle range theory. Nolan and Grant[21] labeled Chenitz's theory of Entry into a Nursing Home as Status Passage as middle range and reported a test of the theory with a respite care sample. Review of Chenitz's theory[22] indicated that it was labeled practice theory by the author even though it may be at the middle range level of discourse. There are other theories that seem to be at the middle range level of discourse but have not been so identified by the primary author. One example is the work of Beck, who has developed a theory of postpartum depression that includes initial quantitative inquiry[23] followed by qualitative study.[24-26]

Although this body of work is at the middle range level of discourse, Beck has not labeled it as middle range theory.

Based on the identified foundation of middle range theory, as the decade unfolded, there appeared to be increased willingness to label theory as middle range. Seven of the theories in Table 35-1 were proposed in the 4-year span between 1988 and 1992 and 15 were proposed in the most recent 4 years of the decade, since 1994, with six middle range theory papers published in 1997 alone. Some of the 1997 proliferation can be attributed to an issue of *Advances in Nursing Science* devoted to middle range theory. Three of the middle range theories listed in 1997 were published in this issue. In her editorial for the issue, Chinn[27] highlighted a shift in nurses' scholarly endeavors to create possibilities for healing science-art as evidenced by the issue's middle range theories, which, she noted, defy a single, limited perspective definition. The question about what constitutes theory at the middle range is not a black and white issue for which a precise and clear definition can be offered. Middle range theory holds to a given level of abstraction. It is not too broad nor too narrow, but somewhere in the middle. It is expected that finding the middle will come as theory in the middle range is spun in the next millennium.

Naming the Theory

Theory, especially at the middle range, is known to practitioners and researchers by the way it is named. It is essential that theories at the middle range be named in the context of the disciplinary perspective and at the appropriate level of discourse. Figuring out the name is a process of creative conceptualization that moves back and forth between putting together and pulling apart until the right name is found. Implicit in naming is a search for a conceptual structure as the theorist remembers and relives practice and research experiences, reflecting on proposed meaning in relation to the literature. This is a creative, energy-demanding process intended to uncover the heart of the theory. The central theory core is molded by the conceptual structure that exposes it and is articulated at the middle range level of abstraction as the name of the theory.

A theory name was accessible in each of the papers in Table 35-1, although some names were more accessible than others. A few theorists announced the presentation of a middle range theory and provided a name in the title of the paper,[7,15,28-31] while others embedded the name in the body of the paper. Facilitating Growth and Devel-

TABLE 35-2 Middle Range Nursing Theories by Level of Abstraction

High Middle	Middle	Low Middle
Caring	Uncertainty in Illness	Hazardous Secrets and Reluctantly Taking Charge
Facilitating Growth and Development	Unpleasant Symptoms	Affiliated Individuation as a Mediator of Stress
	Chronic Sorrow	Women's Anger
Interpersonal Perceptual Awareness	Peaceful End of Life	Nurse Midwifery Care
	Negotiating Partnerships	Acute Pain Management
Self-Transcendence	Cultural Brokering	Balance between Analgesia and Side Effect
Resilience	Nurse-Expressed Empathy and Patient Distress	Homelessness-Helplessness
Psychological Adaptation		Individualized Music Intervention for Agitation
		Chronotherapeutic Intervention for Post-Surgical Pain

opment[32] and Affiliated Individuation[33] both emerge from Modeling and Role-Modeling theory.[34] While each is described as a model at the middle range level of abstraction, distinguishing the unique name from the parent theory was difficult. The challenge of naming a middle range theory resides in determining the middle as sufficiently abstract to allow a breadth of application yet narrow enough to permit guidance in research and practice. Table 35-2 organizes the existing middle range theories into the high-middle, middle, and low-middle level of abstraction, using the theory name. The theories were grouped, relative to each other, based on the generality or scope of the theory indicated by the name. Using the theory name to distinguish the level of abstraction has inherent limitations because the name may not reflect theory content. However, the theory name is its guiding label and this analysis highlights the importance of the theory name. It also highlights the existence of multiple levels of abstraction within the middle range, a fact introduced by Lenz,[12] for further recognition and development. To name a middle range theory is to locate it at an appropriate level of abstraction and to commit to a conceptual structure. Capturing a conceptual structure and expressing theory at the middle range level of abstraction will enable 21st century scholars to recognize, use, and critique the theory for practice and research applications.

Inclusion of a Model

Chinn and Kramer[35] define theory as "a creative and rigorous structuring of ideas that projects a tentative, purposeful, and systematic view of phenomena."[35(p106)] They include purpose, concepts, definitions, relationships, structure, and assumptions as components of theory suggested by their definition, noting that purpose and assumptions may be implicit rather than explicit. So, concepts with their definitions—and relationships expressed as structure—are the core components expected to be made explicit regardless of the theory's level of abstraction. One of the criteria for theories in the foundation list was the presentation of concepts. The relationship and structure components were evaluated by determining whether the theorist included a diagrammed model in the paper. Of the 22 theories in the foundation list, only 5 did not diagram a model.[18,19,32,36,37] Three[18,19,36] did not explicitly address relationships between concepts. One[37] specified relationships through propositions; one[32] described middle range relationships between concepts of a parent theory. All middle range theories since 1995 have included a diagrammed model.

 ## Approaches for Generating Middle Range Theory

Lenz[12] has identified six approaches for generating middle range theory; these were used to categorize the methods used by the creators of the 22 theories identified in the foundation. The categories are not mutually exclusive because theorists often used more than one approach. Lenz's approaches are

1. Inductive theory building through research,

2. Deductive theory building from grand nursing theories,

3. Combining existing nursing and nonnursing theories,

4. Deriving theories from other disciplines,

5. Synthesizing theories from published research findings, and

6. Developing theories from clinical practice guidelines.

A review of the foundation theories indicates that fourteen* appeared to use inductive theory building through research. Three derived the theory from grand nursing theory,[20,29,43] two combined nursing and nonnursing theories,[30,37] four derived theories from those of other disciplines,[20,28,37,44] and two[16,45] developed theory from practice guidelines. The approach of synthesizing theories from published research identified by Lenz was difficult to determine when categorizing the theories. No middle range theory was cited that was generated only by published research. Even when not stated explicitly, there were implicit indications that every theory had referred to published research when generating the theory. Two theories[32,46] fit into none of the approaches described by Lenz. Ruland and Moore[46] recently have proposed using standards of care to generate middle range theory and Kinney[32] describes a practice example to demonstrate a middle range model. Including Kinney, seven theories[7,15,32,36,37,40,42,44] explicitly cited personal practice experiences as contributing to middle range theory development. Only four[7,15,36,40,42] of the seven also described research threads, thus enabling the spinning of research with practice in the building of middle range theory.

The analysis of approaches for generating middle range theory suggests that Lenz's listing generally is comprehensive. The elimination of the approach noting synthesis from published research findings may be appropriate, and an expansion of "clinical practice guidelines" to "practice guidelines and standards" will cover the recent work by Ruland and Moore.[46] Inclusion of the practice thread is critical for 21st century spinning. Therefore, the following five approaches are proposed for middle range theory generation in the new millennium:

1. Induction through research and practice;

2. Deduction from research and practice applications of grand theories;

3. Combination of existing nursing and nonnursing middle range theories;

4. Derivation from theories of other disciplines that relate to nursing's disciplinary perspective; and

5. Derivation from practice guidelines and standards rooted in research.

It is unlikely that any of these theory generation approaches will stand alone as nursing moves into the

*References 7, 15, 18–20, 28, 29, 31, 33, 36, 38–42

next century. Each will need to be combined to most effectively guide the discipline. Guidance for the new millennium is most likely to emerge from theories that spin research and practice to focus on the human developmental potential of health and healing.

Juxtaposition with Grand Nursing Theory

As middle range theory is generated for the new millennium, it is essential that it move beyond the polarities often created between it and grand theories. The all-embracing grand theories were espoused by individuals who attempted to create a view of the whole of nursing. Groups have developed into small circles of schools of thought in which an all-or-nothing adherence to the perspective is advocated strongly. This approach has advanced the discipline through generation of scholarly pursuits and offers a grounding for middle range theory. It is not separate nor antithetical to middle range theory development. Merton[4] identifies the following criticisms of middle range theory leveled by those who advocate grand approaches: (1) conceptualizing middle range theory is low in intellectual ambitions; (2) it completely excludes grand theory; (3) it will fragment the discipline into unrelated special theories; and (4) a positivist conception of theory will be the result. There is no evidence that these criticisms have been realized. Nursing's current middle range theory foundation: reflects scholarly work conceptualized at a lower level of abstraction that rises to intellectual challenge; builds on grand theory that continues to offer a foundation for development; and projects a historical context to begin the millennium with theories at the middle range in the perspective of the discipline.

Disciplinary Perspective of the Middle Range Theory Foundation

An association between the existing middle range theory foundation and the disciplinary perspective synthesized as a caring, healing process in which the human developmental potential for health and transformation emerge[2,3] is depicted in Table 35-3. Through the reflective process of dwelling with the essence of the disciplinary perspective and the middle range theories as named, two themes surfaced. These themes were caring—healing processes and transforming struggle-growth. These themes offer a view of the existing middle range theory foundation in

TABLE 35-3 Middle Range Theories by Disciplinary Themes	
Caring—Healing Process	**Transforming Struggle—Growth**
Caring	Self-Transcendence
Facilitating Growth and Development	Resilience
Interpersonal Perceptual Awareness	Psychological Adaptation
Cultural Brokering	Uncertainty in Illness
Nurse-Expressed Empathy and Patient Distress	Unpleasant Symptoms
Nurse Midwifery Care	Chronic Sorrow
Acute Pain Management	Peaceful End of Life
Balance between Analgesia and Side Effects	Negotiating Partnerships
Individualized Music Intervention for Agitation	Hazardous Secrets and Reluctantly Taking Charge
Chronotherapeutic Intervention for Post-Surgical Pain	Affiliated Individuation as a Mediator of Stress
	Women's Anger
	Homelessness-Helplessness

the context of a disciplinary perspective as well as an integrated paradigm for spinning middle range theory in the new millennium.

The Future: Where Does Nursing Theory Go From Here?

In conclusion, a lot of thoughtful spinning of middle range theory has been done in the past decade; and although knots and tangles have been created along the way, one must remember that spinning theory is a creative human endeavor that can best be described as a work in progress. It is expected that the knots and tangles will be sorted out with the spinner's persistence and careful attention to creating and combining fibers. Based on the description and analysis of the current middle range theory foundation, several recommendations are presented for developing middle range theory in the future. The recommendations are that the creators of middle range theory:

1. Take care to clearly articulate the theory name and approaches used for generating the theory;
2. Strive to clarify the conceptual linkages of the theory in a diagrammed model;
3. Give deliberate attention to articulating the research-practice links of the theory;
4. Create an association between the proposed theory and a disciplinary perspective in nursing; and
5. Move middle range theory to the front lines of nursing practice and research for further analysis, critique, and development.

Twenty-first century theorists are offered the challenge of these recommendations. The challenge is to move nursing theory forward by spinning research and practice in the creation of middle range theories congruent with the current historical context. It is this forward movement that will give substance and direction to the discipline. Middle range theory will create the disciplinary fabric of the new millennium as nurse theorists spin and twist fibers from the past-present into the future.

REFERENCES

1. Anderson TA. Post modern person. *Noetic Sciences Review.* 1998;45:28–33.
2. Watson J. Postmodernism and knowledge development in nursing. *Nurs Sci Quarterly.* 1994;8:60–64.
3. Reed PG. A treatise on nursing knowledge development for the 21st century: beyond postmodernism. *ANS.* 1995;17:70–84.
4. Merton RK. On sociological theories of the middle range. In: *Social Theory and Social Structure.* New York: Free Press: 1968.
5. Smith MJ, Liehr P. Attentively embracing story: a middle range theory with practice and research implications. *Sch Ing Nurs Prac.* In press.

6. Suppe F. Middle range theory—Role in nursing theory and knowledge development. In: *Proceedings of the Sixth Rosemary Ellis Scholar's Retreat, Nursing Science Implications for the 21st century.* Cleveland. OH: Frances Payne Bolton School of Nursing, Case Western Reserve University: 1996.

7. Lenz ER, Suppe F, Gift AG, Pugh LC, Milligan RA. Collaborative development of middle-range nursing theories: toward a theory of unpleasant symptoms. *ANS.* 1995;17: 1–13.

8. Reed P. Toward a nursing theory of self-transcendence: deductive reformulation using developmental theories. *ANS.* 1991; 12:64–74.

9. Fawcett J. *Analysis and Evaluation of Nursing Theories.* Philadelphia, PA: F. A. Davis: 1993.

10. Morris D. Middle range theory role in education. In: *Proceedings of the Sixth Rosemary Ellis Scholar's Retreat, Nursing Science Implications for the 21st century.* Cleveland, OH: Frances Payne Bolton School of Nursing, Case Western Reserve University; 1996.

11. Jacox A. Theory construction in nursing: an overview. *Nurs Res.* 1974;23:4–12.

12. Lenz E. Middle range theory—Role in research and practice. In: *Proceedings of the Sixth Rosemary Ellis Scholar's Retreat, Nursing Science Implications for the 21st century.* Cleveland, OH: Frances Payne Bolton School of Nursing, Case Western Reserve University; 1996.

13. Dluhy NM. Mapping knowledge in chronic illness. *J Adv Nurs.* 1995;21:1051–1058.

14. Jenny JJ, Logan J. Caring and comfort metaphors used by patients in critical care. *Image.* 1996;28:349–352.

15. Lenz ER, Pugh LC, Milligan RA. Gift AG, Suppe F. The middle range theory of unpleasant symptoms: an update. *ANS.* 1997;19:14–27.

16. Good M, Moore SM. Clinical practice guidelines as a new source of middle range theory: focus on acute pain. *Nurs Outlook.* 1996;44:74–79.

17. Good M. A middle range theory of acute pain management use in research. *Nurs Outlook.* 1998;46:120–124.

18. Powell-Cope GM. Family caregivers of people with AIDS: negotiating partnerships with professional health care providers. *Nurs Res.* 1994;43:324–330.

19. Swanson KM. Empirical development of a middle range theory of caring. *Nurs Res.* 1991;40:161–166.

20. Levesque L, Ricard N, Ducharme F, Duquette A, Bonin J. Empirical verification of a theoretical model derived from the Roy Adaptation Model: findings from five studies. *Nurs Sci Q.* 1998;11:31–39.

21. Nolan M. Grant G. Mid-range theory building and the nursing theory-practice gap: a respite care case stud y. *J Adv Nurs.* 1992;17:217–223.

22. Chenitz WC. Entry into a nursing home as status passage: a theory to guide nursing practice. *Geriatric Nurs.* 1983; Mar/Apr: 92–97.

23. Beck CT, Reynolds MA, Rutowski P. Maternity blues and postpartum depression. *JOGNN.* 1992;21:287–293.

24. Beck CT. The lived experience of postpartum depression: a phenomenological study. *Nurs Res.* 1992;41:166–170.

25. Beck CT. Teetering on the edge: a substantive theory of postpartum depression. *Nurs Res.* 1993;42:42–48.

26. Beck CT. Postpartum depressed mothers' experiences interacting with their children. *Nurs Res.* 1996;45:98–104.

27. Chinn P. Why middle range theory? *ANS.* 1997;19:viii.

28. Auvil-Novak SE. A mid-range theory of chronotherapeutic intervention for postsurgical pain. *Nurs Res.* 1997;46: 66–71.

29. Olson J, Hanchett E. Nurse-expressed empathy, patient outcomes, and development of a middle-range theory. *Image.* 1997;29: 71–76.

30. Polk LV. Toward a middle range theory of resilience. *ANS.* 1997;19:1–13.

31. Eakes GG, Burke ML, Hainsworth MA. Middle-range theory of chronic sorrow. *Image.* 1998;30:179–184.

32. Kinney CK. Facilitating growth and development: a paradigm case for modeling and role-modeling. *Issues Ment Health Nurs.* 1990;11:375–395.

33. Acton GJ. Affiliated-individuation as a mediator of stress and burden in caregivers of adults with dementia. *J Holistic Nurs.* 1997;15:336–357.

34. Erickson HC, Tomlin EM, Swain MAP. *Modeling and Role-Modeling: A Theory and Paradigm for Nursing.* Englewood Cliffs, NJ: Prentice-Hall; 1983.

35. Chinn PL, Kramer MK. *Theory and Nursing: A Systematic Approach.* St. Louis, MO: Mosby; 1995.

36. Thompson JE, Oakley D, Burke M, Jay S, Conklin M. Theory building in nurse-midwifery: the care process. *J Nurs-Midwifery.* 1989;34:120–130.

37. Reed PG. Toward a nursing theory of self-transcendence: deductive reformulation using developmental theories. *ANS.* 1991;13:64–77.

38. Mishel MH. Uncertainty in illness. *Image.* 1988;20:225–232.

39. Burke SO, Kauffmann E, Costello EA, Dillon MC. Hazardous secrets and reluctantly taking charge: parenting a child with repeated hospitalizations. *Image.* 1991;23:39–45.

40. Jezewski MA. Evolution of a grounded theory: conflict resolution through culture brokering. *ANS.* 1995;17: 14–30.

41. Tollett JH, Thomas SP. A theory-based nursing intervention to instill hope in homeless veterans. *ANS.* 1995;18:76–90.

42. Gerdner L. An individualized music intervention for agitation. *J Am Psych Nurs Assoc.* 1997;3:177–184.

43. Brooks EM, Thomas S. The perception and judgment of senior baccalaureate student nurses in clinical decision making. *ANS.* 1997;19:50–69.

44. Thomas SP. Toward a new conceptualization of women's anger. *Issues Ment Health Nurs.* 1991;12:31–49.

45. Huth MM, Moore SM. Prescriptive theory of acute pain management in infants and children. *JSPN.* 1998;3:23–32.

46. Ruland CM, Moore SM. Theory construction based on standards of care: a proposed theory of the peaceful end of life. *Nurs Outlook.* 1998;46:169–175.

THE AUTHORS COMMENT

Middle Range Theory: Spinning Research and Practice to Create Knowledge for the New Millennium

We wrote the Spinning article because we were entrenched in making sense of middle-range theory. Our graduate students repeatedly told us that it was challenging to attempt to figure out what theory was middle range. When sent to the literature in search of meaningful middle range theory, the students returned with questions and quagmire. We thought it was important to make some sense of the existing literature on middle range theory if the discipline ever expected to use it as a base for practice and research. We believe that middle range theory offers a promising direction for the next generation of nursing scholars. We have published a coedited book, Middle Range Theory for Nursing, which extends the knowledge developed in the Spinning article and describes eight middle-range theories useful for nursing practice and research.

PATRICIA LIEHR
MARY JANE SMITH

7 Characteristics and Criteria of Nursing Theories

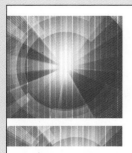

The chapters in this unit address some key characteristics of scientific nursing theory. Knowledge of these characteristics is useful not only for building theory but for building *good* theories—theories that meet evaluation criteria.

There is an exemplary chapter on a contemporary view of nursing theory as related to nurses' theoretical thinking, research, and practice. Another chapter uses theoretical substruction to expose more clearly the components of a theory and the relationships among the conceptual variables. Substruction is also a means for translating abstract concepts into measurable terms that can be used in practice and research. The Hardy chapters present a classic view on theory evaluation criteria that continue to be widely used across disciplines, including nursing. Fawcett and Parse outline criteria that, in addition to criteria used to evaluate theories across disciplines, target evaluation of nursing theories in particular. The classic article by the two philosophers, Dickoff and James, provides a historical perspective on what makes a theory a *nursing* theory. It is still widely cited today and a foundational reading for all nurses.

This unit and others in this book demonstrate that *nursing theory* has advanced beyond the original set of conceptual nursing models that once defined the realm of nursing theory. In general, the term *nursing theory* refers to a wide variety of theories developed in nursing, most of which are mid-range in scope and abstraction. However, as more nurses participate in knowledge development, other types of theories (eg, situation-producing theories, situation-specific theories, micro-theories) may be generated. These theories can enrich the fund of nursing knowledge for healthcare.

QUESTIONS FOR DISCUSSION

- What characteristics distinguish nursing theories from other theories?
- What characteristics do all theories share?
- What characteristics of theory are especially helpful in practice?
- What characteristics of scientific theory may limit its usefulness in practice unless it is translated for practice?
- What role does theory evaluation have in knowledge development?
- What are some new criteria that you think should be included in determining good theories?

Theories: Components, Development, Evaluation

MARGARET E. HARDY, RN, PhD, FAAN

T*he roles of concepts, statements of relationship, and models in theory development are examined. Criteria for evaluating theories are outlined, and the tentative nature of theories is discussed.*

Although nurses in their everyday work are expected to evaluate health conditions of persons under their care, usually little thought is given to evaluating the soundness of the theory and knowledge which guides their action. If the theory is poorly suspended by evidence (i.e., the theory is not "true"), the health of the persons for which nurses are responsible may be severely jeopardized. As health professionals, nurses need to be able to make sound judgments about the rationale for various treatments, therapies, and care. It is often assumed that because an idea is in print (particularly if in a textbook or professional journal), it must be true. Many of the theories on which health professionals base their activities, however, are open to severe criticisms. With the speed with which new ideas are published, nurses now more than ever need to keep abreast of the development of relevant knowledge and be able to evaluate that knowledge in order to make informed judgments.

Unless nurses can assess the knowledge generated in such diverse areas as stress, systems, decision making, leadership, self-concept, body image, family, groups, body systems, they cannot use that knowledge wisely and constructively. Failure or inability to assess knowledge relevant to her area of work means the nurse must function as a technician, depending on others to interpret the knowledge-base which guides her actions. If nurses intend to direct their own actions in a responsible manner, they must become well informed on developing knowledge, they must be able to evaluate critically the knowledge developed, and they must make informed judgments based on this knowledge. They also must learn to function optimally as generalists. A competent practitioner really does not have the luxury of concentrating her efforts in a restricted area (psychiatry is currently under attack for the narrowness of its activities), but must take into account a wide variety of phenomena which have bearing on her clients.

Our comprehension of the world around us is based on the use of concepts, hypotheses, and theories. Nurses, as practitioners in the health field, apply and use knowledge generated from theories. In spite of the pervasiveness of theories in guiding and controlling our everyday life, the literature on theory development is diverse and confusing, and it generally is little related to the activities of practitioners. This article attempts to identify the structure of theory, to differentiate between different types of theoretical statements, and to identify criteria for evaluating theories.

Concepts

Concepts are labels, categories, or selected properties of objects to be studied; they are the bricks from which theories are constructed. Concepts are the dimensions, aspects, or attributes of reality which interest the scientist. Patients, illness, cardiovascular diseases, nurses, or physicians are examples of concepts used in health-related fields on which research may be based. The scientist constructs theories in his domain of interest by linking concepts of one class or attribute to concepts of other classes or attributes. When he has a set of interrelated statements or hypotheses concerning the relationships between concepts (i.e., when he has filled between the bricks with mortar), he has a theory. Concepts are the basic elements of theory. A major part of the evaluation of a theory is the identification and assessment of the concepts.

Components and Structure of Theory

A theory may be viewed from a variety of perspectives. For the purpose of exploring the structure of a theory,

ABOUT THE AUTHOR

MARGARET E. HARDY was born in Edmonton, Alberta, Canada, in 1938. She received her BSN in 1960 from the University of British Columbia in Vancouver, Canada; her MA in 1965 from the University of Washington School of Nursing, with a major in community mental health; and her PhD in sociology in 1971 from the University of Washington. Her employment includes a faculty position at Boston University from 1971 to 1985, where she held a joint appointment in the School of Nursing and the Department of Sociology. From 1985 to her early retirement in 1993, she was a Professor at the University of Rhode Island School of Nursing. Her major contribution to nursing evolved serendipitously as a result of her teaching assignment at Boston University; development of courses for the graduate program led to the publication of her award-winning books *Theoretical Foundations for Nursing* and *Role Theory*, as well as a book *Research Readings*. Through her publications and teaching hundreds of graduate students throughout New England during the 1970s and 1980s, Dr. Hardy provided foundational knowledge on metatheory and inspired many to initiate theory development for nursing. Dr. Hardy enjoys watercolor painting, reading, walking, hiking, traveling, and camping in the mountains with her husband and two dogs.

one may view theory as a language (Rudner, 1966). Like any language, theory consists of elements, formulations, and a set of definitions, i.e., it is comprised of syntax and semantics. When an investigator studies a scientific theory, he is interested in the logical structure or the relation between the elements (concepts) of the theory (the syntax) and the meaning given to the elements (the semantics). Syntax, then, is concerned with the occurrence of concepts in the axioms, postulates, or hypotheses of a theory and the relationship between the concepts and between the hypotheses of a theory, while semantics is concerned with the specific meaning attributed to the concepts. When a theory is made explicit or is formalized, one can examine the syntax and determine if the structure of the theory is consistent with the rules of logic.

The Semantics of Theory

Theories consist of two types of elements or terms. One set, the *derived* terms, are specifically introduced through definition whereas the other set, the *primitive* terms, remain undefined (Hempel, 1952). The primitive terms (or concepts) are the primary building blocks of theories from which new terms are derived. Both primitive and derived terms appear in a theory's axioms and postulates and give meaning to an otherwise uninterpreted or formalized system.

Concepts are defined and their meanings are understood only within the framework of the theory of which they are a part. Much conceptual confusion exists in theoretical areas upon which nurses draw. Concepts are often vaguely defined; the same concept may be defined and described many different ways (each writer providing his own definition). For example, within the area of role theory the concepts of role, status, and role behavior overlap and are often used interchangeably. Concepts develop as part of theory and are altered and refined as a body of knowledge grows. The concern for clarifying concepts involves a dilemma of trying to achieve consistency in meaning without premature closure of theories. Conceptual confusion and vagueness in theories appear to be a necessary and an important condition for creativity in science as elsewhere. Persons in the more applied professions often find this state of confusion difficult to cope with.

The refinement of concepts (improving the bricks) is a continuous process which involves not only sharpening of theoretical and operational definitions, but also modification of existing theory. Theories and concepts are reformulated by relating the theoretical world to the empirical, by organizing a great many concrete items into a small number of classes (regrouping the bricks), and by relating diverse concepts within a more general system of concepts.

General or Abstract

Concepts may be ordered on the basis of their level of abstractness. A specific occurrence, such as a patient's chest pain, is treated as a special case of a more general condition, such as heart disease. Heart disease, in turn, is a special condition of the more general area, the circulatory system.

Concepts are also appraised for their degree of generality; they are assessed according to the extent they change or vary. Concepts which refer to classes or categories of phenomena may be called *nonvariable* (Hage, 1972). Such concepts are found in typologies in which classes are clearly defined; an observation either fits or does not fit into a given category, depending upon the presence or absence of the property of interest, e.g., male, female. Concepts which are used to order phenomena according to some property or concepts which refer to dimensions of phenomena are called *variables* (Hage, 1972). When the results of observations fall on a continuum, the property being observed is a variable concept, e.g., 27 years, 82 years. It has been argued (Hage, 1972) that concepts that have a continuum should be utilized more frequently in conceptualizing and theory construction because such concepts facilitate theory development, are not restricted to time and place, and are more subtle for description and classification. The following illustrates the difference between nonvariable and variable concepts: Schizophrenia, manic depression, phobic reactions, and passive-aggressive traits are nonvariable concepts; they are bound by culture. The following general variable concepts are not so bound: anxiety, the degree of depression, intensity of affect, extent of contact with reality, frequency of phobic reactions. These general variable concepts may be utilized to describe the specific mental disorders listed above as well as other normal and abnormal mental states, whereas the nonvariable concepts (disease entities) are specifically either-or types of abnormal phenomena. By using both abstract and variable concepts, the scientist is able to develop laws and theories which have a wide range of applicability.

Theoretical or Operational

Concepts, whether nonvariable or variable, may have both a theoretical definition and an operational definition. The theoretical definition gives meaning to the terms in context of the theory and permits any reader to assess the validity of that definition. The operational definition tells how the concept is linked to concrete situations. An operational definition, which is used in the process of giving experiential meaning to the concept of a theory, describes a set of physical procedures which must be carried out in order to assign to every case a value for the concept. For example, the concept of level of aggression may be operationally defined as the number of times a child hits another child during an hour of play. How adequately the operational definition reflects the theoretical concept is another matter for consideration. That is, not only do concepts need operational definitions but the operational definition must be a valid reflection of the theoretical meaning of the concept. In this example, the operational definition certainly permits an observer to assign a level of "aggression" to each child observed. The level of aggression score for a child, however, may not reflect the theoretical meaning of the concept. The operational definition does not take into account the intent of the child, aggressive acts other than hitting, or the intensity of the act. The dilemma encountered in trying to link observable events to theoretical constructs is that the more concretely concepts are defined, the more restricted is the scope of the theory and the less useful is the theory. In spite of the difficulty in developing operational definitions, it is necessary to define theoretical terms in a way that the concepts can be measured. Only through developing measurements of concepts can hypotheses and, in turn, theories be tested.

Operational definitions are a necessary part of theory construction. Operational definitions permit the validity of concepts to be assessed. They permit hypotheses to be tested and the empirical relevance of a theory to be assessed. They also permit other scientists to replicate the study. Operational definitions, which form the bridge between the theory and the empirical world, are modified over time as both theoretical and technological knowledge grow.

Theoretical concepts only make sense when considered within the framework of the theories of which they are a part. Such concepts may be examined on the basis of the degree of observability of their referent. Observable concepts (concepts that refer directly to observable objects) are likely to be found in derived theorems which are to be tested, whereas nonobservable concepts are found in axioms. Nonobservable concepts—intervening variables or hypothetical constructs—are derived on the basis of inferences from observable referents. Intervening variables are concepts that are based on inferences from observations. To illustrate this point, consider the following: A state of anxiety is often inferred on the basis of observations of increased heart rate, sweaty palms, and nausea. Anxiety per se is not observable.

Hypothetical concepts are more abstract than intervening variables. Belief in their existence is based primarily on theoretical support, and only indirectly on supporting empirical data. The id and the unconscious are examples of hypothetical constructs. The distinctions between intervening variables and hypothetical constructs are not at all clear. In one theory, a concept may be a hypothetical construct; in another theory, the same concept may be an intervening variable.

Attributes of Concepts Utilized for Evaluation

Concepts are abstractions from concrete events; concepts themselves can have a varying degree of abstraction. As one moves up the level of abstraction in order to develop systematic explanations of general phenomena, one is faced with the problem of relating back from the symbolic concepts to concrete phenomena. Part of the difficulty in doing this is dependent on the adequacy of the rules of correspondence (or the links one is able to make) between the theoretical concepts and their empirical referents. The generality (abstraction) of concepts and the relationship between the concepts and the empirical referent (testability) are criteria used to evaluate a theory. Examination of the semantics of a theory provides another means for evaluation. This may, in part, be examined by assessing the intersubjectivity of meaning. The intersubjectivity of the meaning of concepts refers to whether the concepts are given a meaning similar to the meaning used by other scientists in related areas (Reynolds, 1971, p. 16).

Nature of Relation[1]	Meaning
Symmetrical	If A, then B; if B, then A
Asymmetrical	If A, then B; but if no A, no conclusion about B
Causal	If A, always B
Probabilistic	If A, probably B
Time order	If A, later B
Concurrent	If A, also B
Sufficient	If A, then B, regardless of anything else
Conditional	If A, then B, but only if C
Necessary	If A and only if A, then B

[1]The relations are not all mutually exclusive

Figure 36-1 *Relationships between concepts.*

Statements of Relationships Between Concepts

Syntax of Theory

If a theory is formalized or made explicit, the syntax, or relationship, between concepts can be examined and the logical adequacy of the theory can be assessed. In assessing a theory's logical structure, the meanings of the concepts themselves are not taken into consideration. That is, symbols may be used to represent the concepts. This facilitates the examination of the logical structure without confusing the issue by considering the explicit meaning of the concepts. For example, the statement that social stress "results in" heart disease can be expressed symbolically. If social stress is represented by X, heart disease by Y, and results in by $\rightarrow$ then the statement social stress results in heart disease can be expressed by $X \rightarrow Y$. A formalization of statements like this and other interrelated statements in a theory facilitate the examination of the structure of a theory.

Types of Relationships

To analyze the structure of a theory it is necessary to identify the relationships between concepts. Some types of relationships and their meanings are summarized in Figure 36-1. Relationships listed are not mutually exclusive. Some of the relationships between concepts may be illustrated by using Selye's (1956) theory of stress. This stress formulation indicates that stressors result in a physiological syndrome identified as General Adaptive Syndrome (GAS). If in this formulation the relationship between stressors and GAS is determinate, then this implies that the concepts are *time-ordered* (stressors occur prior to the development of GAS), *sufficient* (if stressors occur, then GAS occurs regardless of anything else), and *necessary* (if stressors and only if stressors occur, then GAS occurs). The

determinate relationship between stressors and GAS is asymmetrical (if stressors occur, then GAS occurs; if no stressors occur, then no conclusions may be reached about the occurrence of GAS) rather than symmetrical (if stressors occur, GAS occurs; if GAS occurs, then stressors occur). It is possible, however, that the relationship between stressors and GAS is not determinate but probabilistic (if stressors occur, there exists a 90 percent chance that GAS will occur) or conditional (if stressors occur, then GAS occurs, but only if specific physiological condition W exists). For clarity in theoretical formulations, it is necessary to specify the type of relationships between concepts. Although the identification of causal relationships in the health sciences is the reason for considerable success in disease prevention, relationships which are stochastic and relationships which are conditional are valuable in the prediction and control of disease-related events and hence should be identified rather than ignored.

Sign of the Relationship

An additional characteristic of the relationship between concepts is the sign ($\pm$) of the relationship. Concepts may be either positively (+) or inversely (−) related. The sign of relationships, though being discussed here in the context of theory development, really relates to the concept of measures of association or correlation. Thus, in the postulates—the greater X, the greater Y, and the greater Y, the greater Z—a positive relationship is implied between concepts as measured by some measure of association. Knowing that Y increases with X and Z increases with Y, it can be logically deduced that Z increases with X. The sign of the relationship between X and Z depends upon the sign of the relationships between the concepts X and Y, and Y and Z in the postulates. The sign rule has been summarized from work by Zetterberg (1963); Costner and Leik (1964) stated that the sign of the deduced relationship is the algebraic product of the signs of the postulated relationships. If Y is positively correlated with X and Z is positively correlated with Y, then it can be concluded by deduction and the sign rule that Z is positively correlated with X. This process of deduction may be expressed as:

$$
\begin{array}{ll}
\text{If} & X \xrightarrow{\;+\;} Y \\
\text{and} & Y \xrightarrow{\;+\;} Z \\
\hline
\text{then} & X \xrightarrow{\;+\;} Z
\end{array}
$$

It is still an empirical question as to whether this logically deduced relationship actually exists. A relationship which is true according to logic is not necessarily true empirically.

Formalizing and Examining a Set of Statements

This discussion has emphasized that the evaluation of a theory's structure is facilitated if the concepts and the relationships between the concepts are formalized. The following stress formulation will be utilized to illustrate ways of assessing the syntax of theory: Social stress results in emotional tension whereas cognitive dissonance and social stress are inversely related; emotional tension results in somatic dysfunctioning. These statements may be formalized and displayed diagrammatically or in a matrix (Figure 36-2). The matrix used here is an adaptation of a data correlation matrix. The

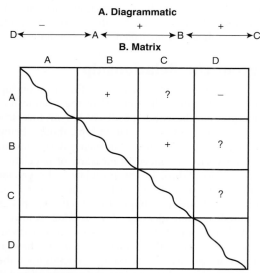

Concepts: Social stress, A; emotional tension, B; somatic dysfunctioning, C; cognitive dissonance, D.
Sign of the relationship: Positive, +; inverse, –; unspecified, ?
Relationships between concepts: Symmetrical, ←→; asymmetrical, —→.

Figure 36-2 *Representation of stress formulation: concepts and their relationships.*

visual representation of the formalized model makes it relatively simple to examine the theory's structure. The diagram shows the relationship between the concepts while the matrix readily displays the completeness and logical consistency of the formulation. Discontinuities in the stress formulation are evident in both the diagram (lack of connections between the concepts) and the matrix (empty cells). Deductions can be made from the postulates stated. Using the sign rule and the deduced relationship, we may conclude that A and C are positively associated. That is, an increase in social stress is associated with an increase in somatic dysfunctioning. From this deduction the formulation is made more complete; no logical inconsistencies exist. The formalization of a theory to facilitate an evaluation of it will be discussed later.

Types of Statements

Although "postulates," "proposition," "hypothesis," "axiom," "laws," "principles," and "empirical generalizations" refer to different types of statements, they have a common characteristic in that they link together two or more concepts. A theory is made up of a set of interrelated propositions, theorems, or hypotheses derived from axioms, initial hypotheses, or postulates. Hypotheses refer to facts that are as yet unexperienced; they are corrigible in view of fresh knowledge. Principles and empirical generalizations are statements about data and are generally believed to be true. The distinguishing characteristic between empirical generalizations and hypotheses is that a hypothesis may be formulated in the absence of data, while an empirical generalization summarizes empirical evidence. Statements differ in their degree of generality and degree of empirical support. Empirical generalizations, since they summarize data, are closer to reality than are hypotheses. However, hypotheses, because they are at a higher level of generalization, are invaluable in aiding our understanding of events which have not yet been systematically tested.

Scientific hypotheses are more or less *grounded* on previous knowledge, i.e., they are partially supported (or at least not refuted) by empirical evidence and by theory. Hypotheses are developed from a rationale; they are not wild, groundless guesses. They should show reasonable conjecture—not fly in the face of existing knowledge.

Laws are well grounded; they have strong empirical support. They state a constant relation among two or more variables, each representing (at least partly and indirectly) a property of concrete systems. An example of a law is $E = Mc^2$. In the psychosocial area few, if any, laws exist. Laws are propositions that assert universal connections between properties.

Statements on the highest level of generality are laws and axioms. Statements on a lower level of generality (propositions, theorems, hypotheses) can be deduced from laws. The purpose of deduction is to test the general statements. In a deductive system, high-level statements can be falsified by the falsification of lower-level (deduced) statements. In any hypothetico-deductive theory, the less universal statements or lower-level statements are themselves still, strictly speaking, universal statements; they are empirical generalizations and must have the character of hypotheses. Postulates, axioms, and laws are primitive statements about an infinite universe, whereas hypotheses and empirical generalizations are statements about a finite universe.

The following examples may illustrate the difference between laws and hypotheses A law in physiology is: Cardiac output = heart rate × stroke volume. This statement is true under *all* conditions (i.e., for all human hearts regardless of time or culture and also for nonhuman hearts). An hypothesis in physiology is: Resting potentials in nerve and muscle cells depend only on the difference in potassium ion concentration across the cell membrane. The statement has not reached the status of a law. Although there is reasonable evidence to support this statement, experimental evidence suggests that other ions may affect resting potentials. The generalization holds true for most muscle and nerve cells rather than for all cells. An hypothesis in social psychology is: In any task-oriented group, inequality in task activity among group members occurs and results in role differentiation. This generalization has mixed empirical support. Some experimental studies corroborate this hypothesis, while other experimental studies identify conditions under which role differentiation in task-oriented groups does not occur. The generalization may only apply under specific conditions and only in the American culture.

 Models

Although a scientific theory is considered to be a deductive system, the relationship between variables may best be expressed in terms of a model. That is, an investigator may formalize a theory, identify its postulates, identify or derive the remaining propositions, and then decide that the problem of relationships is best represented by a model. A model is a simplified representation of a theory or of certain complex events, structures, or systems. Constructing a model forces the theorists to specify the precise relationship between components.

Models, like theories, are isomorphic systems; they are selective representations of the empirical world with which the scientist is concerned; crucial aspects of the phenomena are identified and aspects not considered important are ignored. Models are descriptive; they simplify the area of concern and can help the scientist grasp key elements and the relationships between these elements. The distinction between theories and models is not always clear. For example, what is considered a well-established theory in one academic area may be used as a model to represent phenomena in another area. Modeling is a technique used to describe and explain as well as to generate ideas and predictions.

Types

One type of model is an *analog* model, or an analogy. This model directs attention to resemblances between theoretical entities and familiar subject matter (Kaplan, 1964). For example, a nurse may use the analogy of a mechanical pump to explain to a patient the workings of his heart. In doing this, the nurse is using properties of the pump (an entity with which the patient is familiar) to explain characteristics about the heart (an entity with which the patient is unfamiliar). A problem which is difficult to understand may be made more comprehensible by the use of an analogy. The study of social organizations has been based on an organic model, e.g., Parsons' (1951) description of social systems, and social interactions have been described in terms of economic exchanges (Blau, 1964). Because the model is "true" in one area of science, however, does not mean that it will be true or hold up on another area. The model must be tested for its validity in each area of application. Although many characteristics of the organic model are inappropriate for describing social systems, the organic model has been a useful starting point for the study of social phenomena.

Iconic models are used if a direct representation of the subject is wanted (DiRenzo, 1966). The model may vary as to the number of properties represented and the level of abstraction. A kidney machine, for example, although it does not resemble the kidney in appearance, does represent relatively accurately some of the kidney processes. A model of the heart (built to scale), a scaled model of a DNA molecule, an organizational chart of a hospital, and a miniature social system depicting the hierarchical structure and communication processes in an organization are examples of iconic models. These models represent the original phenomena but in another form. Such models are useful to the extent that they increase our sense of understanding of the entity. This type of modeling has been utilized more perhaps in the physical sciences than in the social sciences. The usefulness of iconic models for understanding social phenomena may be directly related to our ability to identify key variables and to abstract these characteristics. For many persons it is easier to accept a plastic model of the heart as a useful model than it is to accept a three-person decision-making network as a useful model of a social organization. The value of models is dependent upon the extent to which they increase understanding, explain phenomena, or give us a sense of what is going on and why.

Another type of model is the *symbolic* model which represents phenomena figuratively (DiRenzo, 1966). A set of connected symbols, objects, or concepts may be used to represent a problem of interest. The relationship between concepts may be represented diagrammatically to facilitate conceptualization and understanding.

Use

Although models have proved to be extremely helpful in theory construction, they should be used carefully. Models have no truth value themselves. There is no guarantee that a model that has been successfully used in one area of study will be useful in another area. A major question to consider is the extent to which the model faithfully represents the phenomena of interest. There may be a tendency to overlook the differences between the phenomena of interest and the model since the scientist is more interested in the similarities. The differences, however, may completely negate the usefulness of the model. Models are tools for understanding reality which should be used judiciously and be replaced or modified when outmoded or inappropriate.

Criteria for Evaluating Theories

Theories are sets of interrelated hypotheses which are subject to reformulation and refinement. The development of adequate theories to describe, explain, predict, and control phenomena is a slow process and requires the cooperative effort of many persons. Knowledge is not acquired by one person in isolation but results from the cumulative efforts of many persons over a long period of time. Various writers, primarily philosophers, have suggested criteria to assist in the evaluation of theory. A theory may be evaluated in terms of its logical adequacy, abstractness, testability, empirical adequacy, and pragmatic adequacy (Schrag, 1967). These criteria are not meant to hinder the development of theories but to provide guidelines.

Theories are developed to help describe, explain, predict, and control phenomena in the world around us whether the theory is concerned with the area of astronomy, genetics, physics, chemistry, psychology, sociology, physiology, or biology. Implicit in the discussion of theories is the assumption that a theory can be evaluated according to certain universal standards. Regardless of the content of the theory, an investigator examines the underlying assumptions, the validity of the concepts and of the general perspective, the degree of generality of the theory, the soundness of the reasoning, the testability of the hypotheses, the empirical support for the hypotheses, the ability to control and manipulate the phenomena, and the degree of accuracy with which predictions can be made.

Meaning and Logical Adequacy

That few theories successfully meet all these criteria does not mean that theories should not be evaluated. A first step in evaluating theory is to identify basic assumptions (these may not be stated), the concepts, and the relationships between the concepts and to consider the validity of the assumptions, the validity of the meaning attributed to the concepts (are the concepts defined in a manner similar to that used by other scientists in the area?), and the logic of the theoretical system.

When an investigator has reached a conclusion about the validity of the concepts and proposed theory, he can assess the logic of the argument. In doing this, the scientist is concerned with the reasonableness of the argument. The logical adequacy of a theory can be evaluated by formalizing the theory and examining it for discontinuities, discrepancies, and contradictions. In the example cited earlier (Figure 36-2), discontinuities in the theory were evident. When the theory was formalized, it was apparent that nothing was said about the relationship between social stress and somatic dysfunctioning or about the relationship between cognitive dissonance and emotional tension and cognitive dissonance and somatic dysfunctioning. From the postulates and using the sign rule, it was deduced that A and C are positively associated. Since D is related (inversely) only to A, nothing can be said about its relationship to B or C. Because the relationships between A and B and B and C are asymmetrical $(A \rightarrow B, B \rightarrow C)$, the conclusion that A is positively correlated with and results in C is logical. Had the relationship between the variables been symmetrical $(A \leftrightarrow B, B \leftrightarrow C)$, then the conclusion that A is related to C might not hold up. The relationship between A and B, for example, says that A and B vary together; the relationship is not necessarily causal. A and B may be related because of their common relationship to another variable, i.e., the relationship could be spurious.

Likewise, the symmetrical relationship between B and C might be spurious. If either or both of the relationships in these postulates are spurious, then the relationship between the concepts in the deduced proposition is open to question. No contradictions were evident in the stress formulation. Formalizing a theory increases the probability that discontinuities and contradictions will be identified.

Operational and Empirical Adequacy

Next, the theory can be assessed for its testability. To be testable, a theory must have operationally defined concepts. Since Bridgman's (1927) introduction of the phrase, "operational definition," scientists in all areas have been concerned with identifying adequate operational definitions for their concepts. When operational definitions for theoretical concepts have been established, the theory can be tested. Assessing the operational adequacy of a theory requires consideration of (a) whether the concepts can be measured and (b) how accurately the operational definitions reflect the theoretical concepts.

In testing a theory, it can be subjected to falsification (be found false) rather than to confirmation (Popper, 1959). If a sincere attempt is made to refute a theory and the theory stands up, the theory is considered supported or tentatively confirmed. Terms such as "confirmation," "verification," "support," "corroboration," "disconfirmation," "falsification," "failure to support," relate to the empirical base for a theory. Hypotheses may not be proved true, verified, or falsified by limited evidence, but evidence gathered over time from a variety of sources may tend to support, bear out, corroborate, or be in accord with an hypothesis, and thus be confirming evidence. If the evidence does not support the hypothesis, the evidence may be viewed as disconfirming rather than falsifying; the hypothesis is not "proved false." The use of the term "evidence" and the terms "disconfirming," "supporting," and "corroborating" suggests that one recognizes the status of the hypothesis as tentative—awaiting further testing. An hypothesis is not an absolute statement or a truth statement; it should be stated in a way that it can be tested and refuted. For data from any one study and for cumulative evidence from numerous studies, the question of the empirical adequacy of the theory is raised, i.e., how well does the evidence support the theory?

Over time, evidence that both supports and fails to support a theory accumulates. When the relative strengths of the evidence are evaluated, some conclusion about the empirical adequacy of a theory may be reached. Assessing the empirical adequacy of a theory requires the determination of the degree of congruence between the theoretical claims and the empirical evidence.

Generality

Another criterion used to evaluate a theory is the degree of generality or the degree of abstractness which characterizes it. The more general a theory, the more useful it is. A theory of the grieving process which can be applied to persons of all ages, to persons in any culture, and to losses of any object is more useful than a theory of grieving which can be applied only to middle-aged persons who lose a spouse.

Contribution to Understanding

A theory may be assessed as to how much it increases understanding. Does it describe the phenomena and give a sense of insight? Does it suggest new ideas and a new way of looking at the phenomena? The scientist constantly looks for theories that will increase his understanding of phenomena, which are relatively simple explanations, and which suggest new lines of reasoning and new avenues of exploration.

Predictability

Another criterion used to assess theory is the extent to which predictions can be made. A theory may describe a process, may increase the understanding of the process, but it may not assist in making any predictions about the outcomes of that process. A theory, for example may permit a description and explanation of a process after it has occurred; i.e., it is possible to look at a family which has suffered a "loss" and describe the family behavior in terms of adjustment to a crisis, but it may not be possible to predict accurately the behavior of family members in response to this crisis before the crisis occurs.

Pragmatic Adequacy

Since the purpose of a theory is to explain, predict, and control, the ability to control phenomena of interest is one means for assessing a theory. This criterion is pragmatic adequacy (Schrag, 1967). A theory may permit explanation and accurate prediction, but the theory may not permit the scientist to control the phenomena of interest.

The business of the applied professions (nursing, engineering, social work, medicine, architecture, political science) is to make *use* of existing theory to predict certain processes or outcomes and to control "events" in such a way that desired outcomes are achieved. The usefulness of a theory (pragmatic adequacy) for changing conditions is of major importance to the health professions. In the biological sciences many theories enable scientists or professionals to control outcomes; e.g., disease control, (prevention) of degenerative process in the body, and control or replacement of defective body parts. Although it is recognized that science has as its goal the production of knowledge for predicting and controlling phenomena, the ethics of using this knowledge is only now being examined in detail. Some of the decisions as to whether man should use the knowledge he had generated to control and alter the forces around him are being questioned more in some areas than in others, i.e., few question the use of vaccines to prevent disease, but the use of abortions to prevent overpopulation has been severely attacked by some segments of the population. Although there are relatively few theories (particularly in the area of social behavior) which permit the scientist to control phenomena, the development of such theories is likely to increase. The problems associated with the use of these theories by the applied professions will also increase.

 ## Tentative Nature of Theories

Although rules and guidelines can be postulated to aid in the development and evaluations of theories, theories are tentative. With new knowledge, old facts are subject to different interpretations, and different data are brought to light. The development of theory is man's attempt to establish structure and meaning in his world. In assessing existing knowledge, one needs to take into account the culture of the scientific community as well as the values of society in general. The values of both communities come into play in many aspects of the process of establishing knowledge.

The selection of problem areas and the development and use of concepts involve arbitrary choices. The theories that develop reflect the interests of the scientific community and of society and do not necessarily represent the areas that are in most need of examination.

REFERENCES

Blau, P. M. (1964). *Exchange and power in social life*. New York: John Wiley & Sons.

Bridgman, P. W. (1927). *The logic of modern physics*. New York: Macmillan.

Costner, H. L., & Leik, R. K. (1964). Deductions from axiomatic theory. *American Sociological Review, 29*, 819–835.

Di Renzo, G. J. (Ed.). (1966). *Concepts, theory and explanation in the behavioral sciences*. New York: Random House.

Hage, J. (1972). *Techniques and problems of theory construction in sociology*. New York: John Wiley & Sons.

Hempel, C. G. (1952). Fundamentals of concept formation in empirical science. In *International encyclopedia of unified sciences*. Chicago: The University of Chicago Press.

Kaplan, A. (1964). *The conduct of inquiry*. San Francisco: Chandler.

Parsons, T. (1951). *The social system*. Glencoe, IL: Free Press.

Popper, K. (1959). *The logic of scientific discovery*. New York: Basic Books.

Reynolds, P. D. (1971). *A primer in theory construction*. Indianapolis: Bobbs-Merrill.

Rudner, R. S. (1966). *Philosophy of social science*. Englewood Cliffs, N.J.: Prentice-Hall.

Schrag, C. (1967). Elements of theoretical analysis in sociology. In L. Gross (Ed.), *Sociological theory: Inquiries and paradigms* (pp. 220–253). New York: Harper & Row.

Selye, H. (1956). *The stress of life*. New York: McGraw-Hill.

Zetterberg, H. (1963). *On theory and verification in sociology (A much revised edition)*. Totowa, NJ: Bedmeister Press.

THE AUTHOR COMMENTS | Theories: Components, Development, Evaluation

The motivation for writing this article was the need for students to have an organizing framework for selecting one theory over another when faced with a clinical situation, regardless of clinical specialty or unit of study, from the physiologic to the organizational. Students also needed to link theoretic areas, which, at the time, often included the concepts of stress, crisis, and adaptation. To do this, students had to know the characteristics and components of a theory and the criteria for selecting and evaluating theory. This metatheoretic knowledge was and still remains a necessary prerequisite for comparing and selecting theories for nursing practice, as well as for evaluating one's own theories. At the time this article was written, there was no literature published on this topic. This article, along with the book publications, forged new and important territory in knowledge development for nursing.

MARGARET E. HARDY

From Practice to Midrange Theory and Back Again
Beck's Theory of Postpartum Depression

GERRI C. LASIUK, RN, PhD

LINDA M. FERGUSON, RN, PhD

This article presents a brief overview of theory as background for a more detailed discussion of midrange theory—its origins, the critical role for midrange theory in the development of nursing practice knowledge, and the criteria for evaluating midrange theory. We then chronicle Cheryl Tatano Beck's program of research on postpartum depression (PPD) and advance the thesis that her theory of PPD, titled "Teetering on the Edge" is an exemplar of a substantive midrange nursing theory. We demonstrate Beck's progression from identification of a clinical problem to exploratory-descriptive research, to concept analysis and midrange theory development, and finally to the application and testing of the theory in the clinical setting. Through ongoing refinement and testing of her theory, Beck has increased its generalizability across various practice settings and continually identifies new issues for investigation. Beck's program of research on PPD exemplifies using nursing outcomes to build and test nursing practice knowledge.

In today's world of *evidence-based nursing* and *knowledge utilization,* few question the centrality of theory to nursing knowledge development and the importance of that process to the ongoing evolution of the discipline. Although even Florence Nightingale knew that the practice of nursing requires specialized, discipline-specific knowledge,[1] it would he several decades before the science of nursing had evolved sufficiently to systematically develop that knowledge. In the early part of the last century, nursing practice knowledge took the form of "rules, principles, and traditions"[1(p34)] derived from experience and taught by rote. The competent practitioner needed only a caring disposition coupled with a handful of technical skills, which were taught in hospital-based apprenticeship-training programs. The little-theoretical knowledge that did exist in nursing was co-opted from other disciplines.

This situation began to change when the public health movement took hold in the Western world. By 1913, the National League for Nursing Education in the United States recognized that the increasing scope and complexity of nursing practice required a broader knowledge base that must include "some knowledge of the scientific approach to disease, causes, and prevention ...."[2(p60)] The social upheaval that accompanied two world wars and the intervening Depression years spawned major shifts in the social order; changes to the delivery of healthcare; and a growing demand for skilled nurses. In response, national governments invested new resources into the study of nurse education and work life. This was a critical juncture for the discipline because it presented both an opportunity and an imperative for nurses to articulate the nature of the discipline, to define its domain, and to set a course for future development. Consideration of these weighty issues precipitated a cascade of events that culminated in a consensus about the need for a body of distinctly nursing knowledge, developed and tested through research (for reviews, see references 1 and 3).

The importance of theory to nursing knowledge development received official sanction in 1965 when the American Nurses Association (ANA) issued a position paper declaring theory development to be the primary goal of the profession.[3] Nursing scholars responded and the earliest nursing theories went to press in the late 1960s and through the 1970s. These highly abstract grand theories and conceptual models defined the boundaries of the discipline and established the theoretical foundations for nursing curricula.[1,3,4] While many practicing nurses saw them as having little direct relevance to their work, their articulation was a necessary precondition for subsequent phases in nursing knowledge development.[4] In their seminal article, Dickoff et al[5] reiterated the theory-practice gap and sketched out a course for the development of research-based knowledge to guide nursing practice. At the same time, the sociologist Merton[6] introduced the notion of middle-range

From G. C. Lasiuk & L. M. Ferguson, From practice to midrange theory and back again: Beck's theory of postpartum depression. Advances in Nursing Science, 2005, 28(2), 127–136. Copyright © 2005. *Reproduced with permission of Lippincott Williams & Wilkins.*

ABOUT THE AUTHORS

GERRI LASIUK was born and grew up in Saskatchewan, Canada, where the subtle beauty of the flat prairie landscape is juxtaposed against the glorious drama of wide-open skies. She is an Assistant Professor in Nursing Faculty at the University of Alberta. Her interest in women's health and health research stems from her clinical nursing practice with individuals across the life span and from a range of geographic, social, economic, and cultural backgrounds. Through first-hand experience, she came to appreciate the profound and far-reaching impact that women's health has on families and on society as a whole. In particular, she is interested in the health effects of interpersonal violence and other severe stressors. Her doctoral research focused on the experience of pregnancy and birthing of women with histories of childhood sexual abuse. Other scholarly contributions include participation in a multidisciplinary, multisite study on the sensitive healthcare of individuals with histories of childhood sexual abuse; a three-part examination of the sufficiency of the posttraumatic stress disorder construct to capture the range of human responses to trauma; and contributions to the first Canadian psychiatric nursing textbook.

LINDA FERGUSON was raised in Saskatchewan, Canada, and has worked as a Nurse Educator for most of her career. She teaches obstetrical nursing in a baccalaureate nursing program at a major medical-doctoral university and has always been affected by those young women for whom birth and the care of a young family have been difficult. The emotional responses to the demands of childbirth and parenting are significant and need to be addressed within the biosocial events of birthing. Beck's work as a midrange theory is fundamental to how healthcare providers interact with these women. She also has a focus on nursing education research and is committed to the development of the science of nursing education. To this end, she is a Professor and the Director of the Center for the Advancement of the Study of Nursing Education and Interprofessional Education (CASNIE) at the University of Saskatchewan. Her funded research focuses on preceptorship and mentorship in nursing, and the epistemology of nursing as it relates to the development of practice knowledge and clinical judgment by new nurses entering practice.

theory as a means to guide empirical inquiry and to test that discipline's organizing theories. Jacox[7] would later endorse middle-range theory development as an important vehicle for the development of practice knowledge needed in nursing.

By the late 1980s, nursing was primed to respond to Meleis[8(p123)] impassioned plea for a "reVisioning" of the goals of nursing scholarship. For the discipline to go forward, she said, it must refocus its efforts on developing substantive nursing knowledge built on concepts grounded in practice. This marked the entry of nursing into the current era, one in which the main thrust is toward the generation and testing of midrange and situation-specific theory.

This article opens with a brief review of theory as a way to create a context for a more detailed discussion of midrange theory—its origins, the critical role for midrange theory in the development of nursing practice knowledge, and criteria for evaluating midrange theory. We then chronicle Cheryl Tatano Beck's program of research on postpartum depression (PPD) and advance the thesis that her theory of PPD, titled *Teetering on the Edge,* is an exemplar of a substantive

midrange nursing theory. We demonstrate Beck's progression from identification of a clinical problem, to exploratory descriptive research,[9-12] to concept analysis[13] and midrange theory development,[14] and finally to the application and testing of her theory in the clinical setting.[15-18] Through ongoing refinement and testing of the theory, Beck has increased its utility and applicability across various practice settings and continually identifies new issues for investigation. This research program on PPD exemplifies of using nursing outcomes to develop practice knowledge through midrange theory development.

Theory: A Primer

Chinn and Kramer describe theory as the "creative and rigorous structuring of ideas that projects a tentative, purposeful, and systematic view of phenomena."[1(p91)] More specifically, it consists of concepts and the relationships among those concepts, for the purpose of describing and explaining the phenomenon, predicting outcomes, or prescribing nursing actions.[3,19,20]

Theory serves to organize disciplinary knowledge and to advance the systematic development of that knowledge.[6] It may also identify the parameters of a discipline; provide a means for addressing disciplinary problems; furnish a language with which to frame ideas of interest to a discipline[3]; and provide unifying ideas about phenomena of interest to a discipline.[20]

By its nature, theory is abstract and does not exist in the material world per se; rather, it is a mental conception or an idea that represents things or events in that world. Because it is abstract, theory does not necessarily represent a particular thing or event, but may refer more generally to a class of similar things or events. In contrast, something that is concrete does exist in material form and "is embodied in matter, actual practice, or a particular example."[21] In elucidating the nature of a particular theory, we might construct an imaginary line or continuum (an abstraction in itself!) anchored on one end by things or events that are *concrete* and on the other by things or events that are *abstract*. Theories that are relatively more abstract are broader in scope and can be generalized to a greater number of things or events, whereas those that are more concrete are narrower in scope and applicable to a smaller range of phenomena.

A concept is "a complex mental formulation of experience."[1(p61)] It is the totality of a phenomenon, as it is perceived and—if it is empiric—can be verified by others. Like theories, concepts also exist at varying levels of concreteness and abstractness. A concept such as "biological sex" is more concrete (or empiric) because we can directly observe evidence of it. On the other hand, phenomena that can be measured only indirectly (such as depression) are somewhat more abstract and exist somewhere in the middle of our continuum. At the other end of the scale are highly abstract concepts like "self esteem" or "social support." Measurement of these concepts is also done indirectly, via agreed-upon indicators. The relationships between and among the concepts of a theory are stated as *propositions*.[1] These are "postulates, premises, suppositions, axioms, conclusions, theorems, and hypotheses,"[1(p266)] each of which reflects the proposition's purpose, type of logic used in its construction, and the context in which the propositions occurs.

Types of Theory

Having described key elements of theory, we can begin to label theories on the basis of their nature and purpose. Here we will consider metatheories, grand theories, midrange theories, and situation-specific theories.

Metatheory is global in nature and stipulates, in the broadest terms, the phenomena of interest to a discipline. Because of its high degree of abstraction, metatheory does not lend itself to empirical testing. This level of theory furnishes the concepts and propositions that are epistemological building blocks for disciplinary knowledge development. To a lesser degree than metatheory, *grand theory* is also very abstract. It offers conceptual frameworks, which define and organize disciplinary knowledge into distinct, though still broad, perspectives.[1]

The sociologist Merton[6] introduced the notion of *middle range theory* as a tool for empirical inquiry. He described it a "limited set of assumptions from which specific hypotheses are logically derived and confirmed by empirical investigation."[6(p68)] Midrange theories are less abstract and more limited in scope than grand theories. They involve fewer concepts, have clearly stated propositions, and readily lend themselves to the generation of testable hypotheses.[3]

Situation-specific or microtheories focus on specific phenomena in a particular setting. They are very limited in scope and are not intended to transcend time, place, or social-political structure.[3] Two such nursing theories are Gilliland and Bush's[22] theory of social support for family caregivers and Im and Meleis'[23] theory of Korean immigrant women's menopausal transition.

Midrange Theory

A major limitation of grand-theory is that its concepts are too broad and abstract for empirical testing. In contrast, situation-specific or single-domain theories[3] contribute little to building a cohesive and unified body of disciplinary knowledge because they are very concrete and too narrow in scope. Merton[6] argues that middle range theory circumvents both of these problems. To his way of thinking, efforts to explicate a unifying grand theory in sociology had just the opposite effect. That is, they resulted in the proliferation of a "multiplicity of philosophical systems in sociology and, further, led to the formation of schools, each with its cluster of masters and disciples."[6(p3)] Merton believes that sociology's advance as a discipline rests on the development of middle-range theory whereas continued focus on total sociological systems (ie, grand theories) impede that progress. In nursing, early efforts to define the parameters of nursing's domain and to identify its phenomena of interest led to the development of metatheory and grand-theory. While these did serve to differentiate nursing from other disciplines and explicated the discipline's ontological values, they provided little direction for nursing research to say nothing of the day-to-day practice of nursing.

According to Merton,[6] middle range theory can be developed from grand-theory (deductively) or from empirically grounded concepts (inductively). He emphasized, however, that the strength of middle-range theory is its capacity to describe, explain, and make predictions about concrete phenomena of interest to a discipline. The range of theoretical problems and testable hypotheses generated by middle range theory potentates its utility and productivity. While Merton believes that the larger conceptual schemes of the discipline should evolve from the conceptual consolidation of tested middle-range theories, he does not advocate exclusive focus on them.

Early nursing advocates of midrange theory[24] envisioned that a particular midrange theory might support a single or multiple grand-theories, thus cohering nursing knowledge. As well, Cody[25] suggests that midrange theory testing provides a way to analyze the adaptability of nonnursing theories to nursing practice. On a cautionary note, however, he adds that researchers and clinicians must first determine whether this *borrowed* theory is consistent with the ontological values of nursing. If it is not, he warns, it will not advance nursing science.

Evaluating Midrange Theory

In a 1993 address to the ANA's Council of Nurse Researchers Symposium, Suppe proposed that midrange theory is identifiable by its scope, level of abstraction of the concepts, and testability.[26] The scope or generalizability of a theory refers to the range of phenomena to which the theory applies[1] or to the number of situations addressed by a particular theory.[3] Because midrange theory is more concrete than grand theory—but less so than situation-specific theory—it applies across several client populations and practice settings, but not to all.[1,18,26] The concepts of a midrange must be clearly delineated and sufficiently concrete as to be testable.[19,20,26–28] Testability requires that these concepts can be coded objectively, as operational definitions, empirical measures, or hypothesized relationships, and that researchers can test the relationships between and among these concepts under different conditions.[19,26,27]

In the following section, we examine Cheryl Tatano Beck's theory of PPD. Our method for doing this is adapted from an approach to theory analysis described by Meleis[3] and on the more specific criteria for analysis and evaluation of midrange theory proffered by Whall.[29] Meleis' approach encourages attention to the theorist's background and important life influences; the paradigmatic origins of the theory; as well as analysis of the theory's rationale, scope, goal, and system of relations among other factors. This provides a context for the theory, locates the theorist in the larger scientific community, and fosters an understanding of where their work resides within the disciplinary knowledge structure. On the other hand, Whall's approach to theory evaluation is more directly oriented to an analysis of whether or not a theory bears the characteristics of a midrange theory. The latter considers (1) the assumptions underlying the theory; (2) the relationship of the theory to philosophy of science; (3) any loss of information due to concepts not being interrelated via propositions; (4) presence/absence of internal consistency and congruence among all components of the theory; (5) empirical adequacy of the theory; and (6) evidence as to whether it has been tested in practice and/or through research and has held up to that scrutiny.

Teetering on The Edge: Is It a Midrange Nursing Theory?

Beck's Background and Life Influences

According to her curriculum vitae.[30] Beck received a bachelor's degree in nursing in 1970 from Western Connecticut State University. Two years later, she earned a master's degree in both maternal-newborn nursing and nurse-midwifery from Yale University. She specifically chose the Yale program because of this blend of research training and clinical specialization (written communication, November 25, 2002). A decade later, in 1982, Beck completed a doctorate in nursing science from Boston University. During that time, we see foreshadowing of Beck's later interest in PPD. The first of these is an article[31] examining the contributions of role conflict and learned helplessness to women's depression The second comes during her doctoral research (involving time perception during labor and delivery) when she is intrigued to discover a link between depression and alterations in time sensibility (written communication, November 25, 2002). Ten years later, in an analysis of maternal-newborn nursing literature published between 1977 and 1986.[9] Beck concluded that nurse researchers need to aim for methodological congruence in their choice of research designs; that the reliability and validity of instruments employed in maternal-child research must be evaluated; and that maternal-child nurse researchers need to identify areas of potential research.

Paradigmatic Origins of the Theory

Beck's initial study in the area of PPD explored early discharge programs in the United States through a literature review and critique, in which she identified a significant gap in maternal care. She wrote:

> What has not been given equal priority in post-partum follow-up care, however, is the mother's psychological status, more specifically, the phenomenon of maternity blues. Early discharge mothers are at home when the blues usually occur during the first week after delivery. Specific assessments for maternity blues should routinely be part of the nurse's assessment of these mothers during home visits.[10(p137)]

The next year, she reviewed the existing literature on maternity blues[11] and began clarifying the differences among the concepts of *postpartum psychosis, postpartum depression,* and *maternity blues.* She also identified the need to improve the instruments employed in this area and called for "both qualitative and quantitative research designs ... to completely investigate the phenomenon of the blues."[11(p298)]

Beck[32] takes exception to the notion that qualitative research belongs exclusively to the early stage of a research program. She contends that at the outset of a research program it is impossible to predict its trajectory. Rather, she says, the "path of a nurse scientist's research program is truly determined by the state of knowledge that is known at each juncture when the research questions for the next study are being determined."[32(p266)] In response to Morse's[33] caution against investigators moving back and forth between inductive and deductive research approaches at the expense of methodological rigor, Beck counters that researchers can acquire the knowledge and skills about a variety of research methods through continuing education and/or via collaboration with others who have the methodological expertise needed for a particular study. In her rejection of the incommensurability of different inquiry perspectives, she provides the basis for her program of research: the need to address the question that arises with the most appropriate research method.

Philosophical Foundations

Beck reflects characteristics of a postmodern philosophy of science. Many postmodernists are also constructivists who believe that each of us constructs an understanding of the material world on the basis of our perceptions of it. Because observation and perception are fallible, these understandings are invariably incomplete. Our best hope for approximating a full understanding of phenomena of interest, is through systematic research employing multiple methods. According to Beck, "Each successive research project should be guided by the previous research study. The objective of this systematic, continuous inquiry is the cumulative production of new knowledge in a substantive area of nursing."[32(p265)]

Scope of the Theory

In 1992, Beck[13] published a phenomenological study of the lived experience of PPD. Data for the study were the text of transcribed interviews with women attending a PPD support group, which Beck cofacilitated for a number of years. From those, Beck identified 45 significant statements about the women's experience of PPD and clustered them into the following 11 themes, which explicate the "fundamental structure of postpartum depression"[13(p170)]:

1. Unbearable loneliness
2. Contemplation of death provides a glimmer of hope
3. Obsessive thoughts about being a bad mother
4. Haunting fear that "normalcy" is irretrievable
5. Life is empty of all previous interests and goals
6. Suffocating guilt over thoughts of harming their infants
7. Mental fogginess
8. Envisioning self as a robot, just going through the motions
9. Feeling on the edge of insanity due to uncontrollable anxiety
10. Loss of control of emotions
11. Overwhelming feelings of insecurity and the need to be mothered

The next year Beck[13] extended those findings into a grounded theory of PPD, titled *Teetering on the Edge.* She chose a qualitative approach to the topic because she believed that the Beck Depression Inventory (BDI),[34] a widely used instrument to detect depression, failed to accurately capture the 'horrifying experiences' (written communication, November 25, 2002) of PPD that she saw in her clinical practice. Research evidence corroborated Beck's observations,[35,36] calling into question the content validity of the BDI for PPD and identified a need for further investigation.

Beck's grounded theory inquiry involved a purposive sample of women attending her PPD support group. Data were collected over a period of 18 months and included field notes from the support group meetings and transcriptions of in-depth interviews with 12 of the group's participants. Through constant comparative analysis, Beck identified the core variable or basic psychological problem in PPD as being *loss of control,* which the women experienced as teetering on the edge of insanity. Participants' attempt to cope with PPD through 4 stages— *encountering terror, dying of self, struggling to survive,* and *regaining control* (Fig. 37-1).

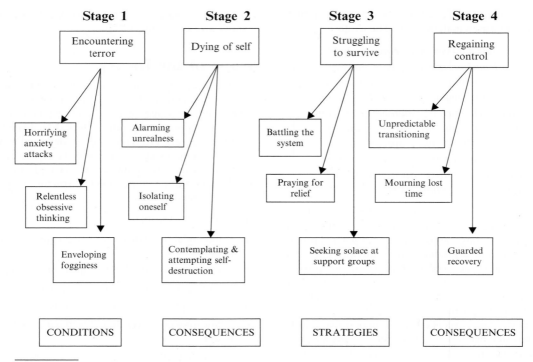

Figure 37-1 *The 4-stage process of Teetering on the Edge.*

In the first stage of PPD, *encountering terror,* the women live with horrifying anxiety, relentless obsessive thinking, and enveloping fogginess. During the stage of *dying of self,* they experienced alarming unrealness, isolation, and thoughts/attempts at self-harm. The third stage of PPD, *struggling to survive,* reflects the women's attempts to survive by praying for relief, battling the system, and seeking solace in support groups. In the final stage, *regaining control,* participants experience unpredictable transitioning, mourning of lost time, and guarded recovery. These 4 stages of PPD subsume the 11 themes generated in Beck's earlier phenomenological study,[13] which, according to Beck,[14] extends and enhances the trustworthiness of her conceptualization of PPD.

Internal Consistency

The major concepts in Beck's theory of PPD (*loss of control, encountering terror, dying of self, struggling to survive,* and *regaining control*) are moderately abstract and relatively narrow in scope. All of the important concepts in Beck's theory are clearly identified, as are the propositions that explicate the relationships among them. The author explains each of the concepts and supports them with direct quotes from participants. With respect to the concept of *dying to self,* Beck

furnishes[14(p44)] a partial audit trail illustrating how she derived the concept from the data. The fact that the 11 themes from her phenomenological study[13] readily subsume into the codes in her grounded theory study[14] indicates a high degree of transferability, dependability, and congruence of results between the studies. Not only is information not lost, but the findings from a prior phenomenological study[13] are integrated into Beck's[14] ground theory research project. This suggests a high degree of internal consistency and congruency among elements of the theory.

An assumption underlying Beck's theory is that PPD is a significant women's health problem that not only affects individual women but also has deleterious effects on their children's health and development.[37-40] Despite the fact that PPD had received considerable research attention by 1993, little of it was qualitative in nature. That being the case, Beck believed that some aspects of the experience of PPD remained underexplored. As well, because previous studies had never demonstrated an unequivocal link between PPD and the physiological changes associated with pregnancy and childbirth, there were undoubtedly other factors at play (eg, psychosocial, environmental, etc).

Other assumptions supporting Beck's theory of PPD are those embedded in the qualitative inquiry paradigm, which is consistent with nursing's values. Participants in qualitative research are viewed as competent *knowers* of their own experience and, as such, are collaborators in the inquiry process. In this tradition, there is emphasis on understanding phenomena by attending closely to participants' lived experience. Furthermore, because qualitative research is discursive in nature and emergent in design, the researcher examines data for patterns of meaning with the aim of objectifying those patterns for scientific inquiry, while at the same time endeavoring to remain true to the participants' construction of their experience. Qualitative research arises from traditions of human science inquiry in which the intent is to construct a holistic and ecological understanding of the phenomenon in question.

Empirical Adequacy and Testing

The empirical adequacy of Beck's theory of PPD becomes apparent in her subsequent work. She went on to develop the Postpartum Depression Predictors Inventory[16] (PDPI), a tool to identify women at risk for developing PPD. The PDPI is a checklist of 8 risk factors, determined through 2 meta-analyses[39,41] to relate to PPD. These factors include prenatal depression, prenatal anxiety, history of previous depression, social support, marital satisfaction, life stress, childcare stress, and maternity blues. The PDPI is used in clinical settings across North America and in Iceland.[42] In 2002, Beck published a revised version of the PDPI—the PDPI-R, which incorporates the results of another, more recent meta-analysis.[16]

Beck has also collaborated with Gable[15,17,18] to develop the Postpartum Screening Scale (PDSS) for detection of PPD. The PDSS is a 35-item, Likert-type, self-report instrument whose psychometric properties are supported in the literature and by content experts.[15] Confirmatory factor analysis of the scale supports the existence of its 7 hypothesized dimensions. Analyses of the 5-point response categories supported meaningful score interpretations and the internal reliability ranged from 0.83 to 0.94. Recently Beck[43] published a Spanish version of the PDSS.

Beck's research program clearly adopts a holistic approach to understanding the experience of PPD, consistent with the perspective and values of nursing. She explores views about women as whole beings operating in the context of a person-health-environment-nursing complex. In all of her writing, Beck discusses the implications of the work for nursing care. At the same time, her work resonates with those in other clinicians and researchers who work in the area of PPD. We find evidence of this in the congruence between Beck's theory with the work of Sichel and Driscoll (cited in reference 18) "earthquake model" of PPD. The latter explains that a woman's vulnerability to PPD reflects her unique genetic, hormonal, and reproductive makeup in the context of her life stressors. Depression, like an earthquake, can erupt when pressures increase at already highly stressed points of the system.

 ## Conclusion

This article reviewed the basic elements of theory and chronicled the development of *Teetering on the Edge*. Cheryl Tatano Beck's theory of PPD.[14] We argue that Beck's theory is an exemplar of substantive midrange nursing theory. Through ongoing refinement and testing of her theory of PPD, Beck has increased its generalizability across various practice settings and continually identifies new issues for investigation. Beck's program of research on PPD represents a significant contribution to nursing practice knowledge through midrange theory development, which, in turn, advances the discipline of nursing.

Midrange theory has the potential to address the theory-practice gap that continues to plague nursing and to develop the substantive practice knowledge needed to advance nursing as a discipline.

REFERENCES

1. Chinn PL. Kramer MK. *Integrated Knowledge Development in Nursing*. 6th ed. St Louis. Mo Mosby 2004.
2. Gortner SR. Knowledge development in nursing our historical roots and future opportunities *Nurs Outlook*. 2002:48:60–67.
3. Meleis Al *Theoretical Nursing: Development and Progress*. 3rd ed. Philadelphia: Lippincott Williams & Wilkins: 1997.
4. Blegen MA. Tripp-Reimer T. Implications of nursing taxonomies for middle-range theory development. *Adv Nurs Sci*. 1797: 19:37–49.
5. Dickoff J. James P. Wiedenbach E. Theory in a practice discipline. Pt I: practice oriented theory. *Nurs Res*. 1968: 17:415–435.
6. Merton RK. *Social Theory and Social Structure* New York: The Free Press: 1968.
7. Jacox A. Theory construction in nursing an overview *Nurs Res*. 1974:23:4–13.
8. Meleis Al. ReVisions in nursing knowledge development: a passion for substance. In Nicoll LH. ed. *Perspectives on Nursing Theory* 3rd ed. Philadelphia Pa: Lippincott Williams & Wilkins 1997:123–132.
9. Beck CT. Maternal-newborn nursing research published from 1977 to 1986. *West J Nurs Res*. 1989:11:621–626.
10. Beck CT. Early postpartum discharge: literature review and critique. *Women and Health*. 1991:17:125–138.
11. Beck CT. Maternity blues research: a critical review. *Issues Mental Health Nurs*. 1991:12:291–300.
12. Beck CT. Postpartum depression a meta-synthesis. *Qual Health Res*. 2002:12:453–472.
13. Beck CT. The lived experience of postpartum depression: a phenomenological study. *Nurs Res*. 1992:41:166–170.
14. Beck CT. Teetering on the edge: a substantive theory of postpartum depression. *Nurs Res*. 1993:42:42–48.

15. Beck CT, Gable RK. Postpartum Depression Screening Scale: development and psychometric testing. *Nurs Res.* 2000:49:272–282.

16. Beck CT. Predictors of postpartum depression an update. *Nurs Res.* 2001:50:275–285.

17. Beck CT, Gable RK. Further validation of the Postpartum Depression Screening Scale. *Nurs Res.* 2001:50:155–164.

18. Beck CT, Gable RK. Comparative analysis of the performance of the Postpartum Depression Screening Scale with two other depression instruments. *Nurs Res.* 2001:50:242–250.

19. Fawcett J. *Analysis and Evaluation of Contemporary Nursing Knowledge: Nursing Models and Theories.* Philadelphia FA Davis: 2000.

20. Walker LO, Avant KC. *Strategies for Theory Construction in Nursing.* 3rd ed. Norwalk Conn: Appleton & Lange; 1995.

21. Oxford University Press. *Oxford University Dictionary.* Available at http://dictionary. oed.com/. Accessed April 16, 2005.

22. Gilliland MP, Bush HA. Social support for family caregivers: toward a situation-specific theory. *J Theory Constr Testing.* 2001:5:53–62.

23. Im E, Meleis AI. Situation-specific theories: philosophical roots, properties, and approach. *ANS.* 1999:22:11–24.

24. Suppe F, Jacox AK. Philosophy of science and the development of nursing theory. *Ann Rev Nurs Res.* 1985:3:241–267.

25. Cody WK. Middle-range theories: do they foster the development of nursing science? *Nurs Sci Q.* 1999:12:9–14.

26. Higgins PA, Moore SM. Levels of theoretical thinking in nursing. *Nurs Outlook.* 2000:48:179–183.

27. Lenz ER, Suppe F, Gift AG, Pugh LC, Milligan RA. Collaborative development of middle-range nursing theories: toward a theory of unpleasant symptoms. *ANS.* 1995:17:1–13.

28. Lenz ER, Pugh LC, Milligan RA, Gift A, Suppe F. The middle-range theory of unpleasant symptoms: an update. *ANS.* 1997:19: 14–27.

29. Whall AL. The structure of nursing knowledge analysis and evaluation of practice, middle-range, and grand theory. In: Fitzpatrick JJ, Whall AL, eds. *Conceptual Models of Nursing: Analysis and Application.* Stamford, Conn: Appleton & Lange: 1996: 13–25.

30. Cheryl Tatano Beck's Web Page. Available at: http://www. nursing.uconn.edu/FACULTY/CherylT.html. Accessed April 6, 2005.

31. Beck CT. The occurrence of depression in women and the effect of the women's movement. *J Psych Nurs Mental Health Serv.* 1979:17:14–16.

32. Beck CT. Developing a research program using qualitative and quantitative approaches. *Nurs Outlook* 1997:45: 265–269.

33. Morse J. Qualitative nursing research: a free for all? In: Morse J. ed. *Qualitative Nursing Research: A Contemporary Dialogue.* Newbury Park Calif: Sage; 1991:14–22.

34. Beck AT, Ward CH, Mendelson M, Mock J, Erbaugh J. An inventory for measuring depression. *Arch Gen Psychiatry.* 1961:4:561–571.

35. O'Hara MW, Neunaber DJ, Zekoski EM. Prospective study of postpartum depression prevalence course and predictive factors. *J Abnorm Psychol.* 1984:93:158–171.

36. Whiffen VE. Screening for postpartum depression a methodological note *J Clin Psychol.* 1988:44:367–371.

37. Beck CT. The effects of postpartum depression on maternal-infant interaction: a meta-analysis. *Nurs Res.* 1995:44: 298–304.

38. Beck CT. Postpartum depressed mothers experiences interacting with their children. *Nurs Res.* 1996:45:98–104.

39. Beck CT. A meta-analysis of the relationship between postpartum depression and infant temperament. *Nurs Res.* 1996:45:225–230.

40. Beck CT. Maternal depression and child behavior problems: a meta-analysis. *JAN* 1999:29:623–629.

41. Beck CT. A meta-analysis of predictors of postpartum depression. *Nurs Res.* 1996:45:297–303.

42. Stefansdouir H. Eiriksdouir IK. Karlsdouir S. Ingolfsdouir E. *How Do Icelandic Women Express Their Feelings During the Last Trimester of Pregnancy?* [Unpublished BS dissertation]. University of Iceland: 2000.

43. Beck CT. Postpartum Depression Screening Scale (Spanish version). *Nurs Res.* 2003:52:296–306.

THE AUTHORS COMMENT
From Practice to Midrange Theory and Back Again: Beck's Theory of Postpartum Depression

This article evolved from an assignment in a graduate-level nursing theory course that challenged us to examine the scholarship of a nursing theorist and decide whether it meets the criteria for midrange theory. We both chose to explore the work of Cheryl Tatano Beck, and through independent analysis, we concluded that her theory of postpartum depression (*Teetering on the Edge*) exemplifies a substantive midrange nursing theory. Beck's theory reflects a holistic approach to understanding women's experience of postpartum depression that is consistent with the values of nursing and demonstrates nursing praxis in action. Beck's other midrange theories diminish the theory–practice gap and advance nursing into the 21st century through development of empirically grounded practice knowledge.

GERRI C. LASIUK
LINDA M. FERGUSON

Theoretical Substruction Illustrated by the Theory of Learned Resourcefulness

ABIR K. BEKHET, RN, PhD, MSN

JACLENE A. ZAUSZNIEWSKI, RN-BC, PhD, FAAN

This article describes the process of theoretical substruction and uses this process to examine the significance of Rosenbaum's resourcefulness theory for nursing research and practice. The article discusses relocation as a phenomenon of interest to geropsychiatric nurses working with elders who have relocated to retirement communities, illustrated by the theory of learned resourcefulness. The literature was reviewed to assess the congruence between the theoretical and operational systems suggested by Rosenbaum's resourcefulness theory. A model of learned resourcefulness is presented that includes middle-range concepts, relational statements, and propositions derived from the research literature. Theoretical substruction provides a mechanism for testing middle-range theories that may contribute to nursing knowledge development. **Key words:** *theory, substruction, learned resourcefulness, relocation*

Science, as a body of knowledge, refers to "cumulative theory and research findings that are generic, re-researchable, valid, and generalizable" (Hardy & Conway, 1988, p. 3). Nursing theories and conceptual frameworks are thus essential to advance nursing science (Frederickson, 1992; Schoenhofer, 1993; Zauszniewski, 1995a). However, they reflect highly abstract constructs (Hodnicki, Horner, & Simmons, 1993; Zauszniewski, 1995a). Theoretical substruction provides a logical picture that can clarify models, guide research, and allow theory testing (McQuiston & Campbell, 1997); it is a hierarchical model that progresses from the abstract to the concrete, relating key concepts, propositions, and operationalization (McQuiston & Campbell, 1997). In theoretical substruction the researcher identifies the major variables in a study, analyzes the level of abstraction of the variables, and identifies hypothesized relationships among variables, thus connecting the theory to the methodology (Beattie & Algase, 2002; Dulock & Holzemer, 1991; Dunn, 2004). It is a dynamic thinking process (Wolf & Heinzer, 1999) that enhances the researchers' ability to assess the congruence between theoretical and operational systems in a research design (Dulock & Holzemer, 1991).

Substruction is the opposite of construction; therefore it can be used to reevaluate models and make the results of theory testing explicit (McQuiston & Campbell, 1997). It is especially important for graduate students and new researchers because it helps them rely on their knowledge of infrastructure and reconstruct details when needed (Bruner, 1963). When Wolf and Heinzer

(1999) surveyed students about their experiences with a substruction assignment, the students indicated that the assignment was difficult, challenging, confusing, and even frustrating; however, they finally "got it." They called for more friendly literature on the phases and elements of substruction but admitted that although challenging, the substruction process stimulated their critical thinking (Wolf & Heinzer, 1999).

Doctoral students have shared the same experience in terms of the challenges of theoretical substruction. However, they would also agree that theoretical substruction stimulates critical thinking and helps them formulate, clarify, and better understand their research. The process is particularly challenging where research is scarce or completely absent. This article examines the process of theoretical substruction and illustrates use of the process to examine the significance of Rosenbaum's resourcefulness theory for nursing research and practice.

The Research Example

The process of theoretical substruction isolates concepts, relational statements, and propositions from an existing theory and arranges them into a diagram that has vertical and horizontal configurations representing theoretical and operational systems (see Figure 38-1) (Dunn, 2004) to assess the congruence between the theoretical and operational definition in a research design and to identify the theoretical relationships among the variables of interest (Zauszniewski, 1995a).

ABOUT THE AUTHORS

ABIR K. BEKHET was born in Alexandria, Egypt. She received her BSN and MSN from Alexandria University, Egypt, and her PhD in 2007 from Case Western Reserve University, Cleveland, Ohio. She is currently an Assistant Professor at Marquette University, Milwaukee, WI. Dr. Bekhet has been recognized nationally and internationally for her funded research and scholarship on effects of positive cognitions and resourcefulness in overcoming adversity. Her awards include Outstanding Paper by the Western Journal of Nursing Research and an MNRS Mentorship Grant. She is also certified as a Holistic Stress Management Instructor by the National Holistic Nurses' Association. She enjoys diving, fishing, traveling, and music with her husband and her three children.

JACLENE A. ZAUSZNIEWSKI received a BA in Psychology/Interpersonal Communication from Cleveland State University, an MA in Human Services/Counseling from John Carroll University, and an MSN in Psychiatric and Mental Health Nursing and her PhD from Case Western Reserve University, Frances Payne Bolton School of Nursing in Cleveland, Ohio. She is currently the Kate Hanna Harvey Professor in Community Health Nursing, Professor and Associate Dean for Doctoral Education, and Director of the PhD in Nursing Program at the Frances Payne Bolton School of Nursing, Case Western Reserve University. Her areas of scholarship include funded studies and publications in the areas of resourcefulness in chronically ill older adults, informal caregiving, and depression across the life span.

In this article, theoretical substraction is used to examine the significance of Rosenbaum's (1980) theory of learned resourcefulness for nursing theory and practice. The adapted theoretical substraction process outlined by Zauszniewski (1995a) provided the framework for the analysis (Figure 38-1).

Certain variables were derived and operationalized from Rosenbaum's theory of learned resourcefulness. Table 38-1 summarizes the theoretical and operational definitions of the phenomenon of interest to geropsychiatric nurses working with elders who have relocated to retirement communities. The derivation of the study variables from learned resourcefulness theory is discussed below under the definition of the model components. The operational system includes measurement of the study variables.

Definition of the Model Components

The theoretical system comprises the theoretical construct, concepts, and subconcepts identified as the phenomenon of interest (Zauszniewski, 1995a).

Constructs are highly abstract notions that can be partially defined (Dulock & Holzemer, 1991; Gibbs, 1972; Zauszniewski, 1995a). Four constructs comprise the model used here: situational factors, process regulating cognitions (PRC), self-control behaviors, and the target behavior (Figure 38-1). Situational factors are the combination of circumstances that occur at a given moment (*The American Heritage dictionary of the English language*, 2000). According to Rosenbaum (1990), situational variables determine how much pressure will be put on a person at a given time. Process regulating cognitions (PRC) are defined as cognitive processes that provide reference mechanisms for perception, evaluation, and self-control behaviors (Rosenbaum, 1990). Self-control behaviors are internal cognitive and behavioral efforts that enable individuals to cope with adverse life experiences (Rosenbaum, 1990). Target behaviors are the consequences of the self-control process and are referred to as health-related behaviors (Rosenbaum, 1990). The relational statements, or horizontal axis, describe the relationships between the constructs and are called axioms (Dulock & Holzemer, 1991; Dunn, 2004; Zauszniewski, 1995a) (see Figure 38-1).

Concepts are words that express a mental image of the phenomenon of interest (Dulock & Holzemer, 1991; Fawcett & Downs, 1986; Zauszniewski, 1995a). Linkages between concepts and theoretical constructs are described in relational statements called postulates (Dulock & Holzemer, 1991; Zauszniewski, 1995a) (Figure 38-1). Each vertical configuration represents a descending level of abstraction of each concept from the theory (Dunn, 2004). Four concepts were derived from four constructs in the proposed model of Rosenbaum's theory of learned resourcefulness. The construct situational factors include relocation as a concept, which is defined as "a change in environment when one moves from one location to another, experiences a change in life situation, and adjusts to new surroundings; it is a disruptive emotional experience that can cause anxiety, loss, pain, anger, and isolation" (Gaylord & Symons, 1986, p. 32; Remer & Buckwalter, 1990). More recently, Lutgendorf et al.

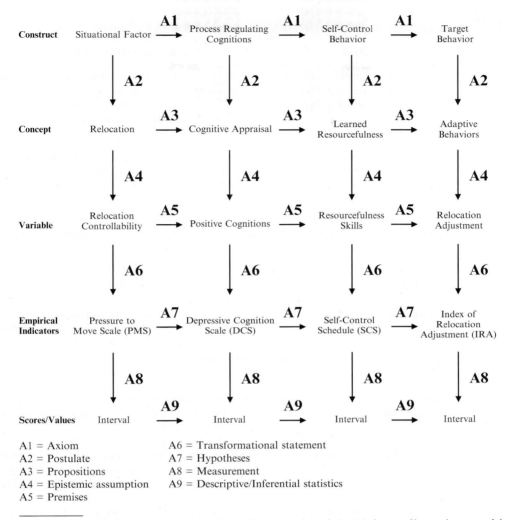

Figure 38-1 *The substruction diagram derived from Rosenbaum's (1990) theory of learned resourcefulness.*

defined relocation as "a stressful life event in the life of older adults because it is frequently accompanied by major losses such as changes in possessions, social support systems, self-perception and mobility" (Lutgendorf et al., 1999, p. 553).

Cognitive appraisal represents an aspect of the larger construct, process-regulating cognition. Cognitive appraisal is defined as the cognitive process by which people evaluate things or events subjectively with regard to their worth or significance (Lazarus & Folkman, 1984).

The construct of self-control behavior includes learned resourcefulness, a concept that represents a dimension of the larger construct. Learned resourcefulness has been defined as an intraindividual coping resource (White, Tata, & Burns, 1996) and as a personal characteristic acquired through interactions with

others and demonstrated in the ability to independently manage daily activities (Zauszniewski, 1995a).

Finally, the concept adaptive behavior is derived from the construct of target behaviors that are health-related; it represents many dimensions of daily living and refers to the ability of the individual to behave in an appropriate manner within the person's social roles and to carry on self-care activities in a psychologically stable manner (Zauszniewski, 1997a, 1997b).

Propositions make up the horizontal axis that represents relational statements between concepts (Figure 38-1) (Dunn, 2004; Zauszniewski, 1995a). The model of Rosenbaum's theory identifies the following propositions: Humans use cognitive appraisal and learned resourcefulness in achieving adaptive behaviors, and the effects of relocation on adaptive behavior can be modified by cognitive appraisal and learned

TABLE 38-1	Conceptual and Operational Definitions of Study Variables	
Variable	**Conceptual Definition**	**Operational Definition**
Relocation controllability	"The extent to which elders decided to move while they were still in control of the move and the extent to which they participated in choosing to move."	Reflect the extent to which the respondent felt that he or she was being pressured by others or by circumstances, as measured by the Pressure to Move Scale (Smider et al., 1996).
Positive cognition	"A collection of specific positive thinking patterns that are thought to enhance one's ability to effectively manage daily activities and promote mental health (Zauszniewski et al., 2002).	Hopefulness, purposefulness, meaningfulness, as measured by the Depressive Cognition Scale (Zauszniewski, 1995a).
Resourcefulness skills	A behavioral repertoire of cognitive skills that minimize the disturbing effects of thoughts and feelings on daily activities and adjustment (Rosenbaum, 1980).	Self-control skills, problem solving, and belief in one's coping effectiveness, as measured by the Self-Control Schedule (Rosenbaum, 1980).
Relocation adjustment	Adaptation to a particular condition, which is in this case the movement from one location to another (Smider et al., 1996).	The physical integration of self, psychosocial, and cultural belonging, independence, and maintenance of a sense of continuity, as measured by the Index of Relocation Adjustment (Prager, 1986.)

resourcefulness. Cognitive appraisal and learned resourcefulness thus affect the attainment of adaptive behaviors.

Variables refer to dimensions of phenomena (Hage, 1972) and are used to order phenomena according to some property (Zauszniewski, 1995a). Variables are, in fact, subconcepts derived from more global concepts (Fawcett & Downs, 1986; Zauszniewski, 1995a). Four variables were derived from Rosenbaum's theory of learned resourcefulness: relocation controllability, positive cognitions, resourcefulness skills, and relocation adjustment (Table 38-1). Bekhet and colleagues have investigated the relationships among these four variables in 104 elders who relocated to retirement communities (Bekhet, Zauszniewski, & Wykle, 2008).

Relocation controllability is the extent to which elders decide to move while they are still in control of the move and the extent to which they participate in choosing to move (Lutgendorf, Vitaliano, Reimer, Harvey, & Lubaroff, 1999).

Positive cognitions are defined as "a collection of specific positive thinking patterns that are thought to enhance one's ability to effectively manage daily activities and promote mental health" (Zauszniewski, McDonald, Krafcik, & Chung, 2002, p. 733).

Resourcefulness skills constitute a behavioral repertoire of cognitive skills that minimize the potentially disturbing effects of thoughts and feelings on daily activities and adjustment. These skills include self-control, problem-solving skills, and a belief in one's ability to cope effectively with adverse situations (Zauszniewski, 1995a).

Relocation adjustment is adaptation to a particular condition that is the movement from one location to another. Relocation adjustment includes two integrally related dimensions of adjustment: congruence and continuity. The congruence of adjustment includes the physical integration of the self, the experience of psychosocial and cultural belonging, and the maintenance and maximization of control and independence in interactions with situational stimuli. Continuity reflects the need of the individual undergoing relocation to maintain a sense of connection with his or her past (Prager, 1986).

As shown in the diagram (horizontal arrows), the relationships among the variables are premises (Figure 38-1) (Jacox, 1974; Zauszniewski, 1995a). However, in the vertical configuration, the relationships between concepts and variables are described as epistemic assumptions (Northrop, 1947; Zauszniewski, 1995a) (Figure 38-1).

Our study in progress, "Milieu change and relocation adjustment in elders" (Bekhet et al., 2008), has several premises that reflect the relationships among study variables. These premises, supported by theoretical writings from nursing and other related disciplines, are discussed below.

The relationship between voluntary/involuntary relocation and adjustment is supported by the premise that those who moved voluntarily had better adjustment than those who moved involuntarily (Schultz & Brenner, 1977). The relationship between resourcefulness skills and positive cognitions is supported by Rosenbaum's (1983) theory of learned resourcefulness, which posits that those with high resourcefulness will not be affected by disturbing thoughts and feelings. Furthermore, highly resourceful individuals will use positive cognitive skills to function independently and continue daily activities with better adjustment.

Lewinsohn and Alexander (1990) found that resourcefulness skills were significantly related to satisfaction with social relationships. More specifically, greater resourcefulness skills were related to greater satisfaction with social relationships, suggesting that resourcefulness skills may also be related to adjustment to new situations involving changes in social relationships, such as relocation to retirement communities.

Operational System

Empirical Indicators

The operational system includes empirical indicators, scores, values, and measures of study variables (Zauszniewski, 1995a). Empirical indicators are actual instruments or experimental conditions (Dulock & Holzemer, 1991; Zauszniewski, 1995a). Scores and values are units of measurements (Dulock & Holzemer, 1991), and *measurements* are the means of assigning units (Dulock & Holzemer, 1991). Transformational statements represent the relationships between variables and empirical indicators, which are logically derived (see Figure 38-1) (Dulock & Holzemer, 1991; Zauszniewski, 1995a). In our study of the adjustment of elders relocating to retirement communities, empirical indicators were identified from reliable and valid measures. The scores derived from these four instruments represent the operationalization of study variables.

The empirical indicator for relocation controllability is the Pressure to Move Scale (PMS) developed by Smider, Essex, and Ryff (1996). This scale consists of nine items that reflect the extent to which the respondent feels that he or she was pressured or pushed to relocate by others or by circumstances. The response options are set up as a 6-point continuum, with anchors of "1" "not at all" and "6" "very much." There are no specific descriptors associated with the numbers 2 to 5. Subjects are asked to select a number that best describes where they put themselves on the continuum.

The empirical indicator for positive cognitions is the Depressive Cognition Scale (DCS), developed by Zauszniewski (1995b). When DCS measures depressive cognitions, scoring is reversed because the items are phrased in a positive direction (Zauszniewski, Chung, Krafcik, & Sousa, 2001). However, in this study,

scores are not reversed and therefore measure positive cognitions. The scale has also been used in this way in previous research (Zauszniewski, McDonald, Krafcik, & Chung, 2002). The 6-point Likert scale ranges from 0 "strongly disagree" to 5 "strongly agree" to indicate the degree to which a particular statement describes the respondent's current thoughts. Strong agreement with a specific item indicates presence of a positive cognition.

The empirical indicator of resourcefulness skills is the Self-Control Schedule (SCS; Rosenbaum, 1980). The SCS is a well-known and accepted self-report measure that assesses individual tendencies to apply resourcefulness skills to solve behavioral problems (Rosenbaum, 1990). The SCS consists of 36 Likert-type items answered using a 6-point scale. Respondents indicate the degree to which each item describes their behavior, ranging from "0" (very characteristic of me) to "5" (very uncharacteristic of me).

The empirical indicator for relocation adjustment is the Index of Relocation Adjustment Scale (IRA; Prager, 1986), a six-item, 4-point Likert-type scale with item responses ranging from completely agree to completely disagree. The six items reflect two related dimensions of adjustment: congruence and continuity. The physical integration of the self, the experience of psychosocial and cultural belonging, and the maintenance and maximization of control and independence in interaction with one's situational stimuli are suggested by the first three items. The last three items reflect the need to relocate individuals to maintain a sense of continuity with their past.

Hypotheses are relational statements between empirical indicators (Dunn, 2004; Zauszniewski, 1995a) (Figure 38-1). In the current study, several research hypotheses were tested. Measures of relocation controllability (PMS), positive cognitions (DCS), and resourcefulness skills (SCS) were expected to positively affect the measure of relocation adjustment (IRA). In addition, the measure of relocation controllability (PMS) was expected to affect the measure of relocation adjustment (IRA) through the measures of positive cognition (DCS) and resourcefulness skills (SCS).

Scores Obtained

To calculate the score for the Pressure to Move Scale, four items are reverse coded. The scores on individual items are then summed. Scores may range from 9 to 54. Higher scores reflect greater pressure to move. On the Depressive Cognition Scale, scores on individual items are summed; the scores may range from 0 to 40, and the higher the score, the greater the number of positive cognitions. On the Self-Control Scale, items are scored from 0 to 5 (Zauszniewski, 1994, 1995a; Zauszniewski & Wykle, 1994) and scores range from 0 to 180, with higher scores (after reverse scoring 11 negatively worded items) indicating greater use of resourceful-ness skills (Rosenbaum, 1990; Zauszniewski, 1997a). Finally, on the Index of Relocation Adjustment Scale, the score for each item ranges from 0 to 3, and scale scores range from 0 to 18, with higher scores (after reverse scoring three items phrased negatively) indi-cating better relocation adjustment.

Descriptive and inferential statistics were used to examine the relationships between the scores on meas-ures of the study variables (see Figure 38-1) (Dulock & Holzemer, 1991; Zauszniewski, 1995a). Analytical strategies included descriptive statistics (i.e., means, standard deviations), correlational analyses, and hier-archical multiple regression.

 ## Conclusion

Theoretical substruction addresses consistency between the theoretical and the operational aspects of a study design (Beattie & Algase, 2002; Dulock & Holzemer, 1991) and facilitates determination of testable research hypotheses that are consistent with the study's theoretical underpinnings (Zauszniewski, 1995a). Substruction, then, can be used to examine theoretical models and plan a study in such a way to ensure that the theoretical and empirical systems are linked (Dulock & Holzemer, 1991). Theoretical sub-struction thus provides an invaluable guide for theory testing research in nursing (McQuiston & Campbell, 1997), which, in turn, contributes to nursing science and knowledge development (Hardy & Conway, 1988). This article has used Rosenbaum's (1980, 1990) theory of learned resourcefulness to illustrate the articulation and consistency between the theoretical and empirical dimensions of research.

In summary, the theoretical substruction includes highly abstract concepts, relational state-ments, and propositions from theory. It also includes new middle-range concepts, relational statements, and propositions derived from the research literature. Then, configurations are completed with the integra-tion of empirical indicators (Dunn, 2004). The testing of hypothesized relationships among measures of the study variables following theoretical substruction pro-vides a mechanism for testing middle-range theories that may contribute to nursing knowledge develop-ment (Zauszniewski, 1995a).

REFERENCES

The American Heritage dictionary of the English language (4th ed.). (2000). Boston: Houghton Mifflin.

Beattie, E. R., & Algase, D. L. (2002). Improving table-sitting behavior of wanderers via theoretic substruction. *Journal of Gerontological Nursing, 28*(10), 6–11.

Bekhet, A., Zauszniewski, J. A., & Wykle, M. (2008).Midwest nursing research society sage best paper award: Milieu change and relocation adjustment in elders. *Western Journal of Nursing Research, 30*(1), 113–129.

Bruner, J. S. (1963). *The process of education.* New York: Vintage.

Dulock, H. L., & Holzemer, W. L. (1991). Substruction: Improv-ing the linkage from theory to method. *Nursing Science Quarterly, 4*(2), 83–87.

Dunn, K. S. (2004). Toward a middle range theory of adaptation to chronic pain. *Nursing Science Quarterly, 17*(1), 78–84.

Fawcett, J., & Downs, F. (1986). Analysis of theory. In J. Fawcett & F. Downs (Eds.), *The relationship of theory and research* (pp. 13–52). Norwalk, CT: Appleton-Century-Crofts.

Frederickson, K. (1992). Research methodology and nursing research. *Nursing Science Quarterly, 5*(4), 150–151.

Gaylord, M., & Symons, E. (1986). Relocation stress: A definition and a need for services. *Employee Assistance Quarterly, 2*(1), 31–36.

Gibbs, J. (1972). *Sociological theory construction.* Hinsdale, IL: Dryden.

Hage, J. (1972). *Techniques and problems of theory construction in sociology.* New York: Wiley.

Hardy, M. E., & Conway, M. E. (1988). *Role theory: Perspectives for health professionals* (4th ed.). California: Appleton & Lange.

Hodnicki, D., Horner, S., & Simmons, S. (1993). The sea of life: A metaphorical vehicle for theory explication. *Nursing Science Quarterly, 6*(1), 25–27.

Jacox, A. K. (1974). Theory construction in nursing: An over-view. *Nursing Research, 23*(1), 4–13.

Lazarus, R. S., & Folkman, S. (1984). *Stress, appraisal, and coping.* New York: Springer Publishing.

Lewinsohn, P. M., & Alexander, C. (1990). Learned resource-fulness and depression. In M. Rosenbaum (Ed.), *Learned resourcefulness: On coping skills, self-control, and adaptive behavior* (pp. 203–217). New York: Springer Publishing.

Lutgendorf, S. K., Vitaliano, P. P., Reimer, T. T., Harvey, J. H., & Lubaroff, D. M. (1999). Sense of coherence moderates the relationship between life stress and natural killer cell activity in healthy older adults. *Psychology and Aging, 14*(4), 552–563.

McQuiston, C. M., & Campbell, J. C. (1997). Theoretical sub-struction: A guide for theory testing research. *Nursing Sci-ence Quarterly, 10*(3), 117–123.

Northrop, F. (1947). *The logic of the sciences and humanities.* New York: Macmillan.

Prager, E. (1986). Components of personal adjustment of long distance elderly movers. *The Gerontologist, 26*(6), 676–680.

Remer, D., & Buckwalter, K. (1990). Decreasing relocation stress. *Continuing Care, 26*, 42–50.

Rosenbaum, M. (1980). A schedule for assessing self-control behav-iors: Preliminary findings. *Behavior Therapy, 11*, 109–121.

Rosenbaum, M. (1983). Learned resourcefulness as a behavior repertoire for the self-regulation of internal events: Issues and speculations. In M. Rosenbaum, C. M. Franks, & Y. Jaffe (Eds.), *Perspectives on behavior therapy in the eighties* (pp. 54–73). New York: Springer Publishing.

Rosenbaum, M. (1990). *Learned resourcefulness on coping skills, self-control, and adaptive behavior.* New York: Springer Publishing.

Schoenhofer, S. O. (1993). What constitutes nursing research? *Nursing Science Quarterly, 6*(2), 59–60.

Schultz, R., & Brenner, G. (1977). Relocation of the aged: A review and theoretical analysis. *Journal of Gerontological Nursing, 32*(3), 323–333.

Smider, N. A., Essex, M. J., & Ryff, C. D. (1996). Adaptation to community relocation: The interactive influence of psychological resources and contextual factors. *Psychology and Aging, 11*(2), 362–372.

White, R., Tata, P., & Burns, T. (1996). Mood, learned resourcefulness, and perceptions of control in type I diabetes mellitus. *Journal of Psychosomatic Research, 40*(2), 205–212.

Wolf, Z. R., & Heinzer, M. M. (1999). Substruction: Illustrating the connections from research question to analysis. *Journal of Professional Nursing, 15*(1), 33–37.

Zauszniewski, J. A. (1994). Health seeking resources and adaptive functioning in depressed and non-depressed adults. *Archives of Psychiatric Nursing, 8*(3), 159–168.

Zauszniewski, J. A. (1995a). Operationalization of a nursing model for psychiatric nursing research. *Western Journal of Nursing Research, 17*(4), 435–447.

Zauszniewski, J. A. (1995b). Development and testing of a measure of depressive cognition in older adults. *Journal of Nursing Measurement, 3*(1), 31–41.

Zauszniewski, J. A. (1997a). Evaluation of measure of learned resourcefulness for elders. *Journal of Nursing Measurement, 5*(1), 71–86.

Zauszniewski, J. A. (1997b). Teaching resourcefulness skills to older adults. *Journal of Gerontological Nursing, 23*(2), 14–20.

Zauszniewski, J. A., Chung, C. W., Krafcik, K., & Sousa, V. D. (2001). Psychometric testing of the Depressive Cognition Scale in women with type 2 diabetes. *Journal of Nursing Measurement, 9*(1), 61–72.

Zauszniewski, J. A., McDonald, P. E., Krafcik, K., & Chung, C. W. (2002). Acceptance, cognitions, and resourcefulness in women with diabetes. *Western Journal of Nursing Research, 24*(7), 728–741.

Zauszniewski, J. A., & Wykle, M. L. (1994). Racial differences in self-assessed health problems, depressive cognitions, and learned resourcefulness. *Journal of National Black Nurses Association, 7*(1), 3–14.

Acknowledgments. The authors wish to acknowledge the editorial assistance of Elizabeth M. Tornquist of the University of North Carolina at Chapel Hill.

THE AUTHORS COMMENT

Theoretical Substruction Illustrated by the Theory of Learned Resourcefulness

I wrote this article as a PhD candidate under the mentorship of Dr. Jaclene Zauszniewski. When I started to write my dissertation and identified my concepts, it was really challenging because few publications on the topic existed and none were recent. It was an attempt from a PhD candidate to PhD students and researchers to update the literature on this area. The theoretical substruction stimulated my critical thinking and helped me formulate, clarify, and better understand relationships among the conceptual variables that were of interest to me; it helped me to be a successful researcher. Now, I have over 20 publications; two of them were recognized as Outstanding Papers by the Western Journal of Nursing Research. Although this article focuses on a theory of resourcefulness, it serves an exemplar to guide future researchers in establishing consistency and congruence between the theoretical and operational components within their study design as well as in developing testable research hypotheses. As researchers and clinicians continue to evaluate the utility and applicability of middle-range theories from within nursing and related disciplines, the process of theoretical substruction provides a means for translating highly abstract theoretical notions into measurable terms that are both meaningful and useful for future research and practice in the 21st century and beyond.

ABIR K. BEKHET
JACLENE A. ZAUSZNIEWSKI

39

A Theory of Theories: A Position Paper

JAMES DICKOFF, PhD
PATRICIA JAMES, PhD

This paper takes a position on two important issues: first, on the issue of what a theory is; then, on the issue of what a nursing theory should be. Even more fundamentally, the position is taken that the difficulty in identifying and developing nursing theory stems in important part, on the one hand, from a conceptual muddle as to what theory is in any of its manifestations and, on the other hand, from the tendency in nursing, or in any discipline or individual, to grasp any structural security—even one that vitiates the basic purpose of individual or discipline—rather than to rest without security or even to brave fumbling toward a more significant security.

The Position in Four Theses

The position taken can be seen in outline through four theses:

1. Theory is a conceptual system or framework invented to some purpose; and as the purpose varies so too must vary the structure and complexity of the system.

2. Professional purpose requires a commitment beyond mere understanding or describing.

3. Significant nursing theory must be theory at the highest level—namely, so-called situation-producing theory.

4. A profession or practice discipline has built-in advantages that facilitate theory development for that discipline.

A major part of this paper was also presented by Doctors Dickoff and James at the Fourth Inter-University Faculty Work Conference of the New England Council on Higher Education for Nursing, held in Chatham, Massachusetts on June 18–23, 1967, and is also published in their report, Physical-Biological Bases for Nursing Care: Implications for Newer Dimensions in Generic Nursing Education, *under the title, "Putting the Biological Sciences in Their Place(s)."*

These four theses will be elaborated and then the third thesis—that significant nursing theory must be theory at the highest level, must be *situation-producing* theory— will be presented as the thesis most central to the position taken.

What Is Theory?

In some nebulous way we all know what theory is. But if we want to deal with theory at close quarters—if we want to develop, criticize, or use theory—then a more explicit awareness or agreement is needed as to what is meant by theory, at least within the context of any given discussion. Our claim is that a real advance in clarity and potential usefulness is made if we view theory in this perspective: A theory is a conceptual system or framework invented to some purpose.

To emphasize theory as a *conceptual* device is to urge careful discrimination of theories and theoretical entities from things or reality, on the one hand, and from the inarticulate and incommunicable mental awareness, on the other hand. Theory is essentially verbalizable and hence communicable; but theory is a structuring proposed as a guide, control, or shaper of reality, and is not itself reality. Things, situations, matters of fact, histories—all these are to be distinguished from conceptual entities that are or go to make up theories. Entities on the conceptual or theoretic level are *concepts, propositions, laws, set of propositions* (and sometimes the linguistic expression of these conceptual entities are considered as theoretic entities). The question of the relation to reality of theoretical entities either in isolation or as systematically interrelated is the question of validation for theories. But, as we will urge later, no such simple-minded notion as isomorphism or mirroring exhausts or even helps much with the question of this relation—particularly in the higher reaches of theory.

Ontologically, then, theory is an entity at the conceptual level. But what is the structure of this "conceptual entity?" Practically speaking, no concept in

From J. Dickoff and P. James, A theory of theories: A position paper. Nursing Research, 1968, 17(3), 197–203.
Copyright © 1968. Reprinted with permission of Lippincott Williams & Wilkins.

ABOUT THE AUTHORS

At the time this article was reprinted in the 3rd edition (1997) of *Perspectives on Nursing Theory*, JAMES DICKOFF and PATRICIA JAMES were Professors of Philosophy at Kent State University in Kent, Ohio.
DR. DICKOFF had been teaching at Kent State since 1970 and was Chair of the Department of Philosophy. He studied philosophy at Washington University, where he received a BA in 1954. He continued his study of philosophy at Yale, where he received an MA in 1958 and a PhD in 1962. He worked with nurses and wrote

about nursing for many years. Dr. Dickoff is deceased as of June 2005. Dr. James, his widow, is retired and living in Ohio.
DR. JAMES graduated from the University of Detroit in Michigan with a BS in mathematics in 1955. She was a Fulbright Scholar in Belgium and then studied at Yale, where she obtained an MA in 1958 and a PhD in 1962. She was a Visiting Professor at the Oregon Health Sciences University School of Nursing. She collaborated with Dr. Dickoff in writing many articles on nursing, education, and healthcare ethics.

isolation and rarely any proposition or law in isolation is deemed a theory, though strictly speaking even such single-element systems might be proposed as theories. Speaking most generally, a theory is a *conceptual system or framework*. That is, a theory is a set of elements in interrelation. All elements of a theory are at the conceptual level, but theories vary according to the number of elements, the characteristic kind and complexity of the elements, and the kind of relation holding between or among the theory's elements or ingredients. The factor (or concept) is the simplest element; a proposition or law is a certain relation among concepts. Theory at one level might be a coordinate set of factors or a coordinate set of propositions. But theory at its highest level has elements that are not merely coordinate, elements that differ from one another in level of complexity and even some elements that contain whole theories as elements.

A theory, then, is a conceptual system—but a conceptual system invented to some purpose. To emphasize that theory is invented rather than found in, or discovered in, or abstracted from, reality calls attention not only to the conceptual status of theory but also to the necessity for imagination and risk-taking in the proposing of a theory. Reality is not prefactored; and even more obviously, no relation among factors comes automatically noted or automatically labeled.

Though theory is no mere picture of reality, neither is theory an invention that is a mere fancy. Rather theory is a conceptual system invented to some purpose. And a good theory—or in perhaps more familiar terms a true or valid theory—is a theory that in fact fulfills the purpose for which the theory was proposed or invented. As the purpose of the theory varies, the structure or level of the theory varies—and so also will vary the mode of validating and even of proposing the theory. Theory whose purpose is prediction is the most familiar kind of theory, and the most developed methodology is that for testing the "goodness" of such a theory (or at least of the component elements of such

a theory). But the position is taken here that important types of theory are presupposed by predictive theory and that moreover a more sophisticated kind of theory exists within which predictive theory functions as an element of an element of the theory. Nursing theory is of this elaborate kind.

What Is a Professional Purpose?

To consider what kind of theory is needed for a professional discipline requires articulating professional purpose. A true professional as opposed to a mere academic is action-oriented rather than being a professional spectator or commentator. But a professional as opposed to a mere technician is a doer who shapes reality rather than merely a doer who merely tends the cogs of reality according to prescribed patterns. A true professional—as opposed to a mere visionary—shapes reality according to an articulate purpose and in the light of means conceptualized in relation not only to purpose but also in relation to existent reality. In short, a professional cannot just watch, cannot just do, and cannot just hope or dream. The position taken here is that a theory for a profession or practice discipline must provide for more than mere understanding or "describing" or even predicting reality and must provide conceptualization specially intended to guide the shaping of reality to that profession's professional purpose.

What Would Constitute a Nursing Theory?

If nursing is a profession, then, the position taken here is that nursing must have an action orientation that aims to shape reality, not hit or miss, but by a conception of ends as well as means. This conception of ends and means is based somehow on conceptual awareness deemed adequate to take into account reality in its structure, course, and potential. A proper nursing theory, then, would be a conceptual system invented to serve the requisite purpose. Given the purpose, quite clearly the conceptual apparatus wanted is necessarily more elaborate than any merely predictive theory. The position taken here is that nursing theory must be theory at the fourth or highest level—namely, situation-producing theory. Situation-producing theory is called fourth-level theory because it presupposes the existence of three prior levels of theory, where predictive theory is a kind of third-level theory.

Situation-producing theory is called highest level theory because each of the other levels of theory exists in part at least to allow or provide basis for the next level of theory. But situation-producing theory is not as such developed for the sake of producing a theory of more elaborate structural level but rather for the production of or shaping of reality according to the situation-producing theory's conception. In plainer terms, situation-producing theory is produced to guide action to the production of reality. The major contention here is that all theory exists finally for the sake of practice (since in a sense every lower level of theory exists for the next higher level and the highest level exists for practice) and that nursing theory must be theory at the highest level since either the nursing aim is practice or else nursing is no longer a profession as distinct from some mere academic discipline.

How Could Nursing as a Profession or Practice Discipline Hope to Produce so Sophisticated a Theory?

On the surface it seems unreasonable to expect that a discipline newly dedicated to producing its own theory should have the capacity to produce a theory whose structural sophistication is necessarily greater than the sophistication of, say, physics, psychology, or biochemistry. But the position taken here is that nursing—like any practice discipline—has certain built-in advantages that could, if properly exploited, facilitate theory development within the discipline. As one level of theory presupposes another, so theorizing itself presupposes prior nontheoretical awareness (and prior activity other than theorizing). The privileged and habitual intercourse with empirical reality carried on in a practice discipline—often within the bounds of rote-like or carefully specified procedures—is a rich source of such preconceptual awareness. In the terms of "the father of empiricism" Francis Bacon, nursing or any profession is richly endowed with so-called "polychrest instances"—i.e., without artifice a "night watch" can be taken on highly complex phenomena and patterns of behavior and other changes.[1]

Not only is there a privileged and nonartificial field of observation at any present instance but also—thanks to the unity and history of the profession—there is a fund of practical wisdom passed on now often by word of mouth or apprenticeship. This wisdom could, if properly viewed, be precipitated and surveyed with keener scrutiny not just as a guide to the immediate practice of the scrutinizing individuals but for the sake of being put into more communicable, more stable, more generalized, and hence more amendable form. Not only is nursing rich in nonthetic awareness since its "professionals" engage habitually in practice and so encounter reality at least nonconceptually; nursing possesses also certain regularized patterns of behavior which are inherited and persistent over time—a built-in body of accepted practice, if not a body of knowledge in some other sense. That is, nursing has at the very least some awareness of the basis from which a constructive criticism should start. Moreover, not all this "basic wisdom" remains at the preconceptual level. Within nursing practice and tradition there is a certain abundance of written sources—among these the lowly or mighty procedure books—which could constitute a veritable gold mine of "incipient theory," recoverable and refinable given appropriate tools, energies, and aims.

In the pursuit of a scientific body of knowledge, nursing or any profession must be on guard against the two-fold temptation: 1) on the one hand, of a too quick contempt for anything already possessed or developed before the newest phase within the profession, or developed without or independently of skills newly acquired and hard won by current leaders in the profession; and 2) on the other hand, the temptation of embracing seemingly safe procedures from any other discipline, without very critical scrutiny of what those procedures have done for that discipline, let alone what they might do for nursing.

What must be admitted is the complexity and difficulty of producing a nursing theory in accordance with the position taken here. The temptation will be to do something easier, even though perhaps useless to nursing; to do something less novel and more in keeping with rigid stereotypes of researchers and theorists in natural and social sciences; to do what will make an acceptable doctoral thesis, whether or not useful to nursing; to do what is fundable, whether or not useful to nursing. These are temptations to which succumbing is easy, resistance difficult. But recognizing that to succumb is to sell your birthright as a nurse may

---

[1]Bacon, Francis. New Organon Book II, especially Aphorisms 50 and 41.

give the impetus, and energy needed: 1) to entertain the proposed notion of theory with the burden of its detail; 2) to persist in nursing inquiry despite the allurements of smoother sailing and quicker payoff in status and funds to be found in repetition or imitation of inquiry in a more academic discipline; and 3) to exploit the advantages, history, and special peculiarities of nursing toward an appropriate bias within nursing inquiry.

Nursing Theory as Situation-Producing Theory

The four theses explored, let's sketch out what we take to be the levels of theory and some of the distinctive features of theory at each level. We but sketch these levels and features here for two reasons. First of all, too much detail here on these matters moves the focus away from the four-thesis position taken by this paper. The more detailed consideration of these matters is offered in a paper "Theory in a Practice Discipline"—a paper basic in a sense to the present discussion, written by us with Ernestine Wiedenbach, and to be published in a forthcoming issue of *Nursing Research*.[2] Secondly, the task of the present paper is in part to create the need for that more detailed consideration. Unless there is some awareness of the practical import of seeing the relation of professional purpose to the mode of theorizing, exploring in depth levels and structure of theory could constitute just one more academic distraction for nursing. The point here is to emphasize the structure of fourth-level or situation-producing theory, so as to render somewhat more concrete the kind of structure we deem any viable nursing theory should have. Without initial awareness, awareness of the needed structure of theory, it is hard to see how any progress can be made in assessing any purported theory as to its adequacy or in deciding: 1) where work is already done; 2) where work must be done; and 3) how to guide in economical and feasible ways the time, energies, and talents at nursing's disposal so that the inquiry made will neither founder in despair nor constitute a mere status search or distraction.

The Kinds or Levels of Theory

A severe limitation in many current notions of theory stems from the oversimple view that takes as theory only sets of causal laws, so that the only conceptual systems regarded as theories are those that allow

prediction on their bases. We have suggested that we can profitably see as theory conceptual frameworks which allow something less than prediction (for example, theories of classification or more simply systems or even conventions for naming or marking off significant elements) as well as conceptual frameworks that go beyond mere prediction.

It seems to us that careful attention to the structure of predictive theory suggests three things: 1) predictive theory presupposes the prior existence of more elementary types of theory; 2) predictive theory is not the only kind of theory dealing essentially with relations conceived as between states of affairs; and 3) there is a type of theory which presupposes and builds on theories at the level of relations between states of affairs.

The point of emphasis here is that in addition to factor-isolating and depicting theories (presupposed by predictive theories) and to predictive or causal theories (including what we elsewhere call promoting or inhibiting theories), there does or could exist another kind of theory which presupposes and builds on these other levels of theory. This fourth-level of theory can be called prescriptive theory, goal-incorporating theory, or perhaps most graphically, situation-producing theory. Situation-producing theories are not satisfied to conceptualize factors, factor-relations, or situation relations, but go on to attempt conceptualization of desired situations as well as conceptualizing the prescription under which an agent or practitioner must act in order to bring about situations of the kind conceived as desirable in the conception of the goal.

In "Theory in a Practice Discipline," (section on "The Four Levels of Theory"), the lands of theories are charted thus:

I. Factor-isolating theories

II. Factor-relating theories (situation depicting theories)

III. Situation-relating theories

   A. Predictive theories

   B. Promoting or inhibiting theories

IV. Situation-producing theories (prescriptive theories)

Situation-Producing Theory

A theory is here viewed as a conceptual framework invented to some purpose, and since the purpose of a situation-producing theory is to allow for the production of situations of a desired kind, the three essential ingredients of a situation-producing theory are: 1) goal-content specified as aim for activity; 2) prescriptions for activity to realize the goal-content;

[2]Cp. especially the sections on "What is Theory?" and "What is Nursing Theory?"

and 3) a survey list to serve as a supplement to present prescription and as preparation for future prescription for activity toward the goal-content. The goal-content specifies features of situations to be produced; the prescriptions give directives for activity productive of such situations; the survey list calls attention to those aspects of activity and to those theories at whatever level deemed by the theorist relevant to the production of desired situations but not (or not yet) explicitly or fully incorporated into goal-content or prescriptions.

We suggest that six aspects of activity fruitful to highlight as well as to use to organize a theory's survey list are these:

1. Agency
2. Patiency
3. Framework
4. Terminus
5. Procedure
6. Dynamics

In "Theory in a Practice Discipline" these ingredients and organization of situation-producing theory are charted as follows:

Ingredients of a Situation-Producing Theory

Goal content
Prescriptions
Survey list (organized, e.g., as follows)
1. Agency (explored, e.g., with respect to)
    a. Dimensions of the aspect (here agency) deemed especially relevant
        (1) External resources of agents
        (2) Internal resources of agents
        (3) Factors of agency proposed as significant in the statement of the theory or for acting under the theory
    b. Theories from other disciplines (at whatever level) deemed relevant
2. Patiency
    a. Relevant dimensions or realities
    b. Relevant theories
3. Framework
    a. Relevant dimensions or realities
    b. Relevant theories
4. Terminus
    a. Relevant dimensions or realities
    b. Relevant theories
5. Procedure
    a. Relevant dimensions or realities
    b. Relevant theories
6. Dynamics
    a. Relevant dimensions or realities
    b. Relevant theories

The Structure of Nursing Theory

Our contention is that any practice-minded nursing theory must be a theory at the situation-producing level. Looking at the ingredients typical of a situation-producing theory and at a survey list organized along the suggested dimensions is a first step toward rendering the contention plausible. Once initial plausibility is granted, the further investment of energy in the articulation of such theory becomes less academic and moves us one step closer to seeing whether practice bears out the contention.

What is the point of calling attention to goal, prescription, and survey list as essential ingredients of any nursing theory in a context where we are emphasizing the explicit conceptual nature of theory and the practical orientation of theory for any professional discipline? Emphasizing goal as a theoretical entity has three advantages: we dare or deign to become articulate about the explicit features of what we desire to produce; secondly, we see goals as giving explicit practical direction rather than merely emotional tone; and thirdly, we see the essential and respectable function of professional bias in the formulation of a practice theory. That is, goals become speakable—and hence communicable and alterable, functional, and finally viewable as professional rather than personal prejudices.

Calling attention to prescription as an essential ingredient of nursing theory, first of all, stresses the extra-academic features of a professional and of his situation-producing theory. Demand for prescriptions toward the realization of stated goals furnishes not only a stimulation to practical thought but also an antidote to the "beautiful soul" syndrome of the self-righteous reformer who won't sully ideals in any interplay with demands of practice. More specifically, a call for prescriptions constitutes a demand for bringing into the practical realm—in terms of real personnel and circumstances—the ideally desirable.

Presence of the survey list is a healthy reminder that the basis of professional judgment is incredibly complex and probably at no time fully articulate rather than something mysterious, ineffable, or inborn. The suggested six-fold organization pattern for the survey list gives at least one mode of rendering more manageable the admittedly wide and rich and deep scope of nursing activity. Any suggested patterning would provide an initial basis of exploration or command of this scope. The six-fold analysis suggested—along the dimensions of Agency, Patiency, Framework, Terminus, Procedure, Dynamics—brings the mind to bear on certain features of nursing which though perhaps noted dumbly in practice are often unnoted in theory or actively repressed from theory.

Considering Agency—or the question, Who or what performs the activity?—could be useful in at least bringing up for theoretical consideration the practical value of considering as agents of nursing activity not just registered nurses but also other professionals and nonprofessionals who might be directed or exploited to contribute to realization of nursing goal. Shouldn't a nursing theory take theoretical account of the proper function of at least, say, licensed practical nurses and aides? And is the sick person ever an agent? With similar generality, considering the aspect of Patiency (Who or what is the recipient of the activity?) makes us realize that even if we consider only the registered nurse as agent her activity is received or "suffered" by many others in addition to the sick "patient." And realizing that sometimes inanimate things such as charts or machines "receive" a registered nurse's activity might broaden the conception of both agent and patient not just beyond the registered nurse and the sick but also to include things other than persons. But what's the purpose of so irreverent an extension of agent and patient? Perhaps this: seeing their analogy to inanimate things may increase the theoretical sensitivity to the limits of elasticity and of repertoire and to the need for upkeep and fuel-input not only for immediate service but for any long-range expectation of serviceability.

Attending to Framework makes less plausible the insistence on registered-nurse-sick-patient dyad functioning in isolation as the sole focal point of a viable nursing theory. Part of professional purpose may in fact be to support or maintain not only the "patient" but also the profession and its supporting institutions. Practice would never deny this; why does theory not note it?

Emphasis on the aspect of Terminus (What is the end point of the activity?) calls for not recipes for service but apt characterizations of practical units of work. Conceiving these practical units might stimulate articulation of alternative modes of realization. But perhaps more importantly, considering Terminus calls attention to the function of the mode of conceptualizing activity as a possible contributor to the ease of doing or receiving the activity in question.

Giving explicit status to the Procedure aspect of activity requires attending to the safety, economy, and controlled performance that constitutes some of the virtues of rote, ritual, and policy: and seeing procedures as distinct from terminus demands an attempt at integrating appropriate detail with appropriately sensed direction.

Focusing on Dynamics (What is the energy source for the activity?) brings up for specific consideration, for example, psychological input, and makes discussable in theoretical terms the question of the appropriate place of, say, motivation other than service motivation in the rendering of professional services. Moreover, the very multiplicity of the noted dimensions makes

evident the need to consider in theory as well as in practice the mutual interaction of these dimensions and their relation to prescription and to goal.

Given this general notion of nursing theory as a situation-producing theory with the three characteristic ingredients and with the survey list ingredient organized along the lines of the six distinguished aspects of activity, now it might be proper to ask where particular theories of biology, psychology, and sociology, to name a few, would fit within a nursing theory? Any one of these theories—or some specific part of any one of them—might (considering only structural demands) be a cited theory under any heading of the nursing theory survey list. More generally, a nursing theory is a situation-producing theory which presupposes the existence of many lower level theories. Natural and social science theories are likely to be important contributors for these lower level theories of prediction, correlation, and terminology. But to say that nursing science or theory is merely applied biology, or applied psychology, or applied anything is misleading if it makes us overlook that conceptualization at a very sophisticated level constitutes the integration of the so-called pure sciences into nursing theory. These theories are building blocks, so to speak, in the mansion of nursing theory. This remark is not meant to demean the importance of these supporting theories, but to call attention to the mighty labor needed to exploit these basic sciences intelligently toward the nursing function.

 ## This Theory of Theories—Its Novelty and Its Viability: An Immodest Proposal

Novelty alone is no reason to accept a theory or anything else. To the timid or conservative the tinge of novelty may in fact be reason sufficient to reject any proposal. Nonetheless, for two special reasons we point out what are the novel aspects of the position offered here. First of all, to label as inappropriate—before it appears—a rejection of the position offered on the mere grounds that the position differs from certain currently accepted theories of theory. This reason for rejection, though inappropriate, is the more likely to appear the more recently acquired is the awareness of other theories of theory and the more pain spent in acquiring that awareness. Secondly, to emphasize that no apology is made for the novelty—quite the contrary.

The first point of novelty to be urged is the contention that nursing or any so-called applied theory is more, rather than less, conceptually sophisticated than are so-called "pure" theories. To exclude the possibility of specific conceptual guidance in the attempts to put to use descriptive theories of reality is to confuse the present state of theory production with the theoretic possibilities for theory production. This remark leads to the main point of novelty claimed. We suggest that proposing a theory of theories that sees theory as a conceptual system invented to some purpose—when seen in its full consequences—has revolutionary possibilities. The proposal allows at last for theory to be viewed as a proper tool to man even in his role of providing himself with purpose. But how is the novel related to the old? As Einstein's theory of relativity is to the Newtonian physician, so is our theory of theories to the, shall we say, classical theories of theory. The theories of Hempel, Carnap, Toulmin, Nagel, and so on, are special cases of the broader theory proposed here; these earlier views are not wrong so much as they are overly restrictive, concentrating only on one kind of theory without backing up to inquire as to theoretic activity itself and without seeing that one kind of theory—predictive—in relation to other possible kinds.[3]

The theory of theories offered here may be novel; but is it correct? To answer this question requires answering whether or not the proposed position

constitutes a fruitful view of theory. It is important to realize that—whether the domain be nursing or theory—the theory of that domain must be invented rather than "discovered" from a hidden store of truth or "abstracted" somehow from the real. But consulting empirical reality is an important way of assessing fruitfulness. Reality may be so consulted by carefully controlled experiments with all action on the basis of the questioned theory postponed until research results are in and interpreted. But sometimes action cannot and should not wait on such niceties: the face validity, so to speak, of a theory or hypothesis may be sufficient to lead us to the acceptance of a conceptual framework as a tentative guide to action, with the resolution to note the results of following the guide so as to be prepared for needed amendments or to be sure of knowing how to repeat the happily followed path. For—as will be clear in our remarks on research—sometimes time, money, or energy demands make research narrowly defined too costly a mode of reassurance. And more importantly, there are some things about which we seek reassurance but for which research narrowly conceived can never be justly expected to constitute a reliable guide.

THE AUTHORS COMMENT | A Theory of Theories: A Position Paper

"Our conception of theory for nursing evolved from our interaction with nurses. It was fashioned in response to two things: (1) our philosophically educated awareness and enthusiasm for possibilities of concepts as guides for action and (2) our intensive work with nurses involved in enhancing nursing research, nursing practice, and nursing education by developing the conceptual dimension of nursing" (p. 108). "As philosophers, our interest centered on 'concepts as they mattered for action.' Within philosophy, we had concentrated on normative philosophy, including ethics but especially

logic; even in the more speculative parts of philosophy, we gravitated to problems of action-oriented thought …" (p. 111). "Our conception of theory was a purposive and innovative move—a reconception of theory itself" (p. 109).

JAMES DICKOFF
PATRICIA JAMES

Note: J. Dickoff and P. James, A Theory of Theories: A Position Paper, in L. Nicoll, Ed., (1986). *Perspectives on Nursing Theory (pp. 101–116)*, Boston: Little, Brown, and Co.

[3]For example : HEMPEL, C. G. Fundamentals of concept formation in empirical science. IN *International Encyclopedia of Unified Science*, ed. by Otto Neurath and others. Chicago, Ill., University of Chicago Press, 1952, Vol. 2, No. 7; Hempel, C. G. *Philosophy of Natural Science.* New York, Prentice-Hall, 1966; CARNAP, R. Methodological character of theoretical concepts. IN *Foundations of Science and the Concepts* *of Psychology and Psychoanalysis*, ed. by H. Feigl and M. Scriven. (*Minnesota Studies in Philosophy of Science*, Vol. 1) Minneapolis, University of Minnesota Press, 1956; TOULMIN, S. E. Philosophy of Science. London, Hutchinson & Co., Ltd., 1953; NAGEL, ERNEST. *Structure of Science.* New York, Harcourt, Brace, 1961.

40

Perspectives on Nursing Theory

MARGARET E. HARDY, RN, PhD, FAAN

In recent years, the discipline of nursing has invested considerable time and effort in developing knowledge about theories, models and conceptual frameworks in order to direct nursing practice and establish the boundaries of its knowledge. Nursing conferences, journals and graduate curricula reflect this interest and concern. Nurses are now asking: What is nursing theory? What theory can nurses use? What is a theory as opposed to a conceptual framework? Although some of us may at times be dissatisfied and impatient at the speed with which these questions are being answered, we can perhaps gain a better understanding of theory development by looking at the total process objectively. Furthermore, the evaluation of nursing theory may be more appropriate and useful if the evaluator is aware of the stages of scientific development.

Stages of Scientific Development

Paradigms and Preparadigms

The dissent and confusion about "what is theory" and "what is nursing theory" may be typical of the early stages of scientific development in any discipline. Kuhn (1970), in *The Structure of Scientific Revolutions,* presents a fascinating thesis on the development of scientific knowledge; some of his points may shed considerable light on nursing's present concern with theory. Kuhn points out that the early stage of scientific development, the preparadigm stage, is characterized by divergent schools of thought which, although addressing the same range of phenomena, usually describe and interpret these phenomena in different ways. Nursing appears to be now in this preparadigm stage.

Kuhn challenges the commonly held belief that scientific knowledge advances through slow and steady increments; he proposes that while accumulation of knowledge plays a major role in the advances

of scientific knowledge, progress occurs as a result of scientific revolution. Kuhn's model of the development of scientific knowledge may be represented as given in Figure 40-1. In each revolution, a prevailing paradigm with its associated theories, concepts and research methods is overthrown when anomalies in the accumulating data cannot be accounted for. Then a new paradigm with its own theories, concepts and methods, which more fully accounts for the anomalies, replaces the prevailing paradigm. If a paradigm is to prevail in a discipline, it must attract an enduring group of adherents away from competing scientific orientations, and it must be sufficiently open-ended to leave all sorts of scientific problems to solve (Kuhn, 1970, p. 19).

The paradigm of interest in this article is the *metaparadigm.* This is a gestalt or total world view within a discipline; it provides a map which guides the scientist through the vast, generally incomprehensible world. It gives focus to scientific endeavor which would not be present if scientists were to explore randomly.

The metaparadigm is the broadest consensus within a discipline. It provides the general parameters of the field and gives scientists a broad orientation from which to work. A more restricted type of paradigm is the *exemplar.* This paradigm is more concrete and specific than a metaparadigm (Kuhn, 1970, p. 175). A discipline may have several exemplar paradigms which direct the activities of scientists. For example, in the field of social psychology scientists may group according to their agreement on the model of human nature: noble (Maslow), hedonist (Skinner) and cognator (Mead). This discussion of the metaparadigm and the exemplar paradigm will make the reader aware that the two types of paradigms exist, differentiated primarily on their level of abstraction; a metaparadigm may subsume several exemplar paradigms.

In summary, the metaparadigm or prevailing paradigm in a discipline presents a general orientation or total world view that holds the commitment and consensus of the scientists in a particular discipline. In general the paradigm: (1) is accepted by

From M. E. Hardy, Perspectives on Nursing Theory, Advances in Nursing Science, *1978, 1(1), 37–48.*
Copyright © 1978. Reproduced with permission of Lippincott Williams & Wilkins.

ABOUT THE AUTHOR

MARGARET E. HARDY was born in Edmonton, Alberta, Canada, in 1938. She received her BSN in 1960 from the University of British Columbia in Vancouver, Canada; her MA in 1965 from the University of Washington School of Nursing, with a major in community mental health; and her PhD in sociology in 1971 from the University of Washington. Her employment includes a faculty position at Boston University from 1971 to 1985, where she held a joint appointment in the School of Nursing and the Department of Sociology. From 1985 to her early retirement in 1993, she was a Professor at the University of Rhode Island School of Nursing. Her major contribution to nursing evolved serendipitously as a result of her teaching assignment at Boston University; development of courses for the graduate program led to the publication of her award-winning books *Theoretical Foundations for Nursing* and *Role Theory*, as well as a book *Research Readings*. Through her publications and teaching hundreds of graduate students throughout New England during the 1970s and 1980s, Dr. Hardy provided foundational knowledge on metatheory and inspired many to initiate theory development for nursing. Dr. Hardy enjoys watercolor painting, reading, walking, hiking, traveling, and camping in the mountains with her husband and two dogs.

most members of the discipline, (2) serves as a way of organizing perceptions, (3) defines what entities are of interest, (4) tells the scientists where to find these entities, (5) tells them what to expect and (6) tells how to study them (i.e., the research methods available).

What do paradigms have to do with nursing theory? Kuhn's (1970) discussion of paradigms suggests that the metaparadigm and the exemplar paradigm are endorsed by a discipline and its subgroups because of their scientific-empirical support. The existence of a prevailing paradigm facilitates the normal work of science. Research is purposeful, orderly and raises few unanswerable questions.

When a dominant paradigm does not exist, a discipline may be in a crisis situation characterized by competing paradigms or it may be in a *preparadigm* stage with different, ill-defined perspectives that are heatedly argued and defended. In the preparadigm stage of a discipline, there is little agreement among its scientists as to what entities are of particular concern, where to locate these entities or how to study them. Such is the status of nursing today, with energy going into attempts to justify one of several embryonic paradigms rather than into purposeful, orderly research. Confusion prevails as to what exactly nursing should be studying; the research that is conducted is often poorly focused and unsystematic.

Kuhn's theory of paradigms and scientific revolution suggests that the development and evaluation of knowledge in nursing may proceed at a very slow pace, not because nurse-scientists lack the necessary ability to develop empirically-based scientific knowledge but because so much time is being devoted to justifying the various preparadigms. Until there is a prevailing paradigm and exemplar paradigms to give focus to the thinking and work of nurse-scientists, knowledge in nursing will develop slowly and somewhat haphazardly. This leaves the practicing nurse in a difficult position of deciding what knowledge is usable and how it should be evaluated for use.

Nursing as a Preparadigm Science

If Kuhn's conception of science is correct and if nursing is indeed in the preparadigm stage, then the time spent in defending one of the existing nursing conceptualizations (Riehl & Roy, 1974), the present concern with conceptual frameworks, models, theory construction and research methods are all part of an evolutionary process that other disciplines have either experienced already or have yet to face. Although this period of theory development in a discipline is characterized by ambiguity and uncertainty, nurse-scientists can help build the knowledge base that will help formulate an acceptable paradigm. They can do this by being well informed in a substantive area and participating actively in both theory construction and research. Nursing cannot decree that a specific paradigm will be adopted; the adoption of a paradigm will be based on its scientific credence and its potential for advancing scientific knowledge in nursing.

Paradigm₁ ──→ Normal Science ──→ Anomalies ──→ Crisis ──→ Revolution ──→ Paradigm₂

Figure 40-1 *Process of scientific revolutions.*

The preparadigm stage of science is one of confusion and frustration, with much dispute over theory, research and frequent factional power struggles. Nurse-scientists who realize this may be able to raise themselves above the battleground and focus their efforts and skills on developing sound nursing knowledge. Their work to solve very specific nursing-care problems may contribute significantly to developing exemplar paradigms and a predominant paradigm in nursing. The predominant nursing paradigm, when developed, will make it possible for other nurses to define more clearly their own "turf" or subject matter. While working on knowledge for practice, nurse-scientists must at present tolerate loosely constructed theoretical notions. This preparadigm stage of nursing science is difficult not only for those developing theory and research but also for those attempting to evaluate and use nursing knowledge.

 ## The Development of Theory

The Nature of Theory

Before addressing the question of theory evaluation, the term *theory* must be defined. In common usage, the meaning of theory ranges from a hunch or a speculative explanation to a body of established knowledge. Kaplan (1964), in *The Conduct of Inquiry,* elaborates on the process of theorizing, suggesting that theory formation may well be the most important and distinctive attribute of human being. He does not perceive theorizing as a process removed from experience as opposed to brute fact (Kaplan, 1964, p. 294).

In science, the term *theory* refers to a set of verified, interrelated concepts and statements that are testable. In his discussion of the human ability to develop scientific theory, Kaplan says:

> In the reconstructed logic, … theory will appear as the device for interpreting, criticizing, and unifying established laws, modifying them to fit data unanticipated in their formulation, and guiding the enterprise of discovering new and more powerful generalizations. To engage in theorizing means not just to learn by experience but to take thought about what is there to be learned. (Kaplan, 1964, p. 295)

Nurses will do well to remember the vital part that experience plays in theorizing.

Since a theory is a validated body of knowledge about some aspect of reality, it is appropriate that in developing theory nurses should concern themselves with identifying aspects of reality they wish to focus on, developing relevant theory and evaluating the soundness of the knowledge they develop. The scientist, in developing theory, looks for lawful relationships, patterns or regularities in the empirical world. Such relationships between concepts, sets facts or variables are carefully studied in order to identify conditions that modify or alter the original relationship.

Few "theories" in nursing or related disciplines are sufficiently well developed to permit specification of both lawful relationships and the condition under which these relationships vary. One possibility is behavior modification theory, which expresses a lawful relationship between specified behavior and reinforcement. Furthermore, this relationship may alter according to the type of reinforcement schedule employed.

Relationship Between Theory and Practice

Kaplan stresses the interrelatedness of theory and experience. In nursing, scientists and practicing nurses are frequently out of touch with one another. The nurse-scientist is a thinker unconcerned with the practice setting, while the practitioner is a provider of nursing care and is sometimes referred to as a technician. But it is from the practice setting that the nurse-scientist should derive ideas, and it is for the nurse in the clinical setting that ideas are developed. If the nurse-scientist is to be the major developer of theoretical knowledge, the practitioner must be in a position to provide the nurse-scientists with research-worthy problems and, at the same time, must be able to evaluate the knowledge generated for its soundness and applicability. A similar symbiosis has been highly successful in other fields. For instance, the theoretical physicist develops ideas and the engineer applies those ideas for the practical benefit of human beings.

Nursing has a mandate from society to use its specialized body of knowledge and skills for the betterment of humans. The mandate implies that knowledge and skills must grow in such a way as to keep up with the changing health goals of society. Furthermore, nursing must regulate its own practice, control the qualifications of its practitioners and implement *newly developed knowledge.*

The majority of nurses are clearly "doers" or practitioners. However, the discipline must also include scientists dedicated to generating knowledge. These scientists must be committed to finding things out, to obtaining an understanding and explanation of phenomena in their world and to identifying means for controlling significant phenomena. Nursing practice and nursing science, as pointed out earlier, are not antithetical; each depends on the other. It is important that theory be useful and encompass significant concepts and conditions that can be applied and favorably altered in the clinical setting.

Drawing on Work in Other Disciplines

Nursing draws on theories and knowledge from the disciplines of psychology, sociology and physiology. This is entirely legitimate; there is no reason for nurse-scientists to spend years of hard work duplicating knowledge that already exists but is housed in other disciplines. However, theory from another discipline must first be empirically validated to determine if its generalizations are applicable to nursing and its particular problems and needs. For example, generalizations from cognitive dissonance theory should be assessed to see if they can be used by nurses in practice settings; it is conceivable and, in fact likely, that modifications will first be necessary.

A large number of hours has been expended by social scientists in developing empirically based theoretical frameworks on role and social exchange. If nurses and nurse-scientists wish to employ these two sets of knowledge, they will need to determine how, when and where the concepts and empirical generalizations are applicable. In making this evaluation, they are likely to identify conditions unique to nursing practice which alter the social scientists' generalizations; they may also find they need to expand the original theory.

Types of Theory: Grand Versus Circumscribed

If the discipline of nursing is indeed in the preparadigm stage, consideration must be made for the level of theory development. Given a set of criteria for evaluating theory, the evaluator must make a decision as to what can be considered to be theory. A body of knowledge which is in the preparadigm stage cannot be evaluated as rigorously as a theory, nor can formulations which are "grand theories" or philosophies about nursing. They provide neither solid nor practical foundations for nursing practice; they are difficult to evaluate for their scientific value.

A theory in the early stage of development is characterized by discursive presentation and descriptive accounts of anecdotal reports to illustrate and support its claims. The theoretical terms are usually vague and ill defined, and their meaning may be close to everyday language. A paradigm at this embryonic stage is very readable and provides a perspective rather than a set of interrelated theoretical statements. This type of formulation *lacks empirical support;* the empirical illustrations accompanying it are not tests of the theoretical perspective.

This type of formulation, the "grand theory" or "general orientation," is aimed at explaining the totality of behavior (Merton, 1957). Grand theories tend to use vague terminology, leave the relationships between terms unclear and provide formulations that cannot be tested. Examples of grand theory might be Parsons's theory of Social Systems, Rogers's (1970) formulations of nursing theory, crisis theory, and some of the stress formulations. All present unique ways of looking at reality, but their ill-defined terms and questionable linkages between concepts make them impossible to put into operation and test empirically—and testability of a theory is one of the most important conditions a formulation must meet (Gibbs, 1972).

In addressing the problem of grand theories, Merton (1957) makes a plea for scientists to move into the study of partial theories. Since this plea, social scientists seem to have been successful in developing and testing partial or circumscribed theories. These circumscribed formulations may become exemplar paradigms; the move from grand formulations to circumscribed theory may take a discipline from a preparadigm stage to a paradigm stage with exemplar paradigms.

Circumscribed theories focus on selective aspects of behavior such as communication, social exchange, role behavior and self-consistency. In time, these formulations may lead to explication of theoretical terms and hypotheses which can be tested by carefully designed studies. The cumulative research and resulting theory is sound. Of the paradigms developed, one may eventually predominate, several may combine into a new paradigm which will address a larger part of reality, and several may coexist as exemplar paradigms.

The circumscribed theories on which scientists focus may seem irrelevant and unimportant when compared to the complex day-to-day problems confronted by nurses. Yet nurses must recognize that such complex problems cannot be solved quickly—as is evident in the enormous number of hours this country has spent trying to determine what cancer is and how it develops. Complicated scientific problems usually must be broken down into smaller, more manageable parts and tackled one by one. The scientific process for developing knowledge is slow, but it is the only sure one we have.

The norms that guide scientific activities seem to be universal; they are not specific to a discipline or country (Hardy, 1978). These norms include the need for public discourse on knowledge; the need for establishing the validity of scientific work; the need for critical assessment of both theory and research; and the need for empirical, objective work which can be replicated by others. It is in a milieu influenced by these norms that knowledge is generated and theory is developed; thus the outcome of the scientific process, the scientist's major goal, is achieved. If theory application is to contribute to the advancement of knowledge and to the professional code of ethics, nurse-scientists must adhere to these norms when developing knowledge.

Evaluation of Theory

Scientists have a variety of criteria for assessing knowledge. They examine their theories for explanatory and predictive power, for parsimony, generality, scope and abstractness (Hage, 1972; Hardy, 1978). For nurse-scientists, there is also a subset of criteria relating to the application of a particular theory in clinical practice. The following questions might be asked for such a theory: Is it internally consistent or *logically adequate?* How sound is its *empirical support?* Does the theory present concepts and conditions which the nurse can actually *modify?* Can the theory be used in bringing about *major, favorable changes?*

Logical Adequacy (Diagramming)

Since a theory is a set of interrelated concepts and theoretical statements, its structure can be analyzed for internal consistency or logic (Hardy, 1978; Rudner, 1966). This involves examining the syntax of the theory rather than its content. If the structure is inconsistent or illogical, then empirical testing may not provide a test of the theory itself but only of unrelated or loosely related hypotheses.

One method for examining a theory's internal consistency involves identifying all the major theoretical terms. These may include constructs, concepts, operational definitions or referents. Once identified, each term can be represented by a symbol. Use of symbols serves to decrease the evaluator's bias and thus lessens the likelihood that substantive meaning will be attributed to the theory when it is not present.

The next step is to identify the relationships or linkages between terms. The linkages are usually expressed as follows: direction, type of relationship (positive or negative) and form of relationship (Hage, 1972). Symbols are used to signify the linkages; if the theory does not specify a linkage, this will become obvious as the structure of the theory is diagrammed.

To illustrate this process, consider the statement "high role conflict experienced by a person results in less communication with coworkers" and the statement "frequent communication with coworkers is associated with job satisfaction." The structure of these two statements would then be as shown in Figure 40-2. Diagramming these statements shows clearly that there are no contradictions in the specified linkages, and that there is no link specified between role conflict and satisfaction. This type of diagramming makes it possible to identify gaps, contradictions and overlaps. Linkages between constructs, concepts and operational definitions can also be diagrammed. (See Figure 40-3.) Diagramming a theoretical formulation will clearly show whether the hypothesis to be tested flows logically from the more abstract theoretical statements.

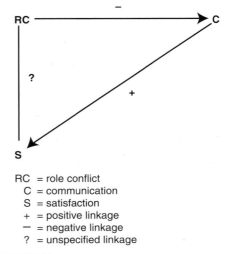

RC = role conflict
C = communication
S = satisfaction
+ = positive linkage
− = negative linkage
? = unspecified linkage

Figure 40-2 *Typical linkage diagram.*

Empirical Adequacy

Empirical validity is perhaps the single most important criterion for evaluating a theory which is to be applied in a practice setting. However, a theory cannot be empirically valid if it is logically inadequate. Many theories are proposed but only a few are testable. Unfortunately, it is all too easy to select a theory which seems plausible or fits our own belief system and then use it in teaching students and working with patients. Among others, popular theories which have such questionable empirical support are psychoanalytic theory, crisis intervention theory and Erikson's theory of developmental crisis.

Assessment of Empirical Support

Assessing the empirical support for a theory is a rigorous but exciting puzzle-solving activity which involves several independent but closely related steps. Suppose an individual is planning to go to a major theoretical work and attempt to identify the key theoretical terms and the linkages between them. This process is identical to the processes used in determining the internal consistency of the theory, and a linkage diagram is used. When the individual has diagrammed the theory and identified predictions and hypotheses, it is necessary to examine the empirical support which actually exists. This requires going to the literature and identifying related studies.

After the pertinent studies have been reviewed, they may be classified according to the strength of their research methodology and the empirical support given to the hypotheses tested. Care must be taken in judging which studies represent valid empirical tests of the theory. Case studies, anecdotal reports

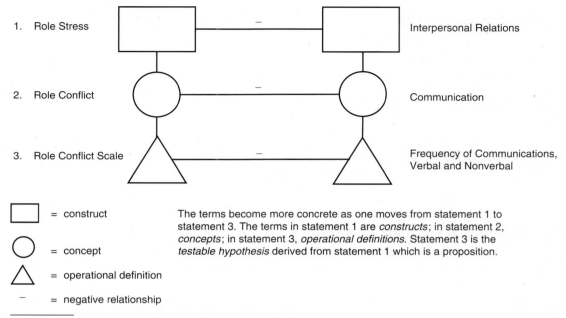

1. Role Stress

Interpersonal Relations

2. Role Conflict

Communication

3. Role Conflict Scale

Frequency of Communications, Verbal and Nonverbal

☐ = construct

○ = concept

△ = operational definition

— = negative relationship

The terms become more concrete as one moves from statement 1 to statement 3. The terms in statement 1 are *constructs*; in statement 2, *concepts*; in statement 3, *operational definitions*. Statement 3 is the *testable hypothesis* derived from statement 1 which is a proposition.

Figure 40-3 *Linkage diagram showing relationships between terms.*

or descriptions of processes presented in discursive accounts of the theory do not constitute empirical tests. Such accounts are generally presented to give the reader the feeling that the theory is plausible and congruent with life events. This type of material may, however, be used to assess the theory's potential scope and generality.

It should not be forgotten that researchers usually have vested interests in their studies and may have introduced biases that alter the interpretation of the findings. During the critical reading, a study's hypotheses and their empirical referents may be diagrammed, as may the empirical relationship found between the concepts. The congruence between theoretical predictions and empirical outcomes can then be readily assessed in a relatively objective manner.

Factors to Consider

In evaluating research, possible changes in meaning of terms and concepts should be kept in mind. For example, in the literature of the 1950s on therapeutic communication theory, the concept of negative feedback may have been defined as derogatory (negative) communication, while in the 1970s, negative feedback has been redefined to mean any communication that alters (increases or decreases) the communication of the other person.

In analyzing a theory and its empirical support, it is necessary to determine that the hypotheses tested are clearly deduced from the theory. If they are not,

the research is not testing that theory. In examining theoretical terms and their corresponding operational definitions, one's immediate concern is with the validity of the operational definitions. A theory may be logically sound—the hypotheses may follow clearly from it and be stated in a form that can be confirmed or rejected—but if the operational definitions do not reflect the meaning of the theoretical concepts, the research is not really addressing the theory and results will have limited or no bearing on it.

To complete the assessment, the entire body of relevant studies must be evaluated in terms of the extent to which it supports the theory, or some part of the theory. This assessment should result in a decision as to whether empirical support is sufficient to warrant the theory's application. The absolute necessity for determining the empirical adequacy of a theory cannot be overemphasized. If nurses are taught "theories" that have little or no empirical support, the nursing care interventions based on such "theories" may have deleterious effects on clients who believe in the nurse's skill, expertise and competence. And indeed there has been a tendency to base nursing actions on tradition, intuition and conceptual frameworks which seem sound but have not been empirically tested. Though they may be creative and may give nurses a sense of security in what they do, these sources of knowledge remain in the realm of myth and nonscientific knowledge.

For example, even if a conceptual framework for crisis intervention makes intuitive sense to a nurse, using it as a basis of action when it does not have sound empirical support is a serious error in judgment and one that has considerable ethical implications. There is a need to develop and use empirically sound scientific knowledge if nursing is to retain its reputation as a profession. And the process of evaluating a theory empirically should be shared with students since they, as practicing nurses, should carry out this same process for the remainder of their nursing careers.

Usefulness and Significance

Since nursing is an applied profession, it follows that relevant theories are those which nurses may use in the clinical setting. After a theory has been identified as having internal consistency and strong empirical support, can it actually be put to use by a nurse? The theory is *useful* to the degree that the practitioner is able to control, alter or manipulate the major variables and conditions specified by the theory to realize some desired outcome. Knowing multiple sclerosis is caused by a virus that lies dormant in a person for 30 years does not provide nurses with a basis for immediate intervention. On the other hand, the awareness of the empirical association between smoking and both lung cancer and heart disease allows the nurse to manipulate variables that can decrease the occurrence and severity of these diseases. Here theoretical knowledge is useful. Inhaling carcinogens from cigarettes is an activity over which the nurse can exert some influence, either through persuading individual patients not to smoke or by assisting in more general public education efforts.

Related to the usefulness of a theory is its *significance*. Given two theories which are internally consistent, have strong empirical support and encompass variables that the nurse is able to modify, what else should influence the choice of which theory to use? Assuming that both are focused on the same nursing problem, presumably the nurse would act on the one which would bring about the *strongest, most favorable outcome*. Take, for example, psychoanalytic

theory and behavioral modification theory, both of which may address the problem of obesity. Although one theory addresses the childhood origins of obesity and the other the environmental factors influencing overeating, both can be used to assist patients to lose weight. However, behavior modification appears to bring about more major and enduring changes in eating habits. In this experiment no comparison is being made of the internal consistency of empirical support of the two theories; the point is to illustrate the efficacy of one theory over another in achieving desired behavioral outcomes.

Nursing as a health profession and as a scientific discipline has come a long way, but it still has much to achieve. As a discipline, it needs to struggle through and beyond the preparadigm stage of scientific development. This will entail challenges and risks, but the process should help create a corps of nurse-scientists able to develop knowledge which reflects sensitivity to problems in clinical practice, and a corps of their clinical counterparts capable of evaluating and using this knowledge.

REFERENCES

Gibbs, J. (1972). *Sociological theory construction*. Hinsdale, IL: Dryden Press.

Hage, J. (1972). *Techniques and problems of theory construction in sociology*. New York: John Wiley & Sons.

Hardy, M. (1978). Perspectives on theory. In M. Hardy & M. Conway (Eds.). *Role theory: Perspectives for health professionals*. New York: Appleton-Century-Crofts.

Kaplan, A. (1964). *The conduct of inquiry*. New York: Chandler Press.

Kuhn, T. (1970). *The structure of scientific revolutions* (2nd ed.). Chicago: University of Chicago Press.

Merton, R. (1957). The bearing of sociological theory on empirical research. In R. Merton (Ed.). *Social theory and social structure*. New York: Free Press.

Riehl, J., & Roy, C. (1974). *Conceptual models for nursing practice*. New York: Appleton-Century-Crofts.

Rogers, M. E. (1970). *An introduction to the theoretical basis of nursing*. Philadelphia: F. A. Davis.

Rudner, R. (1966). *Philosophy of social science*. Englewood Cliffs, NJ: Prentice-Hall.

Note to Readers: From Editors, Reed & Shearer—*This Reactions and Response is printed here to provide historical perspective on Hardy's chapter.*

REACTIONS	Perspectives on Nursing Theory

To the Editor:

… I would like to have Margaret Hardy's explanation, description, or definition of paradigm as a concept before she gives us examples of two classes of paradigms. Incidentally, I found her article most thought provoking and significant…

Betty D. Pearson, RN, PhD
Associate Dean
Graduate Program in Nursing
School of Nursing
The University of Wisconsin
Milwaukee, Wisconsin
1978

Advances in Nursing Science, 1(3), viii-ix.

RESPONSE	Perspectives on Nursing Theory

To the Editor:

This letter is in response to Dr. Betty Pearson's letter … Kuhn's term "paradigm" is central to my article "Perspectives on Nursing Theory" (*Advances in Nursing Science, 1*(1), 37–48). The term paradigm has been used frequently and with a wide variety of meanings by Kuhn (1962, 1970) as he developed his ideas on the growth of scientific knowledge. Although the term paradigm is central to his work, he left it undefined. He does say that the established usage of the term—meaning model or pattern—is not his usage (Kuhn, 1972, p. 23).

Masterman (1970), in an analysis of Kuhn's original work in 1962, identifies paradigm as being used in at least 21 different senses. Masterman clusters these 21 different meanings of paradigm into three groups. One of these, the metaphysical or metaparadigm, is the only type of paradigm that Kuhn's philosophical critics have referred to (Masterman, 1970, p. 65) and it is the type of paradigm central to my ANS 1:1 article. From this article I would like to quote what I consider to be a general definition of a metaphysical or metaparadigm.

The … metaparadigm … is a gestalt or total world view within a discipline; it provides a map which guides the scientist through the vast, generally incomprehensible world. It gives focus to scientific endeavor … The metaparadigm is the broadest consensus within a discipline. It provides the general parameters of the field and gives scientists a broad orientation from which to work. (Hardy, 1978, p. 38).

This definition of paradigm as a gestalt, cognitive orientation or general perspective that has broad consensus within a discipline is based on several descriptive phrases used by Kuhn. Here I will cite phrases referring to the gestalt nature of paradigm. In a recent paper (Hardy, 1979), I focus on the significance of a paradigm having consensus within a discipline. Kuhn (1962), for example, refers to paradigm as a set of beliefs, as a successful metaphysical speculation, as a standard, as a way of seeing, as an organizing principle overriding perception itself, as a map, and as something that determines a large area of reality. Masterman points out that Kuhn's metaparadigm is neither "basic theory" nor a "general metaphysical viewpoint" (Masterman, 1970, p. 61). The metaparadigm is far broader than scientific theory and is prior to it. It is an ideologic, philosophic, and cognitive entity that has gained the consensus of scientists in a discipline.

In response to Dr. Pearson's request, I have gone to considerable length in quoting both Kuhn and Masterman. I have done so because philosophy is not my field of specialization and those with more expertise in this area may make different inferences than I, and secondly, because I think that the meaning of metaparadigm is not easy to grasp, particularly for those of us who are heavily steeped in the tradition of scientific theory, hypothesis testing, and research. Finally, I think it is an important concept for those of us in nursing who are attempting to identify nursing knowledge as opposed to knowledge in the basic and social sciences.

Margaret E. Hardy, PhD
Boston, Massachusetts
1978

Advances in Nursing Science, 2(3), viii-ix.

REFERENCES

Hardy, M. E. (1978). Perspectives in nursing theory. *Advances in Nursing Science, 1,* 37–48.

Hardy, M. E. (1979, April). *Paradigms as tools for structuring the professional science of nursing.* Paper presented at the 1979 Rozella M. Schlotfeldt Lectureship, Case Western Reserve University, Cleveland.

Kuhn, T. (1962). *The structure of scientific revolutions.* Chicago: University of Chicago Press.

Kuhn, T. (1970). *The structure of scientific revolutions* (2nd ed.). Chicago: University of Chicago Press.

Masterman, M. (1970). The nature of paradigm. In I. Lakatos & A. Musgrave (Eds.). *Criticism and the growth of knowledge.* London: Cambridge Press.

THE AUTHOR COMMENTS | Perspectives on Nursing Theory

This article reflects my thinking regarding the knowledge needed by doctoral students to evaluate theories that are germane to nursing. The ideas in this article were first presented at a nursing conference at Case Western Reserve in response to an invitation from Dr. Rosemary Ellis to speak to doctoral students. The notions of metaparadigm and theory development were important metatheoretical ideas for students to understand to effect the status and progress of knowledge in nursing. The ideas in this article, including the often-used diagrammatic model of the structure of a theory, were borrowed from sociology. This diffusion of knowledge from sociology helped launch the explosion of theory development activity that occurred in nursing during the decade this article was written and continues to this day.

MARGARET E. HARDY

Criteria for Evaluation of Theory

JACQUELINE FAWCETT, PhD, FAAN

T his chapter and the next chapter present criteria for evaluation of nursing theories
specified by Jacqueline Fawcett and Rosemarie Rizzo Parse. Fawcett's criteria are
significance, internal consistency, parsimony, testability, empirical adequacy, and
pragmatic adequacy. Some of those criteria are differentiated for grand theories and middle-
range theories but are not differentiated by type of data—qualitative or quantitative—used
to develop the theory. Parse's criteria are structure and process. Structure encompasses
historical evolution, foundational elements, and relational statements. Process encompasses
correspondence, coherence, and pragmatics. Parse's criteria are appropriate for the critical
appraisal of all frameworks and theories, regardless of level of abstraction. Parse also presents a comparison of her own and Fawcett's criteria.

Several different sets of criteria for evaluation of theories have been published (Barnum, 1988; Duffy &
Muhlenkamp, 1974; George, 2002; Marriner-Tomey &
Alligood, 2002; Meleis, 1997; Parse, 1987). Just one set
of criteria, however, differentiates between grand theories and middle-range theories (Fawcett, 2000, 2005).
Although none of the authors of those publications
have indicated that the source of the data for a theory
influences the selection of evaluation criteria, a recent
conversation with a colleague raised the question of
whether theories grounded in qualitative data should
be evaluated using criteria that differ from those used
to evaluate theories grounded in quantitative data.
That conversation resulted in an invitation to Rosemarie Rizzo Parse to engage in a dialogue about what
criteria are appropriate for evaluating grand theories
and middle-range theories and whether those criteria can be applied to theories regardless of the type of
data (qualitative or quantitative) in which a theory is
grounded.

Consensus exists that theories are made up of
ideas called concepts and statements about the concepts, called propositions (King & Fawcett, 1997).
Consensus also exists that components of nursing knowledge, including theories, vary in levels of
abstraction (King & Fawcett). I regard grand theories as more abstract than middle-range theories but
less abstract than conceptual models (Fawcett, 2005).
Accordingly, my framework includes some differences in the evaluative criteria for grand theories and
middle-range theories. I do not, however, differentiate

criteria for evaluation of either grand or middle-range
theories based on the type of data (qualitative or
quantitative) used to develop the theory.

I developed a framework for both the analysis
and evaluation of nursing theories several years ago
and refined the framework twice (Fawcett, 1993, 2000,
2005). Analysis involves objective and nonjudgmental
descriptions of theories, whereas evaluation involves
judgments about the extent to which nursing theories
meet certain criteria. For the purposes of this dialogue, my comments are limited to the criteria for
evaluation of grand theories and middle-range theories. Those criteria are significance, internal consistency, parsimony, testability, empirical adequacy, and
pragmatic adequacy.

The criterion of *significance* focuses on the context of the theory. That criterion requires justification of the importance of the theory to the discipline
of nursing and is met when the metaparadigmatic,
philosophical, and conceptual origins of the theory
are explicit, when antecedent nursing and adjunctive knowledge is cited (Levine, 1988), and when the
special contributions made by the theory are identified. The four questions to be asked when evaluating
the significance of a theory, which are applicable to
both grand and middle-range theories, are listed in
Table 41-1.

The criterion of *internal consistency* focuses
on both the context and the content of the theory.
That criterion requires all elements of the theorist's
work, including the philosophical claims, conceptual

ABOUT THE AUTHOR

JACQUELINE FAWCETT received her Bachelor of Science degree from Boston University in 1964, her master's in Parent–Child Nursing from New York University in 1970, and her PhD in nursing, also from New York University, in 1976. Dr. Fawcett currently is a Professor, College of Nursing and Health Sciences, University of Massachusetts, Boston. She is a Professor Emerita at the University of Pennsylvania. Starting with her dissertation, Dr. Fawcett conducted a program of research dealing with wives' and husbands' pregnancy-related experiences that was derived from Martha Rogers' conceptual system. Subsequently, she undertook a program of research dealing with responses to Cesarean birth derived from the Roy Adaptation Model of Nursing. A third program of research, also derived from the Roy Adaptation Model, focuses on function during normal life transitions and serious illness. Dr. Fawcett is perhaps best known for her metatheoretical work, including many journal articles and several books. Since 1996, Dr. Fawcett has lived in the mid-coast region of Maine with her husband John and a now-tame feral cat, Lydia Dasher. She and her husband own Fawcett's Art, Antiques, and Toy Museum. She swims laps and walks on a treadmill at a fitness center for exercise and relaxation and sails on a windjammer off the Maine coast during the summer.

model, and theory concepts and propositions, to be congruent. The internal consistency criterion also requires the concepts of the theory to reflect semantic clarity and semantic consistency. The semantic clarity requirement is more likely to be met when a theoretical definition is given for each concept than when no explicit definitions are given. The semantic consistency requirement is met when the same term and the same definition are used for each concept in all of the author's discussions about the theory. Semantic inconsistency occurs when different terms are used for a concept or different meanings are attached to the same concept. In addition, the internal consistency criterion requires that propositions reflect structural consistency, which means that the linkages between concepts are specified and that no contradictions in relational propositions are evident. The three questions to be asked when evaluating the internal consistency of a theory, which is applicable to both grand and middle-range theories, are listed in Table 41-1.

The criterion of *parsimony* focuses on the content of the theory. Parsimony requires a theory to be stated in the most economical way possible without oversimplifying the phenomena of interest. This means that the fewer the concepts and propositions needed to fully explicate the phenomena of interest, the better. The parsimony criterion is met when the most parsimonious statements clarify rather than obscure the phenomena of interest. The question to be asked when evaluating the parsimony of a theory, which are applicable to both grand and middle-range theories, is given in Table 41-1.

The criterion of *testability* also focuses on the content of the theory. That criterion frequently is regarded as the major characteristic of a scientifically useful theory. Marx (1976) declared, "If there is no way of testing a theory it is scientifically worthless, no matter how plausible, imaginative, or innovative it may be" (p. 249). Testability typically is regarded as an empirically based criterion. Yet the relatively abstract and general nature of grand theories means that their concepts lack operational definitions stating how the concepts are measured, and their propositions are not amenable to direct empirical testing. Therefore, I identified different criteria for the evaluation of the testability grand theories and middle-range theories.

Description of personal experiences may be used to evaluate the testability of grand theories (Silva & Sorrell, 1992). That approach requires specification of an inductive, qualitative research methodology that is in keeping with the philosophical claims and content of the grand theory and that has the capacity to generate middle-range theories. The product of the descriptions of personal experiences approach is "generalities that constitute the substance of [middle-range] nursing theories" (Silva & Sorrell, 1992, p. 19). In essence, then, evaluation of the testability of a grand theory involves determining the middle-range theory-generating capacity of a grand theory. The criterion of testability is met when the grand theory has led to the generation of one or more middle-range theories. Three questions, which were adapted from requirements proposed by Silva and Sorrell (1992), are asked when evaluating the testability of a grand theory (Table 41-1).

The relatively concrete and specific nature of middle-range theories means that their concepts can have operational definitions and their propositions are amenable to direct empirical testing. Consequently, an approach called traditional empiricism is used to

TABLE 41-1	Fawcett's Criteria for Evaluation of Nursing Theories and Pertinent Questions
Criteria	**Pertinent Questions**
Significance	Are the metaparadigm concepts and propositions addressed by the theory explicit?
	Are the philosophical claims on which the theory is based explicit?
	Is the conceptual model from which the theory was derived explicit?
	Are the authors of antecedent knowledge from nursing and adjunctive disciplines acknowledged and are bibliographical citations given?
Internal Consistency	Are the context (philosophical claims and conceptual model) and the content (concepts and propositions) of the theory congruent?
	Do the concepts reflect semantic clarity and semantic consistency?
	Do the propositions reflect structural consistency?
Parsimony	Is the theory content stated clearly and concisely?
Testability: Grand Theories	Is the research methodology qualitative and inductive?
	Is the research methodology congruent with the philosophical claims and content of the grand theory?
	Will the data obtained from use of the research methodology represent sufficiently in-depth descriptions of one or more personal experience(s) to capture the essence of the grand theory?
Testability: Middle-Range Theories	Does the research methodology reflect the middle-range theory?
	Are the middle-range theory concepts observable through instruments that are appropriate empirical indicators of those concepts?
	Do the data analysis techniques permit measurement of the middle-range theory propositions?
Empirical Adequacy: Grand Theories	Are the findings from studies of descriptions of personal experiences congruent with the concepts and propositions of the grand theory?
Empirical Adequacy: Middle-Range Theories	Are theoretical assertions congruent with empirical evidence?
Pragmatic Adequacy	Are education and special skill training required before application of the theory in nursing practice?
	Has the theory been applied in the real world of nursing practice?
	Is it generally feasible to implement practice derived from the theory?
	Does the practitioner have the legal ability to implement and measure the effectiveness of theory-based nursing actions?
	Are the theory-based nursing actions compatible with expectations for nursing practice?
	Do the theory-based nursing actions lead to favorable outcomes?
	Is the application of theory-based nursing actions designed so that comparisons can be made between outcomes of use of the theory and outcomes in the same situation when the theory was not used?
	Are outcomes measured in terms of the problem-solving effectiveness of the theory?

NOTE: From Fawcett (2005 p. 447–448. Copyright 2005) by F. A. Davis. Adapted with permission.

evaluate the testability of middle-range theories. That approach requires the concepts of a middle-range theory to be observable and the propositions to be measurable. Concepts are empirically observable when operational definitions identify the empirical indicators that are used to measure the concepts. Propositions are measurable when empirical indicators can be substituted for concept names in each proposition

and when statistical procedures can provide evidence regarding the assertions made. The criterion of testability for middle-range theories, then, is met when specific instruments or experimental protocols have been developed to observe the theory concepts and statistical techniques are available to measure the assertions made by the propositions. Three questions, which were adapted from requirements identified by Silva

(1986) and Fawcett (1999), are asked when evaluating the testability of a middle-range theory (Table 41-1).

The criterion of *empirical adequacy* requires the assertions made by the theory to be congruent with empirical evidence. The extent to which a theory meets that criterion is determined by means of a systematic review of the findings of all studies that have been guided by the theory. The logic of scientific inference dictates that if the empirical data conform to the theoretical assertions, it may be appropriate to tentatively accept the assertions as reasonable or adequate. Conversely, if the empirical data do not conform to the assertions, it is appropriate to conclude that the assertions are false. Evaluation of the empirical adequacy of a theory should take into consideration the potential for circular reasoning. More specifically, if data always are interpreted in light of a particular theory, it may be difficult to *see* results that are not in keeping with that theory. Indeed, if researchers constantly uncover, describe, and interpret data through the lens of a particular theory, the outcome may be limited to expansion of that theory and that theory alone (Ray, 1990). Therefore, unless alternative theories are considered when interpreting data or the data are critically examined for both their fit and nonfit with the theory, circular reasoning will occur and the theory will be uncritically perpetuated. Circular reasoning can be avoided if the data are carefully examined to determine the extent of their congruence with the concepts and propositions of the theory, as well as from the perspective of alternative theories (Platt, 1964). In other words, evaluation of a theory always should take alternative theories into account when interpreting data collected within the context of the theory in question.

It is unlikely that any one test of a theory will provide the definitive evidence needed to establish its empirical adequacy. Thus decisions about empirical adequacy should take the findings of all related studies into account. Meta-analysis and other formal procedures can be used to integrate the results of related studies. It is important to point out that a theory should not be regarded as the truth or an ideology that cannot be modified. Indeed, no theory should be considered final or absolute, because it is always possible that subsequent studies will yield different findings or that other theories will provide a better fit with the data. Thus the aim of evaluation of empirical adequacy is to determine the degree of confidence warranted by the best empirical evidence, rather than to determine the absolute truth of the theory. The outcome of evaluation of empirical adequacy is a judgment regarding the need to modify, refine, or discard one or more concepts or propositions of the theory.

The extent to which a grand theory meets the criterion of empirical adequacy is determined by a continuation of the description of personal experiences approach discussed earlier in the section on testability of grand theories. The data used to determine the empirical adequacy of a grand theory may come from multiple personal experiences of an individual or similar personal experiences of several individuals. The extent to which a middle-range theory meets the criterion of empirical adequacy is determined by a continuation of the traditional empirical approach discussed earlier in the section on testability of middle-range theories. The questions to be asked when evaluating the empirical adequacy of grand and middle-range theories are listed in Table 41-1.

The criterion *of pragmatic adequacy* focuses on the utility of the theory for nursing practice. The extent to which a grand theory or a middle-range theory meets this criterion is determined by reviewing all descriptions of the use of the theory in practice. The pragmatic adequacy criterion requires that nurses have a full understanding of the content of the theory, as well as the interpersonal and psychomotor skills necessary to apply it (Magee, 1994). Although that may seem obvious, it is important to acknowledge the need for education and special skill training before theory application.

The pragmatic adequacy criterion also requires that the theory actually is used in the real world of nursing practice (Chinn & Kramer, 1995). In addition, the pragmatic adequacy criterion requires that the application of the theory-based nursing actions is generally feasible (Magee, 1994). Feasibility is determined by an evaluation of the availability of the human and material resources needed to establish the theory-based nursing actions as customary practice, including the time needed to learn and implement the protocols for nursing actions; the number, type, and expertise of personnel required for their implementation; and the cost of in-service education, salaries, equipment, and protocol-testing procedures. Moreover, the willingness of those who control financial resources to pay for the theory-based nursing actions, such as healthcare system administrators and third-party payers, must be determined. In sum, the nurse must be in a setting that is conducive to application of the theory and have the time and training necessary to apply it.

Furthermore, the pragmatic adequacy criterion requires the nurse to have the legal ability to control the application and to measure the effectiveness of the theory-based nursing actions. Such control may be problematic in that nurses are not always able to carry out legally sanctioned responsibilities because of resistance from others. Sources of resistance against implementation of theory-based nursing actions include attempts by physicians and healthcare system administrators to control nursing practice, financial barriers imposed by healthcare institutions and third-party payers, and skepticism by other health professionals about the ability of nurses to carry out the proposed actions (Funk, Tornquist, & Champagne, 1995). The cooperation and collaboration of others may, therefore, have to be secured.

Moreover, the pragmatic adequacy criterion requires that theory-based nursing actions be compatible with expectations for practice (Magee, 1994). Compatibility should be evaluated in relation to expectations held by the public and the healthcare system. If the actions do not meet existing expectations, they should be abandoned or people should be helped to develop new expectations. Johnson (1974) commented, "Current [nursing] practice is not entirely what it might become and [thus people] might come to expect a different form of practice, given the opportunity to experience it" (p. 376).

The pragmatic adequacy criterion also requires the theory-based nursing actions to be socially meaningful by leading to favorable outcomes for those who participate in the actions. Examples of favorable outcomes include a reduction in complications, improvement in health conditions, and increased satisfaction with the theory-based actions on the part of all who participate.

The outcomes of theory-based nursing actions are further judged by use of what Silva and Sorrell (1992) called the problem-solving approach. That approach emphasizes the problem-solving effectiveness of a theory and seeks to determine "whether what is purported or experienced accomplishes its purpose" (Silva & Sorrell, 1992, p. 19). The problem-solving approach is based on the position that theories are developed "to solve human and technical problems and to improve practice" (Kerlinger, 1979, p. 280). It requires deliberative application of a theory. Chinn and Kramer (1995) explained that the application "involves using research methods to demonstrate how a theory affects nursing practice and places the theory within the context of practice to ensure that it serves the goals of the profession … [and] provides evidence of the theory's usefulness in ensuring quality of care" (p. 164). The problem-solving approach can be used with all types of theories but is most effective when applied to middle-range predictive theories. In that case, the application seeks to determine the effects of interventions specified in middle-range predictive theories on the health conditions of the human beings who participate in the interventions (Hegyvary, 1992). The eight questions to be asked when evaluating pragmatic adequacy are given in Table 41-1. Two last two questions, which were adapted from requirements identified by Silva and Sorrell (1992), are asked when evaluating the problem-solving effectiveness of nursing theories.

REFERENCES

Barnum, B.J.S.(1998). *Nursing theory: Analysis, application, evaluation* (5th ed.). Philadelphia: Lippincott.

Chinn, P. L., & Kramer, M. K. (1995). *Theory and nursing. A systematic approach* (4th ed.). St. Louis, MO: Mosby.

Duffy, M., & Muhlenkamp, A. F. (1974). A framework for theory analysis. *Nursing Outlook, 22,* 570–574.

Fawcett, J. (1993). *Analysis and evaluation of nursing theories.* Philadelphia: F. A. Davis.

Fawcett, J. (1999). *The relationship of theory and research* (3rd ed). Philadelphia: F. A. Davis.

Fawcett, J. (2000). *Analysis and evaluation of contemporary nursing knowledge: Nursing models and theories.* Philadelphia: F. A. Davis.

Fawcett, J. (2005). *Contemporary nursing knowledge: Analysis and evaluation of nursing models and theories* (2nd ed.). Philadelphia: F. A. Davis.

Funk, S. G., Tornquist, E. M., & Champagne, M. T. (1995). Barriers and facilitators of research utilization. *Nursing Clinics of North America, 30,* 395–407.

George, J. B. (Ed.). (2002). *Nursing theories: The base for professional nursing practice* (5th ed.). Upper Saddle River, NJ: Prentice Hall.

Hegyvary, S. T. (1992). From truth to relativism: Paradigms for doctoral education. In *Proceedings of the 1992 forum on doctoral education in nursing* (pp. 1–15). Baltimore: University of Maryland School of Nursing.

Johnson, D. E. (1974). Development of theory: A requisite for nursing as a primary health profession. *Nursing Research, 23,* 372–377.

Kerlinger, F. N. (1979). *Behavioral research: A conceptual approach.* New York: Holt, Rinehart, & Winston.

King, I. M., & Fawcett, J. (Eds.). (1997). *The language of nursing theory and metatheory.* Indianapolis, IN: Sigma Theta Tau International Center Nursing Press.

Levine, M. E. (1988). Antecedents from adjunctive disciplines: Creation of nursing theory. *Nursing Science Quarterly, 1,* 16–21.

Magee, M. (1994). Eclecticism in nursing philosophy: Problem or solution? In J. F. Kikuchi & H. Simmons (Eds.), *Developing a philosophy of nursing* (pp. 61–66). Thousand Oaks, CA: Sage.

Marriner-Tomey, A., & Alligood, M. R. (2002). *Nursing theorists and their work* (5th ed.). St. Louis, MO: Mosby.

Marx, M. H. (1976). Formal theory. In M. H. Marx & F. E. Goodson (Eds.), *Theories in contemporary psychology* (2nd ed., pp. 234–260). New York: Macmillan.

Meleis, A. I. (1997). *Theoretical nursing: Development and progress* (3rd ed.). Philadelphia: Lippincott.

Parse, R. R. (1987). *Nursing science: Major paradigms, theories, and critiques.* Philadelphia: Saunders.

Platt, J. R. (1964). Strong inference. *Science, 146,* 347–353.

Ray, M. A. (1990). Critical reflective analysis of Parse's and Newman's research methodologies. *Nursing Science Quarterly, 3,* 44–46.

Silva, M. C. (1986). Research testing nursing theory: State of the art. *Advances in Nursing Science, 9*(1), 1–11.

Silva, M. C., & Sorrell, J. M. (1992). Testing of nursing theory: Critique and philosophical expansion. *Advances in Nursing Science, 14*(4), 12–23.

THE AUTHOR COMMENTS | Criteria for Evaluation of Theory

I developed a framework for analysis evaluation of nursing grand theories and middle-range theories that is a companion to my framework for analysis and evaluation of conceptual models of nursing. Both frameworks are published in my book, *Contemporary Nursing Knowledge: Analysis and Evaluation of Nursing Models and Theories (2nd ed.)*, Philadelphia: F. A. Davis, 2005. I developed the theories framework in an attempt to distinguish theories from the more abstract conceptual models and to convey my belief that grand theories are not the same as conceptual models. The article reprinted here is part of a dialogue with Rosemarie Parse that we undertook in an attempt to clarify whether the same evaluation criteria could be used for theories based on qualitative data and those based on quantitative data. Although the evaluation criteria that I identified were intended for all theories, regardless of the type of data used, the dialogue led me to begin to think about the need for different criteria for theories based on different types of data; I have not yet reached any conclusions.

JACQUELINE FAWCETT

Parse's Criteria for Evaluation of Theory With a Comparison of Fawcett's and Parse's Approaches

ROSEMARIE RIZZO PARSE, PhD, FAAN

I am pleased to share with Dr. Fawcett my criteria for evaluation of theory and a comparison of our work. First, I should clarify my position on middle-range theory, since it is in direct contrast to Dr. Fawcett's. The term middle-range theory is ubiquitous in the nursing literature without any substantive definition. Cody (1999) said that there is "a lack of clarity as to what constitutes middle-range" (p. 10). He raised this question: Are those "working in the middle range on myriad topics … really developing nursing science or merely elaborating the vast patchwork quilt of applied-science nursing" (Cody, 1999, p. 11)? Dr. Fawcett and I generally agree that nursing is a basic science with its own unique body of knowledge and that theory is defined as a set of concepts combined uniquely and written at an abstract level to describe, explain, or predict phenomena (Parse, 1997). My view is that propositional statements written at lower levels of abstraction, often called middle-range theories, are really hypotheses that can be tested only through quantitative research methods using appropriate instrumentation (Parse, 2000). Thus, my comments here do not address middle-range theories and are relevant only to theory as described above.

I set forth criteria for the evaluation of nursing theory in my 1987 book, *Nursing Science: Major Paradigms, Theories, and Critiques*. At that time, I developed a design for critical appraisal appropriate for all frameworks and theories, no matter how they are constructed. I have modified these ideas considerably to be consistent with my current thinking, but I still believe in the basic premise that criteria for evaluation of theory should be broad enough to accommodate all perspectives in the discipline. The two major areas of critical appraisal in my design are structure and process (Parse, 1987). Questions applicable to both areas are listed in Table 42-1.

Structure criteria refer to the physiognomy of the theory, that is, the historical evolution, foundational elements, and relational statements. *Historical evolution* refers to the details of the development of the theory including the philosophical and theoretical antecedents and the changes in the theory over time. *Foundational elements* refer to the philosophical assumptions underpinning the theory and the major concepts of the theory. These are written at an abstract level and are the theorist's beliefs about the phenomenon of concern to the discipline, the human-universe-health process. *Relational statements* refer to the principles that are created from the unique weaving of the concepts into descriptions of the human-universe-health process, and they also are written at an abstract level.

ABOUT THE AUTHOR

ROSEMARIE RIZZO PARSE was born in Pittsburgh, PA. She is a graduate of Duquesne University in Pittsburgh and received her master's and doctorate from the University of Pittsburgh. Dr. Parse is a distinguished professor emeritus, Loyola University Chicago. She is the founder and editor of *Nursing Science Quarterly* and president of Discovery International, which sponsors international nursing theory conferences. Dr. Parse is also the founder of the *Institute of Human Becoming*, where she teaches the ontological, epistemological, and methodo-logical aspects of the human becoming school of thought, including classes on topics such as birthing-dying, suffering, and hope. She has authored many books on her theory and science including *Illuminations: The Human Becoming Theory in Practice and Research; The Human Becoming School of Thought: A Perspective for Nurses and other Health Professionals;* and *Qualitative Inquiry: The Path of Sciencing*. Additional information about Dr. Parse and human becoming can be found at www.discoveryinternationalonline.com.

From R. R. Parse, Parse's criteria for evaluation of theory with a comparison of Fawcett's and Parse's approaches,
Nursing Science Quarterly 2005;18(2):135–137.

TABLE 42-1	Parse's Criteria for Evaluation of Theories and Pertinent Questions
Criteria	**Pertinent Questions**
Structure Criteria	
Historical evolution	How was the theory developed?
	What are the philosophical and theoretical antecedents to the theory?
	What changes have been made since the first publication of the theory?
Foundational elements	Are the philosophical assumptions explicitly stated?
	Are the major concepts explicitly stated?
	Do the philosophical assumptions and major concepts refer to the human-universe-health process?
	How is the human-universe-health process defined?
Relational statements	How are the philosophical assumptions reflected in the principles?
	How do the principles reflect the unique weaving of the basic concepts?
Process Criteria	
Correspondence *Semantic integrity*	Are the meanings of the terms that appear in the assumptions, the concepts, and the principles consistent?
	Does clarity prevail in the descriptions of the assumptions, concepts, and principles?
	Are consistent levels of discourse evident within and among the assumptions, concepts, and principles?
	Are the meanings of words consistent throughout the description of the theory?
	Do the principles interrelate concepts at the same abstract level of discourse to describe, explain, or predict about the human-universe-health process?
	With what paradigmatic perspective does the theory correspond?
Simplicity	Are the descriptions of the assumptions, concepts, and principles clearly written at an abstract level?
	Is the word usage economical?
Coherence *Syntax*	Is there a logical flow from the philosophical assumptions to major concepts to principles?
	Are the foundational elements presented precisely at the same level of discourse?
	Are the relational statements presented precisely at the same level of discourse?
Aesthetics	How is the beauty of the theory expressed?
	Is the theory structured symmetrically?
Pragmatics *Effectiveness*	How is the theory used as a guide for research?
	How is the theory used as a guide for practice?
	What publications and presentations have emanated from the research studies and practice projects?
Heuristic potential	What possibilities for further inquiry arise from the research findings of studies guided by the theory?
	How have the research findings from studies guided by the theory advanced nursing knowledge?
	What new knowledge surfaced from the research studies?
	What possibilities for different practice projects arise from the reports of projects guided by the theory?

The process criteria encompass correspondence, coherence, and pragmatics (Parse, 1987). *Correspondence* refers to semantic integrity and simplicity. *Semantic integrity* is recognized by the consistency of meanings among the terms used to explain the human-universe-health process in the philosophical assumptions and in the definitions of the concepts and principles. Two aspects of semantic integrity are substance and clarity (Parse, 1987). Substance refers to the durability of the meaning assigned to terms, the breadth of the descriptions, and the consistency in levels of discourse within and among the assumptions, concepts, and principles. Clarity refers to the distinctness and mutually exclusive nature of the definitions. *Simplicity* is recognized by the uncluttered abstract descriptions and economy of words used to explain the theory.

Coherence refers to syntax and aesthetics. *Syntax* is recognized by the precision with which ideas are presented, that is, the logical flow in organization and movement of the central ideas from philosophical assumptions to major concepts to principles. *Aesthetics* is recognized in the beauty of the presentation of the theory, that is, the symmetry and harmony present in the descriptions of the major concepts, principles, basic concepts, and the connection of these to the philosophical assumptions.

Pragmatics refers to effectiveness and heuristic potential. *Effectiveness* is recognized by the way the theory is used as a guide to research and practice. This is shown through publications and presentations of research findings and reports of projects related to practice. *Heuristic potential* refers to the possibilities for further inquiry arising from the contributions made through the use of the theory in research and practice. The potential is shown in the ways that the research findings advance knowledge and further develop the theory.

In comparing Fawcett's criteria (Fawcett, 2005) for evaluation of theories with the criteria I set forth,

it is clear that there are similarities and differences. Fawcett's criteria for significance, internal consistency, and parsimony are similar to my criteria for historical evolution, semantic integrity, simplicity, and syntax. The differences arise with Fawcett's criteria for testability, empirical adequacy, and pragmatic adequacy. The language used to describe these criteria is slanted toward validation of theory through quantitative research methods and evidence-based practice. Thus, theories grounded in philosophical assumptions that preclude use of quantitative research methods and predetermined outcomes as evidence for effective practice cannot be fairly evaluated with Fawcett criteria's (see Table 41-1). These would include theories that describe the human-universe-health process as indivisible, unpredictable, and ever changing. Parse's criteria (Table 42-1) are specified to include all perspectives of the human-universe-health process in the discipline of nursing.

I am grateful to have this opportunity to share my views on the evaluation of nursing theory in this column. A diversity of perspectives is essential for the advancement of knowledge of a discipline. This scholarly dialogue sparked by Dr. Fawcett's interest in clarification is one of many dialogues that contribute significantly to the advancement of nursing knowledge.

REFERENCES

Cody, W. K. (1999). Middle-range theories: Do they foster the development of nursing science? *Nursing Science Quarterly, 12,* 9–14.

Fawcett, J. (2005). Criteria for evaluation of theory. *Nursing Science Quarterly, 18,* 131–135.

Parse, R. R. (1987). *Nursing science: Major paradigms, theories, and critiques.* Philadelphia: Saunders.

Parse, R. R. (1997). The language of nursing knowledge: Saying what we mean. In I. M. King & J. Fawcett (Eds.), *The language of nursing theory and metatheory* (pp. 73–77). Indianapolis, IN: Sigma Theta Tau International Center Nursing Press.

Parse, R. R. (2000). Obfuscation: The persistent practice of misnaming. *Nursing Science Quarterly, 13,* 91–92.

THE AUTHOR COMMENTS | **Parse's Criteria for Evaluation of Theory With a Comparison of Fawcett's and Parse's Approaches**

The article was written to offer an alternative to the linear perspective apparent in the language used in the extant published works on the evaluation of nursing theory. The extant works exclude the theories grounded in philosophical perspectives that honor the human–universe process as indivisible, unpredictable, and ever-changing. The criteria set forth in the Parse article allow for the evaluation of theories from all perspectives of the human–universe process in the discipline of nursing.

ROSEMARIE RIZZO PARSE

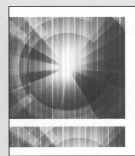

Philosophies of Nursing Practice

This unit focuses on the *ontology* of nursing, that is, the content, focus, or substance of nursing theory and knowledge. This is the flip side of the focus of other Units that address the *epistemology* of nursing, which focuses on the process, methods, and tools of theory and knowledge development. Ontological ideas are found within the concepts, definitions, theoretical statements, and philosophies of a discipline. The chapters in this unit are rich with concepts and statements that define focuses of nursing practice and research. Philosophies and theories also represent a consensus about some of the phenomena of interest within the discipline.

Readers may also excavate the chapters for metaparadigmatic statements about nursing—that is, statements about how nursing is defined and what is its unique disciplinary focus. The chapters also address the meaning of nursing in relation to advanced practice, clients, praxis, art, and science. The section concludes with an overview of paradigms (nursing philosophies) and an approach to making choices across multiple paradigms in nursing.

QUESTIONS FOR DISCUSSION

- In your opinion, what is a key focus of nursing?
- How is this focus distinct from that in other disciplines? How is it similar?
- Can you synthesize some of the concepts presented in this Unit to compose your own metaparadigmatic statement about nursing?
- What philosophic views or paradigms best characterize your beliefs and approaches in nursing research and practice?

The Focus of the Discipline Revisited

MARGARET A. NEWMAN, RN, PhD, FAAN

MARLAINE C. SMITH, RN, PhD, AHN-BC, FAAN

MARGARET DEXHEIMER PHARRIS, RN, PhD, MPH, FAAN

DOROTHY A. JONES, RNC, EdD, FAAN

We have come a long way in explicating the discipline of nursing. We have moved from an implicit acknowledgment of the relationship that constitutes nursing to an explicit designation of the process as *caring in the human health experience*.[1] We recognize that differences in the research ascribed to nursing stem from the philosophical assumptions underlying the methods and practice. When first set forth, the paradigms (labeled particulate-deterministic, interactive-integrative, and unitary-transformative [UT]) were considered separate categories, but as the practice emanating from these points of view was examined more closely, it became apparent that practice is a unified whole that transcends the limitations of each paradigm. The UT paradigm can be looked upon as a meeting place for holistic thinking and problem solving and may include deterministic and integrative thinking. A nurse approaching a patient* from the UT perspective *sees* the whole while attending to the part. As a matter of fact, the nurse enters into the whole through the part. The caring, knowing presence of a nurse taps into what is meaningful for the patient and opens the way for relevant action. This article aims to summarize the progress nursing has made in defining the discipline and to exhort members of our profession to come together in a shared meaning that brings coherence to our practice.

The Process of Knowledge Development

The worldviews that have guided our exploration of knowledge include a traditional scientific approach, a multidimensional evaluation of the interactive milieu, and, more recently, a unitary perspective. The unitary perspective represents a shift from looking at the whole as the sum of the parts to looking at the whole as primary, from seeking to solve a problem to seeking to know the pattern, and from embracing an action-reaction causal approach to realizing the mutuality of the unfolding, rhythmic process through which insight into action arises. Nursing scholars have contributed meaningfully to this knowledge base. The history of nursing epistemology reflects a receptive phase, where nursing knowledge was derived mainly from other disciplines, a self-generative phase, in which knowledge is concentrated on the nursing discipline, and a transformative phase, in which nursing knowledge significantly influences other disciplines as well as nursing practice.[2] Following the prevailing scientific traditions, the early nurse theorists strove to isolate, control, and test relevant variables as a basis for nursing intervention; their work raised questions about interventions of central concern to nursing. Broadening the context, but still emphasizing control and predictability, the next generation of nursing theorists emphasized interactions of multiple factors influencing health; this research inspired nurses to consider the interpersonal approaches that define the nature of the nursing relationship in facilitating health. In 1970, Rogers' revolutionary insight shifted the view to an undivided whole of a mutually unfolding person-environmental field.[3] The theories of *health as expanding consciousness* and *human becoming* emanated from this perspective.[4–8] Theories that originated in the interactive-integrative paradigm on *caring* and *adaptation* have continued to evolve in ways consistent with the UT perspective.[9–17] The collective emphasis of the discipline is on a caring presence that is transforming for both the patient and the nurse in revealing new vision and understanding of the human health experience. Its relevance worldwide directs the profession in meeting global, social, and moral responsibilities.

The shift to a unitary concept of health, in which pathology is relevant but not separate and dominant, along with acknowledgment of patterning as the identifying process of the whole, allowed *relationship* to emerge as the central focus of the discipline. Nursing

---

*The use of the term *patient* is for the sake of simplicity of language and refers to the individual person and a plurality of persons, such as family or community.

ABOUT THE AUTHORS

MARGARET A. NEWMAN received her undergraduate education in nursing from The University of Tennessee Health Science Center, Memphis. Her graduate study included a Master of Science in Nursing from the University of California San Francisco and a PhD from New York University. Her career path included a stint as Director of Nursing for the University of Tennessee Clinical Research Center and graduate teaching appointments at New York University, The Pennsylvania State University, and the University of Minnesota. The major focus of her career has been in the development of nursing theory. In 1978, she first presented her theory of health as expanding consciousness, which was later elaborated in her books, *Theory Development in Nursing* (1978), *Health as Expanding Consciousness* (1986; 1994), *and Transforming Presence: The Difference That Nursing Makes* (2008). She is an avid fan of live theater and orchestral presentations.

MARLAINE C. SMITH is the Helen Karpelenia Persson Eminent Scholar and Dean at the Christine E. Lynn College of Nursing at Florida Atlantic University in Boca Raton, Florida. She was born in Turtle Creek, Pennsylvania, near Pittsburgh, and received her nursing education from Duquesne University, University of Pittsburgh, and New York University. Her contributions to nursing can be clustered in two areas: developing knowledge related to processes and outcomes of healing and analyzing, extending, and applying existing nursing theories. For 20 years, she has been conducting research related to outcomes of touch therapies. She is the co-editor with Marilyn Parker of the 3rd edition of the popular book, *Nursing Theories & Nursing Practice* published in 2010 by FA Davis. Marlaine enjoys reading, yoga, walking on the beach, and cooking Italian food.

MARGARET DEXHEIMER PHARRIS is the Graduate Programs Director in the Department of Nursing at St. Catherine University in St. Paul, Minnesota. She is a co-author (with Carol Pavlish, UCLA) of a Jones and Bartlett 2011 book, *Community-Based Collaborative Action Research: A Nursing Approach*, which situates CBCAR within a unitary participatory paradigm based on Newman's theory of health as expanding consciousness.

DOROTHY A. JONES was born in Brooklyn, New York, and completed her undergraduate work at Brooklyn Hospital and Long Island University. At Indiana University, she was introduced to nursing knowledge and Rogerian Science while achieving her Master's Degree. She received her doctorate at Boston University where she met many nurses educated in Unitary Science at NYU. She continued to participate in the advancement of nursing science, and in particular Margaret Newman's work on Health as Expanding Consciousness, in her teaching, clinical practice, and research. As an example, she co-authored the 2005 book, *Giving Voice to What We Know*, elaborating on applications and significance of Newman's theory. Through writings and presentations, she has had the opportunity to communicate the critical importance of advancing health for all through the integration of nursing science as the essential knowledge of the discipline.

has taken the lead in elaborating relationship-centered care, a concept sought as well by voices outside of nursing. McLeod, citing the work of the Relationship-Centered Care Network, formed by a collaboration of the Fetzer Institute and the Pew Health Professionals Commission, called for a "... culture of caring-of respect for relationship, and optimism for a more balanced and meaningful life" and for "... creating a revolution of the heart by nurturing wholeness-honoring the fundamental role of relationship and connection."[18(pp37–38)]

It is the nature of the nurse-patient relationship that unites the practice of nursing as it occurs in myriad settings throughout the world at every moment of every day. Whether it be a neonatal nurse applying knowledge of highly technical treatments aimed at preserving the life of the baby of the parents before her, a nurse sitting on the cot of a person dying of a chronic illness in a remote village, or a nurse working with community members faced with an epidemic, nursing actions occur within the context of a unified commitment. That commitment is to a caring relationship focused on understanding the meaning of the current situation for the people involved, and appreciating the pattern of evolving forces shaping health, so that appropriate actions can be realized.

The development of nursing knowledge unfolds within a participatory process. Each nurse-patient relationship is unique, formed by the informational patterns of the nurse and the patient. Nurses bring to the situation their personal knowledge and experience as well as the background of liberal and professional education and experience. Patients bring to the situation their personal history and life experience as well as the health concern that of ten is the precipitant for the nurse-patient meeting. The nurse's responsibility is to be fully present, seeking to know what is meaningful to the patient, and allowing the pattern to unfold. The fruitfulness of the encounter is a function of the nurse's commitment to an unconditional caring presence, openness, and perseverance in allowing action possibilities to emerge. The relationship is embedded in a concept of health based on wholeness, evolving pattern, and transformation. Research guided by this perspective has revealed patients' developing understanding and insight regarding their place in the world, a sense that their concerns are being addressed, and enhanced caring relationships.[19,20] Many in the UT paradigm suggest that knowledge develops as nursing praxis, a synthesis of theory, research, and practice. Theory guides and informs the practice experience the research process, and the generation of knowledge. Nursing praxis is not only a pathway to knowledge development, but also the actualization of transformational practice.

The structure of the discipline began by recognizing the similarity of concepts of the various nursing theories.[21,22] These connections fit into a larger pattern of the discipline. Nursing has been through an ambiguous state of multiple, competing, possibly disconnected theories, but now the discipline is at a critical point of an emerging, overarching form that expands beyond the initial links. A consensus statement of philosophic unity was described by a group of international nurse scholars as the basic ontology of the discipline and its relationship to knowledge development and practice.[23] Selected points of convergence reflected by the statement include the following:

- The human being is characterized by wholeness, complexity, and consciousness.

- The essence of nursing involves the nurse's true presence in the process of human-to-human engagement.

- Nursing theory expresses the values and beliefs of the discipline, creating a structure to organize knowledge and illuminate nursing practice.

- The essence of nursing practice is the nurse-patient relationship.

The elaboration that follows builds upon the unifying construct of the nurse-patient relationship and provides a framework for its substantive content. The concepts of health, caring, consciousness, mutual process, patterning, presence, and meaning have been selected to address the essence and dimensions of the nursing relationship. The basis for choosing these concepts was: (1) prevalence in the nursing literature across nursing theories, (2) consistency with knowledge development in other fields, and (3) utility across multiple cultures. There is considerable overlap in meaning as these concepts merge as a unified whole.

 ## Concepts Central to the Discipline

Health: The Intent of the Relationship

Health is central to the focus of the discipline of nursing. Many disciplines and professions commonly use it as the umbrella goal for those who care for people. The meanings of the concept of health abound in of ten ambiguous or inconsistent ways such as: the absence of disease; a continuum from wellness to illness; optimal wellness; integration of body, mind, and spirit; and a holistic phenomenon. Nursing literature reveals great diversity in the explanations of health. Donaldson and Crowley,[24] held to a dichotomous view of health by specifying that nursing is concerned with the actions or processes by which positive changes in health are affected. Wagner,[25(p43)] viewed health as the ability to function independently: "adapting successfully to life stressors," implying that through independent functioning the potential for achieving a full life occurs. Other definitions of health include: health as a dynamic life experience and a way to achieve potential,[26] a state and process of being and becoming,[15] an expression of unity and harmony of body-mind-spirit.[12] From a unitary perspective, the concepts of health and illness are seen as manifestations of rhythmic fluctuations of the life process.[27] This view is the foundation for viewing health as a unitary process moving through variations in order-disorder. From this standpoint, one can no longer think of health and illness in a dichotomous way, that is, health as absence of disease, or health as a continuum from wellness to illness. According to Newman's thesis, health is a transforming process to higher levels of consciousness.[4-6] Health and the evolving pattern of consciousness are the same.[6,20] The evolving pattern of the whole requires a nonfragmentary view of health. Newman referred to Bohm's theory of the implicate order to substantiate her position that both disease and nondisease are expressions of the whole, that is, explications of the underlying implicate order.[5,3,28] Thus disease and nondisease are different points of view of a larger reality. In this way, health may be expressed and revealed in illness. Health in the face of illness derives meaning through a caring nurse-patient relationship.

Caring: The Nature of the Relationship

Caring, also, is one of the defining terms of the discipline and is central to nursing's identity. Newman and colleagues asserted that nursing is about facilitating health, and that caring is the quality of relating that potentiates a transformative connection between nurse and patient.[1] The establishment of caring as a defining attribute of the discipline was recommended in a landmark conference in 1989 convened by the American Academy of Nursing and Sigma Theta Tau. Nursing leaders asserted that the concept "caring" should replace "nursing" in Fawcett's[29] constellation of concepts purported to define the intellectual and social boundaries of the discipline. Leininger[30] was the first to describe caring as the distinguishing focus of the discipline. She argued that care and caring were basic needs essential for human growth and development, and advanced the study of caring by examining it from cultural practices. Watson[11] defined nursing as the art and science of human caring and focused on the relational dimensions of caring and its connection to healing. In more recent writing, she has articulated its commonalities with a unitary perspective.[14,13] Boykin and Schoenhofer[17] asserted that all human beings are caring, living it moment to moment. They defined caring as "an altruistic, active expression of love...the intentional and embodied recognition of value and connectedness,"[31(pp335–336)] but reminded us that it is known by experience and reflection and not by definition.

Other nursing scholars have described caring in various ways: as a fundamental human attribute lived out in relationship, a unique trait possessed by some, an affect, a moral ideal that compels right action, an ethic of practice, an interpersonal process, a therapeutic intervention, and a process of nurturing. Because of these differences, and the lack of precision in use of the word "caring," some have argued that it is not a clarifying concept in delineating nursing's disciplinary focus. It is true that there is ambiguity in the concept of caring that obfuscates the depth of its meaning. For this reason, understanding its meaning within the UT paradigm may bring clarity to its use. Smith[22] identified 5 constituents of caring when viewed within the unitary paradigm: manifesting intention, attuning to dynamic flow, appreciating pattern,[32] experiencing the infinite, and inviting creative emergence. From a unitary perspective, caring is a quality of participative patterning. This way of being is characterized by holding the best intentions for the other and expressing them in thoughts, words, and actions. It is sensing and moving synchronously with the dynamic rhythms of relating, following the lead of the other in the dance of human becoming. This way of being is respecting the unique life story of each person and the diversity of life choices. It is valuing and supporting what matters most to the person, family, or community. Caring is seeing the other and self as interconnected to something more extensive than both. This way of being nurtures growth, and leads to self-discovery, unique self-expression, and new ways of becoming and leading one's life.[22] For some, it is time to adopt the word *love* in describing this quality of relating in nursing.[33,13] Teilhard de Chardin described *love* as the energy of connection that compels relationship. "Love alone is capable of uniting living beings in such a way as to complete and fulfill them, for it alone takes them and joins them by what is deepest in themselves."[34(p265)] In this way, caring enhances or facilitates health and healing and illuminates consciousness.

Consciousness: The Informational Pattern of the Relationship

The concept of consciousness has become central to the nursing discipline. A major shift in the concept of consciousness has occurred during the past 4 decades. International organizations have been formed for the study of consciousness along with scholarly journals created for that purpose.* Whereas in the first half of the 20th century the study of consciousness focused on characteristics of the brain, the current movement opens wide the focus to participatory exploration of the experience of consciousness and beyond.[35] DeQuincey,[36] a prominent spokesperson in this movement, claimed that consciousness must be studied in relationship between persons.

Grounded in a UT worldview of the phenomena of nursing and stimulated by Bentov's[37] thesis that life is a process of expanding consciousness, Newman[4] incorporated this shift in an understanding of the nursing relationship by asserting that health is the expansion of consciousness. This view broadened the old concept of consciousness to include the total information of the field (of nurse-patient-environment). Consciousness, the information of the pattern of the whole[6] includes all forms of information: sensation and physiology as well as intellect, emotion, and intention. A person is identified by a pattern of consciousness, which includes awareness of self within a larger system of consciousness. Arguelles,[38] a noted Mayan scholar, went so far as to say that "in actuality there is only consciousness."[(p56)] The human field is a pattern of consciousness within the

---

*For example, The University of Arizona Center for Consciousness Studies, Institute of Noetic Sciences, *ReVision*.

total pattern of consciousness of the universe. It is constantly receiving and sending information and includes patterns that may appear disruptive as well as those considered harmonious. Jumps in consciousness occur in far from equilibrium states.[39] These critical points may be turning points at which the pattern is transformed and new insights occur. A shift from a matter-based representational focus to a self-organizing field has emerged, particularly in relation to health.

Theoretical elaborations from other nursing scholars support the process of expanding consciousness. Mishel's[40] conceptualization of uncertainty as a growth move through chaos to a higher level of organization supports the transformation of persons facing what appear to be disruptive, immutable situations. Reed's[41] theory of transcendence elaborates the process of human becoming leading to higher consciousness. It describes the potential for persons to go beyond the space-time limitations of their situations to a deeper experience of their lives. Watson[12] coined the term *caring consciousness* to convey a synthesis of the 2 concepts in the nurse's relationship with the patient. Roy[16] has asserted that human consciousness is integral to an evolving, creative universe.

The essence of consciousness is information, and the essence of information is resonance. Rogers[3] included resonancy, the way information is shared, as a principle of the science of unitary human beings. She asserted that the human being "experiences his environment as a resonating wave … uniting him with the rest of the world."[(p101)] This information is accessible to us as feeling and meaning. In attending to feeling, we sense the resonance of incoming information and cocreate a resonant field. The basic way of knowing is through attunement, resonant receptivity, intuition, and revelation—a direct, unfiltered index of communication.[42] All points in space-time have immediate access to a vast storehouse of information. The whole organizes the parts, and any event happening anywhere is immediately available everywhere as information. The fields are conceived as being unbounded by space, time, and matter. This mechanism of information transfer explains the immediacy of transformation. Resonance implies that the transformation is a mutual process.

Mutual Process: The Way in Which the Relationship Unfolds

Nurses are central to creating an environment that fosters relationship and health. This environment is not conceptualized as a linear communication process of sending and receiving. Rather, it is viewed as a simultaneous unfolding, a sharing, moving together. Rogers'[27] principles of homeodynamics included integrality as a continuous mutual process between human and environmental fields. Mutual process occurs in the moment of being fully present with the individual,

family, or community. In mutual process the patient is invited to participate, and through reflection to find opportunities for new awareness, action, movement, and transformation.[43]

In mutuality, the focus is on wholeness, being with and in relationship.[6] The unfolding pattern that emerges within this mutual process occurs as an intentional presence as the nurse and the patient reflect on the meaning in the moment. The process embodies the experience of nurse and other over time, and through this process, pattern is revealed. True reality behind the appearance of separate, distinct entities, consists of wave-like, oscillating possibilities, waiting to become actualities. These possibilities become actualities once we engage in practice.[12(p121)]

Each interaction with the nurse and patient offers in mutual process the potential for discovery and choice. In mutual process the unfolding of meaningful events and relationships in people's lives is manifested in pattern. The mutual process with another is enhanced by the nurse's authentic presence. The purposeful invitation by the nurse to dialogue invites trust and fosters relationships within a caring partnership.[20,44] In mutual process the self and other are engaged in an experience that promotes awareness of self and other, and potentiates insight with new choices and actions.

The idea of human unfolding, emergence, and evolutionary transforming is significant within a number of nursing theories sharing the emergent unitary paradigm.[3,6-8,11,13,14,17] Rogers[3] asserted that "The capacity of life to transcend itself, for new forms to emerge, for new levels of complexity to evolve, predicates a future that cannot be foretold."[(p57)] The mutual process of human becoming is unpredictable, but always reflects growing complexity.

A centerpiece of Parse's school of thought, human becoming is described as a rhythmical process lived in relationship, expressed through values, and "transcending with the possibles."[8(pp19-20)] Van Kaam,[45(p10)] described the human as both potentiality and emergence. Multiple potentialities are present, and through choice, these potentialities are actualized in each moment. The mutual process of human becoming is not imposed on the other but is always happening. Teilhard de Chardin[34] stated that the direction of human becoming is toward increasing complexity, centration, interiority, and consciousness. This path is illuminated in relationship, and the pacing and direction of the journey on the path is personal. When one trusts this force, he or she relinquishes any false sense of external control, having confidence that each person knows his or her own way. There is no predetermined health outcome that is preferable for each person. The preferred outcome emerges in the person-environment mutual process, through choice. Action possibilities arise in the context of recognizing the pattern of person-environment interactions.

Patterning: The Evolving Configuration of the Relationship

Attention to pattern is a central aspect of nursing practice and research. Descriptions of patterning in the nursing literature include the following: *(a)* each person exhibits distinguishing characteristics and a unique pattern of interactions between self and environment[3,5,32,46];*(b)* pattern is a characteristic of wholeness and gives insight into life meaning[6];*(c)* patterning provides deep insight and understanding of the whole, and detailed comprehension of the uniqueness of the life process; *(d)* contrast and time are essential to the identification of pattern; *(e)* patterning is unpredictable and creative[3]; and *(f)* the process of pattern recognition reveals insights into action, an expanding horizon, and increasing connectedness.[6,47] The purpose of attention to pattern in nursing has evolved with the explication of the knowledge of the discipline-moving from diagnosis of illness and disorder to exploration of meaning, appreciation of the whole, and recognition of new possibilities for health. Pattern conveys connections of a meaningful whole.

The focus of pattern in nursing has changed overtime. Ever since Florence Nightingale developed the *pie chart* to examine patterns of disease distribution in the environment, patterning has been a central concern and unifying concept of nursing. Many nursing theories contain frameworks through which nurses can assess patterns in patients' lives to better plan nursing care. For example, in the Neuman's *systems model* nurses identify the pattern of interaction between the client system and the environment to determine the impact of environmental stressors on the client system, and to plan prevention and intervention strategies to maintain system stability.[21] The theory of *cultural care diversity and universality* guides nurses to assess patterns relating to social structures and geoenvironmental factors to plan culturally congruent care.[9] In the interactive-integrative paradigm, patterns are assessed through attention to categories or modes and are used to guide the selection of nursing interventions. As the worldview shifted to an awareness of the dynamic mutually evolving nature of the person-environment pattern, the Roy *adaptation model*, for example, was modified to express the foundational view of persons as coextensive with their social and physical environments, with an emphasis on meaning and consciousness in the mutual relationship between people and their environment.[15] As nursing theories have evolved, they have focused less on patterns of illness and disorder as a basis for intervention, and more on patterning as a way of partnering with people as they grasp the meaning of the wholeness of their life, gaining insight into new possibilities for health.

Rogers[3] identified pattern as a unifying concept in nursing and as ever-evolving in the direction of increasing complexity, with each repatterning being a revision of the immediately preceding pattern: "At each point in space-time, man [*sic*] is what he has been becoming but he is not what he has been. Moreover, he cannot go back to what he has been."[(p98)] People's lives go on through various permutations of order and disorder; after periods of chaos, their lives reorganize at a higher level of organization.

Newman described pattern as a characteristic of wholeness: "Pattern is information that depicts the whole, understanding the meaning of all the relationships at once. It is a fundamental attribute of all there is and reveals unity in diversity."[6(p71)] It reveals the meaning of life. Pattern is dynamically related with one's environment, both human and nonhuman.[6] When engaging community members in dialogue, centered on representations of individual and family patterns, it is possible to see the pattern of the community and envision possibilities for transformation in the health of the community.[48]

Patterning reveals the evolving nature of the whole. As nursing embraced holism as a central tenet of human existence, better ways to understand and respond to the whole were needed. Newman uses a process of pattern recognition that focuses on the evolving pattern of meaningful relationships and events in people's lives, stressing that meaning characterizes pattern. The process provides insight into potential actions.[6] Cowling[46] described a similar process of pattern appreciation that is creative, receptive, and responsive to individual uniqueness; gives "primacy to the voices of those seeking care"; and provides "a context for human flourishing."[(p94)] The practice of healing from this perspective focuses on appreciating the wholeness that resides within the pattern[32] and enhances nurses' ability to be attentive to their patients.

Presence: The Resonance of the Relationship

The concept of presence has been described as genuine dialogue, commitment, full engagement and openness, the core element of nursing activity, free-flowing attentiveness, transcendent togetherness, and transcendent oneness.[49] It demonstrates the uniqueness of the patient-nurse relationship: connecting with patients' experience, sensing the current moment, going beyond scientific data, knowing what will work and when to act, and the sine qua non of being with the patient.[50] Presence is a nonsensory prehension of the being of the other. Being fully present is central to the relational process of nursing:

> "... *authentic presence' between patient and nurse ... [is] a transformation of both. Presence is a matter of consciousness and is reflected in the holistic beings that are both nurses and patients.*[51 (p323)]

Melnechenko[52] described Parse's concept of true presence as a way of being that values the other's dignity and freedom and concluded that "true presence creates the opportunity for nurses to go where the patient is in life, to learn about the experience of health as it is defined and lived, and to work with patients as they choose the meaning of the situation."[(p23)] Koerner[53] stressed the importance of active receptivity as an essential aspect of nursing presence, stating, "Guided by the intent to support what is in the highest good for the person and family, we create an empty space of open expectancy, which allows individuals to connect with their inner wisdom and innate power to heal."[(p9)]

The epistemology of presence focuses on a trust that understanding deepens exploration in relationship. The emphasis is on engagement rather than on measurement, on meaning rather than on mechanism.[36] DeQuincey pointed out that "being intensely engaged in relationship with another … is, perhaps, the most vital manifestation of consciousness." It requires a shift from a world of subjects-objects, to a "view, which sees relationship as fundamental."[(p173)]

Transforming presence is becoming one with the other. This involves letting go of time constraints, putting everything aside and focusing completely on the patient, that is, being with the individual (family or community) with all aspects of oneself.[54] One must let go everything else and be fully present in the moment. Being fully present goes beyond pattern identification and is the evidence of transformation. Becoming one with the patient through presence focuses the nurse on what is meaningful to the patient.

Meaning: Importance of the Relationship

Caring presence and intentional resonance focus nurses on what is meaningful in the lives of patients. Searching for meaning and its message for the future is the primary motivation in people's lives,[55] and thus is of primary importance to nurses. The focus on meaning shifts the nurse's purpose from objective problem-solver to sojourner in discovery, interpretation, and revelation. Bohm[56] described meaning as a dynamic process. Through reflection on meaning, new meanings emerge. This process deepens with additional perspectives and expands as contexts change. Meaning arouses, organizes, and gives direction to energy.[56] As nurses and patients reflect on the unfolding pattern of meaningful interactions and events in patients' lives and on the meaning of presenting situations and the context, in which they occurred, new perspectives and deeper insights evolve. Through this process, new meanings give birth to new possibilities. Concentration on meaning in the life of the patient brings forth and directs energy into healing that is uniquely appropriate to the patient, demonstrating the centrality of a resonant, caring presence focused on meaning in people's lives.

Several nurse theorists have asserted that nursing springs from a focus on meaning in peoples' lives—nursing care cannot be predescribed or routinely applied in the same manner across clients. Travelbee[57] asserted that nurses must go beyond helping people cope with illness and suffering, to helping people explore the unique meaning they find in their experiences and predicaments. Parse[58] described meaning as being illuminated and structured multidimensionally through a cocreative process between the nurse and the patient. She pointed to the importance of dialogue, in which values are expressed to identify what is cherished and imagine what is possible. Parse,[58(p7)] stated, "One cocreates meaning, and the meaning changes with experiences as new images arise, expanding possibilities. People live their treasured beliefs in the process of evolving."

In her theory of *meaning*, Starck[59] emphasized the importance of engaging different perspectives to more fully understandable meaning, realizing that patterns of meaning may be manifest not only through verbal reflection, but also through spiritual and somatic experiences. This realization focuses the nurse-patient relationship on the meaning of all that the patient is experiencing as relevant at the moment. Meleis[60] attributed grasping meaning to "perceptions rather than intellect; it depends on observations, feelings, imagination, and understanding that go beyond description—it depends on inner experiences and is holistic in nature."[(p97)] Watson[61] invited nurses to return from the outer world of technology where meaning has been stripped, to the inner world of healing and meaningful "human-to-human connections and caring moments."[(p913)] Koerner[53] defined meaning as "the way in which we use a life experience to grow and deepen as human beings;" she called nurses to use "slower wisdom" which she defined as "longitudinal examination of issues over time"[(p208)] to remove the veil of confusion from complex situations so that meaning can be revealed. Newman[62] has demonstrated that it is in attending to the unfolding pattern of patients' lives that the meaning of the whole can be fully comprehended. Pattern and meaning are central to nursing care and give insight, one into the other.

Meaning differs from person to person and from time to time. There is no universal definition of meaning, but rather it is uniquely manifest as each individual searches for it. "The meaning of life differs from man to man [sic], from day to day, and from hour to hour. What matters, therefore, is not the meaning of life in general, but rather the specific meaning of a person's life at a given moment."[55(p108)] Clarke[63] reported that the quest for meaning is the most commonly occurring attribute of spirituality found in the nursing literature.

Drawing on the work of theologian Paul Tillich, Clarke described meaning as ultimate concern, and exhorted nurses to focus with patients on what is at the depth of their being, rather than simply on superficial concerns. Henery[64] rejected the relevance of a hierarchical notion of what is most meaningful, stressing that nurses should not place judgment on what patients perceive as meaningful. Sometimes what seems to be a superficial act or concern can open a window that sheds light on deeper meaning and insights for action. Newman[65] gave the example of walking into a patient's room, noticing that the patient is reading a newspaper, and saying, "Reading the want ads, huh?" This led directly to a dialogue about the patient's unemployment situation and its meaning in the patient's life. The caring, resonant presence of the nurse creates the context, in which the dialogue can go deeper still. Further reflection and dialogue opens a door to deeper meaning. Newman demonstrated the importance of entering into the interaction where the patient is and riding the wave of caring presence and resonance into the center of what is meaningful, trusting that the process will illuminate the direction toward health.[5,6]

The Task Before Us

An issue facing the nursing profession is the question of what knowledge will direct our practice. From our perspective, nursing practice must be first and foremost grounded in the discipline as defined by the concepts presented here, while at the same time incorporating relevant knowledge from other disciplines. The patient and the nurse both need access to the best evidence in making decisions about patient care. The UT perspective expands the notion of evidence and situates its relevance within the unique meaning and pattern of patients' lives.

Peat[66] offered a philosophy of wholeness that is consistent with the UT perspective in nursing and warned, "If we are to move toward a more holistic and healthy world, then we must discover a way of unifying the statements of objective science with our personal vision of the world, and we must do this without diluting the authenticity of either approach."[(p47)] Watson added, "Thus, an expanded and evolved disciplinary-professional view of health, healing and quality of life/living will not allow one level of evidence or technology to privilege itself over the human condition and humanity itself. The evolved future becomes large enough to hold the paradox of both side by side."[67(p14)]

Bohm,[68] in writing about meaning as the root of our whole being warned, "Without meaning, our society will fall apart."[(p150)] For nursing, "Knowing who we are in the context of society and other related disciplines is essential for our own health and well-being,

and essential to our ability to serve others."[69(p14)] Without a clear sense of our nursing identity and the meaning of our mission to society, we have no value or purpose other than to support and promote the practice of medicine. Nurses are thirsting for a meaningful practice, one that is based on nursing values and knowledge, one that is relationship-centered, enabling the expression of the depth of our mission, and one that brings a much needed, missing dimension to current healthcare. What is missing in healthcare is what nursing can provide when practiced from a disciplinary perspective. Realizing this goal begs for consensus in the collective consciousness of the nursing profession.

REFERENCES

1. Newman MA, Sime AM, Corcoran-Perry SA. The focus of the discipline of nursing. *Adv Nurs Sci.* 1991;14(1):1–6.
2. Perry DJ, Gregory KE. Global applications of the cosmic imperative for nursing knowledge development. In: Roy C, Jones D, eds. *Nursing Knowledge Development and Clinical Practice.* New York: Springer Publishing; 2007:315–326.
3. Rogers ME. *An Introduction to the Theoretical Basis of Nursing.* Philadelphia: Davis; 1970.
4. Newman MA. *Theory Development in Nursing.* Philadelphia: FA Davis; 1979.
5. Newman MA. *Health as Expanding Consciousness.* New York: NLN Press; 1986.
6. Newman MA. *Health as Expanding Consciousness.* 2nd ed. Sudbury, MA: Jones and Barlett (NLN Press); 1994.
7. Parse R. *Man-Living-Health: A Theory of Nursing.* New York: John Wiley & Sons; 1981.
8. Parse RR. *The Human BecomingSchoolof Thought.* Thousand Oaks, CA: Sage; 1998.
9. Leininger M, McFarland MR. *Culture Care Diversity and Universality: A World Wide Nursing Theory.* 2nd ed. Sudbury, MA: Jones and Bartlett; 2006.
10. Leininger M. Theoretical questions and concerns: response from the theory of culture care diversity and universality perspective. *Nurs Sci Q.* 2007;20(1):9–15.
11. Watson J. *Nursing: Human Science and Human Care.* Stamford, CT: Appleton-Century-Crofts; 1985.
12. Watson J. *Postmodern Nursing and beyond.* London: Churchill-Livingstone, 1999.
13. Watson J. *Caring Science as Sacred Science.* Philadelphia: FA Davis; 2004.
14. Watson J, Smith MC. Caring science and the science of unitary human beings. *J Adv Nurs.* 2002;37(5):452–461.
15. Roy C, Andrews HA. *The Roy Adaptation Model.* 2nd ed. Stamford, CT: Appleton & Lange; 1999:145–161.
16. Roy C. Knowledge as universal cosmic imperative. In: Roy C, Jones DA, eds. *Nursing Knowledge Development and Clinical Practice.* New York: Springer; 2007.
17. Boykin A, Schoenhofer S. *Nursing as Caring: A Model for Transforming Practice.* Sudbury, MA: Jones and Bartlett Publishers; 2001.
18. McLeod BW. Relationship-centered care. *IONS Noetic Sci Rev.* April-July 1999:37–42.
19. Newman M. *Transforming Presence: The Difference That Nursing Makes.* Philadelphia: FA Davis; 2008.

20. Picard C, Jones D. *Giving Voice to What We Know: Margaret Newman's Theory of Health as Expanding Consciousness Nursing Practice, Research and Education.* Boston: Jones and Bartlett; 2005.

21. Neuman B, Fawcett J. *The Neuman Systems Model.* 4th ed. Upper Saddle River, NJ: Prentice Hall; 2002.

22. Smith MC. Caring and the science of unitary human beings. *Adv Nurs Sci.* 1999;21(4):14–28.

23. Roy C, Jones DA eds. *Nursing Knowledge Development and Clinical Practice.* New York: Springer Publishing; 2007.

24. Donaldson S, Crowley D. The discipline of nursing. *Nurs Outlook.* 1978;26(2):113–120.

25. Wagner J. Nurse scholar's perceptions of nursing's metaparadigm. Dissertation, Ohio State University. Cited In Thorne et.al. Nursing's metaparadigm concepts: Disimpacting the debates. *J Adv Nurs.* 1998;27:43.

26. King I. *A Theory for Nursing Systems, Concepts, Processes.* New York: Wiley; 1981.

27. Rogers ME. The science of unitary human beings: current perspectives. *Nurs Sci Q.* 1994;7:33–35.

28. Bohm D. *Wholenss and the Implicate Order.* London: Routledge, 1980.

29. Fawcett J. The metaparadigm of nursing: current status and future refinements. *Image J Nurs Scholarsh.* 1984;16:84–87.

30. Leininger M. *Transcultural Nursing: Concepts, Theories and Practices.* New York: John Wiley and Sons; 1978.

31. Boykin A, Schoenhofer S, Anne Boykin, Savina O. Schoenhofer's nursing as caring theory. In: Parker M, ed. *Nursing Theories and Nursing Practice.* Philadelphia: FA Davis; 2006:334–348.

32. Cowling WR III. Healing as appreciating wholeness. *Adv Nurs Sci.* 2000;22(3):16–32.

33. Ray MA. Illuminating the meaning of caring: unfolding the sacred art of divine love. In Roach MS, ed. *Caring From the Heart: The Convergence of Caring and Spirituality.* New York: Paulist Press; 1997:163–178.

34. Teilhard de Chardin P. *The Phenomenon of Man.* New York: Harper & Row; 1959.

35. Harman WW. Toward an adequate science of consciousness. *Noetic Sci Rev.* 1993;77–78.

36. DeQuincey C. *Radical Knowing: Understanding Consciousness Through Relationship.* Rochester, VT: Park Street Press; 2005.

37. Bentov I. *Stalking the Wild Pendulum.* New York: Dutton; 1977.

38. Arguelles J. *The Mayan Factor: Path Beyond Technology.* Santa Fe, NM: Bear & Co; 1987.

39. Prigogine I, Stengers I. *Order out of Chaos: Man's New Dialogue With Nature.* Boulder/London: New Science Library (Shambhala); 1984.

40. Mishel MH. Reconceptualization of the uncertainty in illness theory. *Image.* 1990;22(4):256–261.

41. Reed P. Toward a nursing theory of self-transcendence: deductive reformulation using developmental theories. *Adv Nurs Sci.* 1991;13(4):64–77.

42. Arguelles J. *Earth Ascending: An Illustrated Treatise on the Law Governing Whole Systems.* Santa Fe, NM: Bear & Co; 1984.

43. Jones D. Health as expanding consciousness. *Nurs Sci Q.* 2006;19(4):330–332.

44. Jonsdottir H, Litchfield M, Pharris MD. Partnership in practice. *Res Theory Nurs Pract Int J.* 2003; 17(1):51–63.

45. Van Kaam A. Existential crisis and human development. *Humanitas.* 1974;10(2):109–126.

46. Cowling WR III. Despairing women and healing outcomes: a unitary appreciative nursing perspective. *Adv Nurs Sci.* 2005;28(2):94–106.

47. Litchfield M. Practice wisdom. *Adv Nurs Sci.* 1999;22(2): 62–73.

48. Pharris MD. Coming to know ourselves as community through a nursing partnership with adolescents convicted of murder. *Adv Nurs Sci.* 2002;24(3):21–42.

49. Smith TD. The concept of nursing presence: state of the science. *Scholarly Inquiry Nurs Pract Int J.* 2001;15(4):299–322.

50. Doona ME, Chase SK, Haggerty LA. Nursing presence: as real as a Milky Way bar. *J Holistic Nurs.* 1999;17(1):54–70.

51. Chase SK. Response to "The concept of nursing presence: state of the science." *Scholarly Inquiry Nurs Pract Int J.* 2001;15(4):323–327.

52. Melnechenko KL. To make a difference: nursing presence. *Nurs Forum.* 2003;22(2):18–24.

53. Koerner JG. *Healing Presence: The Essence of Nursing.* New York: Springer; 2007.

54. Frankl V. *Man's Search for Meaning.* 4th ed. Boston: Beacon Press; 2006.

55. Miller MA, Douglas MR. Presencing: nurses commitment to caring for dying persons. *Int J Hum Caring.* 1998;2(3): 24–31.

56. Bohm D. *Unfolding Meaning.* London: Routledge; 1985–1995.

57. Travelbee J. *Interpersonal Aspects of Nursing.* Philadelphia: FA Davis; 1966.

58. Parse RR, ed. *Illuminations: The Human Becoming Theory in Practice and Research.* New York: NLN; 1995.

59. Starck P. The theory of meaning. In: Smith MJ, Liehr PR, eds. *Middle Range Theory for Nursing.* New York: Springer Publishing Company; 2003:125–144.

60. Meleis AI. *Theoretical Nursing: Development and Progress.* 3rd ed. Philadelphia: Lippincott; 1997.

61. Watson J. Guest editorial: what, may I ask is happening to nursing knowledge and professional practices? What is nursing thinking at this turn in human history? *J Clin Nurs.* 2005;14:913–914.

62. Newman MA. Experiencing the whole. *Adv Nurs Sci.* 1997;20(1):34–39.

63. Clarke J. A discussion paper about "meaning" in the nursing literature on spirituality: an interpretation of meaning as "ultimate concern" using the work of Paul Tillich. *Int J Nurs Stud.* 2006;43:915–921.

64. Henery N. Comment on "A discussion paper about 'meaning' in the nursing literature on spirituality." *Int J Nurs Stud.* 2006;44:645–646.

65. Newman MA. Identifying and meeting patients' needs in short-span nurse-patient relationships. *Image.* 1966;5(1): 76–86.

66. Peat FD. *The Philosopher's Stone: Chaos, Synchronicity, and the Hidden Order of the World.* Bantam Books; 1991.

67. Watson J. Theoretical questions and concerns: Response from a caring science framework. *Nurs Sci Q.* 2007;20(1): 13–15.

68. Bohm D. Science, spirituality, and the present world crisis. *Revision.* 1993;15(4):147–152.

69. Chinn PL. Looking into the crystal ball: positioning ourselves for the year 2000. In: Hein EC, Nicholson MJ, eds. *Contemporary Leadership Behavior: Selected Readings.* Philadelphia: Lippincott; 1994:429–437.

THE AUTHORS COMMENT   **The Focus of the Discipline Revisited**

This article is a follow-up and extension of the previous publication, "The Focus of the Discipline" (Newman, Sime & Corcoran-Perry, 1991), which sought to define the nature of nursing knowledge. Having collaborated with Marlaine Smith, Margaret D. Pharris, and Dorothy Jones on explication of theory, education, and practice within the unitary-transformative paradigm, Newman sought

their help in synthesizing basic concepts from a variety of prominent nursing theories. This contribution strengthens the foundation for continuing development of the discipline.

MARGARET A. NEWMAN
MARLAINE C. SMITH
MARGARET DEXHEIMER PHARRIS
DOROTHY A. JONES

An Ontological View of Advanced Practice Nursing

CYNTHIA ARSLANIAN-ENGOREN, APRN, PhD, BC, CNS
FRANK D. HICKS, RN, PhD
ANN L. WHALL, RN, PhD, FGSA, FAAN
DONNA L. ALGASE, RN, PhD, FAAN

*I*dentifying, developing, and incorporating nursing's unique ontological and epistemological perspective into advanced practice nursing practice places priority on delivering care based on research-derived knowledge. Without a clear distinction of our metatheoretical space, we risk blindly adopting the practice values of other disciplines, which may not necessarily reflect those of nursing. A lack of focus may lead current advanced practice nursing curricula and emerging doctorate of nursing practice programs to mirror the logical positivist paradigm and perspective of medicine. This article presents an ontological perspective for advanced practice nursing education, practice, and research.

The profession and discipline of nursing has struggled for decades to define and refine its disciplinary focus and unique contributions to health care. Although multiple theoretical perspectives exist to assist in guiding practitioners and scientists in their respective work, we continue to be hindered in fostering a unifying framework that is helpful to all of nursing's varied practitioners. Across the globe, nurses are pursuing advanced education to keep up with the demands of an ever-expanding knowledge base and the omnipresent need for effective health care services. Graduate nursing education has been prevalent in the United States for more than 50 years. Yet, trends in nursing education in the US may not necessarily be headed toward an advancement of nursing knowledge or nursing practice if these programs are based on a medical model that has as its main goal the transmission of medical knowledge. With the multiplicity of educational entrees to nursing at the graduate level, it is more crucial than ever to define the unique perspective of nursing and its relation to health care. The purpose of this article, therefore, is to explicate an ontological view of nursing that may be helpful to advanced practice nurses (APNs) and nurse scientists. Advances in developing nursing knowledge are synthesized into a coherent framework, and suggestions presented for nurses to incorporate into clinical practice.

The Case for a Disciplinary Focus

Identifying, developing, and incorporating nursing's unique ontological and epistemological perspective into APN practice places priority on delivering care based on knowledge derived from the disciplinary perspective of nursing. Moreover, practicing from a strong nursing perspective that is theoretically grounded and steeped in specialized knowledge assists our efforts to gain recognition and respect as a profession and an academic discipline. Without such grounding, the very future of the profession and discipline is at stake. It is imperative that APNs be able to delineate their unique contribution and perspective to health care delivery. For without a clear distinction of our metatheoretical space, we risk blindly adopting the practices, views, and values of other disciplines (Whall, 2005), which may not necessarily reflect those of nursing. A lack of disciplinary focus may lead current APN curricula and emerging doctor of nursing practice (DNP) programs in the US to mirror the logical positivist, reductionistic paradigm and perspective of medicine.

Equally disturbing are national certifications that may embrace a medical focus, thus neglecting the nursing focus that should be inherent in APN programs. The question that must then be asked is: Does the current system of educating APNs mirror the focus of medicine (i.e., laboratory data interpretation, medication management, and medical diagnoses) or nursing? A review of such educational content should include an emphasis on nursing diagnoses, questions that address the metaparadigm of nursing, and inquiries that address holistic, patient-centered care. If national examinations for advanced practice nursing are limited in scope to medical phenomena of

ABOUT THE AUTHORS

CYNTHIA ARSLANIAN-ENGOREN was born and raised in Detroit, MI. She earned her BSN from Wayne State University in Detroit, MI; her MSN in Adult Health Nursing as a Clinical Nurse Specialist from the Medical College of Ohio, Toledo, OH; and her PhD in Nursing from the University of Michigan. Currently, she is Associate Professor at the University of Michigan School of Nursing. Dr. Arslanian-Engoren's scholarship focuses on nurses' cardiac triage decisions and the treatment-seeking decisions of women with symptoms suggestive of acute coronary syndromes.

FRANK D. HICKS was born and raised in Hammond, IN. He has a BSN from Indiana University and an MS and PhD in Nursing Science from the University of Illinois at Chicago, and he completed a 2-year Postdoctoral Fellowship at the University of Michigan School of Nursing. Currently, Dr. Hicks is Associate Professor and Director of Generalist Education at Rush University College of Nursing. His scholarly foci are decision making, self-management behaviors, and theory development. He enjoys cooking, reading, coffee, and his dog, Alex.

ANN L. WHALL is currently holding the Allesse Endowed Chair in Gerontological Nursing at Oakland University School of Nursing, in Rochester, Michigan. She is also Visiting Professor at the University of Cork, Republic of Ireland, and Professor Emerita at The University of Michigan, Ann Arbor. Ann is active in her program of research in the targeting of behavioral treatments for the nursing care of older adults with dementia. She also teaches doctoral level philosophic foundations of nursing theory classes in several invited venues.

DONNA L. ALGASE is Associate Dean for Research and Evaluation at the University of Toledo, Ohio. She received a diploma from St. Vincent Hospital School of Nursing in Toledo, OH; her BSN from the University of Toledo; an MSN from the Medical College of Ohio at Toledo; and her PhD from Case Western Reserve University in Cleveland, OH. She is the Editor of the outstanding journal, *Research and Theory for Nursing Practice*. Her scholarly work and research focus on behavioral issues in dementia and Alzheimer's disease, particularly wandering behavior, and therapeutic use of the environment. She also writes on complex measurement issues, observational methods, and theory development and testing. Dr. Algase has developed and published an instrument, the *Wayfinding Effectiveness Scale*, and on its use in the understanding and effective management of wandering behavior.

interest, these examinations will not reflect the essence or values of nursing. Failing to differentiate the practice of APNs compared to physicians and physician assistant colleagues further blurs the essential nursing core of disciplinary knowledge that should be inherent in any advanced nursing degree program. While diagnostic reasoning processes are essential to all health care professions, the questions, data, and clinical labels applied in these processes are specific to each profession and reflect knowledge generated through related research in the discipline.

Advanced Practice Nurses and Knowledge Development

By virtue of their education and experience, and the emphasis on holistic care and health promotion, APNs are in a prime position to provide affordable, expert, and efficient health care to diverse populations. Moreover, as clinical experts, APNs have a unique and significant part to play in advancing the development of nursing knowledge. Often believed to be the sole responsibility of academicians, clinical practice in essence is *the field* for knowledge development, for it is in the practice arena that nursing's phenomena of interest are encountered. Indeed, there is a largely untapped source of nursing knowledge embedded within nurses' daily practice (Benner, 1984; Benner, Tanner, & Chesla, 1996). By virtue of their exposure and participation in clinical nursing, APNs are in a prime position to add to and shape the body of nursing knowledge from a nursing perspective.

Knowledge development from a unique nursing perspective defines the boundaries of nursing and delineates the nature and application of nursing knowledge that explicates nurses' unique contribution to the health care team. Without this, nurses merely interpret what other disciplines have come to know. Without a unique and clearly articulated body of knowledge, nursing will never truly achieve the independence and stature of a profession. Thus, nursing practice will depend upon others to legitimate and guide it.

If knowledge is power, then nursing knowledge is the power base of the profession and its development is the responsibility of both practicing and academic nurses. Many nurses are daunted by the prospect of developing knowledge and often feel ill-prepared to assume this charge and actualize this process. Such feelings are understandable if one considers there may be a lack of attention paid to nursing knowledge and its development in today's APN nursing education programs. Given the emphasis on medical care and the medical approach taken in many graduate nursing curricula, it may be unlikely that the nursing knowledge embedded in clinical practice can ever be realized by today's APN.

Developing a Worldview: Philosophy, Science, and Nursing Science

A philosophy of science is the umbrella under which all science emerges. Its importance is especially noted in the formation of a worldview that influences the work of scientists and, ultimately, nursing clinicians. A worldview seeks to answer two types of philosophical questions fundamental to knowledge development. The first, the ontological question, seeks answer to the nature of phenomena (i.e., What is this thing?). The second, the epistemological question, seeks an answer to how the phenomena are known (i.e., How do we come to understand this thing?). As a means of looking at the world and interpreting its experiences, a worldview contains both explicit and implicit assumptions, beliefs, and values about the world and how one goes about gaining an understanding of it. Moreover, a worldview identifies phenomena worthy of attention and investigation, ultimately affecting the focus of nursing practice, education, and research (Whall & Hicks, 2002).

Nursing philosophers and scientists who have articulated their ontological and epistemological views include Rogers (1970, 1990), Parse (1981, 1998), and Watson (1985, 1995). Each has a unique way of viewing the world and nursing's place in it. These views have had a significant influence on the way nurses investigate phenomena and practice their profession, and have even influenced the ways in which some nurses have been educated. Over the last 50 years, common themes have emerged that form the basis of nursing's disciplinary identity. These themes sometimes known as the "metaparadigm," common to all nursing theory, and extremely important in today's education, include person, environment, health, and nursing. The way these themes are explicated, however, varies greatly among theorists. For example, Neuman (2002), Parse (1981, 1998), and Rogers (1990) view humans as unitary beings that cannot be divided into parts; whereas Roy (1995) and Orem (1991) view them as holistic beings comprised of several facets of human experience (e.g., psychosocial, physiological). For Rogers (1970, 1990) the environment and person are in constant mutuality, whereas Nightingale (1860/1969) viewed the person and environment as separate entities that influence one another. Health is sometimes viewed as an objectified phenomenon by some theorists, whereas Rogers (1990) viewed health as a culturally defined and socially enforced concept, and Neuman (2002) conceptualized it as a state of consciousness. While individual theorists have added or interpreted concepts from their worldview (King, 1971, 1995; Orem, 1991; Roy, 1995; Watson, 1985,1995), their resulting theories and frameworks clearly reflect nursing's historic metaparadigm concepts and our holistic view. Therefore, it is especially important that existing APN programs and emerging DNP programs align themselves with the historic paradigmatic approach of nursing to deliver theory-based, culturally relevant, holistic care. To ignore nursing's scholarship is to deprive an emerging generation of practitioners and scientists of nursing's foundational knowledge and to impair the further building of knowledge that is so crucial to professional discipline and its related science.

Diversity in ontological approaches, while positive and exemplary of our scholarship, has led to divisions among nurse scientists and clinicians, resulting in a multiplicity of perspectives within the discipline that further confuse nursing's purpose and place in the world. A common complaint among graduate nursing students is that these multiple views make it impossible to understand and articulate the common nature of nursing. There is, however, an ontological perspective that synthesizes and unites these various views.

A New View: Nursing Processes

According to Reed (1997), the nature and substance of nursing derives from the fact that *nursing is* the substantive perspective of our discipline. That is, nursing is concerned with the human processes of well-being that are inherent among all human systems, whether individual, family, or community. However, that is not to dismiss the existence of sickness or pathology. Rather, we integrate knowledge of pathology into a view of and interaction with the person who, as a whole, is striving for well-being. On the other hand, medicine often tends to *disease-ify* normal health processes, such as birth or sleep. Nurses strive to help people to *health-ify* themselves, including overcoming disease or adapting to or integrating the limits imposed by irreversible pathologies.

Nursing processes emanate from persons, groups, and communities and are by their nature relational, contextual, and transformative. These processes are known by the intersection of complexity, integration, and well-being, and are manifested by changes in complexity and integration that generate well-being. Our quest as nurses is to "understand the nature of and to facilitate nursing processes in diverse contexts of health experiences" (Reed, 1997, p. 77).

Within this ontological perspective, individuals are open, living systems, intrinsically active, innovative, and capable of self-organizing. Self refers to the entire system, generating qualitative change out of ongoing events of life processes and the context (environment) in which they are situated. Complexity occurs when human systems experience or express variables (e.g., life events, physiologic events) as parts, separated from the whole, rather than as patterns of the whole. Complexity provides diversity, specialization, and depth of experiences. Increasing complexity brings quantitative, not qualitative change. Integration is the system's ability to synthesize and organize experiences or phenomena that results in a change in form, and is dependent upon a certain level of complexity. Integration is transformative and involves qualitative change, providing organization, coherence, and breadth.

Well-being arises out of the intersection of complexity and integration, which are rhythmical in creating change. According to Reed (1997), well-being occurs when the particulars of a life experience are brought together and synthesized in a coherent way. Without this synthesis, people feel *dis*-integrated, *dis*-associated, and *dis*-organized, in other words, *dis*-eased. Promoting well-being through a perspective of inherent processes of complexity and integration is distinctly nursing. If nursing is viewed as inherent human-environment processes that lead to well-being vis-à-vis complexity and integration, then it follows that the focus of nursing science should be on understanding those processes, while nursing practice assists those processes. Thus, instead of seeing nursing as something exterior to the patient/client/system, nursing is viewed as intrinsically inherent to the patient/client/system; something to be developed and nurtured in human systems. Within this ontological view, the approach to understanding nursing processes is achieved with sensitivity to the contextual and holistic nature of the human system. Thus, nurses need to strive to understand and teach the complexities involved in human life processes as they influence and are influenced by well-being. The unique role of the nurse, then, becomes one that assists the human system in integrating the dynamic complexities that evolve from human-environment interactions and is thusly important in clinical practice.

Reed's (1997) view of nursing not only provides a unique perspective, but it also raises interesting philosophical and scientific questions, and presents a novel approach to nursing practice. The exciting ideas contained within this ontology hold promise for unifying and articulating the age-old questions of: What is nursing, and what do nurses do?

Application to Advanced Practice Nursing

Nursing's philosophic views and beliefs have led to a unique perspective that distinguishes APNs from other health care providers. The importance of this understanding cannot be underestimated. Grounding practice within this perspective, nurses will find it easy to understand their own contribution to health care as well as to articulate this to other members of an interdisciplinary team. A lack of understanding of the essence of nursing will threaten the existence of nursing as is now known and understood by society. The social contract between nursing and the public will be jeopardized and it will be difficult to ascertain the role of nurses as compared to other health care providers. Nursing has a service to offer that has been historically understood by society. Not recognizing this unique nursing perspective and philosophic view will jeopardize nursing existence. This perspective should underpin APN education, practice, and research.

APN Education

As specialty curricula are developed and implemented for the education of APNs and nurses with DNP degrees, ontological and epistemological perspectives necessary to actualize these roles must be carefully considered. While not negating the importance of natural, biological, organizational, and social science knowledge (e.g., pathophysiology, statistics, and psychology), commonly found within APN curricula, these alone do not provide the student with the advanced skills and knowledge necessary to deliver high-quality, advanced practice nursing. Indeed, many theoretical foundations shared with the medical discipline are used to prepare expert clinical practitioners. However, what distinguishes APNs from medical health care providers is the unique contribution of nursing's ways of knowing and holistic approach to the delivery of patient care. The clinical care provided by APNs focuses on the whole of a person's health and illness experiences (American Association of Colleges of Nursing, 1996). APN education, therefore, must focus on educating nurses to understand the essential nursing processes inherent in the human conditions, and teach students to analyze the relationship of complexity, integration, and well-being. The mission of advanced practice nursing, "to provide expert, quality, and comprehensive nursing care to clients" (American Nurses Association, 1996, p. 1) must be grounded in the ontological and epistemological perspectives of the nursing discipline and reflected in professional competencies unique to nursing's pattern of knowing (Vinson, 2000).

APN Practice

The clinical practice of APNs must actualize the values and beliefs inherent within the discipline of nursing. Therefore, it is imperative that APNs who address the health care needs of patients do so from an advanced nursing perspective. APNs must not limit the focus of their care to just the differential medical diagnoses and prescribed pharmacological therapy. Instead, APNs must be mindful to include the integration of the family, the environment, and the human response to health and illness in the provision of health care, for this is what sets APNs apart from other health care professionals.

APNs must begin to reconceptualize their practice and endeavor to examine the multiplicity of patterns that evolve from the intersection of complexity, integration, and well-being. As such, the discernment of human health patterns may be able to capitalize on the existing nursing diagnosis taxonomy. Delineating and incorporating relevant nursing diagnoses into the plan of care illuminates the nursing component of APN practice. Firmly rooted in the epistemological and ontological values of the discipline, nursing diagnoses represent the essence of nursing; its focus, function, and future at an advanced practice level.

APN Research

Another available means to accentuate the nursing perspective within APN practice is through the utilization and generation of nursing research. Conceptual and philosophic consistency is obtained when scientists work under an overarching ontologic worldview. If nurse scientists and APNs both operated from this ontologic worldview, incorporating empirical knowledge with diverse ways of knowing, it would facilitate a richer and more holistic approach to patient care. Moreover, the application of nursing research to APN clinical practice anchors the delivery of care within a nursing perspective and communicates the value and importance of nursing investigations to clients, families, communities, and other health care professionals. The generation of nursing knowledge through scientific research advances the science of nursing from which APNs practice.

Conclusion

As the discipline of nursing continues to develop, the direction will be set by the philosophy and theories selected and the values espoused. To truly practice professional nursing at an advanced practice level requires a vast repertoire of skills coupled with a mastery of conceptual, empirical and clinical knowledge of nursing. Embracing a paradigmatic perspective that unifies the values of the discipline of nursing will advance the profession, direct clinical practice, and enhance our understanding. Ignoring the complexity of nursing phenomena will lead to an incomplete nursing science (Whall & Hicks, 2002) that fails to serve its members or the public's health care needs.

REFERENCES

American Association of Colleges of Nursing. (1996). *The essentials of master's education for advanced practice nursing.* Washington, DC: Author.

American Nurses Association. (1996). *Scope and standards of advanced practice registered nursing.* Washington, DC: Author.

Benner, P. A. (1984). *From novice to expert: Excellence and power in clinical nursing practice.* Menlo Park, CA: Addison-Wesley.

Benner, P. A., Tanner, C. A., & Chesla, C. A. (1996). *Expertise in nursing practice: Caring, clinical judgment and ethics.* New York: Springer Publishing Company.

King, I. M. (1971). *Toward a theory for nursing.* New York: Wiley.

King, I. M. (1995). The theory of goal attainment. In M. A. Frey & C. L. Seiloff (Eds.), *Advancing King's systems framework and theory of nursing* (pp. 23–33). Thousand Oaks, CA: Sage.

Neuman, B. (2002). *The Neuman systems model* (4th ed.). Upper Saddle River, NJ: Prentice Hall.

Nightingale, F. (1969). *Notes on nursing: What it is and what it is not.* New York: Dover Publications. (Original work published 1860)

Orem, D. E. (1991). *Nursing: Concepts of practice* (4th ed.). St. Louis: Mosby Year Book.

Parse, R. R. (1981). *Man-living-health: A theory of nursing.* New York: Wiley.

Parse, R. R. (1998). *The human becoming school of thought: A perspective for nurses and other health professionals.* Thousand Oaks, CA: Sage Publications.

Reed, P. G. (1997). Nursing: The ontology of the discipline. *Nursing Science Quarterly, 10*(2), 76–79.

Rogers, M. E. (1970). *An introduction to the theoretical basis of nursing.* Philadelphia: F. A. Davis. Rogers, M. E. (1990). Nursing: Science of unitary, irreducible human beings. Update 1990. In E. A. M. Barrett (Ed.), *Visions of Rogers' science-based nursing* (pp. 5–11). New York: National League for Nursing.

Roy, C. L. (1995). Developing nursing knowledge: Practice issues raised from four philosophical perspectives. *Nursing Science Quarterly, 8*(2), 79–85.

Vinson, J. A. (2000). Nursing's epistemology revisited in relation to professional educational competencies. *Journal of Professional Nursing, 16* (1), 39–46.

Watson, J. (1985). *Nursing: Human science and human care.* Norwalk, CT: Appleton-Century-Crofts.

Watson, J. (1995). Postmodernism and knowledge development in nursing. *Nursing Science Quarterly, 8*(2), 60–64.

Whall, A. L. (2005). "Lest we forget": An issue concerning the doctorate in nursing practice (DNP). *Nursing Outlook, 53*,1.

Whall, A., & Hicks, F. D. (2002). The unrecognized paradigm shift within nursing: Implications, problems, and possibilities. *Nursing Outlook, 50,* 72–76.

THE AUTHORS COMMENT | **An Ontological View of Advanced Practice Nursing**

The genesis of this article was a conversation between Drs. Arslanian-Engoren and Hicks about the lack of a nursing theoretical base in many advanced practice nursing (APN) programs. From our years of studying and teaching nursing theory, we believed that there was a wealth of information to be gleaned from nursing theory. Our purpose in writing this article was to begin to explicate that belief and show that nursing theory has a place in APN.

We were thrilled when Drs. Whall and Algase, mentors and supporters of nursing theory, agreed to assist us in writing this article. We hope that this article will serve as a resource and an inspiration for others who wish to emphasize nursing in APN.

CYNTHIA ARSLANIAN-ENGOREN
FRANK D. HICKS
ANN L. WHALL
DONNA L. ALGASE

CHAPTER 45

Nursing: The Ontology of the Discipline

PAMELA G. REED, RN, PhD, FAAN

*The purpose of this article is to contribute to clarifying the ontology of the discipline by extending existing meanings of the term **nursing** to propose a substantive definition. In this definition, nursing is viewed as an inherent human process of well-being, manifested by complexity and integration in human systems. The nature of this process and theoretical implications of the new nursing are presented. Nurses are invited to continue the dialogue about the meaning of the term and explore the implications of nursing, substantively defined, for their practice and science.*

Distinguishing the term *nursing* as a noun from its use as a verb was put forth most profoundly by Rogers (1970), whose vision extended the scholarship of earlier nursing theorists to thrust nursing forward to be recognized as both a scientific discipline as well as a professional practice. It is time, however, to push back the frontier once again, beyond these two important understandings of nursing, by proposing a new meaning of nursing. With this new meaning, the term itself represents the nature and substance of the discipline. In other words, *nursing* is the ontology of the discipline.

The ideas put forth here are done so in the spirit of accepting Watson's (1995) "postmodern challenge" to exploit the climate of deconstruction of nursing (see Rampragus, 1995; Reed, 1995) to extend and, by some degree, reconstruct current understandings of nursing. Smith's (1988a) article outlined the ongoing dialogue about two meanings of nursing, as a verb and a noun. This dialogue is revisited here for the purpose of further clarifying what is the ontology of the discipline, long considered a crucial question by seminal thinkers in nursing (Ellis, 1982; Rogers, 1970; Roy, 1995).

Continuing the Dialogue: Nursing as a Process of Well-Being

It is proposed here that there exists a third and perhaps most basic definition of nursing in which nursing represents the *substantive* focus of the discipline. Disciplines are characterized by their substantive focus: archaeology is the study of the archaeo, or what is ancient and primitive; astronomy is the study of the astro, astronomical phenomena such as the motion and constitution of celestial bodies; biology is a branch of knowledge about biol, or living matter; chemistry deals with the processes and properties of chemical substances; physics is the study of physical properties and processes; psychology is the study of the psyche, referring to mental processes and activities associated with human behavior; and nursing, the discipline, is proposed here to be the study of nursing processes of well-being, inherent among human systems.

This meaning of nursing, as an inherent process of well-being, derives in part from the root word, nurse, defined as a process of nourishing, of promoting the development or progress of something. The meaning also derives from synonyms of nurse meaning to heal, to foster, to sustain (Laird, 1971; *Webster's New Collegiate Dictionary*, 1979). These descriptions signify that nursing involves a process that is developmental, progressive, and sustaining, and by which well-being occurs.

The Inherent Nursing Process

The theme of human beings' inherent nursing processes as the substantive focus of the discipline is supported in nursing theorists' works from Nightingale in 1859, to the mid-20th century writings of Henderson, to the contemporary turn-of-the-century ideas of Schlotfeldt. Nightingale (1859/1969) wrote about the person's "innate power" and the inner "reparative process." Henderson (1964) eloquently symbolized the power of the nurse within, describing nursing as "the consciousness of the unconscious, the love of life of the suicidal, ... the eyes of the newly blind, a means of locomotion for the infant, ... the voice for those too weak or withdrawn to speak" (p. 63). Watson (1985) referred to

ABOUT THE AUTHOR

PAMELA G. REED is Professor at the University of Arizona College of Nursing in Tucson, where she also served as Associate Dean for Academic Affairs for 7 years. She is a three-time graduate of Wayne State University in Detroit, receiving a BSN, an MSN (with a double major in child–adolescent psychiatric mental health nursing and teaching), and her PhD with a major in nursing (focused on life span development and aging) from there in 1982. Dr. Reed pioneered research into spirituality and well-being with her doctoral research with terminally ill patients. She also developed a theory of self-transcendence and two widely used research instruments, the *Spiritual Perspective Scale* and the *Self-Transcendence Scale*. Her publications and funded research reflect a dual scholarly focus: spirituality and other facilitators of well-being in life-limiting illness, and nursing metatheory and knowledge development. Dr. Reed also enjoys time with her family, reading, classical music, swimming, and hiking in the mountains and canyons of Arizona.

"self-healing processes," and Schlotfeldt (1994) stressed human beings' "inherent ability and propensity to seek and attain health." In addition, this nursing process is not necessarily based upon a reversal of a disease process, but more upon a moving forward, to gain a sense of well-being in the absence or presence of disease.

The discipline's understanding of how a nursing process is manifested is shifting away from the mid-20th century mechanistic conception of nursing as a process external to patients and conducted by the nurse, that is, the old nursing process. The process of nursing is viewed now more from a relational perspective, congruent with contextual and transformative conceptions of the world (see Newman, 1992; Pepper, 1942). Nursing is a participatory process that transcends the boundary between patient and nurse and derives from a valuing of what Rogers (1980, 1992) described as human systems' inherent propensity for "innovation and creative change."

"Human systems" refers to an individual or a group of human beings (Rogers, 1992, p. 30). As such, human systems, whether in the form of individuals, dyads, groups, or communities, emanate and participate in nursing processes. Nursing processes may be manifested, for example, in the grieving that an individual experiences, in the caring that occurs among people and their families and nurses, in the healing practices shared by a culture, or in many other as yet undiscovered patterns of nursing. Today, these patterns may be described as intentional or unconscious, automatic or contemplative, relational or chemical, or simply unknown. Nevertheless, with continued nursing research, education, and practice, nursing processes can be learned and knowingly deployed to facilitate well-being. Murphy's (1992) visionary book, for example, addresses some of these possibilities. He proposes a future wherein people are more aware of their innate healing potential and employ it to more purposefully enhance health.

Nightingale did not invent nursing, described here in terms of an inherent propensity for well-being. Just as earthquakes existed before geologists and photosynthesis before botanists, nursing processes existed in human beings, ultimately described by Nightingale (1859/1969) as that which nurses were to facilitate by placing the patient in the best situation possible. It follows, then, that nursing does not belong exclusively to certain groups of people, such as "well" persons or professional nurses; it belongs to human nature.

Defining the substance of the discipline of nursing in terms of a well-being process inherent among human beings does not negate the importance of knowledge of factors that interface with nursing to influence well-being and healing. Examples of these factors, often the focus of study in ancillary professions and disciplines, include the environmental, financial, cultural, surgical, and pharmacological. However, any sense of well-being involves, most basically, a nursing process. The quest for nursing is to understand the nature of and to facilitate nursing processes in diverse contexts of health experiences.

The Nature of Nursing Processes

What is the nature of nursing processes that distinguishes them from other human processes? It is proposed that the intersection of at least three characteristics—complexity, integration, well-being—distinguishes human processes as nursing; specifically, nursing processes are manifested by changes in complexity and integration that generate well-being. Importantly, other distinguishing characteristics of nursing processes may be identified as the dialogue continues beyond this article.

This new understanding of the nature of nursing processes derived from various theorists' work, such as von Bertalanffy's (1981) systems view of human beings; Rogers' (1970, 1992) science of unitary human beings; Lerner's (1986) developmental contextualism; and complexity theory (see Kauffman, 1995; Waldrop, 1992). While the translation of these theorists' ideas may not be entirely congruent with those presented here, their ideas nonetheless can help inform development of a new nursing ontology.

Human beings are viewed as open, living systems and not as passive but intrinsically active and innovative. As an open system, human systems are capable of self-organizing, where *self* refers to the system as a whole. Self-organization is an inherent capacity for generating qualitative change out of ongoing events in the life of a system and its environment.

In his seminal work on development, Werner (1957) explained this process of qualitative change as his "orthogenetic principle," which posits that living organisms change over time from lower to higher levels of differentiation and integration. Werner (1957) called this change "development," in contrast to mechanistic processes of change, which are not developmental.

Similarly, Rogers' (1980) principles of homeodynamics describe the inherent innovative patterning of change that occurs in open systems, both environmental and human. Her three principles of helicy, resonancy, and integrality together depict the nature of qualitative change in human beings in terms of ongoing movement from lower to higher levels of diversity.

Complexity theorists (for example, Kauffman, 1995; Waldrop, 1992), and developmentalists (for example, Lerner, 1986; Werner, 1957) in particular have clarified a distinction between quantitative and qualitative change, both of which are necessary for development; contrasting terms such as complexity and order, and differentiation and organization, depict this distinction. Similarly, two distinct forms of change can be identified in Rogers' (1980, 1992) works, namely diversity and innovation (Reed, 1997).

Because of the articulation between quantitative and qualitative change, human systems are not simply complex systems (SCS) but rather are complex innovative systems (CIS) (see Stites, 1994). In the context of nursing, then, nursing processes entail at least two forms of change, complexity and integration.

Complexity. Complexity refers to the number of different types of variables that can be identified in a given situation. A variable is simply something that varies (*Webster's*, 1979). Complexity occurs when human systems experience or express variables (for example, life events, physiologic events) as parts, separated from the whole, rather than as patterns of the whole. So, for example, complexity is evident when loss of a loved one or chronic illness introduces many new and seemingly disconnected variables into an individual's life, on various levels of awareness. Increasing complexity means change in quantity (size or number) not change in quality of the whole; this would become chaotic were it not accompanied by corresponding changes in integration.

Integration. Integration refers to a synthesizing and organizing of variables such that there is a change in form, not just change in size or number of events. A certain level of complexity is needed for integration to occur. Integration is evident, for example, when people construct meaning or identify a pattern in the variables or events experienced. Integration may also occur on levels of awareness that are not yet so readily apparent. Integration is trans*form*ative, involving qualitative change in form.

Well-Being

While changes in complexity and integration may be used to explain many facets of human development and systems' changes, this process may also be used to understand health, healing, and well-being. The rhythm between complexity and integration is proposed here to be a means by which innovative change occurs, as a manifestation of the underlying process called nursing. Thus, well-being may be explained in part by changes in complexity that are tempered by changes in integration. Complexity provides life with diversity, specialization, and depth in experiences, whereas integration provides organization, coherence, and breadth.

Examples of nursing processes are abundant. For example, groups incorporate new attachments or children into an organization called family. Persons with spinal cord injuries develop different pathways that link together shattered parts of life and bodily functions. Premature infants' behaviors become more innovative as they organize the complexity of their environment. Adults reminisce to integrate past life events and inevitable death. Healing after the loss of a loved one or the occurrence of chronic illness requires an integration of what seem like disjointed events and experiences, including memories of the past, future dreams, altered rhythms and routines, physical pain and other bodily symptoms, sadness, anguish, and self-doubt. Further, Sachs (1995) depicted what can be called nursing processes, through his stories about people with various maladies, such as a colorblind painter and a surgeon with Tourette's syndrome. These people were able to create a new organization that fit with their altered needs and world. These health events, in all their initial complexity and heartbreak, gave way to metamorphoses and innovation. Regardless of whether there is a "cure" that can reverse a particular ailment, well-being occurs when the particulars of a life experience are brought together and synthesized in a coherent way. Any less, and people risk feeling disintegrated, disassociated, disorganized.

While the centrality of well-being as a focus in nursing has been established, other disciplines also may be concerned with well-being and its correlates. However, promoting well-being based upon a perspective of the inherent process of complexity and integration is distinctly nursing.

Challenging the Status Quo: Nursing Reconstructed

The definition of nursing proposed here is that of an inherent process of well-being, characterized by manifestations of complexity and integration in human systems. The substantive focus of the discipline, then, is not how *nurses* per se facilitate well-being but, rather, how *nursing processes* function in human systems to facilitate well-being. The focus is, in a very basic sense, how nurses can facilitate nursing.

Refocusing the Lens

This new construction of nursing provides another lens of focus for nursing researchers and practitioners. Smith (1988b) wrote metaphorically about three different camera lenses used to view human wholeness. One in particular, the motion lens, focuses on process and rhythmic flow, and requires a "creative leap" to identify this process. Nurses typically encounter people in motion, in dynamic flow with their environment, whether in life-threatening experiences or perceived memory loss, chronic illness or acute pain.

The creative leap necessary for formulating the motion lens of nursing inquiry may be to address the rhythmic processes of complexity and integration that enhance well-being across these health experiences. From premature infants to dying adults and their families and communities, it is proposed that human systems have nursing processes, that is, inherent resources for well-being based on a capacity to integrate their complexities.

Debates on holism and on what represents the critical focus of nursing may be enlivened by including a new ontology of nursing—an ontology that transcends debates about part versus whole, person versus environment. Nursing processes are not necessarily bound by dimensions such as biologic, environmental, or social. Instead, the lens is focused on any human process that manifests complexity and integration related to well-being. Looking through this new lens, researchers and practitioners may identify a myriad of human manifestations of wholeness, whether they be labeled physiologic, phylogenic, or philosophic, that are integral to well-being.

Nursing as a Metaparadigm Concept

Given this reconstructed view of nursing, as a substantive focus of the discipline, the term *nursing* should be a central concept in the nursing metaparadigm. In the past, for good reason, some have suggested the elimination of the term nursing from the metaparadigm (Conway, 1985). However, rather than remove the term nursing from the metaparadigm, this fin-de-siècle may be the time in nursing history to consider renaming the discipline to something other than a verb, to better distinguish the disciplinary label from the substantive focus of the science and practice.

To help clarify this distinction, a term such as Paterson and Zderad's (1976) "nursology," or another disciplinary label with the "nurs" prefix could be developed, while reserving the term nursing as the *process* word and verb that it is, for the metaparadigm. By identifying nursing as a substantive, metaparadigm concept, nurses can better claim their unique focus and clarify the ontology of their discipline.

Approaching the Frontier

Rogers (1992) explained that one could not push back the frontier of knowledge until one approached it. This article has not been about maintaining the status quo, but about approaching a frontier so that others might join in a dialogue that pushes back the frontier a bit more. In this era of healthcare reform, the discipline must define nursing as nurses truly envision it and not necessarily as others would have it be defined. Nurses may decide against renaming the discipline as was suggested here. Nevertheless, within a broadened and partially reconstructed view of the discipline that embraces nursing at its most fundamental meaning, new understandings that blend with the old can emerge to present a fuller picture of the discipline.

Nursing (as practice and praxis) is a way of doing that creates good actions that facilitate well-being. Nursing (as syntax and science) is a way of knowing that creates goods in the form of knowledge. And nursing (the substance and ontology) is a way of being that creates patterns of changing complexity and integration experienced as well-being in human systems.

Nurses are invited to try on the substantive definition of nursing to see how it fits within the context of their practice and science. Ongoing philosophic dialogue about the ontology of the discipline will help ensure that nurse theorists are theorists of nursing in its fullest sense, and likewise, that nurse researchers are researchers of nursing, and nurse practitioners are practitioners of nursing.

REFERENCES

Conway, M.E. (1985). Toward greater specificity in defining nursing's metaparadigm. *Advances in Nursing Science, 7* (4), 73–81.

Ellis, R. (1982). Conceptual issues in nursing. *Nursing Outlook, 30*(7), 406–410.

Henderson, V. (1964). The nature of nursing. *American Journal of Nursing, 64*(8), 62–68.

Kauffman, S. (1995). *At home in the universe: The search for laws of self-organization and complexity*. New York: Oxford University Press.

Laird, C. (1971). *Webster's new world thesaurus* (rev. ed.). New York: Simon and Schuster.

Lerner, R.M. (1986). *Concepts and theories of human development* (2nd ed.). New York: Random House.

Murphy, M. (1992). *The future of the body: Explorations into the further evolution of human nature*. New York: J.P. Tarcher.

Newman, M. (1992). Prevailing paradigms in nursing. *Nursing Outlook, 40*, 10–13.

Nightingale, F. (1969). *Notes on nursing: What it is and what it is not*. New York: Dover (Original work published 1859)

Paterson, J.G., & Zderad, L.T. (1976). *Humanistic nursing*. New York: Wiley.

Pepper, S.P. (1942). *World hypotheses: A study in evidence*. Berkeley: University of California Press.

Rampragus, V. (1995). *The deconstruction of nursing*. Brookfield, VT: Ashgate.

Reed, P.G. (1995). A treatise on nursing knowledge development for the 21st century: Beyond postmodernism. *Advances in Nursing Science, 17*(3), 70–84.

Reed, P.G. (1997). The place of transcendence in nursing's science of unitary human beings. In M. Madrid (Ed.), *Patterns of Rogerian knowing* (pp. 187–196). New York: National League for Nursing Press.

Rogers, M.E. (1970). *Introduction to the theoretical basis of nursing*. Philadelphia: F.A. Davis.

Rogers, M.E. (1980). A science of unitary man. In J.P. Riehl & C. Roy (Eds.), *Conceptual models for nursing practice* (2nd ed., pp. 329–337). New York: Appleton-Century-Crofts.

Rogers, M.E. (1992). Nursing science and the space age. *Nursing Science Quarterly, 5*, 27–34.

Roy, C.L. (1995). Developing nursing knowledge: Practice issues raised from four philosophical perspectives. *Nursing Science Quarterly, 8*, 79–85.

Sachs, O. (1995). *An anthropologist on Mars: Seven paradoxical tales*. New York: A. Knopf.

Schlotfeldt, R. (1994). Resolving opposing viewpoints: Is it desirable? Is it practicable? In J.F. Kikuchi & H. Simmons (Eds.), *Developing a philosophy of nursing* (pp. 67–74). Thousand Oaks: Sage.

Smith, M.J. (1988a). Nursing: What's in a name? *Nursing Science Quarterly, 1*, 142–143.

Smith, M.J. (1988b). Perspectives of wholeness: The lens makes a difference. *Nursing Science Quarterly, 1*, 94–95.

Stites, J. (1994). Complexity research on complex systems and complex adaptive systems. *Omni, 16*(8), 42–50.

von Bertalanffy, L. (1981). *A systems view of man* (P.A. LaViolette, Ed.). Boulder: Westview Press.

Waldrop, M.M. (1992). *Complexity: The emerging science at the edge of order and chaos*. New York: Simon and Schuster.

Watson, J. (1985). *Nursing: Human science and human care*. Norwalk, CT: Appleton-Century-Crofts.

Watson, J. (1995). Postmodernism and knowledge development in nursing. *Nursing Science Quarterly, 8*, 60–64.

Webster's new collegiate dictionary. (1979). Springfield, MA: G. & C. Merriam Co.

Werner, H. (1957). The concept of development from a comparative and organismic point of view. In D.B. Harris (Ed.), *The concept of development* (pp. 125–148). Minneapolis: University of Minnesota Press.

THE AUTHOR COMMENTS | Nursing: The Ontology of the Discipline

It struck me that nursing is so much more than we typically assume it to be; it is more than the practice that nurses engage in and more than a disciplinary body of knowledge. In this article, I propose that nursing is a basic process of well-being that occurs within and among human beings. It is a natural process, like biologic or geologic processes for example, that defines the disciplinary focus of our particular discipline. And there are many processes of well-being that nursing practitioners and researchers can study, appreciate, and facilitate for human welfare. I invite readers to reflect on how their work in some way addresses a human process of well-being.

PAMELA G. REED

The Power of Wholeness, Consciousness, and Caring
A Dialogue on Nursing Science, Art, and Healing

W. RICHARD COWLING, III, RN, PhD, AHN-BC, APRN-BC, FAAN

MARLAINE C. SMITH, RN, PhD, AHN-BC, FAAN

JEAN WATSON, RN, PhD, AHN-BC, FAAN

Wholeness, consciousness, and caring are 3 critical concepts singled out and positioned in the disciplinary discourse of nursing to distinguish it from other disciplines. This article is an outgrowth of a dialogue among 4 scholars, 3 who have participated extensively in work aimed at synthesizing converging points in nursing theory development. It proposes a unified vision of nursing knowledge that builds on their work as a reference point for extending reflection and dialogue about the discipline of nursing. We seek for an awakening of a higher/deeper place of wholeness, consciousness, and caring that will synthesize new ethical and intellectual forms and norms of "ontological caring literacy" to arrive at a unitary caring science praxis. We encourage the evolution of a mature caring-healing-health discipline and profession, helping affirm and sustain humanity, caring, and wholeness in our daily work and in the world. **Key words:** *caring, caring science, consciousness, healing, nursing discipline, nursing knowledge, unitary science, wholeness*

Wholeness, consciousness, and caring are 3 critical concepts that are evident throughout much of nursing's disciplinary discourse. Each has been singled out as having relevance for distinguishing nursing from other disciplines. Three prominent nursing scholars have strategically positioned these concepts in their theoretical perspectives on nursing science and art.[1-5] They have also developed creative syntheses of nursing theories that incorporate these concepts. This article grew from a dialogue among these 3 scholars and a fourth scholar with the intention of extending previous theoretical discourse and reaching for an expansion of previous syntheses. The dialogue was aimed at creating deeper reflections on the significance of wholeness, consciousness, and caring to inform the discipline of nursing.

Theoretical Perspectives and Syntheses

Newman[1-3] has consistently called for a reexamination of nursing theory and knowledge development. In particular, she has sought to reconcile the differences and explore the commonalities of nursing theories. In 2003, she set forth a detailed description of "the transcendent unity of the theories of nursing knowledge,"[(p243)] using quotes from several nursing scholars. Newman built a case for unity using literature supporting "the synthesis of caring and health with underlying concepts of wholeness, pattern, mutual process, consciousness, transcendence, and transformation."[(p243)]

Likewise, Smith and Watson have proposed perspectives that encompass the commonalities of unitary and caring theoretical frameworks.[4,5] In 2002, they presented a "case for the integration, convergence, and creative synthesis"[(p452)] of caring science and the science of unitary human beings. In their "trans-theoretical discourse in theory and knowledge development in nursing science,"[(p459)] Watson and Smith pointed to philosophical and theoretical convergence and proposed integration and extensions around 7 specific commonalities.

The purpose of this article is to expand the discourse on the nature of nursing science, art, and healing through exploration of these perspectives. Our aim is to suggest a disciplinary vision of nursing knowledge grounded in a view of human life and healing—a vision that integrates wholeness, consciousness, and caring. The points of convergence between various perspectives are synthesized to create a picture

From W. R. Cowling, M. C. Smith, and J. Watson, The power of wholeness, consiousness, and caring:
A dialogue on nursing science art, and health, Advances in Nursing Science, 31(1), E41–E51.

ABOUT THE AUTHORS

W. RICHARD COWLING, III, is currently Professor and Director of the PhD Program in Nursing at the University of North Carolina Greensboro and Editor of the *Journal of Holistic Nursing.* The accomplishments that he is most proud of in relation to nursing are in the areas of research and practice relevant to women's survivorship of childhood abuse and depression. He has sought to integrate theory, research, and practice from a unique holistic and unitary perspective. Outcomes of the work include the creation of innovative practice and research methods, implementation and support of research, conception of a theory of healing, and formulation and implementation of a practice model for intervention with women who have experienced abuse in childhood. He is certified as an advanced practice nurse in both mental health and holistic nursing. In 2008, he was awarded a Department of Health and Human Services' grant to support a PhD program focused on health disparities and health promotion. He was named the 2008 Holistic Nurse of the Year by the American Holistic Nurses Association. Dr. Cowling was inducted as a Fellow in the American Academy of Nursing in 2010. His hobbies and personal interests revolve around the activities with his partner, daughter, and granddaughters who add immeasurable joy to his life.

MARLAINE C. SMITH is the Helen Karpelenia Persson Eminent Scholar and Dean at the Christine E. Lynn College of Nursing at Florida Atlantic University in Boca Raton, Florida. She was born in Turtle Creek, Pennsylvania, near Pittsburgh, and received her nursing education from Duquesne University, University of Pittsburgh, and New York University. Her contributions to nursing can be clustered in two areas: developing knowledge related to processes and outcomes of healing, and analyzing, extending, and applying existing nursing theories. For 20 years, she has been conducting research related to outcomes of touch therapies. She is the coeditor with Marilyn Parker of the 3rd edition of the popular book, *Nursing Theories & Nursing Practice* published in 2010 by FA Davis. Marlaine enjoys reading, yoga, walking on the beach, and cooking Italian food.

JEAN WATSON was born in West Virginia. Her RN preparation occurred at the Lewis Gale School of Nursing in Roanoke, Virginia. Her undergraduate and graduate degrees (BSN, MSN, PhD) are from the University of Colorado. She holds an Endowed Chair in Caring Science at University of Colorado Denver, College of Nursing, where she is also Distinguished Professor, the highest academic standing in the university. Her work in Caring Science and Theory and Practice of Human Caring is studied worldwide. She holds 9 honorary doctorates, 6 international, and has been distinguished lecturer in universities and professional programs around the world. She has received numerous awards and other international/national honors. She is the author of more than 14 books on caring and over 100 publications. Her most recent position is founder of Watson Caring Science Institute, a nonprofit foundation, established to further the work in Caring Science in nursing around the world.

of nursing knowledge expressed in 8 emerging and evolving elements.

The article also responds to the call for what the scholars refer to as a nursing "mandate" and "imperative" to arrive at a more distinctive and clearer focus of the discipline of nursing. A model of caring from a unitary perspective is offered to guide the praxis of nursing, and essential competencies are delineated that are fundamental to the nature of caring-healing praxis.

Wholeness

The ontological view presented in the writings of Newman and Watson and Smith characterizes a universe of human existence that is essentially and inherently whole. This is expressed in a variety of ways. Newman[3] proposes a world of no boundaries and wholeness as the starting point for nursing, arguing that this perspective should guide nursing as well as a conceptualization of health that incorporates the facets of illness, wellness, well-being, and disease into a larger whole. She proposes that healing is realizing inherent wholeness in the form of patterning.

Watson and Smith[5] place the frameworks of both transpersonal caring science and the science of unitary human beings under the umbrella of a unitary-transformative paradigm reflecting the "universal oneness and connectedness of all."[(p459)] Although they do not refer to wholeness in their explication of a synthesized view, they refer to the unitary nature of the universe, which is congruent, if not synonymous, with wholeness. They acknowledge "the unitary, transpersonal, evolving nature of humankind, both immanent and transcendent with the evolving universe."[(p459)] They speak of a unitary caring science that is deeply relational, transcending duality and invoking the infinite. In addition, they refer to a type of consciousness—transcending time, space, and physicality—that is "open and continuous with the evolving unitary consciousness of the universe."[(p459)]

Consciousness

Consciousness is a central concept in both Newman's and Watson and Smith's views of nursing knowledge. Newman[3] refers to the enduring concept of expanded consciousness in her synthesized view, and Watson and Smith[5] refer to caring consciousness. Newman[2] sees consciousness as information in the form of pattern and meaning and refers to meaning and consciousness as constitutive of person-environment integration. Specifically, Newman[2] subscribes to the notion of nursing as a dialogue that involves interpenetrating consciousness and uniqueness of meaning in nurse-patient experiences.[6] Watson and Smith[5] discuss consciousness and energy as integrated features of a unitary caring science. This integration "affirms a deep relational ethic and spirit, which transcend all duality, thus invoking the infinite, which in turn invites the sacred to return to our profession and our practices."[(p459)] Furthermore, they speak of "the universal field of cosmic consciousness energy."[(p459)]

Newman[3] sees caring and health as dialectic and merging with an expanding consciousness characterized by deepening meaning, insight, and new ways of relating to self and others[7]; she also refers to self-transcendence and personal transformation.[8] Watson and Smith[5] make 2 references to caring consciousness. One is a form of consciousness in which the nurse expresses a higher frequency human-environmental wave pattern than someone who is in an ordinary state of consciousness. The potential for caring consciousness is explained by integration of the principles of energy and resonance. Furthermore, caring consciousness is characterized by a transcendence of "time, space, and physicality and is open and continuous with the evolving unitary consciousness of the universe."[(p459)]

Caring

Newman[3] proposes that caring is the process through which the wholeness of human beings should be addressed—starting with wholeness in caring as a moral imperative. While historically caring has been seen as a means to a curing end, Watson and others have noted that caring is not just a means to an end, but an end in itself, thus being the highest ethical commitment one can make to self and society.

As noted earlier, caring is considered dialectically related to health and merging with expanded consciousness. For Watson and Smith,[5] the mutuality of human process is the core of caring that "potentiates the emergence of a new human-environmental energy field pattern."[(p459)] They emphasize the potential for a human-environment field pattern that is "co-created with the one-caring and the one cared-for."[(p459)] Just as caring is related to expanding consciousness, Watson and Smith[5] suggest that there is a consciousness associated with caring that transcends the perceived limits of time, space, and physical reality, and reveals a universe that is open and evolving in a unitary way. Consciousness and energy are integrated in what Watson and Smith refer to as a unitary caring science that is relational, unified, infinite, and sacred.

Newman[3] and Watson and Smith[5] also share common perspectives that include the concepts of pattern, transcendence, and transformation. They all refer to some process of relationship in describing their views, using terms such as dialogue, dialectic, relational, and mutual process or mutuality. Newman[3] places particular emphasis on meaning, although that is not evident in the synthesis suggested by Watson and Smith.[5]

Pattern

Newman[3] accepts the notion that pattern is central to nursing and congruent with the concept of wholeness. She has developed a nursing praxis that integrates theory and action in a process of pattern recognition, facilitating transformation. Pattern and meaning are the forms in which the information of consciousness expresses itself. Watson and Smith[5] refer primarily to the human-environmental energy field or wave pattern potentials for transformation, transcendence, and innovation associated with caring and caring consciousness. Pattern is viewed as a cocreation of the caring enterprise.

Transformation and Transcendence

Both Newman[3] and Watson and Smith[5] use the concepts of transformation and transcendence to describe their synthesized perspectives. They are not, however, seen as synonymous. Pattern recognition spurs transformation through the dialectics of theory and action. Newman has clearly differentiated transformation and transcendence in her writings. Transformation implies a changing of form in a literal sense, as in seeing things from a different angle. Transcendence goes above and beyond this, involving a shift to another dimension. Newman[3] subscribes to the idea that nursing has "the capacity to shift experience into a different realm,"[9(p83)] "to step into another reality"[(p85)] as in aesthetic knowing. Her writings suggest a potential relationship between personal transformation and self-transcendence occurring in expanded consciousness but they are distinct as phenomena.

Watson and Smith[5] refer to a unitary caring science that evolves from frameworks fitting within the unitary-transformative paradigm. They also differentiate between transformation and transcendence in their description of a caring moment as potentiating a new human-environmental field pattern arising from a mutual process. They depict humankind as transformative in nature and a unitary caring science that transcends all duality.

Relationship

Both Newman's[3] synthesis and Watson and Smith's[5] synthesis place emphasis on a relational ontology. For instance, Newman describes transformation as occurring with pattern recognition through the dialectics of theory and action. She refers to nursing as a mutual process manifested as dialogue. Dialogue has to do with the relationship of consciousness and meaning, which are inseparable as evidenced in encounters between nurses and patients.[6] Similarly, Watson and Smith[5] explicate a unitary caring science that "affirms a deep relational ethic and spirit."[(p459)]

Meaning

Newman[3] views meaning and consciousness as aspects of person-environment integration and considers life as essentially transcendent meaning. Nursing meanings are portrayed as unique expressions of nurse-patient encounters that interpenetrate with consciousness. Nursing connects with meaning, which is a form of informational consciousness; deepening meaning is a feature of expanded consciousness.

Expanding the Discourse

From these 2 syntheses, converging points and expanding points may be integrated into a new perspective. The picture of nursing knowledge draws on the following emerging and evolving elements:

- Nursing knowledge is grounded in the wholeness of human life, with a focus on patterning.
- Attention to consciousness in its many forms and varieties as a source of information and knowledge is requisite to recognizing and appreciating patterning.
- Caring is the process through which wholeness is addressed and which potentiates the emergence of innovative patterning and possibilities.
- Nursing science that accounts for wholeness, consciousness, and caring supports creative nursing practice centered on infinite human potentials.
- The primary goal of nursing is healing—the facilitation of transformative and transcendent life patterning consistent with wholeness and human flourishing.
- Transformation and transcendence reflect relational, dialogical, and dialectical processes congruent with a unitary, participatory world.
- The science, art, and politics of nursing call for a unitary, participatory consciousness that appreciates the wholeness of life, the reconciliation of boundaries, and the power of purpose and meaning.
- Integration of the science, art, and politics of nursing is characterized by affirmation of unitary, participatory knowing, transcendence of duality, evocation of the infinite, and the worthiness of human aspiration.

Consciousness, Wholeness, and Caring: Common Ground

We invite dialogue about the nexus of concepts emerging across nursing theories to provide a sharper, more defined focus to the discipline of nursing. Though a groundbreaking delineation of disciplinary boundaries for its time, the metaparadigm concepts of person, environment, health, and nursing require greater clarity and specificity for a new era in knowledge development in nursing. We are among others who have dwelled with the shared ideas expressed in both unitary and caring science. Newman and her colleagues'[1] seminal article on the *Focus of the Discipline* was instrumental in situating caring within the definition of the discipline. Other articles by Newman,[2,3] Watson and Smith,[5] Cowling,[10,11] and Smith[4] have noted that caring theories and unitary theories are rooted in a common ground of knowledge. in this article, we continue to dedicate ourselves to exploring and building on this common ground as the praxis of nursing. By dedicating ourselves to this nexus, we are saying that this is the evolving work of the discipline. By exploring it, we are trying to extend the connections already made ... to find deeper meaning. As we build upon it, we are creating structures and growing gardens that will support and nourish the full expression of human health. But as we dedicate, explore, and build we are not erecting fences; there will be no passports required to enter. Newman[3] has reminded us that dissolving the boundaries is a mandate that comes from living on this ground. Other nursing scholars such as Anne Boykin and Savina Schoenhofer (authors of *Nursing as Caring*),[12] Alice Davidson and Dee Ray (complexity science and caring),[13] Mary Jane Smith and Patricia Liehr (middle range theory of embracing story),[14] Chris Johns and Dawn Freshwater (reflective practice),[15] and Richard Cowling, Peggy Chinn, and Sue Hagedorn (Nursing Manifesto)[16] live comfortably here. Many of our colleagues in other disciplines are approaching this ground. Together in a spirit of collaboration we can join, work in concert, and have greater power for transforming health and life. This is the ultimate goal of this work.

Almost 20 years ago, Sarter[17] examined the commonalities across 4 nursing theories: Science of unitary Human Beings,[18] Health as Expanding Consciousness, Man-Living-Health,[20] now Human Becoming,[21] and Transpersonal Caring.[22] At the conclusion of her analysis, she identified 5 themes that constitute the development of a distinctive world view[17(p58)]: evolutionary process that portends constant change and transcendence; health as evolution or transcendence; open systems; nonlinear space-time; and pattern. Sarter noted that "These themes together form a potentially powerful ... metaphysical and epistemological foundation for the further development of nursing theories."[17(p58)] She concluded that this emergent paradigm has the potential to provide a coherent worldview from which other theories might emerge. Similarly, Newman[23] has described the unitary-transformative paradigm as "essential for full explication of the discipline."[(p5)]

In the first section of our article, Cowling took the lead in bringing together the concepts of consciousness, wholeness, and caring as a new synthesis for the discipline— providing a starting point for our dialogue. Nursing is the study of healing through caring. Healing might be described as remembering wholeness, awakening to the essential nature of human being-becoming, or finding our way home. it is grasping our interconnectedness with all there is. This happens through a shift in consciousness, which can be evolutionary or revolutionary. it happens as we discover and cocreate meaning (recognizing pattern) and care and are cared for. caring is both a way to expand consciousness (gain more information) and a reflection of expanding consciousness and the appreciation of our wholeness. These 3 concepts, consciousness, wholeness, and caring, are interrelated in a circle or triangle.

We are essentially whole beings, but our human perceptions get in the way of experiencing and realizing this. Blake said, "If the doors of perception were cleansed, everything would appear ... as it is, infinite."[24] Caring cleanses the doors of perception so that we can see ourselves and others as they are— whole. As we become more aware of this unity, and more aware of and awake to this universal oneness, we grow in caring and love for ourselves, others, and our environment. When we see ourselves as separate from others, we focus more on our differences, and it is easier to judge, label, objectify, fix, advise, intervene, and order. We may be more easily called to intolerance, conflict, apathy, and disrespect. When we see others as whole, we can marvel, appreciate, journey with, partner with, accompany, support, and facilitate. Seeing others as whole is a different ontology and a different ethical starting point. To acknowledge Levinas, we can comprehend that an "ethic of Belonging" is first principle and comes before an ontology of separation.[25] When we see self as integral with all that is, we are more likely to live life with reverence, harmony, and peace.

Caring potentiates the apprehension of wholeness. We develop sensitized ways of knowing that can more readily take in the pattern of the whole and appreciate it.[10] We have no desire to change the other because we respect the other as whole in the moment. Through caring, others can heal or come to recognize their integral nature, who they really are. REMEMBER WHO YOU ARE!!! This is the message of caring for others... remember who you are. I see you are whole ... remember who you are!

There is a synergistic relationship between consciousness and caring. Caring deepens with expanding consciousness, and growth in caring reflects expanding consciousness. Watson and Smith[5] spoke of a unique energy pattern that characterizes the expression of caring as a higher frequency pattern. The vibrational quality is different and perceptible. It has a coherent quality and can entrain other fields. Caring consciousness is characterized by nonjudgment, focus, presence in the now, and wisdom. It can also be noted that as we evolve in our consciousness, we can acknowledge that the highest level of consciousness is love and joy, allowing for a convergence between caring consciousness and love to return to our work and our world.

In 1998, Smith[4] described unitary caring. The concept was developed on the basis of reviewing the philosophical and theoretical literature on caring in nursing, identifying meanings from this body of literature, and classifying and naming them within a unitary perspective. A decade later, it is important to reflect on this anew and begin to develop theory-practice connections for unitary caring. If we embrace a model of caring from a unitary perspective, we need to delineate the essential ontological competencies[19] that emerge from it. The term *ontological competencies* has been used by Watson,[26] who refers to ontological artistry as the creative work in nursing that reflects the sacred acts of caring and healing. Ontological caring competencies are foundational to the expression of the artistry. They are ontological in that they emerge from the fundamental nature of caring-healing praxis. These are authentic nursing competencies.[26(p231)]

Analysis of the concept of unitary caring reveals 5 constituent meanings: manifesting intentions, attuning to dynamic flow, appreciating pattern,[10] experiencing the infinite, and inviting creative emergence. These are discussed below, with the ontological competencies related to them.

Manifesting intention has been defined as creating, holding, and expressing thoughts, images, feelings, beliefs, desires, will, and actions that affirm the possibilities for human betterment or well-being. Intentions reflect our consciousness; they are meaningful energetic blueprints for transformation.[4] What I hold in my heart matters and makes a difference. My thoughts, feelings, and imaginings are shared in a mutual field. From this point of view, the nurse is the healing environment and creator of sacred space.[27] The ontological caring competencies, revealed as "caring literacy," associated with manifesting intention are self-reflection, cultivating stillness, receptivity, imagination and reverie, focusing attention, energetically creating space, recalling the sense of compassion or agape, centering, and expressing intention through touch or energy work. How do we nurture these ontological competencies in education and practice? We invite nurses into and engage them with centering exercises, spiritual practices such as meditation, mantram repetition, wilderness/nature experiences, and artistic forms that are inspirational and evocative. Rituals can embody these intentions so they are structured in the daily work of nursing praxis. For example, Watson[28] describes *hand washing* as a ritual of centering in which the nurse pauses to cleanse herself of anything she is bringing to the room that may interfere with her presence with the person. It is a time to breathe and focus, perhaps using a chosen mantram to focus attention.[29] Nurses might develop rituals for giving report or handing off patient responsibilities that signify the sacred duty to care. Every nurse needs to learn how to connect more deeply to a source of wisdom, love, and compassion that becomes the fountain from which all nursing actions flow.

Appreciating pattern comes from Cowling[10] and Krieger's[30] work. Cowling describes this as discovery in the service of knowing wholeness and essence. It involves valuing the other, being in awe of our infinite diversity and unity, confirming the worth of the person, and seeing the other as perfect in the moment.[10] Cowling describes the process of approaching knowing of the other with gratitude and enjoyment. This contrasts with the clinical, objective approach of searching for problems and pathology for the purpose of labeling and classifying. Appreciating pattern involves knowing the other, using our entire being, our sensory and extrasensory awareness, as instruments to grasp the whole. It is hearing the life story of the other.[14] Pattern is reflected in meaning, so finding out what is meaningful to the other becomes primary in knowing the other's pattern. Perhaps the first question that we ask our patients should be, "What is important to you right now? What matters to you right now?"[31] Rather than beginning and ending with the traditional history, the nurse practitioner might seek to understand the life story of the patient. This is part of the praxis developed by both Cowling[11] and Newman.[2] The ontological literacy competencies for appreciating pattern are pattern seeing, listening, grasping the essence, learning to appreciate the arts, hermeneutic-dialectical interpretation, and valuing diversity. Nurses might be asked to create a patient profile that reflects the wholeness of the person, different from and complementary to the patient history. As advocate for the client, the nurse may be the one responsible for presenting the patient to others as whole. The nurse might request photographs that capture the essence of the person, or brief descriptions of the person from the person or family members; these could be displayed on a bulletin board in the patient's room or in the patient record. Seeing and hearing about patients' unique patterns, hobbies, family, work, etc., make it less likely that they will be objectified or dehumanized and increase the possibility that they will be engaged as partners in care.

Attuning to dynamic flow is dancing to the rhythms within a continuous mutual process. It is the vibrational sensing of where to place focus and attention and involves attuning to the subtleties that present themselves in the moment, being sensitive to self and other. It is following the lead of the other, going where that person is leading. An example of this is presented in the poem by Marilyn Krysl *Sunshine Acres Living Center* [see sidebar]. In this poem, the nurse meets the stubborn, cantankerous Mr Polansky by finding a point of common interest. She is open to the flow, accepting Mr Polansky for who he is and cocreating who they can be together. Attuning is searching for the points of connection to facilitate relationship. Liz Lerman is a choreographer, who does amazing work with a lay dance company in New York that interprets community experiences and stories in dance. When her uncle was dying, Liz was visiting him and her aunt, who was with him in the hospital room.[32] Close to death, he was moving his arms in the air around him in what seemed to be a disorganized, random pattern. Conventional wisdom might have led some to sedate him for agitation. Liz saw the dance and held her uncle's hands, moving her hands with his, following his lead in this dance of transition. She left to go home and later heard of her uncle's death. Her aunt shared with Liz that she had taken over when Liz left, and she danced with her husband through his journey to death.[27] The ontological competencies for this attuning to dynamic flow are sensing, hearing and moving with rhythms, presensing, and focusing. These competencies might be developed through drumming, dancing, singing, listening to and writing poetry, and listening to and reading stories. They involve listening for shifts or pauses, and all forms of language that suggest meaning.

Experiencing the infinite is the pandimensional awareness of coextensiveness with the universe occurring in the context of human relating.[4] It is a transcendence of time, space, and self, and has been described as similar to a mystical experience or a spiritual union. Watson has called it the actual caring occasion when past and future merge in the present moment.[22] Time stands still and the present is experienced as all there is. There is a sense of unity, a lack of separateness of self and environment. The ontological competencies for this are cultivating a spiritual practice or a practice that fosters deep reflection. This could be meditation, prayer, centering, being in nature, walking a labyrinth, or developing rituals that honor the sacredness of nursing practice. At times, we fail to recognize the extraordinary in the ordinary day-to-day practice of nursing. Telling our stories to each other, the mysteries and miracles of a compassionate practice, can help us appreciate and bear witness to their presence.

Inviting creative emergence reflects the transformative potential of caring and faith in expanding consciousness.[4] All exists as possibility, and this way of being illuminates the landscape of possibilities. The nurse becomes a midwife, birthing the emergence of new patterns. The nurse illuminates choices, options, and other ways of being that might never have been considered, or engages the person, family, community in examining options in light of their values. The ontological competencies associated with this include coaching, listening, sharing interpretations, and affirming new growth. These might be nurtured through activities such as gardening, playing, coaching, and making art.

Summary

In summary, this article seeks to bring convergence and coherence to nursing knowledge and praxis. By positing unity of wholeness, consciousness, and caring as both higher order and deeper order concepts, it moves nursing closer to its ethical and ontological foundations. Embedded within these unitary concepts are new horizons for unitary caring practices, informed by the 5 constituent meanings of caring that Smith[4] gleaned from a unitary lens, that is, manifesting intentions, attuning to dynamic flow, appreciating

pattern, experiencing the infinite, and inviting creative emergence.

Within this view of nursing and unitary caring, we invite wisdom and love back into our work and our world. We are reminded again that "what we hold in our heart matters" and informs our intentions and our consciousness.

Thus, we have a new lens or "theoria" "to see differently" through a unitary caring science view of nursing (theoria—Latin for theory; meaning "to see"). Through this new "theoria" lens of unitary caring science, we find ways to cultivate "ontological competencies" or caring consciousness literacy. This new praxis model invites new visions of hope and informed actions.

Ideals and ideas for "ontological literacy" can lead in time to "ontological design practices." These practices see differently—they see and honor the whole person in a way that affirms the possibilities for individuals and humanity; they offer new energetic heartfelt blueprints for transformation and new fields of mutuality, whereby the nurse becomes the healing environment, the creator of sacred space, holding self and other in their wholeness. As noted above, other ontological practices evoke self-reflection, stillness, receptivity, imagination, inner harmony, peace, and even reverie—energetically focusing our consciousness toward caring, compassion, intentional touch, and, yes, an openness to the infinity of love.

Finally, as nursing awakens to this higher/deeper place of wholeness, consciousness, and caring, as it seeks to synthesize new ethical and intellectual forms and norms of "ontological caring literacy," we arrive at a unitary caring science praxis. We evolve as a mature caring-healing-health discipline and profession, helping affirm and sustain humanity, caring, and wholeness in our daily work and in the world.

A Postreview Consideration

Often reviewers direct authors to substantial concerns in the grounding of scholarship that are not given attention in manuscripts. In our case, 2 substantive concerns worthy of consideration were raised in the review process. We appreciate the willingness of the editor of the *ANS* to give us an opportunity to address these concerns in a rather unconventional way.

First, the reviewer pointed out accurately that the current state of the discipline of nursing is one in which major issues of institutionalized racism, classism, ethnocentricity, and extremes of poverty exist. The review challenges what may be considered patronizing and conservative language in our article and posits that clients may be uncomfortable with phrases like nurses being their "healing space," "healing environment," and "creator of sacred space" as well as "higher," "deeper," and "blueprints for transformation." These are valid concerns worthy of thoughtful attention. The reviewer suggests that these choices of language may be inadvertent. We do not feel that we can excuse them in this way. Intentions cannot substitute for action; however, we consider this a serious call for deeper reflection, not a call for automatic change of language to accommodate publication. At the same time, it must be said that much of the pain and suffering from social injustices comes from a lack of consideration of the deeply human connections that unite, rather than separate and divide us: a lack of caring. The convergence of these ideas of "deeper"/"higher" and so forth invites us to honor the human to human-human cosmos connection in which we all dwell for shared existence. As Palmer[33] noted in his description of epistemology as ethic, in our language and worldview we can insert a form of superiority of public domain over the human private, and intimate, inner lifeworld, creating a violence associated with violating the human dignity, the integrity of the other, whether the other is the earth, another human being, another culture, another race, another gender, another lifestyle, living situation, and so on. In our work here we seek to honor our shared humanity, not to turn our face away from others just because they are different, but rather to face these human realities. These concerns require us to take on the issues raised by the reviewer as major points for dialogue to advance our work in line with a more critical and emancipatory position. More will come from this.

A related concern was "what if a client's wholeness does not appear whole as a nurse expects whole to appear." This concern warrants a direct response since a central thesis of our position is that human wholeness is a given—regardless of the form in which it expresses itself. We submit that a lack of acknowledgment of human wholeness as inherent is responsible for many of the injustices made to individuals and groups in the name of "healing as to make whole." We posit that healing is appreciating the wholeness of human life—a position that disrupts the tendency of nurses to limit the possibilities of human choices and expressions of health.

Sunshine Acres Living Center

The first thing you see up ahead is Mr.
Polanski, wedged in the
arched doorway, like he means absolutely
to stay there, he who shouldn't
be here in the first place, put in here
by mistake, courtesy of that grandson
who thinks himself a hotshot, and too busy
raking in the dough to find time for an old

man. If Polanski had anyplace
to go, he'd be out
instantly, if he had any
money. Which he doesn't, but he does have
a sharp eye, and intends to stay in that
doorway, not missing
a thing, and waiting
for trouble. Which of course
will come. And could be
you-you're handy, you look
likely, you have
the authority. And
you're new here, another young
whippersnapper, doesn't know
ass from elbow, but has been given
the keys. Well he's
ready, *Polanski. Mr. Polanski, good
morning*—you say it in Polish,
which you learned a little of
when you were little, and your grandmother
taught you a little song about lambs, frisking
in a pen, and you danced a silly little dance
with your grandmother, while the two of you
sang. So you sing it
for him, here in the dim, institutional
light of the hallway, light which even you
find insupportable, because even those who just
work here, and can leave when their
shift ends, deserve light to
see by, and because it reminds you
of the light in the hallway
outside the room
where, when your grandmother
died, you were three thousand miles
away. So that you're singing the little song
and remembering the silly little dance
to console yourself, and to pay your
        grandmother
tribute, and to try to charm Polanski,
which you do: you sing, and Mr. Polanski,
he who had set himself against the doorjamb
to resist you, he who made of himself
a fist, Mr. Polanski,
contentious, often
combative and always
and finally
inconsolable
hears that you know
the song. And he steps out
from the battlement
of the doorway, and begins to
shuffle
and sing along.

—M. Krysl[34]

REFERENCES

1. Newman MA. Experiencing the whole. *Adv Nurs Sci.* 1997;20(1):34–39.
2. Newman MA. The pattern that connects. *Adv Nurs Sci.* 2002;24(3):1–7.
3. Newman MA. A world of no boundaries. *Adv Nurs Sci.* 2003;26(4):240–245.
4. Smith MC. Caring and the science of unitary human beings. *Adv Nurs Sci.* 1999;21(4):14–28.
5. Watson J, Smith MC. Caring science and the science of unitary human beings. *J Adv Nurs.* 2002;37(5):452–461.
6. Bowers R, Moore KN. Bakhtin, nursing narratives, and dialogical consciousness. *Adv Nurs Sci.* 1997;19(3):70–77.
7. Pharris MD. Coming to know ourselves as community through a nursing partnership with adolescents convicted of murder. *Adv Nurs Sci.* 2002;24(3):21–42.
8. Neill J. Transcendence and transformation in the life patterns of women living with rheumatoid arthritis. *Adv Nurs Sci.* 2002;24(4):27–47.
9. Chinn PL, Maeve MK, Bostick C. Aesthetic inquiry and the art of nursing … including commentary by Johnson JL. *Sch Inq Nurs Pract.* 1997;11(2):83–100.
10. Cowling WR III. A template for unitary pattern-based practice. In: Barrett EAM, ed. *Visions of Rogers' Science-Based Nursing.* New York, NY: NLN Publishing; 1990: 45–65.
11. Cowling WR III. A unitary-participatory vision of nursing knowledge. *Adv Nurs Sci.* 2007;30(1):61–70.
12. Boykin A, Schoenhofer S. *Nursing as Caring: A Model for Transforming Practice.* Sudbury, MA: Jones & Bartlett Publishers; 2001.
13. Davidson AW Ray MA. Studying the human-environment phenomenon using the science of complexity. *Adv Nurs Sci.* 1991;14(2):73–87.
14. Smith MJ, Liehr P. Attentively embracing story: a middle-range theory with practice and research implications … including commentary by Reed PG. *Sch Inq Nurs Pract.* 1999;13(3):187–210.
15. Johns C, Freshwater D. *Transforming Nursing Through Reflective Practice.* London: Blackwell; 2005.
16. Cowling WR III, Chinn PL, Hagedorn S. The nurse manifesto. http://nursemanifest.com. Published 2000. Accessed July 7, 2007.
17. Sarter B. Philosophical sources of nursing theory. *Nurs Sci Q.* 1988;1(2):52–59.
18. Rogers ME. *An Introduction to the Theoretical Basis of Nursing.* Philadelphia, PA: Davis; 1970.
19. Newman MA. *Health as Expanding Consciousness.* Sudbury, MA: Jones and Bartlet (NLN Press); 1994.
20. Parse RR. *Man-Living-Health: A Theory of Nursing.* New York, NY: John Wiley & Sons; 1981.
21. Parse RR. *The Human Becoming School of Thought.* Thousand Oaks, CA: Sage; 1988.
22. Watson J. *Nursing: Human Science and Human Care.* Norwalk, CT: Appleton-Century-Crofts; 1985.
23. Newman MA, Sime AM, Corcoran-Perry SA. The focus of the discipline of nursing. *Adv Nurs Sci.* 1991;14(1):1–6.
24. Blake W. *The Marriage of Heaven and Hell.* London: Trianon Press; 1960.
25. Levinas E. *Totally and Infinitely.* Pittsburgh, PA: Duquesne University; 1969.
26. Watson J. *Postmodern Nursing and Beyond.* Edinburgh, Scotland: Churchill Livingstone; 1999.
27. Quinn JF. Holding sacred space: the nurse as healing environment. *Holist Nurs Pract.* 1992;6(4):26– 36.
28. Watson J. *Caring Science as Sacred Science.* Philadelphia, PA: FA Davis; 2004.
29. Bormann JE, Smith TL, Becker S, et al. Efficacy of frequent mantram repetition on stress, quality of life, and spiritual well-being in veterans: a pilot study. *J HolistNurs.* 2005;23(4):395–414.
30. Krieger D. *The Therapeutic Touch: How to Use the Hands to Help or Heal.* Englewood Cliffs, NJ: Prentice Hall; 1979.
31. Boykin A, Schoenhofer S. Anne Boykin and Savina O. Schoenhofer's nursing as caring theory. In: Parker M, ed. *Nursing Theories and Nursing Practice.* Philadelphia, PA: FA Davis; 2006:334–348.
32. Lerman L. Are miracles enough? Conflict, healing, and the challenge of colliding truths. Paper presented at: Florida Atlantic University; April 18, 2007; Boca Raton, FL.
33. Palmer PJ. The violence of our knowledge: toward a spirituality of higher education. In: *21st Century Learning Initiatives.* Kalamazoo, MI: Fetzer Institute; 2004. http://www.21learn.org/arch/articles/palmer_spirituality.html.
34. Krysl M. Sunshine acres living center. In: *Midwife and Other Poems on Caring.* New York: National League for Nursing; 1989:35–36.

THE AUTHORS COMMENT | The Power of Wholeness, Consciousness, and Caring: A Dialogue on Nursing Science, Art, and Healing

The inspiration for this article arose from a desire to bring together our thinking regarding the nature of nursing grounded in wholeness, consciousness, and caring as recurring contemporary themes in nursing theory. I was joined in a dialogue at a conference with Marlaine Smith, Jean Watson, and Margaret Newman in which I proposed a synthesis of these themes and they responded by illuminating and elucidating the ideas. I believe that the article that emerged from this dialogue contributes to nursing theory in creating a cross-fertilization of ideology arising from conceptual and theoretical viewpoints that have arisen from the extensive work of praxis scholars in nursing. While it does not fully address the scope of nursing science, art, and healing, it serves to evoke dialogue and inspire deeper understanding of the nature of nursing as a healing phenomenon.

W. RICHARD COWLING III
MARLAINE C. SMITH
JEAN WATSON

A Multiparadigm Approach to Nursing

JOAN C. ENGEBRETSON, RN, DrPH, AHN-BC

Nursing theory development has made good progress in differentiating the domain of nursing from medicine; many of these theories are categorized as holistic theories. Nursing classification systems are also being developed to organize extant nursing practice. The dissonance between the two has been one of the most difficult contemporary issues for the leadership of nursing. A framework is proposed that would account for these disparate approaches. This proposed framework for the domain of healing is in keeping with the metaparadigm of health and uses a multiple paradigm approach. Nursing interventions are discussed in relation to the framework. It invites a dialogue in keeping with the scholarship of holism. Practice and scholarship implications are discussed.

Nursing theory has, since the 1960s, sought to define the profession of nursing and to differentiate its scope of practice from that of biomedicine.[1] This search has led to some discrepancies between theory development that differentiates nursing action from biomedical nursing practice, the latter of which uses many nursing actions derived from biomedicine. Differentiating autonomous nursing practice was a necessary step, because historically many nursing functions were derived from biomedicine, since nurses have practiced in biomedically dominated settings.

One primary differentiating feature was holism, which was contrasted with biomedical reductionism. The movement to declare nursing holistic is now well accepted; however, a holistic framework must be inclusive of, not only differentiated from, biomedicine. In alignment with holism, the appropriate construct for the nursing profession is healing. Health is a derivative of healing, or making whole, and part of the metaparadigm of nursing.

Another element of professional evolution is the development of diagnostic, intervention, and outcomes classifications systems. These are often grounded in nursing practice and thus reflect both nursing activities as well as predominant sociocultural ideologies. There is often a disjuncture between the differentiating and defining theories and the more pragmatic classifications systems.[2] In an effort to reconcile grand conceptual models and practice, this article presents a conceptual framework for discussion as a step toward the consolidation of a holistic approach to nursing. The intent is to support both unique autonomous actions and to incorporate medically derived actions. Using the construct of healing, a multiparadigm model is presented to incorporate both the medical model and other cultural healing models on which nurses may ground their actions. This integration is at the level of paradigm, which allows the incorporation of and expansion beyond the biomedical model and avoids the pitfalls of the derivative-differentiation polarity.

Nursing has over the past 30 years made great strides in the development of nursing theories and conceptual models. These activities have been necessary to define the professional domain to its members and to society at large. Theory guides the practice and the activities that are unique to the profession, informs research efforts, and provides direction for future development.[3]

Contemporary Controversies

Despite the progress made, the use of nursing theories in practice has been a matter of controversy. One area of controversy is the dichotomy between medicine and nursing, with many theories focusing on unique nursing functions and in some cases redefining actions associated with medical models. This position has often still held the medical model as the orthodox standard against which nursing defined itself by negation or differentiation, thereby maintaining dependence on the medical model.

Closely related to the nursing-medicine dichotomy is the rupture between academia and practice.

ABOUT THE AUTHOR

JOAN C. ENGEBRETSON was born in Wisconsin, on November 12, 1943, and grew up in Minnesota. She received a BSN from St. Olaf College, an MS from Texas Woman's University, and a DrPH from the University of Texas Health Science Center at Houston School of Public Health. She worked as a public health nurse both in Oakland, CA, and Boston, MA, and has been a faculty member at University of St. Thomas, Houston, TX. In 1985, she joined the University of Texas Health Science Center at Houston and holds a joint appointment at the UT Health School of Public Health. In 2010, she was appointed to the Judy Fred Professorship in Nursing. Her clinical focus has been maternal-child and women's health. Her academic focus includes health promotion, culture, theory, and qualitative methodologies in research. Her research has included the development of a pacifier for low-birth-weight infants, women's anticipations of hormonal therapy for perimenopause, ethnographic studies of healing, clinical trials of Reiki Touch therapy, patient's beliefs and experiences related to chronic diseases, and the incorporation of complementary therapies and approaches to healing. Her primary focus is related to a better understanding of various perspectives and strategies of healing that nurses can incorporate into patient care to promote health throughout the health-illness continuum. Throughout her life, she has developed interests in travel, cooking, reading, and photography.

Academia and much of theory development focused on the autonomous nature of nursing, differentiating it from medicine. Extant nursing practice often eschewed the nursing theories learned in school, and practicing nurses functioned in a more pragmatic manner reflective of the medical model.[4] Many times the praxis of nursing is covertly, if not overtly, aligned with the medical model. This alliance with the medical model is understandable considering the hegemony of the medical bioscientific model in U.S. culture. Barnum[4] noted that normative theory evolves from practice rather than academic theory development and that inconsistencies develop when practice (theory) is not intellectually analyzed and scrutinized according to logical coherence.

A third, related problem area is the disjuncture between nursing theories and the diagnosis, intervention, and outcome classification systems. The two strongest competitors in the theory business are holistic theories and nursing process,[1,4] which often represent opposing philosophies regarding content, methodology, and interpretation. Holistic theories are global, espouse a transcendental view of humans, and are committed to not viewing subject matter as an accumulation of parts.[4]

Nursing process approaches are much more concrete and practice based and have focused on nursing action and classification systems.[5] The International Council of Nurses,[6] the Omaha Project,[7] the Iowa Project,[8] and separate projects by Grobe[9] and Saba[10] have recently developed nursing classification systems.

Recent debates in nursing have also reflected controversies over the usefulness of a unified theory vs multiple theories. Reed[11] proposed an approach that links science, philosophy, and practice in the development of nursing knowledge. She advocated a metanarrative that involves a dialogue of practice and philosophy. This metanarrative provides an excellent format for the development of nursing theory that is holistic in nature and can integrate multiple paradigms from the patient's perspective and from the nurse. It is in this spirit of inviting a dialogue and providing a format for a dialectic discussion between paradigms that the author presents the multiparadigm model.

Holism and Nursing

Grand theory, or the concept level of theory development, has evolved into a metaparadigm with four propositional statements related to the concepts person-health, person-environment, health-nursing, and person-environment-health.[12] The global level defines the frameworks within which the more restricted structures develop.

Consistent with the concept heal—health, the related ideologies for nursing theory development would come from healing, rather than be restricted to medicine. Healing and health stem from the root word *hale*, or to make whole.[13] This etymology grounds the concept heal—health in holism. Barnum[4] identified holistic theories as the fastest growing trend in nursing. Holistic concepts in nursing have been evident since the time of Florence Nightingale and evolved in nursing theories through the influence of Teilhard de Chardin, Jan Smuts, and Ludwig von Bertalanffy.[14] Anthropology, another discipline based on holism, provides another source of information on healing that can inform nurses in the development of holistic theory. Traditionally, in many cultures, healers, shamans, and medicine people reflected the broader concept of healing rather than the science-based concept of cure.

Holistic health has recently become very popular among both lay and professional groups. Characteristics of holistic health have been described in many studies.[15–19] Two common mistakes occur in the analysis of holism from a modernist perspective based in a scientific or reductionistic paradigm. Alster's[15] analysis of holistic health is an example of such an attempt; it reaches the syllogistic conclusion that holistic health cannot be studied scientifically because it is not scientific.

The opposite pitfall is to romanticize traditional or primitive healing systems and unfavorably compare science and biomedicine. This antiscience position is often seen in lay literature that attributes all social ills to scientific–rational thinking while extolling a holistic framework as the alternative. A consistent holistic framework incorporates science but does not hold that paradigm as sufficient for explaining the human experience or for bringing about health or healing. The model proposed in this article recognizes the holistic nature of nursing and expands the domain from disease treatment to the broader concept of health by incorporating several paradigms and their adjunctive ideological perspectives on humans, health, and therapeutic actions.

Historical Context of Western Medicine

Healing systems reflect and influence the cultural values of the parent culture. Contemporary biomedicine has been informed by and influential in the development of modernism. Modernity had its philosophical origins in the 17th century with the emphasis on rationality by the protagonists Galileo and Descartes.[20] Kuhn[21] described the shift of vision that enabled people to see and think about phenomena in a different manner and that he labeled a "paradigm shift." Modernity is characterized by the development of science and technology, the valorization of reason and humanity's dominion over nature. The scientific paradigm of modernity has dominated medicine and health care.

The establishment of the scientific model as the foundation for biomedicine paralleled the development of modernity. The scientific paradigm is characterized by philosophical dualism between the material and nonmaterial, and the corresponding designation of matter as the subject of science and the nonmaterial or metaphysical as the domain of religion. Descartes

is often credited with conceptualizing the mind–body dualism and the corresponding value of the mind–soul as the superior demarcation of the human.

Throughout the following centuries, especially in England, increasing cultural value was placed on the scientific, material, rational, and technical.[22,23] Metaphysical and nonmaterial issues associated with religion were progressively devalued, especially among intellectuals.[24] Medicine, which historically had been based in a metaphysical model and supported by religion, became the domain of science and was severed from its metaphysical and religious roots. This split allowed medicine to make unprecedented technological advances through the application of scientific reason. But a contemporary surge of public interest in alternative healing modalities suggests that the biomedical scientific approach by itself is insufficient for healing.

Development of the Multiparadigm Model

The multiparadigm model was developed from the author's ethnographic work with healers and nurses. Field work, including participant observation, long interviews, free listing, and pile sorts, was used in a study exploring and comparing the conceptual frameworks of health and healing between nurses and healers.[25] A matrix of healing modalities that incorporated biomedicine and examples of alternative models emerging in the United States in the late 1980s and early 1990s was developed to focus the study on healers using healing touch[26] and used to orient nurse practitioners to alternative healing modalities that their clients might be using.[27]

This matrix was then developed into the Heterodox Explanatory Paradigms Model for health practice that incorporated multiple healing modalities.[28] The philosophical coherence of the model and the related positioning of modalities was presented as a framework for developing integrated health care models. Because nurses and healers have similar conceptual frameworks of healing,[25] this model could be adapted for nursing as a possible framework toward a more holistic model.

Philosophical Design

The multiparadigm model (Fig. 47-1) developed from the author's previous work[25–28] represents a multiparadigm approach to healing. Philosophical dualism between the material and nonmaterial is represented on both axes. Four paradigms of healing are incorporated and philosophically arranged from the most

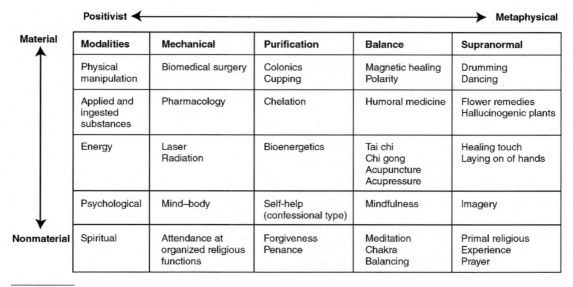

| | Positivist ← | | | → Metaphysical | |

Figure 47-1 *Explanatory paradigms.*

material to the most nonmaterial along the horizontal axis, which represents a philosophical continuum from logical positivism to metaphysics. Consistent with the positivist– metaphysical continuum, the mechanical paradigm is on the extreme left, reflecting the logical positivism of its philosophical scientific foundation. The paradigms are progressively more nonmaterial, ending in the most metaphysical paradigm, supranormal, at the extreme right. The vertical axis represents the Cartesian body–mind dualism in healing activities. Activities that are most material or physical are at the top. Moving down, activities become progressively less material and more psychological or spiritual.

Horizontal Axis

The four paradigms are mechanical, purification, balance, and supranormal. The mechanical paradigm is best represented by examples from biomedicine, which is primarily a mechanistic, materialistic paradigm exemplified by the focus on discovering explanatory mechanisms to understand a healing activity. The positivist philosophy bases knowing on objective, material data perceived by the senses.[29] It is characterized by determinism, mechanism, and reductionism. Disease is assumed to be reducible to disordered body functions and a disease-specific etiology.[30] Treatment and intervention are disease specific.

The purification paradigm has examples cross-culturally and throughout Western history. This paradigm is characterized by healing actions that cleanse or purify. The name of the prestigious English medical journal *Lancet* is a remnant of the bloodletting and purges that dominated Western medicine before

technical advances in surgery and antibiotics in the 20th century. Health and healing activities related to cleanliness or purification either physically or symbolically have been documented in many ritual practices.[31] The hygienic health reform movement of the late 19th century[32,33] incorporated many practices that were understood as cleansing and keeping the body pure.

The balance paradigm is best represented by Eastern or humeral systems. In Eastern systems health–healing is viewed as the proper balance of yin and yang and unimpeded flow of Chi (or Ki or Qi).[34] Humeral medicine, or the balance of vital forces or humors, is evident in Hippocratic, Galenic, and Ayurvedic medicine.[35] Nineteenth-century vitalism also incorporated this approach. Health is attained or maintained by creating a balance in daily living through types of foods, activities, temperature, and so forth. Personality types, environment, and circumstances are considered in determining the corrective balance. One example is the hot and cold classification in Mexican folk medicine. The balance paradigm is on the right half of the model and therefore cannot be fully understood through a materialist mechanistic paradigm.

The supranormal paradigm incorporates all magicoreligious and psychic phenomena used to promote health or create healing. Spiritual, symbolic, and other nonmaterial understandings of healing are in this column. The supranormal paradigm is philosophically the most metaphysical, going beyond physics, sense experience, or any discipline and involving ultimates.[36] This paradigm incorporates psychic, spiritual, and other types of healing such as prayer, distant healing, and other spontaneous healing that cannot be explained by mechanistic models or one of the other paradigms.

(Figure 47-1 table)

Modalities	Mechanical	Purification	Balance	Supranormal
Physical manipulation	Biomedical surgery	Colonics Cupping	Magnetic healing Polarity	Drumming Dancing
Applied and ingested substances	Pharmacology	Chelation	Humoral medicine	Flower remedies Hallucinogenic plants
Energy	Laser Radiation	Bioenergetics	Tai chi Chi gong Acupuncture Acupressure	Healing touch Laying on of hands
Psychological	Mind–body	Self-help (confessional type)	Mindfulness	Imagery
Spiritual	Attendance at organized religious functions	Forgiveness Penance	Meditation Chakra Balancing	Primal religious Experience Prayer

(Material at top of vertical axis, Nonmaterial at bottom)

Vertical Axis

The vertical axis describes types of healing activities that progress along the continuum from body to mind–soul, from material to nonmaterial. The first row contains physical manipulations, and examples are given for each paradigm. Physical manipulation may be performed either by the patient or on the patient by a healer.

In row 2 applied and ingested substances are listed according to each paradigm. Such substances include all foods, herbs, and pharmaceuticals that are ingested, inhaled, or topically applied.

Using energy, the third activity, is a concept that is poorly understood in biomedicine but important in other paradigms. Many healing activities are understood and conducted as an active manipulation of energy. The concept of energy, or the transfer from matter to energy to matter, has been proposed by some scientists (eg, Bohm, Capra[37]) as the basis for quantum physics and as a possible link in understanding the material and nonmaterial worlds. This could be a promising area in linking the material, physical body with nonmaterial thought, spirit, and so on. The concept of energy has been proposed by some nurses as the basis for understanding the benefits of touch therapies.[38–40]

Psychological activities deal with functions of cognition and of the mind. Mind to body medicine has been a rapidly growing area of research. With the discovery of neurotransmitters and hormonal–neural pathways, mechanisms have been discovered by which thoughts and feelings can manifest in physiological changes.[41] Theory has been developed and researched regarding the association of personality characteristics with illness, in particular hostility and heart disease.[42] Psychoneuroimmunology is another promising field where theory is developing. Associations have been demonstrated between various personality characteristics and mortality and morbidity.[43, 44]

Spiritual activities are at the polar opposite of the continuum from physical manipulation. Spiritual actions are distinct from cognitive activities. Spirituality, being the most distant from the physical or material, is the least understood from a modernist perspective. Some studies have found that attendance at religious activities is related to improved health or healing.[45] Attendance at religious activities represents a mechanistic conceptualization of spiritual activity, whereas a primal spiritual experience as described by Cox[46] would be a more metaphysical approach.

The model has, at present, four paradigms, but others could be added along the continuum. Restriction to a two-dimensional format is often interpreted as containing mutually exclusive cells. A more appropriate geographic conceptualization would be as general areas on a double-axis continuum, with no specific boundary between areas. Modalities in the model are examples only, and many other modalities could fit in each location. The modalities describe healing activities only. An individual practitioner–healer could, and often does, use many modalities.

The positioning of modalities according to philosophical continuums also reflects the degree of passivity or activity of the healer. Starting from the upper left corner, where the modalities are most material, the healer is most active and the recipient most passive. Moving diagonally down and across, the person who is healing is progressively more active and the role of the healer increasingly that of facilitator, consistent with healing philosophy, which posits that real healing is done by the "healee."

One area that is a vital part of the nursing metaparadigm and other healing systems is the environment, especially social relationships. Although not specifically addressed in the model, an additional line at the bottom could be added to address social activities.

 ## Application to Nursing

The multiparadigm model is holistic and avoids the medicine-nursing and practice-academia dichotomies by placing the Western biomedical model in context with other paradigms of healing. It speaks to the domain of healing, which is the stated domain of nursing. This model can provide a framework for nursing diagnoses and interventions that easily integrates biomedical model functions with complementary functions that either are autonomous nursing activities or might constitute appropriate referrals. The model also incorporates paradigms that can be useful in understanding cross-cultural healing practices and systems.

 ## Implications for Practice

Operating from a multiparadigm model allows nurses to adapt whatever paradigm or modality fits the situation. This flexibility is helpful in working with patients who practice health- and healing-related activities from other paradigms. A multiparadigm approach that incorporates models of health–healing can help providers better understand beliefs and practices of patients that may be poorly comprehended in the biomedical model.

Most health practices originate in the popular sector,[47] which includes family and social networks. This sector has beliefs about health maintenance and hierarchies of resort that direct types of health–healing activities, healer consultants, and adherence to treatments. The orientation of the popular sector often incorporates other paradigms than the scientific–mechanistic approach of biomedicine. By understanding the explanatory paradigm of health practices, the practitioner is better able to communicate and collaborate with the client and family in the management of health–healing.

Many interventions listed in the various nursing classification systems may be positioned in this model. Examples from one of these systems, the Nursing Interventions Classification (NIC),[8] have been identified in Fig. 47-2, along with other modalities that could be referral sources for the client. Examples are easily placed in the mechanistic and purification paradigms but more difficult to place in the balance and supranormal paradigms. Thus, the model can display areas where nursing has developed actions and where referrals are more appropriate. It is important to note that a holistic paradigm is impossible to implement in its entirety by any one person or discipline; therefore, nurses should be able to understand how other providers fit into an overall plan of care.

By understanding these modalities through the appropriate paradigm, practitioners may select whatever modality is appropriate for the client, either by interventions or referral to other providers. For example, existing NIC actions in the mechanical paradigm for physical manipulation could incorporate positioning, exercise therapy including range of motion, and ambulation. Applied and ingested substances include medication administration of all types. Although energy is poorly understood in the mechanical model, it is present on the NIC as laser precautions. Energy, if better understood, could have potential for much broader use.

Psychological interventions in the mechanical (medical) model include cognitive restructuring and reality therapies. Spiritual interventions may include assisting a patient with religious practices such as attending chapel or praying. This is not specifically listed in NIC but is covered under activity therapy.

Examples of nursing actions in the purification paradigm using physical manipulation include bathing and other hygiene activities. Wound and bladder irrigations are good examples of applied and ingested substances. Many medications have cleaning or purification action, such as emetics, expectorants, and purgatives. Psychological and emotional catharsis are examples of psychological purification. These are not specifically listed, although could be covered under the NIC active listening.

Spiritual purification includes a number of rituals that serve to purify and cleanse the individual, such as confession, seeking of forgiveness, ritual bathing, and use of incense. These would need to be developed or referred because there is no NIC entry related to this.

Nursing interventions are being expanded into the balance and supranormal paradigms through the work of nurses who have expanded their individual practice and those who are using many of the more recent nursing theories, such as Rogers,[48] Watson,[49] Parse,[50] or Newman,[51] to direct their practice. Exercise promotion is listed in NIC and could be expanded and developed with a better understanding of the balance paradigm. Nutritional counseling is based on providing a balance of nutrients and could also be expanded to incorporate use of some herbs for the promotion of health. Approaching these from the perspective

Positivist ◄————————————————————————————► Metaphysical

	Modalities	Mechanical	Purification	Balance	Supranormal
Material ▲	Physical manipulation	Positioning Exercise therapy Joint mobility	Bathing	Exercise promotion	Intuitive body work[†]
	Applied and ingested substances	Medication administration	Wound and bladder irrigation Leech therapy	Nutritional counseling	Homeopathic remedies
	Energy	Laser precautions	Phototherapy	Acupressure Acupuncture[†]	Therapeutic touch
	Psychological	Cognitive restructuring	Active listening[†]	Counseling*	Simple guided imagery
Nonmaterial ▼	Spiritual	Activity therapy*	Forgiveness and purification rituals	Meditation	Spiritual support*

* NIC listed intervention that could be developed with understanding of the paradigm
† No NIC listing and should be considered as a potential referral or potential development for nursing action

Figure 47-2 *Nursing activities and interventions.*

of balance rather than mechanical cure allows for an expansion into health and attention to individual life systems. Acupuncture or acupressure are not on the NIC but could be a source of referral. While currently not part of the balance paradigm, counseling, simple relaxation therapy, or self-modification assistance have the potential for development into that paradigm. Meditation also has potential for development.

Nursing interventions in the supranormal paradigm cluster in the nonmaterial areas. Intuitive body work, if not done by a nurse, could constitute a referral. Likewise, activities using homeopathic remedies or flower essences are included as they are understood to work through the spiritual level.

Therapeutic touch is well developed in nursing and is understood as a supranormal use of energy. Guided imagery is a supranormal psychological technique that is listed in the NIC. Spiritual support, including prayer, could be further developed to fully express this paradigm.

Implications for Research and Scholarship

By constructing a paradigm map with health–healing activities, nurses can determine appropriate paradigms to guide their understanding and research of particular modalities. Locating it on the model can serve as a guide for better understanding a particular modality; it also provides a direction for further scholarship and research. An exploration of both axes can enhance understanding. For example, nursing actions in the mechanical paradigm are often best understood by a better comprehension of the medical—scientific model, and research using the positivist philosophy is often appropriate. Many of the NIC classifications can be understood from this paradigm.

Working with a modality such as guided imagery could be enhanced by exploring both the supranormal paradigm and the psychological literature. Healing touch, a modality with a rich history in nursing, is located at the nexus of energy and the supranormal, the two axes least understood by biomedical science. Nurses who have conducted research using this modality or the existential psychological theories can attest to the frustration in conducting research without documented material and measurable mechanisms of action that are compatible with the mechanical paradigm. Research in these areas can be enhanced by learning more about the approaches of anthropology, theology, some psychology, and other humanity disciplines consistent with the supranormal paradigm. Investigation of energy through quantum physics (energy) and Eastern healing are also proximal areas that can illuminate the understanding of touch therapies.

The model can serve as an agenda for research and scholarship. In some modalities, links have been or can be developed that enable more mechanistic studies. In others, their position invites more qualitative or naturalistic methodologies of inquiry. Nursing theories may develop links that connect modalities for practice. For example, some of the developmental theories may have links across paradigms on the psychological axis. Although methods may be successfully combined, caution must be taken in attempting to link paradigms. Many paradigms are based on contradictory beliefs that are impossible to adhere to simultaneously.[52]

The multiparadigm model provides a holistic approach to bridging the gulf between holistic theories and biomedical nursing praxis. The dialectic method is appropriate scholarship for holistic frameworks.[4,53] In this approach, the whole is seen as governing relationships and providing coherence to the parts. The dialectic process would describe a nursing issue from one position—for example, the mechanical paradigm—and then counter that description with an oppositional position, the supranormal. After debate and dialogue, a third position emerges. This position can, in similar fashion, be refined by the same process. Placing the polar opposites in one model invites a dialectic methodology, appropriate for holistic nursing scholarship. The challenge remains for nurses to continue to develop theory that links modalities and explanatory paradigms. These links are being developed along nursing themes of health, environment, and individual potentials for healing. The model could help to provide a geographic map to locate these dialogues.

REFERENCES

1. Chinn PL, Kramer MK. *Theory and Nursing: A Systematic Approach.* St. Louis, Mo: Mosby; 1995.
2. Fitzpatrick JJ, Whall AL. *Conceptual Models of Nursing Analysis and Application.* 3rd ed. Stamford, Conn: Appleton & Lange; 1996.
3. Newman MN. *A Developing Discipline: Selected Works of Margaret Newman.* New York, NY: National League for Nursing Press; 1995.
4. Barnum BJS. *Nursing Theory: Analysis, Application, Evaluation.* Philadelphia, Pa: Lippincott; 1994.
5. Snyder M. Defining nursing interventions. *Image J Nurs Schol.* 1996;28(2):137–141.
6. International Council of Nurses. *Nurses' Next Advance: An International Classification for Nursing Practice.* Geneva, Switzerland: ICN; 1993.
7. Martin KS, Scheet NJ. *The Omaha System: Applications for Community Health Nursing.* Philadelphia, Pa: W. B. Saunders; 1992.
8. McCloskey JC, Bulechek GM. *Nursing Interventions Classification (NIC).* St. Louis, Mo: Mosby; 1996.

9. Grobe SJ. The nursing lexicon and taxonomy: implications for representing nursing care data in automated patient records. *Holistic Nurs Pract.* 1996;11(1):48–63.

10. Saba VK. The classification of home health nursing. *Caring.* 1992;11(3):50–57.

11. Reed, PG. A treatise on nursing knowledge development for the 21st century: beyond postmodernism. *ANS.* 1995;17(3): 70–84.

12. Fawcett J. *Analysis and evaluation of nursing theories.* Philadelphia, Pa: F. A. Davis; 1993.

13. *Webster's Ninth New Collegiate Dictionary.* Springfield, Mass: Merriam-Webster; 1990.

14. Owen MJ, Holmes CA. Holism in the discourse of nursing. *J Adv Nurs.* 1993;18;1688–1695.

15. Alster, KB. *The Holistic Health Movement.* Tuscaloosa, Ala: University of Alabama Press; 1989.

16. English-Lueck JA. *Health in the New Age: A Study in California Holistic Practices.* Albuquerque, NM: University of New Mexico Press; 1990.

17. Gordon, JS. The paradigm of holistic medicine. In: Hastings AC, Fadiman J, Gordon JS, eds. *Health for the Whole Person.* Toronto, Ontario: Bantam Books; 1980.

18. Lowenberg JS. *Caring and Responsibility.* Philadelphia, Pa: University of Pennsylvania Press; 1989.

19. Mattson PH. *Holistic Health in Perspective.* Palo Alto, Calif: Mayfield; 1982.

20. Toulmin S. *Cosmopolis: The Hidden Agenda of Modernity.* Chicago, Ill: University of Chicago Press; 1990.

21. Kuhn T. *The Structure of Scientific Revolutions.* Chicago, Ill: The University of Chicago Press; 1972.

22. Tarnas R. *The Passion of the Western World: Understanding the Ideas That Have Shaped our World View.* New York, NY: Ballantine Books; 1991.

23. Lavine TZ. *From Socrates to Sartre: The Philosophic Quest.* New York, NY: Bantam; 1984.

24. Johnson P. *Intellectuals.* New York, NY: Harper Perennial; 1988.

25. Engebretson J. Comparison of nurses and alternative healers. *Image J Nurs Schol.* 1996;28(2):95–100.

26. Engebretson J. *Cultural Models of Healing and Health: An Ethnography of Professional Nurses and Healers.* Houston, Tex: University of Texas-Houston, School of Public Health; 1992. Dissertation.

27. Engebretson J, Wardell D. A contemporary view of alternative healing modalities. *Nurse Practitioner.* 1993;18(9): 51–55.

28. Engebretson J. Models of heterodox healing. *Alternat Ther Health Med.* In press.

29. Andrews MM, Boyle JS. *Transcultural Concepts in Nursing Care.* 2nd ed. Philadelphia, Pa: Lippincott; 1995.

30. Freund PES, McGuire MB. *Health, Illness and the Social Body: A Critical Sociology.* Englewood Cliffs, NJ: Prentice-Hall; 1991.

31. Douglas M. *Purity and Danger: An Analysis of the Concepts of Pollution and Taboo.* London, England: Ark Paperbacks; 1989.

32. Brown PS. Nineteenth-century American health reformers and the early nature cure movement in Britain. *Med History.* 1988;32:174–194.

33. Whorton JC. *Crusaders for Fitness: The History of American Health Reformers.* Princeton, NJ: Princeton University Press; 1982.

34. Kaptchuk TJ. *The Web that Has No Weaver: Understanding Chinese Medicine.* New York, NY: Congdon and Weed; 1993.

35. Helman CG. *Culture, Health and Illness: An Introduction for Health Professionals.* 3rd ed. Wolburn, Mass: Butterworth-Heinemann; 1994.

36. Reese WL. *Dictionary of Philosophy and Religion: Eastern and Western Thought.* Atlantic Highland, NJ: Humanities Press; 1991.

37. Horgan J. *The End of Science, Facing the Limits of Knowledge in the Twilight of the Scientific Age.* Reading, Mass. Addison Wesley; 1996.

38. Dossey BM, Keegan L, Guzzetta CE, Kolkmeier LG, *Holistic Nursing: A Handbook for Practice.* Gaithersburg, Md: Aspen Publishers; 1995.

39. Slater VE. Toward an understanding of energetic healing, part 1: energetic structures. *J Holistic Nurs.* 1995;13: 209–224.

40. Slater VE. Toward an understanding of energetic healing, part 2: energetic process. *J Holistic Nurs.* 1995;13:225–238.

41. Rossi E. *The Psychobiology of Mind-Body Healing.* New York, NY: W. W. Norton; 1993.

42. Orth-Gomer K, Schneiderman N. *Behavioral Medicine Approaches to Cardiovascular Disease Prevention.* Hillsdale, NJ: Erlbaum; 1996.

43. Dreher H. *The Immune Power Personality.* New York: Dutton; 1995.

44. Schneiderman N, McCabe P, Baum A. *Perspectives in Behavioral Medicine: Stress and Disease Processes.* Hillsdale, NJ: Erlbaum; 1992.

45. Larson DB. Religion and spirituality—the forgotten factor in public health: what does the research share? Presented at the 12th annual meeting of the American Public Health Association, November 18, 1996; New York, NY.

46. Cox H. *Fire from Heaven.* Reading, Mass: Addison-Wesley; 1995.

47. Kleinman A. *Patients and Healers in the Context of Culture.* Berkeley, Calif: University of California Press; 1980.

48. Rogers ME. *An Introduction to the Theoretical Basis of Nursing.* Philadelphia, PA: F. A. Davis; 1970.

49. Watson J. *Nursing: Human Science and Human Care: A Theory of Nursing.* New York, NY: National League for Nursing.

50. Parse RR. *Man-Living-Health: A Theory of Nursing.* New York, NY: Wiley; 1981.

51. Newman MA. *Health as Expanding Consciousness.* 2nd ed. New York, NY: National League for Nursing; 1984.

52. Nagle LM, Mitchell GJ. *Theoretic Diversity: Evolving Paradigmatic Issues in Research and Practice.* Gaithersburg, Md: Aspen Publishers; 1991.

53. McKeon ZK. *On Knowing the Natural Sciences.* Chicago, Ill: University of Chicago Press; 1994.

THE AUTHOR COMMENTS | A Multiparadigm Approach to Nursing

As a public health nurse, I listened to what people believed about health, disease, and healing, and I became interested in cultural orientations to health. An understanding of these orientations, values, and beliefs that underlie health behaviors is central in working with clients in promoting their health. Conducting fieldwork with lay healers, who incorporated strategies and philosophies from cross-cultural and historical approaches to healing, and exploring related literature from anthropology provided a perspective for the multiparadigm model of healing. This perspective allowed for the development of an integrative healing model that includes the biomedical paradigm as opposed to other approaches that compare all healing methods from the biomedical perspective. Incorporating multiple approaches to healing and understanding the differences at the paradigm level will not only be relevant to providing the best healthcare to a global society but also provide an inclusive model for nursing that incorporates biomedical approaches rather than distinguishing nursing as oppositional to medicine.

JOAN C. ENGEBRETSON

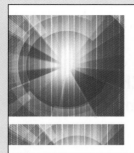

UNIT 9

Future Directions for Nursing Theory

This Unit builds upon the writings from earlier chapters (for example, on ontology, practice-theory links, and theory development) to propose new thinking about the characteristics, concepts, philosophies, and methods associated with nursing theory.

Historical and contemporary events are presented as background for proposing new perspectives.

The chapters interrogate and extend current perspectives on nursing knowledge. Traditional views about nursing science and practice are challenged. New philosophic views are proposed.

Although some of the ideas presented in these chapters are not actively practiced within nursing today, they may find their way into mainstream nursing through the creative translations of students and other readers.

QUESTIONS FOR DISCUSSION

- Which ideas or concepts presented in this Unit should find their way into mainstream nursing? In your opinion, are there any ideas that should not?

- What concepts are central to nursing in terms of clarifying our focus for inquiry and for the public, and distinguishing our discipline from other healthcare disciplines?

- What focuses connect us with other healthcare disciplines?

- Are there ideas embedded in nursing or in the healthcare system that nursing should actively resist?

- Is there any need for a reformation in nursing?

- How might the *participatory paradigm*, with its patient-centered focus on the humanness of the health circumstance, influence or distinguish your approach to practice and research?

- What ideas or experiences have you had that challenge or extend existing perspectives about nursing knowledge?

A Central Unifying Focus for the Discipline

Facilitating Humanization, Meaning, Choice, Quality of Life, and Healing in Living and Dying

DANNY G. WILLIS, RN, DNS, PMHCNS-BC
PAMELA J. GRACE, RN, PhD, FAAN
CALLISTA L. ROY, RN, PhD, FAAN

Nursing has a rich history of knowledge development, yet there remains ambiguity about what is a proper central unifying focus for the discipline. At this time in our history, it is imperative that we clearly define and articulate who we are and what we offer. Confusion about a central unifying focus is a significant problem for practice given the current healthcare environment and global problems affecting health and healing. The authors propose a central unifying focus for the discipline: facilitating humanization, meaning, choice, quality of life, and healing in living and dying. This focus will serve as a basis for our professional identity, strengthen our endeavors, and provide the ontological and epistemological basis for our continuing evolution as a practice profession. **Key words:** disciplinary focus, healing, health, human science, knowledge development, meaning, nursing knowledge, nursing philosophy, nursing practice, ontology

The need for nurses to articulate a coherent philosophical foundation for our practice has never been greater. Contemporary healthcare issues demand that nurses know who they are and what they are about, how to identify and actualize their societal mission and how to communicate it to others.[1(p4)]

Nursing scholars[1-10] have proposed answers to the questions of what is the nature of nursing knowledge and what is a proper central unifying focus for the discipline. Given a variety of nursing conceptual models and theories, disciplinary paradigms such as particulate-deterministic, interactive-integrative, unitary-transformative,[11] and perspectives on knowledge, for example, problem-solving, knowledge as process, and poststructural feminist,[12] can there be a central unifying focus for nursing knowledge development and practice? If not, what does this mean for nursing and those we care for? To answer these questions, the authors engaged in a dialogical process of inquiry over a 2-year period from 2005 to 2007. The purposes were to understand and clarify the current state of the discipline and discern whether it was possible to identify a central unifying focus for the discipline and for undergirding interdisciplinary work.

We came to the conclusion that the answer to the first question is a resounding yes. We believe that nursing's survival as a healing practice discipline may depend on all nurses being able to clearly articulate a central unifying focus. Our notion of a central unifying focus is a clarifying statement. It speaks to the essence or essential nature of the discipline that we believe transcends any one conceptual model or theory or combinations of them. As such, our proposal does not represent a new version of the metaparadigm or a new conceptual model.

In the remainder of this article, we (1) state basic assumptions from which we proceeded in doing our inquiry, (2) describe our process of inquiry, (3) review relevant background information and reasons for caring about a central unifying focus, (4) propose a central unifying focus for the discipline, (5) give our definitions and explanations of the main concepts in the central unifying focus, (6) describe possible linkages among the concepts, and (7) address future directions.

Basic Assumptions

1. Nursing requires a central unifying focus to differentiate its essence from medicine and other health disciplines.

2. Essential themes from nursing knowledge development over the ages are discernible and provide a central unifying focus for the discipline.

From D. G. Willis, P. J. Grace, and C. Roy, A central unifying focus for the discipline: Facilitating humanization, meaning, choice, quality of life, and healing in living and dying, Advances in Nursing Science, *31(1), E28–E40. Copyright © 2008 Wolters Kluwer Health | Lippincott Williams & Wilkins. Reproduced with permission of Lippincott Williams & Wilkins.*

ABOUT THE AUTHORS

DANNY G. WILLIS was born in Tupelo, MS. He received his Bachelor of Science in nursing from the University of Mississippi School of Nursing, and Master of Nursing degree and Doctor of Nursing Science from the Louisiana State University Health Sciences Center School of Nursing in New Orleans. His hobbies include listening to music (jazz, classical, Delta blues), painting, watching modern dance, meditation, cooking, and spending quality time in nature and with loved ones. He currently serves on the faculty at Boston College, William F. Connell School of Nursing. His scholarship has focused on nursing philosophy and science, qualitative research methods, and advancing knowledge about boys' and men's healing and health potentials in the aftermath of traumatic and marginalizing experiences (hate crime, being bullied, witnessing violence, and child abuse). Key contributions to the discipline include advancing a central unifying focus for the discipline of nursing and publications on men's mental health issues after interpersonal abuse, and his current NIH/NINR-funded research focused on describing the phenomenon of healing (1R15NR-011353: Adult Male Survivors Healing from Childhood Maltreatment).

PAMELA J. GRACE was born in Manchester, United Kingdom. After training as a nurse there, she moved to the United States where she worked for many years mostly in critical care areas and eventually pursued a BSN, MSN, and PhD in Philosophy with a concentration in Medical Ethics. Her area of scholarship is nursing philosophy and ethics, specifically the issue of nursing's responsibilities to advocate for individual and social good. She is currently an Associate Professor of Adult Health and Ethics in Boston College's William F. Connell School of Nursing where she collaborates with scholars such as Danny Willis and Sister Callista Roy. She enjoys outdoor activities such as hiking and skiing.

CALLISTA L. ROY is a Professor and Nurse Theorist at the William F. Connell School of Nursing at Boston College. She began her education at Mount Saint Mary's College located in Los Angeles, the city where she was born. Dr. Roy has master's degrees in pediatric nursing and sociology from the University of California at Los Angeles, where she also earned her PhD. Dr. Roy is best known for her work on the Roy adaptation model. Her current research is an intervention study to involve lay study partners in cognitive recovery of patients with mild head injury. Her other scholarly work includes conceptualizing and measuring coping and developing the philosophical basis for the adaptation model and for the epistemology of nursing. She has been named a Living Legend by the American Academy of Nursing and the Massachusetts Registered Nurses Association. She was inducted into the Sigma Theta Tau International Nurse Researcher Hall of Fame in 2010.

3. The central unifying focus reflects the essence of nursing knowledge and practice.

4. The central unifying focus will not change over time if nursing as a discipline continues to exist.

5. Nursing practice (action) and nursing knowledge are interrelated.

6. Nursing practice requires nursing knowledge.

7. Nursing practice shapes nursing knowledge.

8. Future nursing knowledge development and research, utilizing multiple modes of knowing and research methods from philosophic inquiry to bench science, will be grounded in questions that are pertinent to nursing practice and related to the concepts of nursing's central unifying focus.

9. As human beings, one type of being among all other beings, our essential nature is that of the natural world. That is, human beings come into existence in the world, change, and die. Human beings are unitary with the natural world.

10. The essential nature of human beings plus everything that is involved in the evolution of an individual human being in some way and which is influenced by that human being in some way is "the whole."

11. Health and healing are natural and evolving unifications in "the whole."

 ## Process of Inquiry

On the basis of the above questions and assumptions, 4 nurse scholars, with diverse practice and philosophical backgrounds, at Boston College's William F Connell School of Nursing joined together in an ongoing dialogue to identify a central unifying focus for the discipline. From the beginning of our dialogue, it was evident that we are not alone among nurse scholars and practitioners in struggling for coherence and clarity in articulating a central unifying focus. We understood the complexity involved in trying to cogently express and unite the varied and intricate nursing perspectives. Nevertheless, we found it critical to attempt to remedy the situation we saw before us. Three of us decided to write this article as a mechanism for sharing our dialogue with others in nursing. The fourth participant, Dr Dorothy A. Jones, EdD, RN, FAAN, chose not to be involved in writing the article but is acknowledged for her helpful insights during the dialogue. We believe that the results of our inquiry add more clarity and specificity enhancing nursing's ability to clearly articulate both a substantive base for the discipline and a lucid foundation for interdisciplinary collaboration. We believe that a central unifying focus serves as an effective foundation for action and substantive conversations among nursing, medicine, and allied health. A central unifying focus permits nurses to articulate their perspective using essential concepts of the discipline in a manner that is comprehendible and complementary to the perspectives of other disciplines.

At the center of our process of inquiry was sharing with each other our personal experiences as nurses and our substantive nursing knowledge. During the conversations and our review of nursing's knowledge development literature, we reflected on our lives as nurses, educators, philosophers, and researchers. Often our conversations lasted for hours, in which the first author took notes to record significant aspects that would be useful in discerning a central unifying focus. Our dialogues involved discussion of nursing's theoretical base, professional issues affecting nursing knowledge development and nursing practice, and an envisioned future in which all nurses practice "nursing" and are able to clearly articulate the values, mission, and focus of the discipline. Goals were developed during the process of our dialogue. These included (a) unearthing our underlying assumptions, which have been stated earlier in the article, (b) elucidating a fundamental essence and convergence across major nursing theories and paradigms that would guide us in articulating a central unifying focus, (c) constructing a central unifying focus statement, and (d) highlighting the importance of the resulting clarification if we are to meet nursing's goals.

Relevant Background Information and Reasons for Caring About a Central Unifying Focus

Nursing scholars have long attempted to clarify the essence of the discipline. For example, on the basis of

a critique of the metaparadigm concepts of person, health, environment, and nursing[13] as being neither integrated nor sufficient for ongoing knowledge development, Newman and colleagues[4] set out to integrate these and add to the metaparadigm the concepts of "caring" and "human health experience" in a way that was consistent with a unitary-transformative perspective. Their work drew upon the scholarship of nurse leaders/theorists including Patricia Benner, Madeline Leininger, Margaret Newman, Rosemarie Parse, Nola Pender, Martha Rogers, and Jean Watson. They proposed that the disciplinary focus statement for nursing is *caring in the human health experience*.[4] This focus meant that caring, health, and wholeness could be synthesized and that *caring in the human health experience* could be "studied as a unitary-transformative process of mutuality and creative unfolding."[4(p38)] The unitary-transformative paradigm has come to represent, at least for some scholars in nursing, an evolution of nursing theory beyond particulate-deterministic and interactive-integrative views of human and environment to one of an undivided unitary universe in which the whole is already contained in each part. It proposes that human living and dying is an evolutionary unfolding of human-environment integrality that is reflective of the whole, diversification, increasing complexity, and expansion as manifested in human-environmental patterning.

Other scholars have been interested in clarifying a central unifying focus for the discipline. Kim[6] proposed that the metaparadigm should be expanded to include *human living* as a concept, which has integrative appeal. She viewed *human living* as more unifying in nature than the commonly used language of human "states" and human "responses," which seem too fragmentary and stimulus-response in nature. She believed that these more fragmentary concepts have been widely disseminated in nursing language and some nursing theories, leading to a preponderance of technically oriented nursing care in which there is "an artificial interruption in connected human experience."[6(p38)] Jacobs[7] proposed that *human dignity* is the central phenomenon of concern to nursing.

These authors' scholarship should be viewed as pivotal in nursing's evolution toward clarification, integration, and unification in purpose. Still their scholarship cannot mark the end of our search for clarification because many facets of nursing knowledge require further development. Moreover, nursing knowledge needs to relate to the knowledge bases of other healthcare disciplines for the purpose of facilitating human flourishing, health, and healing. Clearly, nursing's evolution at the metatheoretical, theoretical, research, and practice levels is ongoing with the potential for clarifying, reformulating, and honing a central unifying focus that would unite us within the discipline, serve as a basis for our continuing scholarly evolution, and foster interdisciplinary work in which nursing is clearly and substantively visible. Reference to a central unifying focus in which nursing's perspective is clear, distinctive, accessible, and informative allows us to (a) ensure that the goals of human good/human flourishing remain the focus of activity and (b) resist subversion to interests that are not conducive to nursing practice. Congruent with this line of thought, Newman[8,10] calls for a reconciliation of what appears to be opposing perspectives in nursing and healthcare by way of a unitary perspective in which various points of view on health and healing are included in the whole. In fact, other scholars from nursing and related disciplines have criticized nursing as being too insular in its outlook. Nursing has been viewed as self-interested and concerned with legitimizing its standing as a discipline that may have stalled our progress in bringing about needed societal and healthcare reform in the larger sociopolitical world. Because interdisciplinary collaborations are needed for social change, this stance is seen as being at the ultimate expense of nursing's population.[14] This is an important paradox for nursing to keep in mind.

The paradox is that we have had to be somewhat self-protective and insular in order to survive and meet the goal of the discipline, which has been the "human good." But, in doing so, we have distanced ourselves from other disciplines, which we might have joined forces in planning and implementing societal changes needed for human flourishing. Indeed, individual and societal good are interrelated, but our insularity and focus on individuals tend to take us away from collaborative interdisciplinary work that is needed to further societal good. As the discipline of nursing evolves, we do not want to lose sight of the fact that we need to be self-reflective and self-protective as a discipline and also contribute the insights gained to collaborative interdisciplinary work. That is, an emphasis on disciplinary knowledge development is necessary for consolidating our vision and values but this can become dangerous for our population of interest if we do not use the knowledge gained to enrich intra- and interdisciplinary discourse related to common goals of practice.

Now, as Newman[8,10] challenges us, we need to ensure that a central unifying focus is used as a means of communication, uniting healthcare disciplines in fulfilling mutual goals of health and healing but where the substance of the discipline of nursing is clear. Indeed our work in nursing must be unified within an inclusive focus that transcends divisions. This is seen as necessary for an even more useful, relevant, and substantive ground for recognizing a complementary world in which good nursing care and good medical care exist for all who are capable of benefiting from it.[15,16] (M. Newman, oral communication, April 14,

2007). Newman[16] indicates that nursing has already begun to transcend divisions and is evolving toward a "world of no boundaries" in which divisions between disciplines, between nursing art and science, and theory, research and practice are being reconciled. Given this claim, Newman asks, "So what is the transcendent unity of theories of nursing?"[16(p241)]

A nursing focus for guiding practice can be discerned from early in nursing's theoretical development. Since the days of Florence Nightingale,[17] a clear perspective on health protection, restoration, healing, and human flourishing has been seen as necessary. In Nightingale's world and time, she found it critical to define nursing's nature and characteristics in order to guide appropriate actions on behalf of wounded soldiers and society. She researched and articulated what the essential substance of nursing knowledge was to ensure good nursing actions, coordination of services, and procurement of resources necessary to optimize environmental conditions conducive to healing, thus transforming healthcare and human lives. Given the fragmented and uncoordinated healthcare that exist today and radical changes in the delivery environment in the united States and elsewhere that shift the emphasis from human good to the economic bottom line,[18–20] it is time to reexamine these beginning moments in nursing's theoretical history for lessons learned. In order that nursing continues to exist as a force for human and societal good, as it did because of Nightingale, revisiting the question of what is nursing's central unifying focus is both critical and timely at this point in our evolution. We have reached an Archimedean point in which nursing as a discipline is seriously endangered by political forces, uncritical allegiance to interdisciplinary education and work that often fails to acknowledge the distinct bodies of knowledge evolving within disciplines,[21] the medicalization of care, and perspectives that are primarily focused on economic gain and/or cost control at the expense of human welfare.[19,20] Cody[21] noted that "nursing's history includes a subjugation to medicine that has been blatant, at times near-complete, widely if not universally sanctioned, and brutal at times ...."[21(p277)]

Nursing literature points to an apparent disorder within the nursing profession in which there are powerful dynamics at play contributing to role confusion and blurring of nursing and medicine, thereby diluting nursing's disciplinary knowledge and practice.[22–26] Reed[22] has suggested that nursing, even with its rich theoretical heritage dating back to Nightingale, has evolved into a "disintegrated" profession. She opines that nurses, including nurse leaders and executives who identify with medicine at all levels of practice, have cheated nursing of actualizing its full potential. Holmes et al[25] have highlighted the restrictions placed on nursing knowledge development, and its possible disappearance, when nurses uncritically embrace a dogmatic, hierarchical evidence-based notion of validity in nursing knowledge development. They question the power dynamics at play with regard to how knowledge claims within the discipline are validated. They suggest that prevalent notions of evidence-based knowledge, based chiefly in a post-positivistic quantitative perspective, are too restrictive for nursing's multiple ways of knowing and limit what gets recognized as nursing knowledge.

Without a central unifying focus, which allows us to clearly articulate and defend the substantive knowledge and requirements for nursing practice, nursing is in a vulnerable position within the healthcare arena. This vulnerability has implications for humanity and comes from being co-opted and swayed to answer to parties other than nursing. It is imperative that we identify, value, and practice the essence of the discipline to meet our social mandate.

Murphy et al[18] among others,[27-30] suggested that nurses need to go beyond the bedside in their practice to larger social realms in addressing needed social change for human good. Therefore, a central unifying focus for all nursing work is critical. A central unifying focus does not preclude diversity in worldviews, conceptual models, and theories, which are necessary given the myriad ways in which human beings differ on the basis of human growth and development, culture, gender, ethnicity, sexual orientation, religion, life experiences, and socioeconomic and political conditions. A central unifying focus can be thought of as a convergence around the essence or essential nature of the discipline.

A Central Unifying Focus for the Discipline of Nursing

On the basis of our inquiry process, we propose that a central unifying focus for the discipline is *facilitating humanization, meaning, choice, quality of life, and healing in living and dying*. Our proposal builds upon previous work in nursing and represents our interpretation and synthesis/ convergence of ideas espoused in the major nursing conceptual and theoretical works of Leininger,[31,32] Newman,[4,8,10,11,16,33,34] Nightingale,[17] Parse,[35-37] Patterson and Zderad,[38] Peplau,[39] Rogers,[40-42] Roy,[43,44] and Watson.[45-47] These authors have provided the discipline with excellent thoughts about nursing and research related to culture,[31-32] consciousness and pattern,[4,8,10,11,16,33,34] healthy environments and resources,[17] cocreative processes of human becoming and quality of life,[35-37] humanistic existential concerns,[38] interpersonal relationships,[39] irreducible human-environment life processes, pattern, and energy,[40-42] adaptation,[43,44] and caring-healing.[45-47] Our proposal conceptualizes

and operationalizes the focus differently than prior proposals and uses a dialect grounded in nursing practice knowledge that we believe is readily transparent to other healthcare professions such as medicine, social work, and physical therapy. Dialect can be thought of as a socioculturally constructed way of talking that is related to a particular discipline and culture. Our proposal of a central unifying focus addresses unitary human-natural world phenomena of concern in nursing practice and provides a basis for conceptual progress in the discipline.

Definitions and Explanations of the Main Concepts

We believe that transparency in meanings within a central unifying focus is important because lack of it weakens our ability to articulate and stand for who we are and bridge disciplinary dialects, thereby thwarting the fulfillment of common goals for human health and healing. Our definitions and explanations of humanization, meaning, choice, quality of life, healing, and living and dying are given below. We have also included definitions of "nursing" and "health" as we believe they are highly relevant, although they are not specific concepts mentioned in the declarative statement of the central unifying focus.

Nursing is a healthcare discipline and healing profession, both an art and science, which facilitates and empowers human beings in envisioning and fulfilling health and healing in living and dying through the development, refinement, and application of nursing knowledge for practice. Examples of nursing practice include (*a*) engaging in effective, humane relationships grounded in unconditional acceptance of human beings as they are in their whole; (*b*) recognizing, valuing, knowing, supporting, empowering, and nurturing human beings; (*c*) engaging human beings in therapeutic human-to-human, human-to-nature, and nature-to-human interactions; (*d*) helping human beings process the meaning(s) and significance of their life experiences and their health and healing concerns; (*e*) recognizing, welcoming, appreciating, and advocating human beings' personal choices and rights and responsibilities; (*f*) discussing, identifying, respecting, and advocating human beings' ideas about quality of life; and (*g*) ensuring conditions and practices conducive to human beings' humanization, meaning, choice, quality of life, and healing in both living and dying.

Humanization is human beings' careful attending to self and each other as relational and experiential in the whole of the unitary human-natural world with all of our unbroken and broken wholeness as human beings. For example, the whole is the unified human-natural world, involving relating of human-to-human, human-to-nature, and nature-to-human. This includes all types of variable human experiences that are often thought of as opposites but are unifications within the unitary human-natural world. Examples of these unifications include perceptions of pleasure or pain, acceptance or resistance, fearlessness or fear, hope or despair, peace or anxiety, love or hate, respect or disrespect, health or illness, comfort or discomfort, and living or dying.

Humanization, as practiced by nurses, is an open-minded, caring, intentional, thoughtful, and responsible unconditional acceptance and awareness of human beings as they are. Thus, nursing facilitates humanization by engaging experiential human beings in practice and modeling humane relating for other human beings. Humanization, as a nurturing action in nursing practice, is manifested when the nurse works with all human beings grounded in an ontology of human beings as relational, experiential, valuable, respect-worthy, meaning-oriented, flawed, imperfect, vulnerable, fragile, complex, and capable of health and healing even if not capable of being cured. Humanization involves knowing and engaging fellow human beings as human in the unitary human-natural world in which the unifications of opposites are recognized as real, naturally reflective of the whole, and fundamentally meaningful in terms of lived experience. Humanization in nursing practice provides the open space in which human beings have the potential to experience wholeness. Humanizing questions in nursing practice include the following: Who are you as person, as human? What do you value as a person, as human? What are your concerns? What do you understand about what you are going through? What information do you have? What do you need as a person, as human? What is the meaning(s) for you in "this or that" experience? How are you relating to varying aspects of the whole of your life? What are your ideas about your health and healing? Related to your values and notions of health and healing, what would you like to work on? How can I meet you where you are and process with you what you see as choices given your life circumstances, values, beliefs, and meanings? What are your wishes related to quality of life? How can I create an optimal healing environment for you? How can I best support your ideas of quality of life, health, and healing during this experience and beyond? These questions, and others, provide the human-natural world information for processing meaning in relation to one's health and healing.

Meaning is a human's arrived-at understanding of life experiences and their significance that comes from processing those experiences. Constructing meaning(s) in life experiences is a complex dialectic intentional process among multiple unitary human-natural world dynamics whereby understanding and coherence are created from which choice(s) can emerge. Meaning(s) is a basis for human integration of the whole of living and dying and the embodied experience of wholeness. By embodied, we mean that one's existence and living and dying are manifested through the body. The body is the medium through which humans have lived experiences, such as wholeness, and access the world. Humans live and die in their bodies. The process of constructing meaning(s) in life experiences considers the context and particularities of a person's life and results in the emergence of possible choices in relation to particular, circumscribed situations as well as in relation to more global and/or ultimate purpose(s) in one's living and dying. In some situations, individual human beings are involved in the process of constructing meaning(s) in life experiences without reference to the direct, immediate effort of other humans. That is, without reference to other humans, except in the form of the background understandings and meanings that has already been formed in relation to other unitary human-natural world occurrences in the past. An example is being aware of, comprehending, and making sense of human-natural world dynamics in the course of going about everyday living to arrive at meaning(s) and choice(s) based on those meaning(s). Specifically, consider the following: "I am feeling thirsty. I know that there is a water fountain across the room from where I am sitting. Based on my past experiences of drinking water when I am thirsty, I know that the water will quench my thirst. Thus, I am going to drink some water from the fountain."

In addition, the process of constructing meaning(s) in life experiences occurs when human beings engage one another to create understanding and coherence, in which meaning(s) and possible choice(s) emerge that can serve as momentum or leverage for experiencing wholeness and healing. The nurse must remain focused on the question of meaning. The choices of human beings who receive nursing care emerge within the relationship as a result of the intention, purposeful awareness, and humanizing actions of the nurse to know them and engage them in the process of constructing meaning(s) in their life experiences in relation to, and informed by, nursing's knowledge and the self-reflection of both the nurse and the recipient of nursing care. The process of constructing meaning(s) in life experiences may involve the nurse engaging with a proxy on behalf of the recipient of nursing care in situations where the recipient cannot be engaged or dialogue.

Within the context of nursing practice, the process of constructing meaning(s) has at least 3 modes: (*a*) the nurse attending to and helping recipients of nursing care, or their proxies, make sense of health and healing concerns; (b) the nurse constructing meaning(s) related to nursing practice within the larger healthcare and sociopolitical environment, including perceptions of both positive and negative human-natural world conditions, affecting the facilitation of humanization, meaning, choice, quality of life, and healing; and (c) the nurse's reflecting on nursing concepts, ways of knowing, and practical knowledge; the relational use of self and the natural world in forming effective healing relationships; and other healing modalities.

Choice is the human potential for making personally derived decisions, given the developmental and reasoning skills necessary, that are in congruence with one's values, beliefs, and meanings. Choice presupposes intentionality, comprehension, and ability to communicate. Thus, facilitating choice involves both the nurse and the recipient of care making sense of the care recipient's life experiences, envisioned quality of life, and health and healing concerns. One's choices are influenced by one's perceptions and meanings related to quality of life, health, and healing. One's future is influenced by the choices that are or are not made.

Quality of life is the value and significance ascribed by individual human beings to their lives, given their changing unitary human-natural world situations. Individuals' quality of life is based on their values, beliefs, and meanings related to life experiences. For example, what constitutes quality of life is knowable for recipients of nursing care by way of knowing them as human beings. Once what constitutes quality of life for a given individual is known, choice(s) that is congruent can be facilitated. Quality of life is influenced by one's meanings, choices, and health such that optimal quality of life may be synonymous with one's health.

Health is the embodiment of wholeness and integrity in living and dying. That is, health is experienced in the body; it is embodied. Wholeness is the bodily experience of unity, harmony, balance, and integration in the unitary human-natural world, including the integration of what appear to be opposites but are unifications of the whole. For example, wholeness can be experienced in a variety of ways depending on human beings' meanings, choices, and quality of life, and is related to their unitary human-natural world experiences/situations in living and dying. Implicit in health is humanization, meaning-making, choice, quality of life, and healing.

Healing is the multidimensional unitary human-natural world process of restoring bodily experiences (perceptual-physical) of wholeness, meaning, and integrity in living and dying when it is disrupted. This means that healing may or may not occur when a physiological disruption is resolved, such as in congestive heart failure, depending on whether the human being has bodily experiences of wholeness,

meaning, and integrity. Conversely, healing may occur in the absence of resolution of a physiologic disruption, such as cancer, when the human being has bodily experiences of wholeness, meaning, and integrity.

Living and dying is the unitary human-natural world process of coming into existence in a human body in the world and changing until death.

Proposed Linkages Among the Concepts

The linkages among the concepts in the central unifying focus can be thought of as facets in a diamond. That is, the concepts are all interrelated and integrated and reflective of the essence of nursing knowledge for practice. Thus, the relationships among the concepts may be thought of as recursive. Each concept informs and shapes the others and provides a gestalt for thinking about the essential nature of nursing knowledge for practice. The goals and approaches for nursing practice are inherent in the central unifying concepts as described individually and in relation to each other. According to the proposed central unifying focus, the goal of nursing practice, and thus nursing knowledge development, is to *facilitate humanization, meaning, choice, quality of life, and healing in living and dying* for all recipients and potential recipients of nursing care. Nursing knowledge and practice are advanced as we conceptualize our practice within a central unifying focus and use questions, evidence, and interventions from multiple and overlapping modes of knowing—such as empirics, ethics, personal, esthetics,[48] and sociopolitical[49]—to enhance our ways of being with others as nurse healers. Nursing is practiced at the individual, family, community, society, and global levels.

The concept of humanization is prescriptive for nursing practice. As described earlier, it is the foundation for establishing effective, humane relationships in which human beings are known as "human." Thus, knowledge of humanization is a preliminary requisite in nursing practice that is necessary for helping people process their life experiences and construct meaning(s), which necessarily involves them in reflecting on their cherished values, beliefs, and knowledge of self and others. Knowledge and skills related to humanization and our human search for meaning(s) are necessary in healthcare practices that privilege human needs and individualized care. Observations of the human condition over the centuries have revealed that the essential nature of humans is to search for meaning, nurturance, and relationship. While it may seem superficial to claim that humans require meaning, nurturance, and relationship in their lives, the claim is actually profound and it provides us with an opportunity to reflect on the need for these aspects in quality humanistic nursing practice. It seems that nurturing human relationships and meaning are the 2 key aspects of living that we do not fully acknowledge and honor in our own lives as nurses and in contemporary healthcare. Perhaps we take it for granted and pass it over as trivial or not critically important. Or, perhaps it is because envisioning and realizing humanization and meaning are much harder work emotionally than some people are willing to fully engage in. These aspects of human care require an investment in self and others that goes beyond superficiality or just trying to "fix" a problem and hurriedly moving along.

A focus on humanization and the process of constructing meaning(s) in life experiences is prerequisite to facilitating choices that are reasoned, useful, and authentic. Choices that are congruent with a human being's values, beliefs, life context, and meanings emerge from acts of humanization and through discovering and constructing meaning(s). Thus, optimal quality of life cannot be facilitated for humans until the nurse and other clinicians and interested others understand what life experiences mean to an individual. What constitutes quality of life for humans can be understood only through their internal frame of reference. Healing—involving the restoration of bodily experiences of wholeness, meaning, and integrity—can be facilitated for humans when the nurse values, clarifies, and understands their life experiences and the meanings and significance they ascribe to them.

 Future Directions

We have articulated a central unifying focus for the discipline that synthesizes a nursing perspective on human health and healing in living and dying. This focus gives us a strong professional identity and clearly explains the service we offer. We believe that the constituent concepts of the proposed central unifying focus will not change over time if nursing as a discipline continues to exist. Nursing practice will always involve *facilitation of humanization, meaning, choice, quality of life, and healing in living and dying.* For example, meaning will always be an integral concept in nursing practice, but our understanding of the processes of constructing meaning(s) in life experiences and their relationship to choices, decision-making, and healing will be developed and more fully understood with further knowledge development. Given the enduring nature of our proposed central unifying focus, its concepts and their interrelationships will direct nursing education, research, and practice in meeting individual and societal goals for

health and healing, where nursing practice means any action taken to meet nursing's goals. This is nursing's moral/ethical imperative given our proposed central unifying focus.

We believe that the highest priority for advancing nursing practice is that a central unifying focus serves as the linchpin of nursing curricula, other education efforts, and the normative ethic of nursing practice. We believe it is essential that nursing students, at all levels, be exposed to, study, and incorporate the central unifying focus in their practice because this is the most reasonable way to unite us and articulate our substance and service within an interdisciplinary environment. This priority has implications for program outcomes and objectives and for the development of professional values and characteristics that can be nurtured and evaluated.

Nursing exists to serve individual, societal, and global needs for health and healing. Thus, nursing education at all levels, including continuing education, will be shaped by the concepts in the central unifying focus. In nursing curricula, nurses will be steeped in the phenomena of concern to the discipline. As a result of their education, they will be able to clearly articulate nursing's central unifying focus in intra- and interdisciplinary fora for the purpose of facilitating human beings' and societies' health and healing. We believe that nursing's unity around the world would be beneficial and built upon an understanding of the concepts in the proposed central unifying focus. Education within nursing and in interdisciplinary healthcare contexts would emphasize how knowledge from various disciplines is both necessary and complementary in meeting the health and healing needs of humans.

We believe that nurses must lead the discipline forward by knowing what our central unifying focus for practice is, developing it, teaching it, and speaking it, thereby transforming self, other, and the larger healthcare environment. At the highest level of nursing education, doctorally prepared nurses in research and education will be guided by the concepts in the central unifying focus and the disciplines' theories while providing leadership in curriculum design, research, and practice.

While it is clear that answers to the questions of "what is nursing research?" and "what is the relationship between nursing theory and nursing knowledge? are varied and debatable, we believe that knowledge for the development of nursing practice must be grounded in the questions, concerns, and problems that are central to the practice of nursing. That is, nursing research should address questions related to nursing's theoretical base of human care, meanings, choice, quality of life, and healing. As nurses, we need better knowledge about how we can facilitate humans to live more complete, quality, and meaningful lives as envisioned from their implicit frames of reference. We need more knowledge and research about how to be with them in ways that are healing and facilitative of their self-healing and transformation of suffering. We believe that future nursing research should be grounded in questions that are pertinent to practice and related to the concepts in the proposed central unifying focus. Nursing research will include various methodologies including philosophic inquiry, historical, qualitative, quantitative, and mixed methods. In addition, methodological advancements within nursing and other disciplines will contribute to our evolving research and practice. Scholarly endeavors will further develop and refine the knowledge needed for practice. We believe that knowledge development in nursing should span the gamut from philosophic inquiry to bench science, but where the knowledge developed through research has significant relevance and identifiable relationships to the theories and practice of nursing and the meaningful concerns of humans in living and dying. We believe that nurses in practice need knowledge of the physiological, psychological, sociocultural, and spiritual aspects of human living and dying. We endorse evidence-based practice and the use of randomized clinical trials and other forms of evidence as part of the whole, even with their limitations, and envision empirics—as described by Carper[48]—as only one way of developing knowledge within the discipline. We believe, like Fawcett et al[50] that nursing theory (including Carper's multiple ways of knowing), inquiry, and evidence are all interrelated and form the foundation for advancing nursing knowledge development. Within our vision of nursing practice that is grounded in a notion of the unitary whole, there has to be room for all valid ways of knowing. Doctorally prepared nurses will use the concepts and understandings associated with the central unifying focus for developing nursing knowledge related to human-natural world experiences, humanistic and other inquiry methodologies, and practice issues that reflect nursing's ontology. The key in advancing knowledge for nursing practice is that the knowledge produced be related to the important nursing concerns and challenges faced by nurses in providing holistic care to their clients/patients.

At the graduate level of nursing education, the study of nursing theories and the central unifying focus will undergird role preparation of nursing administrators, leaders, educators, and clinical practitioners. At the undergraduate level of nursing education, the study of nursing theory and the central unifying focus will provide a foundation for students in understanding the essence of nursing and engaging in nursing practice that encourages multiple ways of knowing in facilitating humanization, meaning, choice, quality of life, and healing in living and dying.

Other priorities include nursing practitioners', scholars', and leaders' engagement in dialogue, critique, research, practice, and knowledge development to refine concepts in the central unifying focus and others from nursing's theoretical base that are useful and relevant for the goals and purposes of nursing. This is important because the future of nursing practice will be significantly influenced by every nurse's understanding of the discipline as a whole; use of disciplinary philosophies, theories, and practice knowledge; and contributions in meeting the common goals of health and healing across societies and healthcare professions. Responsibilities that are understood as a result of the proposed central unifying focus necessitate addressing health and healing concerns from a broad perspective that transcends divisions and is inclusive of the whole. This is an especially important ethical point in light of nursing's recent weakened sociopolitical influence, which stems in part from their lack of communicating a clear unifying focus for the work of nurses on behalf of humankind. The articulation of a central unifying focus permits the discipline to present a cohesive approach to meeting sociopolitical changes needed for human health and healing contexts. The importance of nursing's contributions in sociopolitical and interdisciplinary work is the addition of a substantive perspective, as articulated in nursing's theoretical base and the central unifying focus, that other professions are unlikely to have developed given their philosophies, interests, roles, and perceived responsibilities.

 ## Conclusion

We set out to identify and clarify a central unifying focus for the discipline of nursing. In the process of doing this, we were able to explain essential concepts and their interrelationships that were derived from our experiences and a synthesis of nursing's theoretical literature. On the basis of the proposed central unifying focus, we addressed implications for future directions in the advancement of nursing practice. We anticipate that our proposal will provoke significant debate and dialogue in nursing aimed at unification in purpose and that nursing will begin to see changes in nursing education, research, and practice.

REFERENCES

1. Cody WK, Mitchell GJ. Nursing knowledge and human science revisited. Practical and political considerations. *Nurs Sci Q.* 2002;15(1):4–13.
2. Donaldson SK, Crowley DM. The discipline of nursing. *Nurs Outlook.* 1978;26(2):113–120.

3. Packard SA, Polifroni EC. The dilemma of nursing science: current quandaries and lack of direction. *Nurs Sci Q.* 1992;4(1):7–13.

4. Newman MA, Sime AM, Corcoran-Perry SA. The focus of the discipline of nursing. In: Newman MA, ed. *A Developing Discipline: Selected works of Margaret Newman.* New York, NY: National League for Nursing Press; 1995:33–42.

5. Silva MC. The state of nursing science: reconceptualizing for the 21st Century. *Nurs Sci Q.* 1999;12(3):221–226.

6. Kim HS. An integrative framework for conceptualizing clients: a proposal for a nursing perspective in the new century. *Nurs Sci Q.* 2000;13(1):37–40.

7. Jacobs BB. Respect for human dignity: a central phenomenon to philosophically unite nursing theory an practice through consilience of knowledge. *ANS Adv Nurs Sci.* 2001;24(1):17–35.

8. Newman MA. The pattern that connects. *ANS Adv Nurs Sci.* 2002;24(3):1–7.

9. Cowling WR. A unitary participatory vision of nursing knowledge. *ANS Adv Nurs Sci.* 2007;30(1): 61–70.

10. Newman MA. The power of one: confidence in our evolving future. *Nurs Sci Q.* 2007;20(3): 204–204.

11. Newman MA. Prevailing paradigms in nursing. *Nurs Outlook.* 1992;40(1):10–13, 32.

12. Jones DA. A synthesis of philosophical perspectives for knowledge development. In: Roy C, Jones DA, eds. *Nursing Knowledge Development and Clinical Practice.* New York, NY: Springer Publishing Company; 2007:163–176.

13. Fawcett J. The metaparadigm of nursing: present status and future refinements. *Image.* 1984;16(3): 84–87.

14. Mechanic D, Reinhard SC. Contributions of nurses to health policy: challenges and opportunities. *Nurs Health Policy.* 2002;1(1):7–15.

15. Roy C. Knowledge as universal cosmic imperative. In: Roy C, Jones DA, eds. *Nursing Knowledge Development and Clinical Practice.* New York, NY: Springer Publishing Company; 2007:145–161.

16. Newman MA. A world of no boundaries. *ANS Adv Nurs Sci.* 2003;26(4):240–245.

17. Nightingale F. *Notes on Nursing: What It Is and What It Is Not.* London: Harrison (reprint, 1957, Philadelphia: Lippincott).

18. Murphy N, Canales MK, Norton SA, DeFilippis J. Striving for congruence: the interconnection between values, practice, and political action. *Policy Polit Nurs Pract.* 2005;5(1):20–29.

19. Miller JF. Opportunities and obstacles for good work in nursing. *Nurs Ethics.* 2006;13(5):471–487.

20. Mechanic D. *The Truth About Health Care: Why Reform Is Not Working in America.* New Brunswick, NJ: Rutgers University Press; 2006.

21. Cody WK. Interdisciplinarity and nursing: "everything is everything," or is it? *Nurs Sci Q.* 2001;14(4):274–280.

22. Reed PG. Nursing reformation: historical reflections and philosophic foundations. *Nurs Sci Q.* 2000;13(2):129–136.

23. Mantzoukas S, Japer MA. Reflective practice and daily ward reality: a covert power game. *J Clin Nurs.* 2004;13(8):925–933.

24. Jones DA. Are we abandoning nursing as a discipline? *Clin Nurse Spec.* 2005;19(6):275–277.

25. Holmes D, Perron A, O'Byrne P. Evidence, virulence, and the disappearance of nursing knowledge: a critique of the evidence-based dogma. *Worldviews Evid Based Nurs.* 2006;3(3):95–102.

26. Parse RR. Nursing and medicine: continuing challenges. *Nurs Sci Q.* 2006;19(1):5.

27. Ballou KA. A historical-philosophical analysis of the professional nurse obligation to participate in sociopolitical activities. *Policy Polit Nurs Pract.* 2000;1(3):172–184.

28. Grace PJ. Professional advocacy: widening the scope of accountability. *Nurs Philos.* 2001;2(2): 151–162.

29. Benner P. Enhancing patient advocacy and social ethics: current controversies in critical care. *Am J Crit Care.* 2003; 12(4):374–375.

30. Spencely SN, Reutter L, Allen MN. The road less traveled: nursing advocacy at the policy level. *Policy Polit Nurs Pract.* 2006;7(3):180–194.

31. Leininger M. Theoretical questions and concerns: response from the theory of culture care diversity and universality perspective. *Nurs Sc iQ.* 2007;20(1): 9–15.

32. Leininger M. *Culture Care Diversity and Universality: A Theory of Nursing.* New York, NY: National League for Nursing Press; 1991.

33. Newman MA. *A Developing Discipline: Selected Works of Margaret Newman.* New York, NY: National League for Nursing Press; 1995.

34. Newman MA. *Health as Expanding Consciousness.* Boston: Jones & Bartlett Publishers; 2000.

35. Parse RR. *Man-Living-Health: A Theory of Nursing.* New York, NY: John Wiley & Sons; 1981.

36. Parse RR. Transforming healthcare with a unitary view of the human. *Nurs Sci Q.* 2002;15(1): 46–50.

37. Parse RR. *The Human Becoming School of Thought: A Perspective for Nurses and Other Healthcare Professionals.* Thousand Oaks, CA: Sage; 1998.

38. Patterson JG, Zderad LT. *Humanistic Nursing.* New York, NY: National League for Nursing Press; 1988.

39. Peplau H. *Interpersonal Relations in Nursing: A Conceptual Frame of Reference for Psychodynamic Nursing.* New York, NY: Springer Publishing Company; 1991.

40. Rogers ME. The science of unitary human beings: current perspectives. *Nurs Sci Q.* 1994;7(1):33–35.

41. Rogers ME. *An Introduction to the Theoretical Basis of Nursing.* Philadelphia, PA: FA Davis; 1970.

42. Rogers ME. Nursing: a science of unitary man. In: Riehl JP, Roy C, eds. *Conceptual Models for Nursing Practice.* New York, NY: Appleton-Century-Crofts; 1980:327–337.

43. Roy C. *Introduction to Nursing: An Adaptation Model.* Englewood Cliffs, NJ: Prentice-Hall; 1976.

44. Roy C, Andrews HA. *The Roy Adaptation Model.* 2nd ed. Stamford, CT: Appleton & Lange; 1999.

45. Watson J. *Nursing: Human Science and Human Care.* Norwalk, CT: Appleton-Century-Crofts; 1985.

46. Watson J. *Caring Science as Sacred Science.* Philadelphia, PA: FA Davis; 2005.

47. Watson J. Theoretical questions and concerns: response from a caring science framework. *Nurs Sci Q.* 2007;20(1):13–15.

48. Carper B. Fundamental patterns of knowing in nursing. *ANS Adv Nurs Sci.* 1978;1(1):13–23.

49. White J. Patterns of knowing: review, critique, and update. *ANS Adv Nurs Sci.* 1995;17(4):73–86.

50. Fawcett J, Watson J, Neuman B, Walker PH, Fitzpatrick J. On nursing theories and evidence. *J Nurs Scholarsh.* 2001;33(2):115–119.

THE AUTHORS COMMENT | **A Central Unifying Focus for the Discipline: Facilitating Humanization, Meaning, Choice, Quality of Life, and Healing in Living and Dying**

I have been intrigued by the similarities among various perspectives on nursing theory and nursing science that have developed since the time of Florence Nightingale. Thus, I was inspired to write this article with my Boston College colleagues Dr. Pamela Grace and Dr. Callista Roy (with feedback from Dr. Dorothy Jones) given our collective beliefs regarding the power that diverse nursing perspectives offer nurses in articulating a disciplinary perspective that facilitates the individual and social good. The central unifying focus allows us to highlight nurses' proper commitments as members of a humanitarian service discipline predicated on a unique body of substantive knowledge. This article makes clear a substantive disciplinary focus that transcends any one nursing conceptual model or theory and is grounded in concepts central to the discipline. At the same time, the focus is transparent and relevant in its meaning to other healthcare professions. We believe the central unifying focus of facilitating humanization, meaning, choice, quality of life, and healing in living and dying provides a way of illuminating the added-value piece that recipients of healthcare are looking for within complex environments of healthcare disparities and advanced biomedical technologies. Additionally, this meets nurses' expressed need for a unifying message about our purpose, aims, and substantive disciplinary knowledge in order to more effectively advocate for and assure individual and societal well-being.

DANNY G. WILLIS
PAMELA J. GRACE
CALLISTA L. ROY

49 Nursing Reformation: Historical Reflections and Philosophic Foundations

PAMELA G. REED, RN, PhD, FAAN

Nursing is in the throes of reform. We are speaking more openly about graduate education as the level of entry for practice, more boldly about the art and spiritual dimensions of nursing care, more matter-of-factly about the necessity of science-based practice, and more creatively about nursing's philosophy and unique methods of building knowledge. Reform means to amend or improve by change of form or removal of faults or abuses (*Webster's New Collegiate Dictionary*, 1993). But will the changes be radical enough to make a positive difference for those within the discipline, those contemplating a career choice, and those who work and are served within healthcare systems?

When we contemplate the roots of professional nursing in reference to contemporary nursing, it is evident that we have not yet mined the full implications of nursing initiated by Nightingale (1859/1969) in the 19th century and carried forward by other visionaries during the 20th century. Nursing has evolved into a disintegrated profession, due largely to factions of variously educated nurses. The purpose of this dialogue is to propose ideas for clarifying philosophic foundations for reforming nursing in the 21st century.

Historical Reflections

There is a need to revive the roots of professional nursing's existence. These roots are found in Nightingale's (1895/1969) emancipatory spirit for nursing and for her patients to not only be well, but to use well every power they have; her spiritual commitment concerning the role of nursing; her clarity of a philosophy for nursing that was both scientific and caring; her revolutionary ideas about formally educating nurses, distinct from other healthcare providers; her pragmatism in addressing the health needs of society; and her vision for nursing as a profession. Despite nurse leaders' revolutionary ideas about health reform, university-based education, theory development, and research during the past 100 years, nursing's roots have not developed the discipline as fully as desired.

Service needs of hospitals and physicians have exploited the nursing vision, twisted its roots and choked potential growth that could have been realized in great part through higher education. There is still a proliferation of technical "nursing" training fostered by political interests and profit-driven employers who quell nursing shortages, and the viability of professional nursing, with employment of nonprofessional "nurses." State boards of nursing, with one exception, maintain an outdated, unenlightened, and dispiriting system of nurse licensure. Furthermore, what occupies too much of state boards' time is implementing disciplinary action against nurses whose most common error, amid all that they do, is the implementation of physicians' (medication) orders. The relentless, dependent activity of passing medications, as well as transcribing, filling, and requesting other orders, sustains the need for undereducated "nurses" and erodes the creativity and autonomy that could be nursing.

Professional nurses, by definition, are morally obligated to work within their field and to have a knowledge base adequate for ordering their own actions, especially for direct patient care, whether ambulating patients, talking with a grieving family, or distributing medications. And physicians must take the responsibility for fulfilling their own orders. Nurses who identify with the oppressor by integrating if not embracing medical practice across nursing roles, whether advanced, basic, or technical, rob from the potential to advance nursing care. So do nurses, as CEOs and directors, academic administrators, and teachers, who have the leadership but lack the vision and expertise to implement nursing models of care in their systems, and who lack the courage to speak the language of nursing in their daily work.

The tangled roots of nursing are due also in part to the entry-into-practice debacle from the 1960s and the so-called diversity in educational offerings. Well-meaning and not-so-well-meaning officials are trying to reframe the diverse and disintegrated condition of nursing preparation today with euphemisms that speak of promoting a continuum of practice and therefore a continuum of education, as though something less than a baccalaureate degree provides a foundation for professional nursing education. This continuum may better serve the hospitals than the science.

ABOUT THE AUTHOR

PAMELA G. REED is Professor at the University of Arizona College of Nursing in Tucson, Arizona, where she also served as Associate Dean for Academic Affairs for 7 years. She is a three-time graduate of Wayne State University in Detroit, receiving a BSN, an MSN (with a double major in child–adolescent psychiatric mental health nursing and teaching), and her PhD (with a major in nursing, focused on life span development and aging) from there in 1982. Dr. Reed pioneered research into spirituality and well-being with her doctoral research with terminally ill patients. She also developed a theory of self-transcendence and two widely used research instruments, the *Spiritual Perspective Scale* and the *Self-Transcendence Scale*. Her publications and funded research reflect a dual scholarly focus: Spirituality and other facilitators of well-being in life-limiting illness, and nursing metatheory and knowledge development. Dr. Reed also enjoys time with her family, reading, classical music, swimming, and hiking in the mountains and canyons of Arizona.

Increasingly, articles from a range of professional nursing journals such as *Journal of Professional Nursing, Nursing Outlook, Image, Western Journal of Nursing Research, Advances in Nursing Science,* and *Nursing Science Quarterly* speak to the invisibility and low profile of nursing, and to the oppression of nurses. Authors ask readers where all the future nurses have gone, or if nursing even has a future. Others ponder whether nursing will become extinct or, more alarmingly, whether it will exist tomorrow.

The force of nursing has waxed and waned since Nightingale's era, in part, because an enormous number of people who call themselves nurses lack knowledge and education to understand the processes of nursing. Their ontology of practice derives from (mostly medical) authority and habit, as well as intuition and experience. But such an ontology is uninformed and unenriched by the science of nursing and by other patterns of knowing that are acquired only through the process of higher education and continued learning. Without this knowledge, what appear to be nursing actions may instead be nursing imitations.

Imitations focus more on what, when, and how to do something, and less on the why, the underlying scientific and moral base. Perhaps, during the first half of the 20th century, there was no urgency to ask why. Wars and medical advances created many employment opportunities for nurses, although these wars weren't used to advance the profession as did Nightingale (1859/1969) in the Crimea. It is regrettable, as Schlotfeldt (1987) reflected, that nursing's early leaders were so preoccupied with preparing sufficient numbers of nurses to meet societal needs. From 1900 to 1926, schools of nursing increased from 432 to 2,155, whereas medical schools decreased from 160 to 79 in response to the Flexner Report. The scientific exploration of Nightingale's Laws of Nursing or Laws of Health was abandoned and the promise of improved nursing practice unfulfilled.

The second half of the 20th century brought more sociopolitical changes and accelerated scientific advancement. The teachings of Peplau (1992), Rogers, (1990), Roy (1997), Newman (1995), Watson (1997), Parse (1995) and others awakened nursing to its scholarly heritage and exposed the dogma of a nursing practice that had been separated from its roots, and lacked its own knowledge base. The relevance of a university-based education for professional nursing, envisioned by historical legends Adelaid Nutting, Lavinia Dock, Richard Beard (Dolan, 1968), and others became more widely recognized. However, this recognition seems fragile in the face of yet another nurses' shortage at the end of this century and the continued proliferation of diploma and associate degree graduates in nursing.

Nursing, regarded most basically as a healing process within human systems, has always existed and will always exist, if only underground at times. Nightingale (1859/1969) formalized nursing in the 19th century by initiating efforts to educate people about the nature and facilitation of this process for the betterment of society. The discipline was born out of nothing less than a learned context, a belief in human potential for healing, and a commitment to serving the welfare of human beings. It is unconscionable that the ontology and epistemology of some if not much of nursing practice is manifested in a dominance of technical knowledge and medical orders. There is a need for nursing reform whereby nursing comes clean of the values and beliefs that have misinformed practice and instead identifies with a new philosophy that reintegrates its diversity for the emancipation of the discipline.

An Integrative Philosophy

Despite the increasing dissatisfaction over the current systems of education, licensure, and healthcare, nurses have not been idle in furthering philosophic development of nursing. What must not be overlooked or underutilized in this time of reform is the direction for change provided by a philosophic basis. In the interest of maintaining this momentum, I propose five theses for dialogue in explicating a philosophic basis for a nursing reformation.

The theses address ontologic and epistemologic areas and derive from the current movement toward an integrative philosophy of nursing. This philosophic perspective more purposely links the art and science of nursing, and closes fissures between practice and science that can be exploited by others and diminish the strength of the profession. It is a philosophy that recognizes nursing as a basic discipline (as distinguished from a basic science or art), with a unique focus, and is collaborative with but not dependent upon the orders or knowledge of other professions to provide the substance and purpose of practice and research.

Thesis 1: Nursing Is a Basic Human Healing Process

Previously, I have described nursing as a process inherent to human systems, characterized by ongoing changes in complexity and integration that generate well-being (Reed, 1997). I proposed this substantive definition of nursing, distinguished from the important meaning of nursing as a disciplinary body of knowledge, to provide a shared focus across nursing theory, research, and practice. This definition was developed in answer to the need for what Peplau (as cited in M. J. Smith, 1988) called a simplified rubric that distinguishes a discipline's phenomena from others. The definition, then, puts forth "nursing processes" as the central concern of nursing.

Nursing processes are manifested in a diversity of health experiences among human systems, on all imaginable levels of the person-environment mutual process (individual, patient-nurse, family, community, etc.) Nursing processes may (or may not) cross boundaries of traditional domains of study, such as the physiologic, psychologic, social, and cultural. As with photosynthesis, pathogenesis, or geologic processes for example, nursing processes can be studied to learn about the patterns and natural laws of, in this case, human well-being. Nursing processes may be elucidated in our theorists' work on pattern recognition, human becoming, adaptation, and knowing participation in change, as well as in other processes discovered to reflect homeodynamic principles of life that generate well-being.

Nursing as process provides a fundamental focus for inquiry and integrates the science and the practice of nursing. This is in contrast to defining nursing primarily as a practice commonly found in the nursing literature (for example, see ANA's, 1995, Social Policy Statement; see also Bishop & Scudder, 1999). Nursing as a "practice" emphasizes the performance and repetition of actions, external to the patient and conducted by someone other than the patient. With the focus on nursing as practice, research logically would delve into the nurse's practice of caring rather than into the patient's potential for healing. Whereas Bishop and Scudder (1999) believe that the "study of nursing should focus on nursing as practiced" (p. 24), I propose that the study should focus on nursing as process, inherent in all human systems.

It is reductionistic and disintegrative to describe nursing primarily as a practice, an art, or a science. The dichotomy between practice and science that is engendered by these descriptors makes the discipline vulnerable to the exploitations that have occurred during the 20th century. It may be more productive to conceptualize nursing first as a healing process, the knowledge of which is developed through the synergy between the science and the art.

Thesis 2: Holism Does Not Define Nursing's Unique Perspective and Contributions

The term *holism* is not adequate for describing what nurses do or what nursing is. Holism is a default term employed too often in place of clearer and more precise language to describe the perspective and unique contribution of nursing. The complexity of meanings and implications regarding holism has made application of the term difficult for both philosophic and practical purposes, despite its intuitive appeal to nursing (Kolcaba, 1997; Owen & Holmes, 1993). Moreover, research into the diffusion of the holistic paradigm in nursing from 1960 to 1990 indicated that the term had various applications in the practice community. Holism referred to a variety of factors including therapeutic modalities, beliefs, and roles of clients and nurses. Moreover, there was no indication of its application in the research community (Johnson, 1990).

As a term, holism is used widely across many disciplines, reflecting various perspectives ranging from mechanistic to unitary (Kolcaba, 1997) and reflecting disparities between written discourse and clinical practice (Owen & Holmes, 1993). The nature of the term is such that qualifying words are often needed to explain holism. For some, holism conjures up vague and sometimes unattainable expectations and stifles attempts to conjecture about nursing phenomena.

It is not inaccurate to describe nursing as a holistic discipline. However, if holism is applicable to only a certain part of the nursing community, as the qualifier in the term holistic nursing implies, then holism is not useful in conveying an integrative perspective for nursing. Alternatively, if the essence of nursing is holism, then use of the term holistic nursing is redundant; the term *nursing* should stand alone. It is more productive to spend our efforts identifying terms that clarify the substance of nursing rather than the substance of holism. These terms will better serve our research and practice endeavors to unite nurses in a deeper understanding of what their discipline is all about.

Thesis 3: Embodiment Is a Core Concept in Understanding Health Experiences

The linguistic focus of postmodernism has emphasized the role of language and discourse in building knowledge. The social, cultural, and political dimensions have garnered recognition of their roles in scientific inquiry. Terms like spiritual, self-transcendence, perception, and consciousness, which tend to emphasize mind over body, have gained increased attention. Nevertheless, embodiment remains a critical context for nursing inquiry into health experiences (Wilde, 1999).

Dewey (1929) addressed the dichotomy in knowledge development found between discursive and nondiscursive experiences, mind and body. He, along with other pragmatists, argued for the importance of nondiscursive experience and he, in fact, posited that nondiscursive experience is foundational to all thinking. Shusterman (1997) extended Dewey's views in a more integrative manner by arguing the need for philosophy to value the somatic as well as the linguistic and rational experience. This was justified, he said, given philosophy's pragmatic goal of not only grounding knowledge but producing a better experience. He proposed, radically, that somatics should be integrated into the discursive practices of philosophy, and in the practices of other disciplines interested in promoting transformation and betterment of life. Similarly, Schneider (1998) called for a revival of romanticism in science and advocated for a more balanced approach to postmodern inquiry that included exploration of peoples' felt impressions, bodily sensations, and existential awareness.

The integration of somatic experience into nursing inquiry helps bridge the gap between the worlds of the patient, the practitioner, and the researcher. The body is an important manifestation of the human being, around which much in nursing revolves. As Gadow (1980) explained, the self is inseparable from the body, and nursing philosophy cannot address human health experiences in abstraction from the existential ground, the body. The quest for nursing knowledge, then, occurs not only through the discursive modes of philosophic inquiry and the research process, but also by attending to the embodiment of health processes and practices.

Thesis 4: Scientific Knowledge Is Transformed into Nursing Knowledge Through Contexts of Nursing Practice

This fourth thesis moves us beyond traditional and disintegrative pathways of developing and distributing knowledge, that is, moving from the top down, from theorist and researcher to practitioner. Putnam (1988), a contemporary philosopher who espouses a pragmatic approach to philosophy, explained that the traditional pathway to epistemologic justification, from the theoretical to the more observable concepts, was only one approach to knowledge development. He proposed that theory development proceed in all directions, in any direction that may be handy. Philosopher Nancy Cartwright (1988) elaborated on this idea in explaining that it is not enough to know a given law of nature and deduce other occurrences from that law, as one would using Hempel's (1966) covering law. That is to say that nature is not so well-regulated and independent of context that events can be determined from a given law. Science, she explained, cannot shut down once a law is put forward. Rather, explanations entail ongoing consideration of data from an integration of various ways of knowing, of which we have identified many in nursing: empiric, personal, ethical, aesthetic, unknowing, and intuition, to mention some. Similarly, philosopher Susan Haack (1996) argued against the received (realist) view of truth and the perceived (relativist) view of truth as being the only options for selecting an approach to developing knowledge in a discipline. Instead, she proposed a new term that represented a synthesis of the two dichotomous views, foundationalism and coherence, which she called "foundherentism." Foundherentism was a better justified and more practical approach to building knowledge, in which both experience and beliefs provided an epistemologic basis.

In realizing the meaning of Carper's (1978) nursing epistemology and other postmodern perspectives, nursing began reforming its traditional top-down approach to building knowledge. More nurses are using approaches that privilege the experiences and beliefs of multiple individuals, including researcher, practitioner, and patient.

Professional nurses are people who, in their practice, ethically and skillfully engage patients and themselves in application and testing of knowledge. This engagement transforms scientific knowledge into nursing knowledge (Reed, 1996). The mutual process between nurses and patients or, more broadly, between persons and their environments provides contexts for both the discovery and confirmation of knowledge.

Thesis 5: Nursing Is a Spiritual Discipline

Spiritual is defined as existing in an intentional community with others where otherness is an unreduced intrusion into the experience of each person (S. G. Smith, 1988). While intentions are shared across the community, the individuals are neither diminished nor supplanted by the community. In applying this interpretation of spirituality in nursing, it can be said that the nurse participates with the patient, sharing intentions about health through the intimacy and skill of touch and talk. Intentions are spiritual, focused on health as experienced wholeness.

A spiritual discipline is distinguished from the psychosocial sciences in that it is not merely descriptive of behaviors but rather poses a normative and pragmatic call to action, which is freely chosen. A spiritual person is said to be "called" or "launched outward to others to inhabit a world that transcends one's own world" (S. G. Smith, 1988, p. 62). The spiritual is directed toward "enabling, supporting, growing, loving, respecting, and appreciating" (Lane, 1988, p. 335). A spiritual person, like a poet, discovers new things and ideas from "beyond the horizon of the self" (S. G. Smith, 1988, p. 71) for the benefit and transformation of others.

Regarding a profession as spiritual enhances the meaning of a profession. It is more than compassion; it requires a sense of self-transcendence, connectedness to others, a desire to promote life, and a sense of freedom in choosing these things (Lane, 1988). This perspective nourishes the aesthetic as well as other ways of knowing required within a discipline.

The spiritual, then, is a philosophic basis for praxis, uniting values and knowledge with actions in accord with patients' needs for healthcare. In so doing, the spiritual is integrative and promotes unity within a discipline.

 Toward Scholarship and Praxis in Nursing

Paradoxically, postmodernism has provided us with an awareness of our freedom to turn toward philosophic foundations to create a possibility for unity within a complex discipline characterized by much diversity. We have come to understand that there is no dichotomy between the theoretical and observable. Kant (1781/1964), Popper (1965), and contemporary philosophers of science have argued convincingly that there is no observation in the absence of theory and values. In nursing, this epistemologic view translates into the realization that some of the distinctions drawn between practitioner and researcher may be reformed in an integrative way to enhance development of nursing knowledge and patient care. This was not so 30 years ago, when Ellis' (1969) idea of practitioner as theorist was dismissed by modernist nurses who regarded science as an endeavor separate from art, values, and practices of nursing.

Contemporary pragmatic approaches to knowledge development diminish the dichotomy between the theoretical and the observable, theory and practice, beliefs and experience. The theses presented here have posited a nursing ontology based upon a relational, embodied, and processual view of health. This view necessitates an epistemology that involves both the scientist's and the practitioner's expertise within what Lerner (1995) called the natural laboratory of the world. Scientific knowledge, which is generated outside of this natural laboratory, is transformed into nursing knowledge by its integration within contexts of nursing practice.

A nursing reformation that derives from an integrated philosophy of nursing is not likely to end in revolt and further divisions. But successful reform will require a type of symbolic home where a diversity of theories and ideas can flourish within a spiritual community of shared values and beliefs. Trainor (1998) distinguished this home from the unshakable foundation of modernism. He described it instead as a home that offers a foundational faith in the connectedness of our ideas to the world and to each other. Nursing reformation will require the participation of theorists, scientists, and practitioners in a shared vision of nursing and of the education needed for nurses to participate in integrated methods of knowledge development. Within this perspective, a reformation may remove faults that divide nurses and may restore the scholarship and praxis to nursing that Nightingale envisioned.

REFERENCES

American Nurses' Association. (1995). *Nursing: A social policy statement* (Rev. ed.). Washington, DC: Author.

Bishop, A. H., & Scudder, J. R. (1999). A philosophical interpretation of nursing. *Scholarly Inquiry for Nursing Practice, 13,* 17–27.

Carper, B. (1978). Fundamental patterns of knowing in nursing. *Advances in Nursing Science, 1,* 13–23.

Cartwright, N. (1988). The truth doesn't explain much. In E. D. Klemke, R. Hollinger, & A. D. Kline (Eds.), *Philosophy of science* (Rev. ed., pp. 129–136). New York: Prometheus.

Dewey, J. (1929). *Experience and nature* (Rev. ed.). Carbondale: Southern Illinois University Press.

Dolan, J. A. (1968). *History of nursing* (12th ed.). Philadelphia: W. B. Saunders.

Ellis, R. (1969). The practitioner as theorist. *American Journal of Nursing, 69,* 1434–1438.

Gadow, S. (1980). Body and self: A dialectic. In S. Specker & S. Gadow (Eds.), *Existential advocacy: Philosophical foundations of nursing* (pp. 86–100). New York: Springer.

Haack, S. (1996). Evidence and inquiry: Towards reconstruction in epistemology. In M. Warnock (Ed.), *Women philosophers* (pp. 273–299), London: J. M. Dent.

Hempel, C. G. (1966). *Philosophy of natural sciences.* Englewood Cliffs, NJ: Prentice-Hall.

Johnson, M. B. (1990). The holistic paradigm in nursing: The diffusion of an innovation. *Research in Nursing & Health, 13,* 129–139.

Kant I. (1964). *Critique of pure reason* (N. Kemp Smith, Trans). New York: Macmillan. (Original work published in 1781).

Kolcaba, R. (1997). The primary holisms in nursing. *Journal of Advanced Nursing, 25,* 290–296.

Lane, J. A. (1988). The care of the human spirit. *Journal of Professional Nursing, 36,* 332–337.

Lerner, R. M. (1995). The integrations of levels and human development: A developmental contextual view of the synthesis of science and outreach in the enhancement of human lives. In K. E. Hood, G. Greenberg, & E. Tobah (Eds.), *Behavioral development* (pp. 421–455). New York: Garland.

Newman, M. (1995). *Health as expanding consciousness* (2nd ed.). New York: NLN.

Nightingale, F. (1859/1969). *Notes on nursing: What it is and what it is not.* New York: Dover.

Owen, M. J., & Holmes, C. A. (1993). "Holism" in the discourse of nursing. *Journal of Advanced Nursing, 18,* 1688–1695.

Parse, R. R. (1995). *Illuminations: The human becoming theory in practice and research.* New York: NLN.

Peplau, H. (1992). Interpersonal relations: A theoretical framework for application in nursing practice. *Nursing Science Quarterly, 5,* 13–18.

Popper, K. R. (1965). *Conjectures and refutations: The growth of scientific knowledge.* New York: Harper.

Putnam, H. (1988). What theories are not. In E. D. Klemke, R. Holllinger, & A. D. Kline (Eds.), *Philosophy of science* (Rev. ed., pp. 178–183). New York: Prometheus.

Reed, P. G. (1996). Transforming knowledge into nursing knowledge: A revisionist analysis of Peplau. *Image: The Journal of Nursing Scholarship 28,* 29–33.

Reed, P. G. (1997). Nursing: The ontology of the discipline. *Nursing Science Quarterly, 10,* 76–79.

Rogers, M. (1990). Nursing: Science of unitary, irreducible human beings: Update 1990. In E. Barrett (Ed.), *Visions of Rogers' science-based nursing* (pp. 5–12). New York: NLN.

Roy, C. (1997). Future of the Roy model: Challenge to redefine adaptation. *Nursing Science Quarterly, 10,* 49–52.

Schlotfeldt, R. M. (1987). Defining nursing: A historic controversy. *Nursing Research, 36,* 64–65.

Schneider, K. J. (1998). Toward a science of the heart. *American Psychologist, 53,* 277–289.

Shusterman, R. (1997). *Practicing philosophy: Pragmatism and the philosophical life.* New York: Routledge.

Smith, M. J. (1988). Perspectives in nursing science. *Nursing Science Quarterly, 1,* 80–85.

Smith, S. G. (1988). *The concept of the spiritual: An essay in first philosophy.* Philadelphia: Temple University Press.

Trainor, B. (1998). The origin and end of modernity. *Journal of Applied Philosophy, 15,* 133–144.

Watson, J. (1997). The theory of human caring: Retrospective and prospective. *Nursing Science Quarterly 10,* 49–52.

Webster's new collegiate dictionary. (1993). Springfield, MA: Merriam-Webster.

Wilde, M. H. (1999). Why embodiment now? *Advances in Nursing Science, 22,* 25–38.

THE AUTHOR COMMENTS — Nursing Reformation: Historical Reflections and Philosophic Foundations

The impetus for this article came from a contributing editor of *Nursing Science Quarterly* who provided me the opportunity to write about what I believed was significant as nursing moved into the 21st century. As an educator and administrator, I was frustrated with the state of nursing practice education; nursing's diverse forms of education often did not prepare nurses to practice independently. I grounded my ideas in historical visions of nursing, still unrealized, in terms of a truly independently functioning profession. I wanted to expose some key philosophic issues (presented as my theses) in reforming nursing from within the discipline to put forth a philosophic basis for professional nursing.

PAMELA G. REED

50 Historical Voices of Resistance

Crossing Boundaries to Praxis Through Documentary Filmmaking for the Public

PAULA N. KAGAN, RN, PhD

This article contextualizes my forthcoming study of a particular instance of resistance in nursing history, the Cassandra Radical Feminist Nurses Network, and examines how nursing history can be produced as public media to advance progressive ideas about nurses and transformative and emancipatory nursing and healthcare. It argues that nurse-generated documentary filmmaking is a natural extension of theory and practice, linking several disciplinary and conceptual fields to support a praxis that is situated at the intersection of nursing, critical theory, and the humanities. **Key words:** *critical studies, digital media, documentary filmmaking, emancipatory inquiry, intersectionality, feminism, nursing history, nursing image, praxis.*

You and I as common people must not pass silently from life. Future historians must have our testimony as their resource. Documentaries are our grassroots visions, not just what was preserved by an elite and its minions.... We can bear witness to these times, reinterpret history, and prophesy the future. The consequences of all this for democracy, and for a richer and more harmonious tapestry of cultures, are incalculable. This is the art and purpose of the documentary film.

—*Michael Rabiger* [1(p15)]

Virginia Henderson once commented, "I wished we had been more independent in our thinking, and had brought people along with us faster. I think the public would be ready to understand what we're doing and support us if they understood, if they knew. But we haven't, I don't think we bothered to try to keep the public with us."[2] There is a real need for nurses to participate in the public sphere to a greater extent than at present. This article seeks to address that gap and create a context in which nurse-generated documentary filmmaking becomes a natural extension of theory and practice. This article connects several disciplinary and conceptual fields to support praxis situated at the intersection of nursing and the humanities. More specifically, this article contextualizes my forthcoming study of a particular instance of resistance in nursing history, the Cassandra Radical Feminists Nurses Network, by examining how that history can be produced as public media to advance progressive ideas about nurses and a healthcare future that is transformative and emancipatory.

Nurses create a transformative future by being with others in life-giving ways as they assist and witness people who are articulating the meaning of lived experience and navigating changes that may be minimal or life altering. Nurses may also foster transformation and emancipation by deploying praxis that affirms human dignity and social justice. To this end, the process of creating visual evidence through documentary filmmaking, in which persons of vision and resistance speak, is essential. Listening to others is fundamentally about participation and it is emancipatory.[3] Listening to the voices, while watching the faces, of those whose influence has been dislocated and rendered invisible can create a powerful effect on the viewing public.

Documentaries have been used for education, propaganda, and promoting social justice issues and activism.[4] Film has the ability to engage the public in unique and powerful ways, emotionally connecting them to ideas that resonate with personal significance. A documentary, in addition to other forms of digital media, can give voice to those marginalized by diverse dimensions of gender, class, color, or sexuality Although nurses today can bring their ideas and perspectives to public discourse in ways not possible in the past, their voices are rarely heard in public health discourse and have been particularly missing from public media sources.[5] Nurses' presence and their characterization in the media were documented in the work of Beatrice Kalisch and Philip Kalisch[6-8] in the 1980s, but the topic has since been paid scant attention by nurse scholars.

A larger, common goal of crafting a vision of a humane, accessible, and outcome-productive

ABOUT THE AUTHOR

PAULA N. KAGAN was raised in Detroit, Michigan, and received her BSN from the University of British Columbia in Vancouver where she lived for many years. While raising her family and working, she earned her Master of Science as a Nurse Scholar in Women's Health from DePaul University and her PhD in Nursing from Loyola University. Dr. Kagan has a background in women's health, psychiatry, substance use, community heath, and health policy. Her scholarship has focused on the experience of feeling listened to, media images of nurses, power in healthcare, nurse activists, and emancipatory nursing. Dr. Kagan is Associate Professor in the Department of Nursing at DePaul University in Chicago, Illinois. A recipient of the Illinois Board of Higher Education Nurse Educator Fellowship Award, Dr. Kagan has also been a DePaul University Humanities Center Fellow for her innovative work on the use of digital media in nursing. She teaches from unitary nursing and critical theory perspectives with an emphasis on social justice and diversity for courses in theory, research, and epidemiology.

healthcare system in the United States will require accessing, documenting, and analyzing multiple voices. Formerly unheard perspectives are needed to, as hooks[9] suggested, "shift the center," from a dangerous and unsuccessful medical model to a holistic one founded on principles of social justice. Shifting the center will require nurses to cross disciplinary and methodological boundaries to make their voices heard.

To counter media invisibility of nurses, I developed a documentary project that seeks to make the publicly invisible voices of self-identified radical nurses accessible beyond the disciplinary literature, moving them into the public sphere. My project looks at a group of nurses who came together in the early 1980s to form the Cassandra Radical Feminist Nurses Network. I focus on their stories of lived experience of resistance, emancipation, and marginalization as these emerge in oral history accounts. I address where, why, and in what form knowledge emerged for the women in the group. I am also interested in the knowledge they generated (and still do), paying particular attention to the potential impact and power of such knowledge to affect public discourse and policy on healthcare. Understanding how nurses are portrayed to the public is essential to an analysis of their power and to enhancing their impact in public matters.

Nurses on Film and Nurses as Filmmakers

Nurses have entered the consciousness of American culture in various ways, primarily through print media, television, and feature fiction films. However, nurses have rarely been decision makers as writers, directors, or producers of these media. Denigrating stereotyping is also rampant in these productions. While it has been difficult for predominantly male filmmakers to "get"

any women authentically on screen, it seems almost impossible for them to imagine and create real and complex *nurses*.

Popular Fiction Television and Film

The genre of fiction television and film is the source of the public's most accessible visual depictions of nurses, some of which have been based on actual persons or events. The obvious inadequacies of these representations point to the need for nurse-generated documentaries and more influence in commercial fiction productions. in the movies, nurses have been represented as virtuous and selfless (*Nurse Marjorie*, 1920); courageous (*Nurse Edith Cavell*, 1930; *The White Angel*, 1936); sexy, smart, and in their underwear (*Night Nurse*, 1931); romantic (*South Pacific*, 1958); sadistic disciplinarian (*One Flew Over the Cuckoo's Nest*, 1975); and sexually objectified (all Roger Corman 1970s "nurse-ploitation" films; MASH, *1970*).[10] Closer to authentic depictions of nurses have emerged more recently, albeit typically in supporting roles. cast often with coded patterns of exploitation, nurses who are black women and gay men support, and frequently take abuse from, white protagonists (*Passion Fish*, 1992; *Miss Evers Boys*, 1997; *Girl Interrupted*, 1999; *Magnolia*, 1999; *Angels in America*, 2003).

In addition, there is a definite gap in the scholarly literature that analyzes nurses in film and television across disciplines. Since the work of Kalisch and Kalisch[6-8] in the 1980s, very little nursing scholarship has emerged that contributes to the foundation they set out for looking at the image of the nurse in the media. These authors consistently found that while physicians were unrealistically represented as overly heroic, scholarly, scientific, and ultra-compassionate individuals, to whom many of nursing's activities were attributed, nurses were depicted as sexy, naïve, unintelligent, and having no particular knowledge base.

With the continuing popularity of television shows such as *ER, Scrubs, House, MD,* and *Grey's Anatomy,* it is all the more imperative for nurse scholars to provide critical analysis of how nurses are portrayed. To date, the most continuous voice advocating for realistic and positive representation of nurses in the media has been *The Center for Nursing Advocacy,* which, with limited resources, calls attention to media incidents unfavorable to the profession.[11] Two studies to note are Bridges' review of images of the nurse and nursing in the media[12] and the Woodhull Study on Nurses and the Media commissioned by Sigma Theta Tau in 1997.[13] Named for the late journalist Nancy Woodhull, founder of *USA Today,* who advocated for appropriate and accurate representation of nurses and nursing in the media, this study demonstrated that nurses are seldom represented as experts in print media.

Addressing the representation of nurses on television from outside the discipline, Lamm[14] provided an excellent analysis of six episodes of the 1960's television series, *The Nurses,* which was aired on *CBS* from September 1962 for 2 seasons. *The Nurses* was the first television show to have 2 women as lead protagonists but, after only 2 seasons, it was revised as *The Doctors and the Nurses.* Two physicians were added in leading roles; however, the show survived only for 1 more season. Lamm argued that the show's excellent writing, direction, and acting contributed to previously unseen explications of the dimensions of gender, class, race, and power. *The Nurses* provided some of the earliest television depictions of social issues, such as abortion, disability, and race relations. I remember watching the show with my mother, a former Lieutenant in the Army Nurse Corps, who considered it a realistic depiction of nursing.

Professional Organization Productions

During the 1980s to 1990s, the National League for Nursing produced videos aimed at nursing audiences and lists more than 30 available through Insight Media. Few are specifically relevant to the purposes and frameworks of my work. However, *Nursing in America: Through a Feminist Lens* (1991) offers a critical account of gender and class in the establishment of medical and hospital dominance in the early 20th century and features, among others, feminist nurse scholars Jo Ann Ashley, Peggy Chinn, and Kathleen McPherson.[15] While the mission of the National League for Nursing is promotion and enhancement of nursing education, Johnson & Johnson produced visual media about nurses, targeting the public with their *Campaign for Nursing's Future.* This campaign has been rightly criticized for continuing a "soft" portrayal of nursing consistent with social stereotyping that

neglects emphasis on nursing knowledge, judgment, decision making, and power.[11] The campaign's advertisements also continue to recognize the hospital as the sole location of nursing practice. Johnson & Johnson also sponsored a short video, *Nurse Scientists: Committed to the Public Trust,* produced by the Friends of the National institute for Nursing Research (2004).[16,17] Clearly showing nurses as researchers and experts on health science and policy who have progressive ideas for making change, this work was not intended for the general public.

Nurse Filmmakers

Nurse-generated and produced documentaries are a rare but important genre. Professional nurses seldom produce, write, or direct documentaries, nor is there a database or comprehensive review in the literature of such efforts. However, several nurses have been moved to tell stories publicly and create documentaries. Examples of nurse filmmakers in the United States include: Margaret (Meg) Carson, *Vietnam Nurses* (2006)[18]; Mukulla Godwin,[19] *A Jewel in History: The Story of Homer G. Phillips Hospital for Colored* (1999); and Claire Marie Panke,[20,21] *A Chance to Grow* (2000). The late nurse, writer, and Canadian filmmaker Marion McMahon's,[22] *Nursing History* (1989), and Australian nurse-producer Nicholas Bird's,[23] *NurseTV* (55 episodes) (2003-2008) are also noteworthy. Other nurses are distinguished as nurse consultants or collaborators such as Jean Waldman,[24] *In Love and War* (1996); Karen Wolf,[25] *Nursing, The Politics of Caring* (1977); and Christine Mitchell,[26] *Code Gray: Ethical Dilemmas in Nursing* (1983). My research continues to locate more nurse filmmakers, nurses who have crossed disciplinary and methodological boundaries to tell a story. Each of these nurses is worthy of discussion; however, I will focus my explication of nurse filmmakers on Carson and Godwin, both of whom I have talked with about their experiences making a documentary.

Mukulla Godwin (oral communication, July 6, 2008) was a nurse working in psychiatry in San Francisco, where she had grown up, when she heard from a friend about an African American hospital in St Louis, Missouri, that was closed the year before amidst tremendous community protest including demonstrations and civil disobedience. That was in 1980, and because of her strong interest in African American activism and Pan-African and black diaspora consciousness, along with her ability to know a good story, she began to visit St Louis. In 1995, Godwin initiated research that would become *A Jewel in History: The Story of Homer G. Phillips Hospital for Colored* almost 20 years later. She said recently, "I tried to make the story of Homer Phillips Hospital as an example of the black hospital experience." She was struck by the story and felt "this is something more people need to know about" as "these community type-based hospitals are gone now" and felt that in some ways health disparities were not as bad then, when the community took care of itself as they are now. Godwin contended that many areas of life in the United States are situated as subsets of mainstream society because of de facto segregation; her personal experiences echoed how "we in the African American community have had to live a separate existence and had to develop our own institutions." The closing of Homer Phillips was also instrumental in changing the community, Godwin maintained, as jobs were lost, professionals such as nurses and doctors moved out, and the area deteriorated. While some clearly gained access to the broader community, for many the hospital's demise was devastating.

Using city archives at Washington University, Godwin created a network of informants and supporters, many of whom recounted fond memories of Homer Phillips. "I felt [being a filmmaker] was activism," Godwin maintained, "a lot of good can come out of nurse activism ...and we need to advocate for what we know will help." She continued, "I had to be motivated to see the film through with some small grants but mostly my own funds because it was a passion." Godwin was particularly motivated when people said, "I didn't know black hospitals existed" and she said, "I was excited to see that this was something I could do." Contributing to black history by facilitating recognition of something important in the African American experience was imperative to Godwin. Feeling an absolute urgency to do so as participants were aging and dying, she brought director Chike Nwoffiah on board.

Together, Godwin and Nwoffiah conducted and edited more than 60 interviews and archival footage before screening the film at the Pan-African Film Festival. Screenings also took place in San Francisco and St Louis. However, in addition to struggling for resources, Godwin faced formidable time constraints; she feels that a lack of both confidence and support has prevented her from pursuing broader distribution of the film. She believes the film is still timely, suggesting, "We should be alarmed" at the inadequate healthcare in marginalized communities. Godwin acknowledged the criticism by some that the film could have been more nurse focused and is planning to reedit the film to emphasize the nursing perspective. Godwin would like *The Jewel* to stimulate future discussions and has made it available to the University of Missouri as part of a symposium on healthcare. Toward the end of our conversation, she said wistfully, "Nurses have allowed others to determine the future" and wished nurses could be heard in the larger dialogue.

Meg Carson's (oral communication, June 28, 2008) experience as a filmmaker is somewhat different from Godwin's, although Carson also spoke about her passion to bring a story to the public on film. Her frustration at feeling the urgency to do so, while having to wait until the time was right, was also similar to Godwin's experience. Carson's film is about a group of former military nurses who participated in her funded research on posttraumatic stress disorder (PTSD). Carson's desire to create a documentary emerged from her study that measured markers for the psychophysiology of PTSD in 173 women who had served as nurses in Vietnam. She was especially struck by their qualitative responses to questions about their experiences during a procedure called script-driven imagery in which the nurses listened to scripts of their actual experiences in Vietnam. As the nurses reminisced about their experiences, Carson felt inspired. "My first reaction," she recalled, "was wow, isn't this a privilege, isn't this a wonderful opportunity... to hear an amazing piece of nursing history," and as time went on, she thought "somehow we have to get this down …. I didn't even formally have a plan at that time." However, Carson believed that "this somehow has to be captured before these nurses are gone."

Carson could not focus on moving forward while her study of PTSD continued. However, when she began to present her findings of that study in public, she included some of the nurses' stories. When she "talked about it to the public there was such a reaction" that "it intensified my desire to have [the film] get done, I made that a purpose in my life." Carson then shifted from making a documentary for nursing audiences to focusing on a film for a public audience. "As my dream broadened" she said, "and expanded, I wanted to show the public the value of nurses and what it is they do, the challenges they face." Carson acknowledged that "nobody knows it like the people who do it" and thus it is difficult to rely on others to represent nurses accurately. "It is important to me that people start to try to get their emotional centers nudged about how valuable nursing is to them," and "media jogs that emotional response from people." She finds many images of nurses in media "troubling" and feels that the "public needs to know not just that nursing is another profession and a good profession but how ultra valuable nursing is," believing that "film and media is a great way to remind people who we are and what we do."

Creative Street Entertainment of Indianapolis produced a pilot with Carson, which was sold to WE television network. At that point David H. Smith (writer/director) and Steven N. Katzenberger (producer) produced the completed film with Carson in which 8 women were featured. Carson is credited as Associate Producer/Consultant. Actress Dana Delany, who starred as army nurse, Coleen McMurphy in the television series China Beach, narrates the film, which won an Emmy Award for Best Editing (Dan Meadows) in 2007.

Carson's advice to nurse filmmakers is to honor their passion and desire to tell a good story and to surround themselves with a supportive team, to have a strong foundation in historical methods or other methods as appropriate, and to make ethics and the protection of participants a priority. She insisted, "there are incredible nurses doing incredible things and why aren't they getting out there?" On crossing disciplinary boundaries, she said, "it is like diving over that abyss into the unknown" but "you have to have a passion for wanting to get it done."

 ## Crossing Boundaries: Nursing, the Humanities, and Resistance

Nurses can create a more productive future for healthcare by resisting the boundaries and limitations of sanctioned modes of knowledge production. They can explicate progressive, socially critical nursing perspectives by looking to history, creating a social justice culture, and utilizing the art of documentary filmmaking. What follows reflects several linkages central to such a process, connecting *science with the humanities, art and aesthetics with nursing, and narrative with resistance.*

Sciences and Humanities

The significance of nurse-generated filmmaking, and its use as a research methodology as well as a dissemination tool, is that it underscores the fundamental connection the humanities have with advancing social and scientific ideas.[4] In the human sciences, such as nursing, memoir and lived narrative can expand the boundaries and limitations of researching and documenting the human experience. Themes underpinning the contexts in which nurses encounter people every day such as suffering, loneliness, compassion, death, love, bravery, confusion, beauty, and alienation, are at the core of the humanities. As filmmakers for social change, nurses can foster a continuous and simultaneous integration of science and the humanities while rejecting compulsory traditional boundaries between disciplines. Nurses can stimulate health systems change through public questioning of the margins and restrictions embedded in the counterproductive health infrastructures that historically and currently operate in the United States.[27]

Nurse documentarians could also provide a comprehensive look at healthcare from an insider's perspective contributing to an intimate understanding of situated frameworks and systems of greed and neglect in addition to proposing solutions that the public may not otherwise realize. Nurses have an obligation to share with the public nursing's contributions to philosophical and scientific foundations that are necessary to support reform of a damaged system. It is the responsibility of the discipline and the profession to inform the public that universal healthcare in the United States cannot occur without significant awareness of the contributions of nurses, elimination of restrictive practice laws, and shifting the center from a medical and biomedical focus on acute care, technology, and cure to multivocal, holistic nurse-directed primary care in the community.

Art, Aesthetics, and Nursing

Mitchell and Cody[28] contended that it is imperative to make the creativity and artistry in nursing visible. Nurse scholars who bridge nursing with the humanities further the use of narrative approaches and other dimensions of aesthetics to both broaden and specify understanding of social and political conditions of healthcare experiences and nursing inquiry and practice. The work of Chinn et al[29] delineated a definition of art in nursing practice as nurses were observed in the rhythm and flow of daily nursing practice. They developed a methodology of aesthetic comprehension and critique in which the movement and narrative of nursing arts surface through analysis of observation, journaling, and photography. In addition, Chinn and Kramer[30] have continued to update their work on aesthetic knowledge in nursing and contend that aesthetic knowledge development provides understanding of instances of the art of nursing in which feelings are evoked and meaning is derived, and that experiences in connection with others are transformative. That is exactly what happens in a documentary, reflecting strong consistency across disciplines and affording an obvious approach for nurses to use when communicating to the public.

Chinn and Kramer,[30] following Johnson's conceptualizations of the art of nursing, delineated 4 assumptions that can be extended to a wide range of living out the artistic processes of nursing. This conceptualization of the art of nursing is an especially applicable framework for nurses working in visual media such as a documentary. I have taken the liberty of adapting these assumptions here from their context of "nurse as artist" in patient care to the concept of "nurse as artist" in documentary filmmaking in order to draw an explicit link between nursing arts and the humanities. Chinn and Kramer[30(pp156-159)] suggested that nursing art demonstrates the ability to grasp meaning in situations, establish meaningful connections, perform skillfully, determine appropriate courses of action, and morally conduct one's practice [praxis]. All of these assumptions underscore the art of the nurse documentarian in the process of historical research utilizing digital media. This will become more apparent in the discussion below of my own project and praxis.

Documenting Historical Narratives of Resistance

Cowling[31] maintained that significant knowledge is developed from narrative accounts of personal knowing. He created a conceptualization of "unitary praxis" in which meaning and understanding emerge from the appreciation of, and in participation with, the lives of others as lived processes of wholeness.[31] This is consistent with my work on persons' lived experience of feeling listened to that showed that people want to feel appreciated and that this appreciation occurs in participatory dialogue with others.[3]

Documentaries are overwhelmingly about how persons' stories emerge in a process of discovery and appreciation and filmmakers' desires to connect with these stories. Filmmakers and subjects together create the visual evidence that is a representation of someone's life. Even if filmed concurrently with present events in real time, documentaries are essentially products of history, in the broadest sense of the word, as soon as they are edited and prepared for presentation to an audience. They are partly historical record and partly interpretation, with many decisions emanating from the director and editor as myriad choices are made toward creating the final product. Narratives of resistance are emancipatory, often articulating marginalized or invisible identities. Narratives of resistance convey transformative critical standpoints while incorporating methods of alternative knowledge production. Support for this is expressed by nurse historian Wall, who argued "for a broad historical approach that takes an interdisciplinary view into consideration when working with, and in the interpretations of, nursing history."[32(p5)] In addition, she supported "forms of expression that look more at power relationships, gender, culture, ethnicity, religion and ideology."[32(p5)]

Nelson,[33] who argued that we are educating nurses who have no connection to historical location and identity, further illuminated the intersection of narration and identity. She contended that nursing theory has replaced nursing history as the "professionalizing discourse" and we are "producing nurses without a historical identity."[33(p181)] I agree that most of nursing theory is ahistorical and the effect is the rendering invisible of social and cultural context and issues of power, gender, color, sexuality, and class. While Nelson argued that analyzing historical data through the lens of history is essential and nursing theory

optional, I suggest that such interpretation requires both a theoretical perspective and a comprehensive understanding of the historical contexts, times, and conditions under study. Finally, consistent with the purposes of this article, Nelson contended that it is important for nurse historians to reach the public and this will more likely occur if nursing history data are appropriately situated in the broader historical context from which they emerge. In the context of this article, narratives of resistance are situated in their social and historical contexts as well as within interdisciplinary critical theoretical frameworks and methods as discussed in the next sections.

Documentary Filmmaking: Praxis for Resistance and Social Activism

Michael Rabiger, filmmaker, educator, and founder of Columbia College's Michael Rabiger Center for the Documentary in Chicago, has suggested that cinematic language is "the 20th century's great contribution to universal understanding."[1(p15)] He and other practitioners and scholars of cinematic arts and science are consistent in voicing the overwhelming social importance of documentaries and their potential to liberate by making both everyday and unique stories widely available.[1,4,34] By illuminating human stories at the margins, usually involving a struggle or conflict, documentaries stimulate the audience to feel and to think. When presented with paradoxes and contradictions along with the familiar, viewers must come to their own conclusions about the human situation explored on film.

Documentaries are embedded with elements of bearing witness to others, conveying meaning and evoking feeling, and uncovering lost or suppressed voices. While varying in quality, documentaries can emerge from literally anyone who sees a good story and can gain access to a camera and the means for postproduction. However, there is a contract with the audience to be fair and honest in representations of actuality.[1,4] This access to broad communication with the public requires accompanying ethical and moral responsibility to protect and respect both subjects and audiences while upholding fidelity to the actual situation. This fidelity can be threatened or fostered by the multitude of production and editorial decisions made by the filmmakers, such as participant selection, what footage is needed to tell the story, constructing interview questions, what to leave in or cut out, and what extra or archival materials to add.

On a broader level there are particular challenges for getting independent documentaries made at all. Their service as vehicles of social change can depend on political and corporate agendas, which can influence funding and distribution. Film scholar Zimmermann,[34] writing from postcolonial and critical feminist perspectives, suggested that we are in a continued "state of emergency" whereby independent documentarians are challenged, confronted, and obstructed by politically conservative administrations, legislation, and corporate media's filtering and vetting processes. She described contemporary battles as the transnationalization of the media corporation fosters an amnesiac and anesthetized global society on one side and the struggle for independent voices of difference emerging and reclaiming the public spheres of communication on the other. Zimmermann called for "oppositional independent documentaries [that] elaborate racialized, gendered, and sexualized discourses that destabilize the homogeneity of the nation with heterogeneity and hybridity" toward "reimagined democracies."[34(pxx)] It is in this spirit that I have undertaken my project.

With the increasing ease of video production and venues for distribution, including Web-based applications,[35] documentaries now not only support but also require a diversity of contributing voices including those of nurses.[34] The content of documentary film scholarship suggests that the disciplines of nursing and documentary filmmaking share many congruent issues, methods, and theoretical standpoints for praxis, critique, and analysis. Barnouw's[36] foundational and definitive history of the documentary and Aufderheide's[4] *Documentary Film: A Very Short Introduction* are excellent starting points for nurses to discover these shared areas.

Praxis in documentary filmmaking and praxis in nursing are strongly parallel. However, while both fields have embedded agendas for critical analysis and social action, nursing sees only a minority of its members intentionally engaged in praxis for social change. Notions of praxis, common to both nursing and documentary filmmaking, are concerned with emancipatory inquiry, concepts of power and of speaking truth to power, resisting dominant discourses, and fostering public awareness.[4,30,34,37,38] These concepts regarding emancipation, transformation, and resistance are significant to both fields and form a synthesis between disciplines that may help guide nurses contemplating praxis in digital media for a public audience. For example, filmmaker Barbara Koppel's *Harlan County, USA* (1973), which she made in collaboration with striking coal miners in Kentucky, incorporates all of these concepts and is an instance of resistance and activism.[4] Filmmakers and nurses working toward social justice value participation in acts of *unhiddenness*, making the invisible visible, as a form of social action aimed at influencing future outcomes that repair the human condition.

Nursing: Praxis for Resistance and Social Activism

The practice applications of nursing and documentary filmmaking are underpinned by theory, some of which is drawn from other disciplines and some of which has been generated within the fields. Both serve to inform praxis in each discipline and shape the forms of "doing" as well as the products and outcomes. Recognizing that theory can be a place of healing, hooks said of theory, "I found a place where I could imagine possible futures, a place where life could be defined differently.'[39(p61)] However, she went on to argue that theory in itself is not active but must be directed to praxis. I propose the following ideas for a praxis that arises out of the nursing literature and emphasizes *emancipatory inquiry and power* and *integration of the humanities and critical studies in nursing education.*

Emancipatory Inquiry and Power

In nursing, Chinn and Kramer[30] added the concept of *emancipatory knowing* to the most recent edition of their classic theory and knowledge development text. They defined emancipatory knowing as the "capacity to critically examine the social, cultural, and political status quo, and to figure out how and why it came to be that way."[30(pp4-5)] Emancipatory knowing, arising from inquiry and analysis, identifies values and beliefs that are constituents of knowledge and knowledge production Emancipatory knowing, with analysis of power dynamics, examines how these elements of knowledge are created, maintained, legitimated, and utilized to support social injustice Chinn and Kramer further claimed that emancipatory knowing emerges from praxis, critical reflection, and social action, and that, "praxis involves the shaping and creating of the future and requires a vision of the future you want to create."[30(p2)]

Similar to notions of emancipation, and central to liberation of nursing knowledge beyond the discipline, are ideas of power. The work of nurse scholar Elizabeth Barrett on power and knowing participation and that of Jo Ann Ashley on power and gender are closely connected.[37] Barrett's theory and practice methodology are about power as knowing participation in change and explicitly about power as participation and emancipation. The theory holds that "power as knowing participation means that awareness and freedom drive what choices a person makes and how they involve themselves in living change."[37(p323)] For Ashley,[38] who made the critical connection between power and gender in healthcare, the notion of power was central. Over 30 years ago, Ashley argued that nurses needed to become politically aware, resistant, and socially active. Ashley "was adamant in her view that nurses utilize creative new forms of research and scholarship in order to explicate mythologies and deceptiveness that undermine the health of the public and ability of nurses to practice nursing."[37(p321)] The work of scholars Barrett and Ashley solicit consideration from nurses to become aware and to take action to create change. Moving nurses forward into the public sphere requires a commitment to underpinning nursing education with such frameworks concerned with power and emancipatory inquiry, pedagogy, and practice.

Praxis in Nursing Education

One particular barrier to nurses' understanding the importance of becoming politically aware and communicating directly to the public is nursing education. Few have the opportunity, in their professional education, to develop critical frameworks of analysis for the social, economic, political, and cultural contexts of healthcare delivery and the structure of healthcare professions. Few consider, from simultaneous positions of privilege (primarily white and professional) and marginalization (by class and gender), how locations along dimensions of gender, class, color, and sexuality operate in healthcare theory and practice. hooks[39(p12)] contended that "the classroom remains the most radical space of possibility in the academy," but that idea seems to be overlooked in nursing education. This is especially troubling considering the strong roots in social and political activism attributed to nursing in the United States. Most nurses today are not educated to reflect critically and intersectionally on the material and social conditions in which healthcare takes place.

Intersectional analysis developed by black feminist scholars in the 1960s focuses on examination of interlocking systems of power, domination, and oppression with attention to racism, sexism, homophobia, and classism.[40,41] This was the framework upon which I developed a graduate nursing course on health and marginality wholly focused on considerations of gender, color, class, and sexuality in healthcare. The syllabus relies on the growing body of nursing scholarship that has emerged from critical studies frameworks over the past decade informed by a wide range of canonical and current interdisciplinary scholarship. These varying approaches to social analysis emphasize aspects of identity, history, language, and the social, cultural, political, economic, and sexual conditions of power and privilege.

Students read, for example, Schroeder[27] on the effect of corporate wealth and globalization and the inability for the united States to create and maintain a viable healthcare system; Reimer Kirkham and Browne's[42] critical analysis of social justice that goes beyond the traditional ideas that emphasize distribution and access to notions that emphasize health outcomes and embrace participation, recognition, and redistribution; and Kirkham et al[43] on postcolonial feminist analysis of evidence-based practice. In addition, readings unlikely to be found in most nursing curricula include those from postcolonial scholar and psychoanalyst Frantz Fanon[44] to transgendered persons such as Kate Bornstein,[45] to feminist scholar Barbara Ehrenreich on class,[46] and critical race theorist bell hooks[47] on race and black rage. Educating the critical-activist nurse, engaged in transgressive and transformative praxis, would require whole curricula to be built upon these intersectional and critical approaches to analysis.

 ## Cassandra Radical Feminist Nurses Network

Similar to Godwin's and Carson's films, my project emerged out of discovery, coming directly out of previous research on feeling listened to and Jo Ann Ashley.[3,37] My documentary project is grounded in the lives, communities, and contributions of a group of nurse activists known as Cassandra Radical Feminists Nurses Network in the 1980s in the United States. The nurses' concerns were documented at a grassroots level in the little remembered news journal *Cassandra*.[48] The film is a major component of a larger project, which aims to articulate and understand the story of these nurse activists through filmed oral histories, textual research, and critical analysis of their activities, concerns, and standpoints relative to those of the broader Women's Liberation Movement, and the current healthcare environment.

Emergence of the Project

The documentary began when I wrote an article commemorating the life and work of Jo Ann Ashley, nurse historian and feminist activist, who died at age 41 in 1980.[37] This set the foundation for the Cassandra film project. Ashley,[38] a nurse full of revolutionary ideas, insisted that nurses retain control over their professional practice to advance the health of the public, a message that has largely been ignored within and outside of the discipline. Ashley's "innovative research uncovered a web of pervasive gender and class bias that continues to resonate [37(p317)] when we examine today's healthcare delivery process that does not serve the public very well. Interviewing several of Ashley's friends and colleagues for the article brought the Cassandra Network to my attention.

My objective in creating this documentary was to create a vehicle for bringing the Cassandra nurses' story to the public. I am continually surprised at how little people know about nurses and the political, social, and economic agendas that structure how healthcare is provided (or for millions of Americans, not provided). While Moore's[49] *Sicko* (2007) presented observations and lay analysis primarily focused on the insurance and pharmaceutical industries, he was not able to provide a comprehensive look at healthcare from an insider's perspective, from a nurse's perspective, and more specifically through a critical feminist and postcolonial lens.

My film will tell the story of what brought these women together, what they hoped to accomplish, how they evaluate their efforts in retrospect, and what they see as the *Cassandra News Journal* and network's legacies. It is a work about seeking and establishing identity, the power of collectivity, and the initiation and implementation of alternative media. This "underground" news journal advanced a strong social critique that ultimately influenced and helped change knowledge production in the discipline. Many in this community of nurse activists went on to become leaders in the discipline and profession of nursing as distinguished scholars, most doctorally prepared, and many designated as Fellows in the American Academy of Nurses. To date, however, there has been very little analysis of the Cassandra group in the literature, and certainly none on film.

Explicating the Historical and Social Context

Cassandra was established in 1982, the year the Equal Rights Amendment met its demise. This pivotal event motivated the women in my study to establish a news journal for voicing their ideas. This community of nurse activists struggled with issues of power, professional control, and the place of women and nurses as workers across a broad range of social divisions.[37] Many in the collective lived within intersections of multiple minority identifications of gender, class, and sexuality. The dimension of race and the location of feminist nurses of color amidst a primarily white group is a part of the analysis and dialogue made obvious by their absence.

Part of the story is how the Cassandra nurses view their experiences of marginalization in the professional and general social milieu of the time. In an environment underpinned by restrictions on the scope of their professional practice, their ability to provide healthcare to the public was limited. Socially restricted by gender, sexuality, and class, these women broke many barriers, taking many personal and professional risks. The discipline of medicine and the hegemony of a biomedical model, as opposed to the humanist holistic model of healthcare they preferred,

dominated their professional lives. Ideas of a nuclear family, women's place in the home, and heteronormativity dominated expectations for their personal lives, as evidenced from their writings in the news journal.[48] The Cassandra nurses, entering the profession a generation after Lillian Wald and Lavinia Lloyd Dock, leaders in the major movements of social justice, women's and human rights, continued traditions of advocacy for the profession and for the health of the public. In contrast, at this time, the majority of nurses were falling into lockstep, supporting an industry whose primary concern emphasized cure and high technology while traditions of care and practice that could improve public health through prevention and health promotion were ignored.

Praxis

My methodology includes filmed oral history interviews, filming of establishing footage for current context, photography, and gathering of collateral visuals such as memorabilia, news reports, relevant videos, home movies, personal photographs, posters, flyers, and illustrations from participants. In addition, I have gathered archival footage and photographs necessary to provide context and meaning. Sources that cover in-depth technical, conceptual, and methodological frameworks and the potential for ambiguities concerning point of view, consent, time, subjectivity, identity, language, interpretation, narrative analysis, and use of archival materials have helped create a foundation for the film.[1,50]

However, filmmaking is a collaborative activity. My participants in Cassandra live across the united States. While I could video and teleconference with them, I am committed to personal meetings and interviews. For me, establishing relationships is a priority for obtaining oral histories and requires extensive e-mailing, "Skyping," telephone conversations, and personal interactions. Relationships with collaborators, participants, and consultants are paramount. My film could not be made without interested and willing others who take the time to participate in interviews, advise me, and work with me in production. A respect for and recognition of the role others have in a documentary production cannot be underestimated. To ensure the protection of human subjects and be in compliance with ethical standards for conducting research, I received approval to conduct oral history research from the DePaul University institutional review board. Having appropriate ethical and legal guidance helps clarify the purposes of the interaction for participants and collaborators. While the institutional review board approved the project and the information sheet for participants, an attorney and production collaborator have assisted with the image and location release forms.

On the technical side, I have found associate producers, camerapersons, editors, and consultants who are interested in this film and its subject matter. The political and social consciousness of collaborators is as important as my own and I try to work with those who share perspectives that are consistent with feminist, critical, and intersectional ideas. Mentoring students in research assistantships has also been a significant part of this project. I have had women's and gender studies, history, and digital cinema students to help me organize materials, begin analysis of the Cassandra news journals, research archival materials, and make production and editing suggestions.

Since identifying the Cassandra Network as the story I wanted to explore, I have been immersed in the specifics of that story and in determining what I wanted to know and how anticipated and unanticipated knowledge might surface. Writing about this project while conducting the research and developing the film has forced me to "live the praxis." For nurses engaged in documentary filmmaking, multiple boundary crossings and challenges to mandatory, traditional disciplinary, and methodological limitations are necessary. The production of nursing knowledge and theory is not naturally limited, but it demands information and analysis from multiple interdisciplinary and methodological foundations. I hope new general and nursing knowledge will emerge from this work that will inform the public and inform health policy and nursing practice, education, and research. This is the power of telling nursing stories and having human stories told by nurses, and it can be emancipatory and transformative.

 Conclusion

This article sets the context for my future analysis of a particular instance of resistance in nursing history, the Cassandra Radical Feminist Nurses Network, by examining the ways in which nursing history can be explicated and produced as public media to advance progressive ideas about nurses and healthcare. I also address a gap in the literature and create a context in which nurse-generated documentary filmmaking seems a natural extension of theory and practice. I have connected several disciplinary and conceptual fields that support praxis situated in the intersection of nursing and the humanities and emphasized the importance the humanities have to advancing social and scientific ideas. Most significantly, this article is about imagination, creativity, and freedom. How can we resist the traditional boundaries imposed on creating the context of freedom as we push toward an imagined future of enhanced health and quality of life for the public? I hope this article will encourage other nurses to resist limiting modes of knowledge production and expand their visions and voices through documentary filmmaking.

REFERENCES

1. Rabiger M. *Directing the Documentary*. 4th ed. Burlington, MA: Focal Press; 2004.
2. Moss L, Moccia P, National League for Nursing. *Nursing Theory a Circle of Knowledge*. New York: Insight Media; 1987.
3. Kagan PN. Feeling listened to: a lived experience of human becoming. *Nurs Sci Q*. 2008;21:59–67.
4. Aufderheide P. *Documentary Film: A Very Short Introduction*. New York: Oxford University; 2007.
5. Buresh B, Gordon S. *From Silence to Voice: What Nurses Know and Need to Communicate to the Public*. Ottawa, Ontario: Canadian Nurses Association; 2002.
6. Kalisch PJ, Kalisch BJ, Clinton J. The world of nursing on prime time television, 1950 to 1980. *Nurs Res*. 1982;31:358–363.
7. Kalisch PJ, Kalisch BJ, McHugh ML. The nurse as a sex object in motion pictures, 1930 to 1980. *Res Nurs Health*. 1982;5:147–154.
8. Kalisch PA, Kalisch BJ. A comparative analysis of nurse and physician characters in the entertainment media. *J Adv Nurs*. 1986;11:179–195.
9. hooks b. *Feminist Theory: From Margin to Center*. 2nd ed. Cambridge, MA: South End Press; 2000.
10. Rasmussen E. Picture imperfect: from nurse ratched to hot lips Houlihan, film/TV portrayals of nurses of ten transmit a warped image of real-life RNs. *Nurse-Week*. May 7, 2001. http://www.nurseweek.com/ news/features/01-05/picture.html. Accessed July 1, 2008.
11. Center for Nursing Advocacy. News on nursing in the media. http://www.nursingadvocacy.org/ news/news.html. Accessed July 5, 2008.
12. Bridges JM. Literature review on the images of the nurse and nursing in the media. *J Adv Nurs*. 1990;15:850–854.
13. Sigma Theta Tau International Honor Society of Nursing. Woodhull study on nurses and the media. 1997. http://www.nursingsociety.org/Media/Pages/ woodhall.aspx. Accessed July 5, 2008.
14. Lamm B. Television's forgotten gems: the nurses. *J Popular Film Telev*. 1995;23:72–79.
15. Ely T, Moss L, Moccia P. *Nursing in America Through a Feminist Lens*. New York: National League for Nursing; 1991.
16. Johnson & Johnson Services Inc. 2008. http://www.jnj.com/. Accessed July 2, 2008.
17. Johnson & Johnson, Friends of the National Institute for Nursing Research (FNINR) Board of Directors. *Nurse Scientists: Committed to the Public Trust*. Washington, DC: Johnson & Johnson; 2004.
18. Delany D, Smith DH, Katzenberger SN, Goodman T. *Vietnam Nurses*. Indianapolis, IN: Creative Street Entertainment; 2006.
19. Nwoffiah, CC, Godwin MJ, Stroud F *A Jewel in History: The Story of the Homer G. Phillips Hospital for Colored, St. Louis, Missouri*. San Francisco, CA: Homer G. Phillips Project; 1999.
20. Panke CM. *A Chance to Grow*. Boston, MA: Fanlight Productions; 2000.

21. Santandrea L. Nursing comes to light. *Am J Nurs.* 2001; 101:87.

22. McMahon M. Nursing histories: reviving life in abandoned selves. *Feminist Rev.* 1991;37:23–37.

23. Bird N. NurseTV. http://www.nursetv.com.au/. Accessed July7, 2008.

24. Field M. On nursing: Hopkins nursing in "Love and War." *The Gazette* [serial online]. January 21, 1997;26(18). http://www.jhu.edu/~gazette/janmar97/jan2197/lovewar.html. Accessed June 28, 2008.

25. Sawyer T, Finck J. *Nursing, the Politics of Caring.* Cambridge, MA: Ilex Films; 1977.

26. Achtenberg B, Sawyer J, Mitchell C. *Code Gray, Ethical Dilemmas in Nursing.* Boston, MA: Fanlight Productions; 1983.

27. Schroeder C. The tyranny of profit: concentration of wealth, corporate globalization, and the failed US health care system. *Adv Nurs Sci.* 2003;26:173–184.

28. Mitchell GJ, Cody WK. Ambiguous opportunity: toiling for truth of nursing art and science. *Nurs Sci Q.* 2002;15:71–79.

29. Chinn PL, Maeve MK, Bostick C. Aesthetic inquiry and the art of nursing. *Sch Inq Nurs Pract: Int J.* 1997;11:83–95.

30. Chinn PL, Kramer MK. *Integrated Theory and Knowledge Development in Nursing.* 7th ed. St Louis, MO: Mosby; 2008.

31. Cowling WR. A unitary participatory vision of nursing knowledge. *Adv Nurs Sci.* 2007;30:61–70.

32. Wall BM. Nursing history: blurring disciplinary boundaries [notes]. *Nurs Hist Rev.* 2007;15:5–8.

33. Nelson S. The fork in the road: nursing history versus the history of nursing? *Nurs Hist Rev.* 2002;10:175–188.

34. Zimmermann PR. *States of Emergency: Documentaries, Wars, Democracies.* Minneapolis, MN: University of Minnesota; 2000.

35. Cohen D, Rosenzweig R. *Digital History: A Guide to Gathering, Preserving, and Presenting the Past on the Web.* Philadelphia, PA: University of Pennsylvania; 2006.

36. Barnouw E. *Documentary: A History of the Non-Fiction Film.* 2nd ed. New York: Oxford University; 1993.

37. Kagan PN. Jo Ann Ashley 30 years later: legacy for practice. *Nurs Sci Q.* 2006;19:317–327.

38. Ashley JA. *Hospitals, Paternalism, and the Role of the Nurse.* New York: Teachers College Press; 1976.

39. hooks b. *Teaching to Transgress: Education as the Practice of Freedom.* New York: Routledge; 1994.

40. McCall L. The complexity of intersectionality. *Signs: J Women Cult Soc.* 2005;30:1771–1800.

41. Schulz AJ, Mullings L. *Gender, Race, Class, and Health: Intersectional Approaches.* San Francisco, CA: Jossey-Bass; 2006.

42. Kirkham SR, Browne AJ. Toward a critical theoretical interpretation of social justice discourses in nursing. *Adv Nurs Sci.* 2006;29:324–339.

43. Kirkham SR, Baumbusch JL, Schultz ASH, Anderson JM. Knowledge development and evidence-based practice: insights and opportunities from a postcolonial feminist perspective for transformative nursing practice. *Adv Nurs Sci.* 2007;30:26–40.

44. Fanon F. *Wretched of the Earth.* New York:Grove Press; 1963.

45. Bornstein K. *Gender Outlaw.* New York: Routledge; 2000.

46. Ehrenreich B. *Nickel and Dimed: On (Not) Getting By in America.* New York: H Holt and Co; 2001.

47. hooks b. *Killing Rage: Ending Racism.* New York: H Holt and Co; 1995.

48. Cassandra Radical Feminist Nurses Network. *Cassandra: Radical Feminist Nurses Newsjournal.* 1982–1989. http://ans-info.net/PLC.htm#cassandra. April5, 2006.

49. Glynn KR, Weinstein H, Weinstein B, O'Hara M, Moore M. *Sicko.* New York: Weinstein Co. Home Entertainment; 2007.

50. Lewenson SB, Herrmann EK, eds. *Capturing Nursing History: A Guide to Historical Methods in Research.* New York: Springer Publishing Co; 2008.

THE AUTHOR COMMENTS

Historical Voices of Resistance: Crossing Boundaries to Praxis Through Documentary Filmmaking for the Public

I was concerned at the lack of nurse experts quoted in print media, interviewed on radio and television, and participating in creating media about health. I was especially dismayed at media portrayals of nurses on television and the preponderance of physicians on news shows to the exclusion of nurse experts. I thought that nurses needed to become more involved in media production in order to have nursing perspectives reach the public rather than only those reflecting dominant medical views in which nurses and their impact on persons' health are absent, invisible, or characterized as limited or ineffectual. While documenting nurse activists, the natural theoretical and practice-as-praxis congruence between documentary filmmaking and nursing emerged. I embarked on seeking out nurse filmmakers and the philosophical connections between film documentarians and nurses for their innate place in creating social change, thus delineating a theoretical framework for research and practice. Scott Erlinder and Jason Berger were extraordinary mentors in documentary filmmaking and digital media.

PAULA N. KAGAN

Unity of Knowledge in the Advancement of Nursing Knowledge

KAREN K. GIULIANO, RN, PhD, FAAN

LYNDA TYER-VIOLA, RNC, PhD

RUTH PALAN LOPEZ, RN, PhD

During the past 20 years, we have witnessed an explosion in nursing knowledge providing the discipline with diverse and multifaceted theoretical frameworks and paradigms. One knowledge theme that pervades the dialogue in the scholarly literature is that of multiple ways of knowing. With the acknowledgement that the fundamental nature of nursing knowledge is grounded in the understanding of human nature and its response to its environment, comes an imperative for a consilience of knowledge. The purpose of this article is to present such a unified worldview by articulating a vision of nursing knowledge, a meaning of unity of knowledge, and a challenge to the discipline to embrace inclusive rather than exclusive ways of knowing.

There are many windows through which we can look out into the world, searching for meaning .... Most of us ... clear a tiny peephole and stare through. No wonder we are confused by the tiny fraction of the whole that we see.

—GOODALL, 2000, p. 10

The explosion in nursing knowledge over the past 20 years has provided the discipline with diverse and multifaceted theoretical frameworks and paradigms. Within this diversity exists disagreement on both the fundamental nature of nursing knowledge and how that knowledge is known. There is some agreement that nursing knowledge should be grounded in the understanding of human nature and its relationship to the environment (Schwartz-Barcott, 1999). In addition, there is some consensus that nursing knowledge should be grounded more practically in the pursuit of describing phenomena, explaining relationships, predicting consequences, or prescribing nursing care (Meleis, 1997). Clearly, these two sets of beliefs are not mutually exclusive, and thus, nursing has come to support the importance of multiple ways of knowing and the value of pluralistic methods of inquiry (Chinn & Kramer, 1999; Forbes et al., 1999). However, simultaneous concern has been expressed that knowledge generated from multiple worldviews or paradigms can ultimately lead to a fragmentation of nursing knowledge (Taylor, 1997). This notion only strengthens the point expressed by Cody and Mitchell (2002) that "the

need for nurses to articulate a coherent philosophical foundation for nursing has never been greater" (p. 4). While the notion of pluralism is certainly widespread in the nursing literature, in most cases this pluralism is seen as relativistic and not as a way of coalescing all nursing knowledge. The purpose of this article is to suggest that the acceptance of pluralism and multiple ways of knowing can be satisfied by embracing Roy's (1997) vision of the unity of knowledge.

The article begins by examining the notion of paradigms and worldviews as currently used in the nursing literature and suggests that the concept of a single paradigm supports a philosophy inconsistent with nursing's goal of building knowledge on the nature of the human response. Next, the strength of plurality in nursing knowledge development, its warrantable evidence, and the concept of a unity of knowledge to support knowledge development and practice is articulated. Finally, the nursing practice implications of this perspective are discussed.

Worldviews and Paradigms

Worldviews and paradigms have been accepted in nursing as essential to researchers' theoretical perspectives, delineation of research questions, and ultimately to the selection of research methods. The search for a nursing paradigm as a means of knowledge

From K.K. Giuliano, L. Tyer-Viola, and R.P. Lopez, Nursing Science Quarterly 2005; 18(3): 243–248.

ABOUT THE AUTHORS

KAREN K. GIULIANO is Principal Scientist at Philips Medical Systems in Andover, Massachusetts. Karen has over 20 years of critical care experience, and her area of research is critical care technology. To her credit, she has numerous publications and national and international conference presentations, which focus primarily on the areas of critical care practice and technology, and creating a more humane critical care environment. Karen's other key contributions to the discipline include publications on statistical methods for nursing research and examining the nature of knowledge of nursing.

LYNDA A. TYER-VIOLA is Assistant Professor of Nursing at Massachusetts General Hospital Institute of Health Professions. Lynda has 25 years of high risk obstetrics experience in multiple level III labor and delivery settings. She is also the Co-Director of the Maternal and Infant Health Initiative for Zambia, a World Health Organization–sanctioned program to address maternal and neonatal mortality. Her program of research is stigma and symptom management for HIV-positive pregnant women. She is an active member of Sigma Theta Tau and contributes to the discipline of nursing by mentoring master's and doctoral students in the clinical setting.

RUTH PALAN LOPEZ was born and raised in Massachusetts. She received her undergraduate nursing education from Boston College, her masters in gerontological nursing from Boston University, and her PhD from Boston College's William F. Connell School of Nursing. She is Associate Professor and Coordinator of the Gerontological Nurse Practitioner Program at the Massachusetts General Hospital (MGH) Institute of Health Professions. Her program of research focuses on the comfort needs of dying nursing home residents and their families. In 2005, she was selected as a 2005 John A. Hartford Geriatric Nursing Research Scholar. She has more than 20 years of experience as a gerontological nurse practitioner during which time she has developed and implemented innovative programs to improve the care of older adults both in hospitals and in long-term care facilities.

development has been extensively reviewed in the nursing literature (Fawcett, 1995; Monti & Tingen, 1999; Newman, Sime, & Corcoran-Perry, 1991; Parse, 1987). Other authors have claimed that nursing knowledge is developed primarily from three slightly different worldviews, postpositivism, interpretive, and critical emancipatory (Jacox, Suppe, Campbell, & Stashinko, 1999). Postpositivism grew out of logical positivism and attempts to identify patterns and regularities and to describe, explain, and predict. The interpretive, humanist, or naturalistic perspective aims to understand meaning. The third worldview, critical emancipatory, strives to address how sociopolitical and cultural factors influence experiences.

The terms *paradigm* and *worldview* are often used interchangeably creating misconceptions regarding their philosophical implications and value. Both terms are used to refer to a cultural group's outlook and beliefs about the world, research traditions, ontology, epistemology, and philosophical perspectives. The terms have also been used in a broad sense to describe a systematic set of beliefs that are held to be true by a scientific discipline (Monti & Tingen, 1999). Worldview can refer to a researcher's general philosophical orientation, belief about the nature of human beings, nursing science, knowledge, and truth (DeGroot, 1988). In addition, worldview can also refer to a point of view from which a field of study is conceptualized, the assumptions that are inherent in those views, and the basis upon which knowledge claims are accepted (Newman et al., 1991). Parse (2000) made the distinction quite clear that "a paradigm is a worldview; it is the philosophical stance about the phenomenon of concern of a discipline" (p. 275).

 ## The Search for a Paradigm

Kuhn (1970) popularized the concept of paradigm in his description of science in *The Structure of Scientific Revolutions.* Kuhn believed that science was not the steady acquisition of knowledge, but instead, revolutionary based on persuasion, major shifts in thinking, and conversion. According to Kuhn, scientific knowledge is generated by preparadigm inquiry, ultimately leading to the endpoint of a defined paradigm, or a period of normal science. The scientific community defines the standards, beliefs, laws, and theory from which all scientists are to conduct themselves. During a period of normal science, all discoveries are focused on supporting the dominant theory. The process of building support for the dominant theory and essentially discarding evidence that does not conform to the matrix of the dominant theory continues until enough refuting evidence becomes apparent that it can no longer be ignored. Once this occurs, there is agreement that something is fundamentally wrong within the existing paradigm, a crisis ensues, and a revolution occurs. This revolution ultimately results in a major shift in thinking and the acceptance of a new paradigm.

According to Kuhn (1970), the new paradigm is so dissimilar from the earlier paradigm that previously accepted tenets are incommensurable with those defined within the newly accepted paradigm. Incommensurable signifies that the set of scientific concepts, propositions, problems, and solutions have changed so dramatically that they no longer have meaning in the new paradigm. Questions once considered as central to the previous paradigm may no longer be questions at all. Incommensurability is manifested as an inability to translate previous ideas into the new language of the new paradigm.

When first published, Kuhn's (1970) ideas were revolutionary and shook the long held view of progressive scientific development that suggests that each stage of knowledge building in science was based on the accomplishments of its predecessors. Each scientific discipline depends on the findings and interpretations of its predecessors, both inside and outside of the discipline. In the spirit of Aristotle, the underlying assumption is that science is a cumulative, rational process in which justified truth is built upon justified truth (Byrne, 1997). New truths, which are temporally and contextually bound, are defined each time something new is discovered. From this perspective, the purpose of science is to amass knowledge about the world and to grow and progress toward the ultimate truth. Nursing is able to embrace this perspective in each nurse-patient encounter by sharing what is known and the possibility of what can be discovered.

Nursing Paradigms

The nursing literature is replete with a variety of classifications of paradigms and worldviews. From a historical and very broad perspective, nursing knowledge can be considered as falling into two paradigms, the received view and the perceived view (Mindy & Beaton, 1983). The received view represents the positivistic-empiricist approach or natural law approach that is based on a belief in the existence of facts. It is the contention of the received view that there is a body of facts and principles to discover and understand as truth that are independent of historical or social context. This view generates knowledge that is disconnected to any process or being that is interactive. In contrast, the perceived view sees science as primarily historical. Thus, the perceived view is based on the belief that facts and principles are embedded in a particular history or cultural setting. Truth from this perspective is dynamic and found only in interactions among people and their sociohistorical contexts. Therefore, it can be said that truth is bound to a person, place and time, yet has meaning as it is communicated in future interactions.

In addition, three philosophical worldviews can be thought of as having influenced the growth of nursing knowledge: rationalism, empiricism, and historicism (Moody, 1990). Rationalism stresses the importance of a priori reasoning as the primary method of knowledge building. Empiricism embraces the notion that scientific knowledge is derived solely from sensory experience. Lastly, historicism argues that scientific progress takes place in intellectual revolutions and emphasizes the influence of history on science.

Nursing has based growth in knowledge primarily on three distinct views of paradigms: totality-simultaneity (Parse, 1987); paniculate-deterministic, interactive-integrative, and unitary-transformative (Newman et al., 1991); and reaction, reciprocal-interaction, and simultaneous action (Fawcett, 1995) with reference to those that are old and new (Cody, 2000). Within each of these views of paradigms lies support or kernels of truth that enrich practice and generate knowledge. Either due to our lack of defined language or possibly in merit to our ability to see more than there is to see in human interactions, the profession of nursing has generated knowledge from each of these paradigms. However, interpreting nursing knowledge from only one view may limit the value of what is known or the possibilities of what can be discovered.

In the totality paradigm (Cody, 1995, 2003; Parse, 1987, 1991), humans are seen as biopsychosocial and spiritual organisms that interact with the external environment and adapt or attempt to control the external environment. Health is a dynamic process that can be assessed objectively by experts, and the goal of nursing is the maintenance and restoration of norms.

In the simultaneity paradigm (Parse, 1987), humans are seen as more than the sum of different parts, they are open and in mutual process with the universe, and they create their own perception of health through personal knowledge and choice. Health is a process that cannot be objectively assessed and is not limited by norms. Health is achieved through a mutual process between the human and the universe, and the goal of nursing is oriented toward quality of life as defined by the living person (Parse, 1991).

In the particulate-deterministic worldview (Newman et al., 1991), phenomena are viewed as isolatable, reducible entities, with definable properties that can be measured and have orderly and predictable connections. The interactive-integrative perspective is an extension of the worldview and incorporates context and experience. Reality is found within the relationship of the properties. The unitary-transformative worldview considers phenomenon as unitary, self-organizing fields, embedded in larger self-organizing fields.

In reciprocal-interaction (Fawcett, 1995), human beings are active holistic beings as well, and their parts are only to be viewed within the context of the whole. Interactions between human beings are reciprocal, and reality is multidimensional, context-dependent and relative. Participants in this process foster the development of trust in experiencing the continuum of human knowledge and creativity and in giving attention to each other's feelings (Green, 1995). Change is probabilistic, and both objective and subjective phenomena are studied. Knowledge is created through empirical observations, methodological controls, and inferential data analysis (Fawcett, 1995).

The lure to define a nursing paradigm is supported by Kuhn's (1970) assertion that the "acquisition of a paradigm and of the more esoteric type of research it permits is a sign of maturity in the development of any given scientific field" (p. 11). In contrast, Meleis (1991) suggested that nursing knowledge has not developed through a revolutionary process as described by Kuhn, but instead has progressed through an integration that accounts for the accommodation of multiple paradigms and theoretical pluralism within the discipline. Meleis proposed that pluralism is important in nursing because of the discipline's focus on the *whole person* and the impact and interaction of people and their evolving environments. To disavow what has been described as knowledge from within the lived experience perspective would be in one sense disavowing the existence of the lived experience. The ideology that new knowledge is incommensurable with existing knowledge as described by Kuhn is counterintuitive to nursing's acceptance that what is known paves the way for what is to be discovered or what can be known.

Pluralism in Nursing

Historically, nursing has embraced many philosophies from other disciplines. Although diversity in approaches to nursing knowledge development is suggestive of vitality, Kim (2001) has also argued that it has created disarray and a disorganized collection of knowledge bits in nursing. Meleis (1991) suggested that it is desirable for knowledge to develop from different

perspectives but that it must be integrated in some way if nursing is to avoid being forever fragmented and divided. According to this view, a unification of methodologies is not what is required, but instead, the acceptance of a broader unifying perspective that allows nurse scholars to integrate and organize different kinds of nursing knowledge under a broader framework.

Kirkevold (1997) believed that full comprehension could be achieved by collection, analysis, and integration of related research findings into a meaningful whole to achieve clarity in practice (Kirkevold, 1997). Hinshaw (2000) supported collectivism as a means of advancing nursing in the 21st century. Hence, according to some contemporary scholars, the discipline of nursing can benefit through the understanding and embracing of multiple perspectives. In addition, there is a strong if not foundational belief throughout most of the contemporary nursing paradigms that the whole of nursing knowledge is greater than the sum of its parts. Variation in theories does not necessarily lead to different bodies of knowledge, but perhaps only to different aspects of a single body (Donaldson & Crowley, 1978). Pluralism of theories promotes productivity and without testing a wide variety of theories, progress toward truth is more difficult to make (Donaldson & Crowley).

What Is Warrantable Evidence for Nursing Knowledge Development?

If one is to accept, as the authors here suggest, that pluralism in nursing is the best path for the development of nursing knowledge, then the notion of what constitutes warrantable evidence must be seriously addressed. It must be clearly understood that acceptance of pluralism does not signify the endorsement of a relativistic perspective. Each piece of new knowledge needs to be scrutinized critically for its merit and credibility within the context of nursing practice and by each practitioner within each patient encounter (Fawcett, Neuman, Walker, & Fitzpatrick, 2001). Evidence should be generated and validated in multiple forms. Rycroft-Malone and colleagues (2004) stated, "The practice of effective nursing, which is mediated through the contact and relationship between individual practitioner and patient, can only be achieved by using several sources of evidence" (p. 81). The multiple bases of evidence are those from the more acknowledged research and clinical experience, and the less informed, patients, clients and providers, and local context and environment (Rycroft-Malone et al., 2004). To assure knowledge development is robust, concerted effort needs to be made to assure that each of these knowledge bases is included and more importantly, evidence from each is examined for its contribution to care and scientific rigor.

To assess the scientific value of knowledge generated from multiple sources, the authors agree with the three common warrants proposed by Forbes and colleagues (1999). The three warrants are scrutiny of findings and methodological strategies, corroboration, and scope of evidence. The *first* warrant rests on the degree to which the research followed procedures accepted by the community of research and the logical derivation of conclusions from the evidence. The *second* warrant is that the evidence can be corroborated and open to public scrutiny. In the quantitative paradigm this may be accomplished by reproduction of research findings. In the interpretivist paradigm, this may be accomplished by corroboration with research participants. Additionally, corroboration is sought from the research and scientific community. The *third* common warrant is whether the scope of evidence is adequate to address the phenomenon under study. More importantly, does the evidence contribute to a greater body of knowledge (including that which is significant or not) by filling a gap, or debunking dogma. Using knowledge developed from multiple sources and methods lends additional scope to knowledge and further supports this warrant.

Roy's Perspective on Nursing Knowledge

If one accepts the belief that pluralism is necessary for the development of knowledge in nursing, how then can nursing synthesize and integrate knowledge from multiple perspectives and worldviews without ending up with an amalgamation of contradictions? The authors believe that Roy's (1996, 2001) vision of knowledge as both unity and diversity provides the necessary theoretical, philosophical and epistemological support to integrate nursing knowledge. Roy's assumptions support multiple theories and research methods and provide nurse scholars with a vast array of possibilities for organizing nursing knowledge. Roy's integrative and cumulative approach offers the position that knowledge is generated from a multidisciplinary perspective and not as divergent paradigms. Two central ideas, unity in diversity and the existence of universal truths, have important implications for the integration of knowledge developed from multiple perspectives.

Unity in Diversity

In 1996, at the Nursing Knowledge Impact Conference, Roy set the stage for the idea of unity of knowledge by exploring the practice issues raised by the philosophical perspectives of realism, relativism, interpretivism, and humanism. Roy's philosophical assumption of unity demonstrates how one can find unity in diversity and is supported by noted philosophers and scientists. Citing Aristotle, she contended that all knowledge is of the universal (Roy, 1996). All things known are in relation to others both before them and to come. Roy asserted that everything is one substance with different attributes creating abroad and unified force. Roy proposed that nursing can find unity in diversity and that knowledge requires a full unveiling of all the diverse ways of seeing the whole (Roy, 1996).

If Roy's conception of unity in diversity can be accepted as central to nursing practice, then it can provide a perspective for uniting seemingly diverse paradigms in nursing. Cody (2003) explored human diversity by explaining human existence as coexistence and how understanding this relationship across diversities leads to "an infinite range of possibilities" (p. 196). Nursing embraces all things known in relation to others by its unique fundamental principle of caring. Cody said it is "not those who are familiar, who are our own or closely resemble our own—but those who are truly different, unfamiliar, and *other* to ourselves" (p. 196). When this perspective of welcoming that which is not familiar is applied to raising one's awareness to a new level in uncovering knowledge, awareness of boundaries dissolves and things become increasingly more unified. In addition, as knowledge boundaries disappear, each smaller level is a reflection of all other levels. Consequently, one can simultaneously possess both unity and diversity. What is seen depends on where one chooses to focus or for whom one chooses to care (Cody). Rawnsley (2003) expressed a similar sentiment in her support for multiple paradigms for nursing as well as her suggestion that nursing has a desperate need for a unifying vision that allows for divergent points of view.

Universal Truths

The idea of the existence of universal truths is fundamental to Roy's conception of knowledge. Roy (1996, 2001) viewed the pursuit of truth as an evolving notion, understood at one moment and undefined at the next. This supports the need for multiple ways of knowing in order to define and understand the whole of nursing knowledge. Knowledge viewed from this perspective provides the middle ground between the positivist who searches for the one true reality and the interpretivist who searches for multiple realities. Roy (1988) suggested that the rationalist bases truth on empirical facts and the relativist knows truth only in relationship to the thinking person. Since the mind of the observer is influenced by perceptions and theoretical presuppositions, taken to its extreme, one could argue that all observations are mind-dependent, influenced by multiple realities, and relativistic.

One of the most compelling aspects of Roy's (1996, 2001) perspective is that it makes room for all knowledge because within the belief in the existence of universal truths is the idea that no simple insight is enough, in and of itself, to disclose the whole truth. From Roy's (1996, 2001) perspective, nursing knowledge is both discipline-specific and open to validation and expansion through multidisciplinary scrutiny. Roy's perspective (1996, 2001) contradicts the view of Fawcett (1999) who proposed that all nursing knowledge should be discipline-specific. Knowledge derived from interdisciplinary inquiry allows the discipline to operate in an open rather than closed system model. Furthermore, it enhances a social responsibility for being open to public scrutiny as well as the goal of further and more widespread understanding. This broadened perspective is what makes nursing's multiple ways of knowing accessible to other disciplines. Finally, while there may be a strong belief that the whole of nursing knowledge is greater than the sum of its parts, scholars have no alternative but to select a small portion of potential truth to examine and a small perspective from which to study it. Because of this limitation in scientific inquiry, it is incumbent upon nurse researchers to recognize that, at best, any knowledge generated from a single episode of inquiry represents only a small piece of knowledge and only a part of a larger truth. As a practical consideration, it is necessary to break knowledge into manageable chunks in order to study it, improve our understanding of what is found, and generate more knowledge for future examination. Therefore, one of the most important tasks of nurse scholars is the responsibility to be honest and explicit with regard to the depth and breadth of the current scope of inquiry, as well as interpretation of the findings within the appropriate scope. The challenge for contemporary nurse scholars is to put the knowledge parts together in a way that is integrative, not simply additive, and not irresponsibly dismissive of opposing views without investing in a full understanding of those views.

Conclusions

It is the authors' contention that nursing knowledge is developed from multiple perspectives and lenses. Nursing knowledge development should not support an epistemology in which empirical knowledge is the pinnacle or *gold standard* for knowledge development. Rather, empirical knowledge simply represents one type of warrantable evidence. This position is critical if scholars are to prevent the devaluation of other types of knowledge so integral to nursing. Plurality of methodological approaches and ways of generating nursing knowledge are necessary to reflect the many facets of nursing science and to illuminate the complex phenomena present in nursing practice situations. No one view is sufficient to embrace or drive nursing knowledge in its totality. As Carper (1978) suggested, nursing must be the discipline that uses knowledge and evidence generated from multiple sources as an integral part of evidence-based nursing recommendations. Nursing's position on evidence for practice should demand that knowledge of a phenomenon include data generated from multiple methods and sources. This approach ensures the most comprehensive and unified view possible, and one that best serves the people. When taken from this perspective, data that refutes dogma, so prevalent in nursing, will illuminate gaps in knowledge and areas in need of further knowledge development.

In conclusion, the worldview of knowledge as unity provides an opportunity for nurses to participate in interdisciplinary research and knowledge development and still retain and emphasize the core dimensions of nursing. Based on the complexity of humans and their response to the environment, wide-ranging development and advancement of nursing knowledge is not possible without the integration and use of multiple ways of knowing.

REFERENCES

Byrne, P. H. (1997). *Analysis and science in Aristotle*. Albany: State University of New York Press.

Carper, B. A. (1978). Fundamental patterns of knowing in nursing. *Advances in Nursing Science, 1*(1), 13–23.

Chinn, P. L., & Kramer, M. (1999). *Theory and nursing: A systematic approach* (5th ed.). St. Louis, MO: Mosby.

Cody, W. K. (1995). About all those paradigms: Many in the universe, two in nursing. *Nursing Science Quarterly, 8,* 144–147.

Cody, W. K. (2000). Paradigm shift or paradigm drift? A meditation on commitment and transcendence. *Nursing Science Quarterly, 13,* 93–102.

Cody, W. K. (2003). Diversity and becoming: Implications of human existence and coexistence. *Nursing Science Quarterly, 16,* 195–200.

Cody, W. K., & Mitchell, G. J. (2002). Nursing knowledge and human science revisited: Practical and political considerations. *Nursing Science Quarterly, 15,* 4–13.

DeGroot, H. A. (1988). Scientific inquiry in nursing: A model for a new age. *Advances in Nursing Science, 10*(3), 1–21.

Donaldson, S. K., & Crowley, D. M. (1978). The discipline of nursing. *Nursing Outlook, 26*(2), 113–120.

Fawcett, J. (1995). *Analysis and evaluation of conceptual models of nursing*. Philadelphia: F. A. Davis Company.

Fawcett, J. (1999). *Theory and research*. Philadelphia: F. A. Davis.

Fawcett, J., Neuman, J. B., Walker, P. H., & Fitzpatrick, J. J. (2001). On nursing theories and evidence. *Journal of Nursing Scholarship, 33,* 115–124.

Forbes, D. A., King, K. M., Kushner, K. E., Letourneau, N. L., Myrick, A. F., & Profetto-McGrath, J. (1999). Warrantable evidence in nursing science. *Journal of Advanced Nursing, 29*, 373–379.

Goodall, J. (2000). *Through a window: My thirty years with the chimpanzees of Gombe.* Boston: Houghton Mifflin.

Green, M. (1995). *Essays on education, art and social change.* San Francisco: Jossey-Bass.

Hinshaw, A. (2000). Nursing knowledge for the 21st century: Opportunities and challenges. *Journal of Nursing Scholarship, 32*, 117–123.

Jacox, A., Suppe, F., Campbell, J., & Stashinko, E. (1999). Diversity in philosophical approaches. In A. S. Hinshaw, S. L. Freeman & J. F. Shaver (Eds.), *Handbook of clinical nursing research* (pp. 3–17). Thousand Oaks, C A: Sage.

Kim, H. S. (2001). Directions for theory development in nursing. In N. L. Chaska (Ed.), *The nursing profession: Tomorrow and beyond* (pp. 273–285). Thousand Oaks, CA: Sage.

Kirkevold, M. (1997). Integrative nursing research: An important strategy to further the development of nursing science and nursing practice. *Journal of Advanced Nursing, 25*, 977–984.

Kuhn, T. (1970). *The structure of scientific revolutions* (2nd ed.). Chicago: University of Chicago Press.

Meleis, A. I. (1991). *Theoretical nursing: Development and progress.* Philadelphia: J. B. Lippincott.

Meleis, A. I. (1997). *Theoretical nursing: Development & progress* (3rd ed.). New York: Lippincott.

Mindy, B. T., & Beaton, J. L. (1983). Toward a new view of science: Implications for nursing research. *Advances in Nursing Science, 5* (2), 27–36.

Monti, E. J., & Tingen, M. S. (1999). Multiple paradigms of nursing science. *Advances in Nursing Science, 21*(4), 64–80.

Moody, L. E. (1990). *Advancing nursing science through research* (Vol. 1). Newbury Park, C A: Sage.

Newman, M. A., Sime, A. M., & Corcoran Perry, S. A. (1991). The focus of the discipline. *Advances in Nursing Science, 14* (1), 1–6.

Parse, R. R. (1987). *Nursing science: Major paradigms, theories and critiques.* Philadelphia: Saunders.

Parse, R. R. (2000). Paradigms: A reprise. *Nursing Science Quarterly, 13*, 275–276.

Parse, R. R. (1991). Human becoming: Parse's theory of nursing. *Nursing Science Quarterly, 5*, 35–42.

Rawnsley, M. (2003). Dimensions of scholarship and the advancement of nursing science: Articulating a vision. *Nursing Science Quarterly, 16*, 6–13.

Roy, S. C. (1988). An explication of the philosophical assumptions of the Roy adaptation model. *Nursing Science Quarterly, 1*, 26–34.

Roy, S. C. (1996, October). *Knowledge as universal cosmic imperative.* Paper presented at the Nursing Knowledge Conference, Boston, MA.

Roy, S. C. (1997). Knowledge as universal cosmic imperative. In D. R. Jones (Ed.), *Knowledge impact 1996: Conference proceedings* (pp. 95–117). Chestnut Hill, MA: Boston College Press.

Roy, S. C. (2001, October). *Knowledge as cosmic imperative and impact on the health care system.* Paper presented at the Knowledge Impact Conference 2001, Newton, MA.

Rycroft-Malone, J., Seers, K., Tichen, A., Harvey, G., Kitson, A., & McCormack, B. (2004). What counts as evidence in evidence-based practice? *Journal of Advanced Nursing, 47*, 81–90.

Schwartz-Barcott, D. (1999). Adaptation as a basic conceptual focus in nursing theories. In H. Kim & I. Kollak (Eds.), *Nursing theories: Conceptual and philosophical foundations* (pp. 9–22). New York: Springer.

Taylor, J. (1997). Nursing ideology: Identification and legitimation. *Journal of Advanced Nursing, 25*, 1365–2648.

THE AUTHORS COMMENT | Unity of Knowledge in the Advancement of Nursing Knowledge

The inspiration for our work emanated from coursework for an epistemology course taught by Sister Callista Roy at Boston College. We were asked to synthesize and critique knowledge for nursing practice. We considered the various ways of developing knowledge for nursing practice, the strengths and weaknesses of various paradigms, and whether knowledge developed from these paradigms with unique assumptions were commensurable. After much debate, we agreed that knowledge to inform nursing practice requires a theoretical framework that integrates and unifies knowledge developed from multiple paradigms. Roy's concept of veritivity, the highest level of knowledge, provides this consilience. This worldview contributes to nursing theory in the 21st century as it provides the discipline with a worldview that unifies diverse and multifaceted theoretical frameworks.

KAREN K. GIULIANO
LYNDA TYER-VIOLA
RUTH PALAN LOPEZ

A Practice Discipline That's Here and Now

MERIAN C. LITCHFIELD, RN, PhD

HELGA JÓNSDÓTTIR, RN, PhD

*T*here is a vacuum for a practice discipline of nursing that would enable nurses to articulate the significance of what they do as an essential thread of contemporary healthcare provision. This article is an effort to develop the meaning and possibilities of a practice discipline for nursing. Tuning into the general shift in thought about our human condition across disciplines and nations, we consider features of a participatory paradigm, which, when refocused on the humanness of the health circumstance, informs our approach to a practice discipline. Knowledge is personal and participatory, evolving in the here-and-now of health systems. Research integral to practice and service innovation illustrates the way of looking and talking about a new phase in discipline development. The discipline is relational and creative in practice, evolving in the forums for dialogue. Each one of us as nurses has responsibility in participation. **Key words:** *dialogue, health circumstance, health experience, humanness, nursing knowledge, nursing practice, participatory paradigm, practice discipline, relational.*

We cannot solve our problems with the same thinking that created them.

Albert Einstein

The escalating problems of providing healthcare in all nations call for new thinking. The shortage of nurses now, as part of the general workforce predicament, is indication of our unsustainable systems. Workplace pressures are constraining the nursing that we as nurses know is needed. As has been so throughout our history, we seek the freedom to nurse. Yet we continue to be hampered by our inability to articulate clearly in the appropriate forums what is essential about nursing that contributes directly to health and society and what conditions are necessary for this given scarce resources. The decades of scholarship in nursing have given us a range of theories, yet the vision—and promise—of a distinct discipline of nursing is not reflected in the strategizing that gives direction to health system reform.

In this discipline vacuum, extensive lists of nurse competencies have just served to portray nursing as a set of activities given meaning as the nurse's work in the health system already defined by the social relevance of medical science. The service mission is rooted in the prevailing health paradigm of prevention, diagnosis, and treatment of disease, its signs, symptoms, and dangers. This obfuscates what nursing knowledge is and how we could be contributing to health in the lives of all people and the nation. The nursing needed

as a professional *practice* is obscure in health policy and system development, while the health missions of service providers/funders define the nature of the work of nurses as employees to be managed as part of their pool of resources.

Health systems are increasingly shaped by the drive to cost-effectiveness in our world of expanding and extravagant possibilities for the cure and control of disease and disability. The challenge is intensifying to articulate our discipline in a way that influences the roles and positions for nurses in the service configuration providing essential healthcare. Our (authors) respective research projects have brought us to the realization that we should be vigorously pursuing the articulation of the discipline of nursing with the scope of research broadened to the health system context—the policies, strategies, service design, and delivery—in which nursing care is inextricably woven. We do not want to just slot practitioners into the workforce; we do want to see them positioned to contribute to changes and to say what needs to happen for healthcare to be socially relevant as well as economically sustainable.

We write this article with the hope for energized dialogue around nursing as a practice discipline, across nations, not with the idea of reaching consensus of what nursing is, which theory is right or best, or what should be achieved. Rather, it is to enliven nursing practice, research, and education in our different ways in different places in the interests of all peoples. We have developed

ABOUT THE AUTHORS

MERIAN C. LITCHFIELD is an academic at large. Since 1999, she has been self-employed as a researcher, consultant, and educator undertaking contracted projects as Litchfield Healthcare Associates with the theme, "Innovation in nursing and healthcare: From idea to operation". She is a citizen of New Zealand where she developed her nursing career, first in pediatric acute care and then as an educator. She completed a Bachelor of Arts degree at Victoria University of Wellington, NZ, under an ICN/3M fellowship, a British Commonwealth Nurses War Memorial scholarship. Under a New Zealand Health Research Council postgraduate scholarship, she studied at the University of Minnesota to earn a master of nursing and PhD. Her focus of study was the nature of nursing practice and the distinct research methodology through which nursing knowledge is developed in practice. Since then, in national and international projects and events, she has worked on building a research foundation for development in healthcare through innovation in nursing practice and roles and a family-oriented service delivery model. Her journal articles and book chapters explore nursing as a contemporary profession and practice discipline, and her books focus on the description, substantiation, and significance of nurse initiatives, and a historical exploration of the nursing research origins in New Zealand.

HELGA JÓNSDÓTTIR received her baccalaureate degree from the University of Iceland and master's and doctoral degrees from the University of Minnesota. She is currently Professor at the Faculty of Nursing, University of Iceland, leading the section for research and development in nursing care for chronically ill adults. She started her research career with studies on the experience of people with chronic health problems, which later developed into a focus on nursing practice for people with chronic diseases, particularly lung diseases, and their families. Holding a joint position at Landspitali University Hospital in Reykjavik, Iceland, she collaborates with practicing nurses on research projects including the restructuring of hospital care for lung patients and the development of theoretical frameworks for out-patient clinics to support smoking cessation and nursing practice for people with advanced lung diseases. Currently, she is the project manager of an interdisciplinary and international study named "Partnership to enhance self-management of people diagnosed with COPD and their families", funded by the Icelandic Centre for Research, the University of Iceland, and the Icelandic Nurses' Association. Her publications include journal articles on experiences and nursing practice for people with various chronic diseases, and on nursing as a contemporary profession and practice discipline in international collaboration. She is the Co-Editor of a new book, *Family Nursing in Action*, from the University of Iceland Press.

our thesis taking account of the historical evolution of the discipline and locate it now within contemporary thought about the human condition to articulate the significance of nursing in its context of healthcare and service delivery. It is intended to contribute among the efforts of many nurses to make sense of our predicament, and as a form of response to the call to "conscience and action" of the Nursing Manifesto project inspired in the United States at the turn of the millenium.[1]

The Call of the Discipline

We see the nursing academy divided into distinct camps of scholarship. In general, the efforts to develop nursing as a discipline have been separated from the pragmatics of nurses' employment as the mainstay of health service delivery—the workforce and allotted work. This division seems inevitable in hindsight. In their seminal 1978 article on "the discipline of nursing," Donaldson and Crowley[2] urged the differentiation of the discipline (development of the body of knowledge) from the activities of practitioners (the profession) to liberate nursing from its vocational status and enable us to claim its social relevance. Clinical practice, they said, is concerned with here-and-now activities, whereas a discipline gives knowledge of its important expansive scope through past, present, and future for use in any place. They recommended "lessening our preoccupation with the process of nursing and pedagogy and placing emphasis on content as substance."[2(p251)]

This distinction must have been a confirmation, perhaps a relief, to the cadre of scholars constructing and evaluating theories. We can now see it as a necessary phase of laying claim to a distinctly nursing knowledge. But, as the often cited theory-practice gap, it created a vacuum for the kind of knowledge that could give identity and value to nursing—as a practice, in practice—that is integral to everyday healthcare, service delivery, and sector development. We see the consequence continuing in the age-old confusion of education and training for nurses. Paradoxically, the division is accentuated in the current drive to *integration* of healthcare when, by default, the disciplinary perspective brought to health assumes medical science as foundational knowledge, privileging the practice of medicine. Medical knowledge has become a generic pool of health knowledge, practiced by physicians and selectively *applied* as the work of nurses.

The division was addressed directly—and most helpfully—in a recent debate published in *Nursing Science Quarterly* between Mitchell and Bournes[3] on one side, arguing that an extant theory is foundational for nurses to even start practicing, and Reed[4,5] and Rolfe[5,6] on the other side, arguing that theorizing is rooted responsively in the pragmatics of everyday activities. We (authors) could both agree and disagree with each side. Neither satisfies the vacuum for a contemporary practice discipline.

We are concerned about the collapse of the vision of professional nursing into the schism between efforts to create a discipline (to date) and the pragmatics of work and workforce. We believe it is timely to juxtapose these seemingly irreconcilable points of view and camps of scholarship, and consider anew what is meant by a practice discipline, looking to a future of globalizing, yet locally attentive healthcare.

The vacuum for a nursing practice discipline has been recognized from outside nursing. Weinberg,[7] a sociologist in the United States, set out to respond to the question "What do nurses do?" She observed the impotence of nurses to claim their share of scarce resources in a tight economic climate. She urged the articulation of nursing in context: "If nurses want to protect themselves and patient care, they cannot wait for interested observers to figure out what is going on.... The first step is to articulate what nurses as professionals do and why the little things are really big things."[7(p43)]

Joining the effort toward a nursing discipline, our (authors') questions are about the coherence of what nursing is about, looking to contemporary wise thinking about the human condition, life, society, and health to give relevance. In the effort to reconcile knowledge and activities in the complex context of health services and workforce, we see that nurses framing nursing as *a practice*—practice wisdom—is the task of discipline development for this era.

An Era of Practice

The political rhetoric is about changing the culture of health systems from a curative/ reactive to a preventive/ responsive orientation. Attention has turned to workforce to achieve it, assuming division of labor according to the generic health/disease outcomes. Yet, we know people need "nursing" not usefully represented in either orientation. For nursing to be recognized in the drive to integration through multidisciplinary projects, the challenge is to be articulate about our own discipline as *practice* in situ: what nurses achieve in relation to other healthcare workers and under what conditions. We see this challenge illustrated in a Canadian Health Services Research Foundation report written by nurses working on policy and mindful of the talk of multitasking and interchangeability of healthcare workers: "The question that must be asked is not 'who *can* do this set of tasks or activities?' but rather 'who *should* and why?' given the context and population."[8(piv)] The question is complex arising in the discipline vacuum.

Methodologies for developing nursing knowledge have derived, often adopted, from other disciplines. They have been useful but found wanting in satisfying the vacuum for a distinct practice discipline. Thorne and colleagues, among many others, explained the inadequacies of both traditional quantitative science and the qualitative tradition for providing the scope and depth of the study needed for the "general knowledge of the sort that enhances particularization in practice."[9(p171)] Swinging to the pragmatic side, they argued that "interpretive description" of health and illness experiences would be more appropriate to bring nursing knowledge into its practice context. The interpretive turn was further reflected in writing about praxis from the 1990s. Connor[10] proposed a time of praxiology entering the new millennium. Doane and Varcoe[11] explained the usefulness of pragmatic enquiry to attend to experience and "ultimately reshape '"reality.'" Methodology is left implicit in whatever the nurse does.

Leaving aside the efforts to develop nursing as a discipline, and with a pragmatic orientation, Liaschenko and Peter found that the current statements of ethics of nursing are outdated in assuming it can be a profession with autonomy in controlling its own work: the statements are "no longer adequate to address the social realities and moral challenges of health care work."[12(p488)] Alternatively, they argued that considering nursing—and medicine too—as "work" would more appropriately accord value in the workplaces of contemporary healthcare; it could achieve the collective ethical responsibility of all healthcare providers to work collaboratively and interdependently. We see this stance as important in our efforts to acknowledge the value of everyday activities of nurses in context, but we are concerned that the social relevance of nursing would continue to be obscured within the hegemony of the current service delivery culture.

Thus, attention has been turning to who the nurse is and moral agency: praxiology has continued to echo in procedures for reflective practice to recognize moral agency. However, reflection on practice remains an ad hoc academic procedure if nurses (as practitioners and educators) do not have the capability of articulating the nature of nursing knowledge in relation to health that signifies the *process* of a practice as part of the whole provision of healthcare. Nursing knowledge is tacit, research framed within the methodologies of other disciplines, nurse employment exploited, and outcomes of healthcare skewed and depleted of essential nursing care.

We acknowledge the pragmatic stance of many nurse scholars. It turns attention to the action of nursing as relational, dynamic, and responsive. But it is the vacuum for a discipline we continue to address, focusing on *practice* as we look for coherence between the pragmatics of nurses as workforce and the evolution of thinking about the nature of nursing knowledge: a *practice* discipline that conveys our ethical foundation.

In the mid 1970s, from their study of the theoretical frameworks for nursing curricula, Torres and Yura[13] identified 4 major concepts: person, society, health, and nursing. With some variations, these have been recognized as the key elements of the discipline.[14] As a member of the theorist group writing at the later end of that era, Margaret Newman[15] took a retrospective look at the trajectory of their emergence. She traced them as a sequential refocusing of theory development to maintain the social relevance of nursing scholarship: "What the theorist chose to examine reflected the needs of that particular time."[15(p29)] She construed the trajectory as environment, nursing (nurse-client process), person (the human being) and, for the 1980s, "health," which she saw was cumulative, giving meaning to all the concepts.

Now we pick up on this historical trajectory to add *practice* as the contemporary integrative theme. We believe, this opens scholarship to exploration of the pragmatic vis-à-vis discipline threads. It has turned us to the nurse-person-environment-health interrelationship as fundamental, and therefore to the process of nursing in relation to content and its social relevance. Our (authors) challenge to find coherence will accord us a practice discipline has brought us to a paradigm that is participatory.

A Participatory Paradigm

We refer to a participatory paradigm that we see is expression of the widespread shift in Western thought about how we understand our human condition now emerging across nations and disciplines. The word participatory orients us to practice as relational; we are prompted to turn our attention to the action of nursing, elaborating beyond just the presence of the nurse with patients/clients, applied knowledge, and a set of activities she or he performs. It is about the self-in-relation, complementarity in our sense of community. This calls for a fresh look at temporality beyond causality, at responsibility and ethics. We see the efforts to develop a nursing discipline resonating within the movement. In this section, we refer to a selective range of authors to point to some features of a participatory paradigm we believe are important for the articulation of nursing as a practice discipline.

Worldview in Nursing

In retrospect, we can see the emergence of a participatory paradigm in the nursing academy unfolding through the last half century. The theorists looked to the great philosophers, sages, and popularizers of contemporary thought about our human world to articulate an ontology of contemporary relevance for nursing, albeit mostly viewed through the lens of other disciplines. It was inevitable that, for a time, methodologies of the respective disciplines and their schools of thought framed the knowledge such that knowledge was abstract to be *applied* by nurses. The theories were *used* and *tested*, mostly *confirmed* as *guides* for nurses.

The ontologies published as grand theories each brought coherence to knowledge in their own frameworks. But the theorists and the practitioners inhabited different worlds of scholarship. Each theory, named to emphasize difference, had its own language for nursing knowledge, its own premises to frame research process and findings, and thus each attracted its own community of scholars. A fragmented discipline has been no match for the coherence of medicine to inform health sector change.

As a second generation from Martha Rogers' articulation of a unique discipline in her "nursing science of unitary human beings," some theories have—separately—intensified an orientation to the engagement of the nurse with patients/clients. They give it significance according to the particular theory. For example, *knowledge* is represented by Parse[16] as cocreated and presented in the language of "human becoming" and by Newman[17] as life patterns recognized through the intersubjectivity of nurse and patient/client and depicted as the expansion of consciousness of each. Newman framed her theory as praxis where "the *form* that nursing research takes is the *form* of practice"[18(p100)] to point to knowledge as—and of—a process through which a transformative change in all participating activities can be achieved. Hence, nurses have been viewed as increasingly knowledgeable as engaged practitioners, even if their methods and "health" ends have been differently construed by each theory.

The theories importantly drew attention to the nurse-patient function, making a difference to the *experience* of people when they are patients/clients, as well as nurses, impacting on their lives.[19] However, what this means for health in relation to service design and delivery has had little attention. Moreover, as forms of knowledge the nurse brings to "what she ought to do," the theories remain as tentative paradigms, coexisting, if not competing, in pockets. Their significance for the employing organization's mission is subtle and fragile. As the workforce, nurses are employed to work in a causal paradigm where knowledge is product—the evidence for discrete interventions. Activities expected of nurses are rooted in the mission of the organization. They continue to be subject to the service boundaries, resources, and conditions that support healthcare within the hegemonic medical cure and control paradigm. The vacuum for the practice discipline of nursing seeks a further turn in a participatory paradigm to move further into the relational nature of nursing—beyond packages of interventions—to bring the coherence of a practice.

Meanwhile, others have been taking an epistemological approach. Benner[20] held her focus on the activities of nurses in their workplaces. She emphasized the embodied moral agency of nurses in caring—socially embedded—and its expression in their expanding capability to practice knowledgeably. The participatory nature of a practice is clear in the depiction of "embodied interdependence" of nurse with patients/clients, as well as in practitioner communities. Doane and Varcoe emphasized the inventiveness of nurses "to create and recreate their knowing in each moment of practice."[11(p89)]

The detour of nursing scholarship through other disciplines and the separate theoretical and pragmatist approaches emerging from it have been important in our consciousness of different paradigms of knowledge in nursing. But although all the leaders of the factions emphasize the importance of communities of scholars, trying to move between them to question and articulate the nature of nursing practice is fraught with misunderstanding. The ontological and epistemological efforts to date call forth new thinking for an inclusive nursing community.

We (authors) have been searching alongside many others for ways of developing the discipline of nursing both for and in practice, such as Boyd,[21] Connor,[22] Doane and Varcoe,[11] Picard and Jones,[19] Reed,[4] and Roy and Jones.[23] Now, as part of this movement, we take our stand in a participative paradigm to look beyond the divisions, while still preserving diversity in how practitioners contribute to "health" in the various places and times of healthcare provision.

A Shifting Worldview

A broad scan of literature reveals a general shift well underway in Western societies in the way we understand our human condition. We refer to some authors to point to features of a participatory paradigm that we believe are of greatest significance for the dialogue in nursing. In particular, we see the significance lies in how we situate ourselves in the world we seek to understand. We are exploring the meaning this lens brings to nursing as a "discipline."

Theological scholars[24-26] have written about a period of transition in human culture over the past centuries from the transethnic world of the great religions to this point of emergence of a global secular world in which we understand ourselves as coparticipants in the creation of lives in our shared places and time, with responsibility for it. Geering writes: "We humans are slowly coming to realize that what each of us inhabits is a world of meaning, which we ourselves have put together."[26(p5)] Cupitt[25] writes about "be-ing" to refer to our here-and-now evolving communal world. All these authors use the term secular to mean attention to *this* world of diverse beliefs and values of the sacred.

Insights from discoveries in the physical sciences have led scientists—and many popularizers—to write about a shift to a paradigm in which observer and observed, knower and known, merge. Schrodinger's cat story of the 1930s has been cited repeatedly to popularize the revelations from quantum physicists: the interrelationship of observer, tools, and observation determine our reality. David Bohm, US/British physicist-turned-philosopher, said: "World views—it's really a self-world-view because it includes yourself."[27(p25)]

In biology, Chilean biologists Maturana and Varela[28] pioneered a "science of cognition," coining the term "autopoiesis" to convey their observations of a dynamic interrelationship of part and whole in cellular systems. They write their insight as: "We live our field of vision … we cannot separate our history of actions—biological and social—from how this world appears to us."[28(p23)] Furthermore, it is relational: "We have only the world that we bring forth with others, and only love helps us bring it forth."[28(p248)]

Lynn Margulis, an evolutionary biologist from Massachusetts, writing with Dorian Sagan,[29] argued the inadequacy of the hegemonic reductionism of evolutionary theory after Darwin, where knowledge is framed as linear and competitive. From another world-view, she reinterpreted observations and drew on recent genome studies to depict evolution as integrative. Conveyed in the term "symbiogenesis," the origins of species, humans included, are explained as ecological interrelationships at the cellular level;

complexity increases through cooperation and new forms of community emerge. This realization led the duo to address the big human question "What is life?" to which they answer (in part) "a question the *universe poses to itself* in the form of a human being … we are only a single theme of the orchestrated lifeform… *our life is embedded*… in the rest of Earth's sentient symphony" (emphasis added).[30(p199)]

M. C. Escher, living and working in western Europe, creatively depicted the participatory thinking in 1956. Choosing to call himself an artisan— "a graphic artist 'with heart and soul,'"[31(p8)] he explored the human capability of representing 3-dimensional reality in 2-dimensional drawings. A drawing called *Print Gallery* shows a man in a gallery looking at a picture in which his "looking at the picture" is an integral part. He described it: "… we come to the logical conclusion that the young man himself also must be part of the print he is looking at. He actually sees himself as a detail of the picture; reality and image are one and the same."[31(p67)]

Historically, tracing ideas of science, theology, and philosophies, Skolimowski, of Polish origin, addressed directly the "new order of reality" as "the participatory mind": "We are woven into the universe we explore."[32(p88)] The world we experience as complex continuously evokes our efforts to simplify: "The patterns and configurations of the world are not there independently of mind, but are the patterns of our knowledge through which our minds work."[32(p88)] Furthermore, "the power of creation is the power of articulation."[32(p14)] A participatory worldview is a new understanding of ontology and epistemology. The meanings of these terms require us to consider them together: "they elicit from each other what they assume in each other."[32(p76)] Knowledge is in process as comprehension, and "to know is to *constitute* the world."[32(p81)]

A proactive ecological philosopher born and based in the United States, Abram[33] also draws on great philosophical writing along with varied depictions of the worlds of indigenous oral peoples and his own experience as a sleight-of-hand magician performing as part of everyday life in many countries. He conveys the participatory thinking inherent in the interrelatedness of human cognition and the natural world. Always, he says, there is an active interplay between the perceiving body and that which it perceives: "We always retain the ability to alter or suspend any particular instance of participation. Yet we can never suspend the flux of participation itself."[33(p59)] We are immersed in a sensuous world. We make sense of this world humanly through our language: "The human mind is not some otherworldly essence that comes to house itself inside our physiology. Rather, it is instilled and provoked by the sensorial field itself, induced by

the tensions and participations between the human body and the animate earth."[33(p262)] "The common field of our lives and the other lives with which ours are entwined … our experience of this field is always relative to our situation in it."[33(p40)]

The participatory thinking has also been emerging in the writing about the general organization of societies and workplaces. The participatory theme has been integral to the women's movement. It shows in Wheeler and Chinn's[34] reframing of group process as community represented by the acronym PEACE: Praxis, Empowerment, Awareness, Consensus, Evolvement. Also in Margaret Wheatley's[35] explanation of transformational leadership for the management of organizations, linking directly to "the participative nature of the universe" emerging from quantum physics. Danah Zohar's experience in childbirth led her to become a popularizer of the new physics revelations with a participatory interpretation. With psychiatrist/psychotherapist Ian Marshall, she is now reaching into the business worlds and corporate culture, elaborating the relational theme of "changing ourselves to change the world."[36]

In these selected but wide-ranging writings, we can see a participatory shift. All authors noted the inadequacy now of our former views of knowledge of past eras. These views have increasingly obscured the humanness of living our lives—experience, spirituality, sentience, and mystery. But this participatory view does not negate previous ways of thinking, nor even transcends them. Everything just looks different. Cupitt[25] uses the terms "contingency," "immanence," and "outsidelessness" to refer to our humanness.

All authors bring coherence to their reasoning with reference to community and love. We are participants in a creative world in the moment, constantly evolving as participants in it and together making sense of it in our own particular ways. Our spirituality is our interrelationship, as participants, in the sensuousness and communion of our living universe. We seek to understand, see patterns, find order, and theorize, knowing we are ourselves inside what we write about. Temporality moves beyond the linear; we live and act in the here and now: "always in the middle of things," Cupitt says.[25(p64)] The meaning of the past-future is unfolding and enfolding in the moment of "holomovement," Bohm[27] says. Hence we are brought to the realization of our vulnerability and our responsibility in action.

Expressing these features, a participatory worldview has language at its core. Geering explains language as evolving meaning, "Language is the collective product of the powers of human imagination and creativity," where words to syntax to stories construe our cultural heritage, such that "by means of stories we create the world we live in."[26(pp18,41)] Abram views language as evolving from and expressing the participatory nature of the universe: "The sensuous, perceptual life-world, whose wild, participatory logic ramifies and elaborates itself in language … a vast, living fabric continually being woven by those who speak."[33(pp83–84)] Bohm's[27] physics led him to focus his thinking about language on the dialogic nature of our human world of unfolding meaning where "meaning is active," making sense of things; culture construes language, and dialogue is a form of "social meditation" unfolding among us in what we attend to.

In the academy of social sciences, John Heron and Peter Reason[37] have been elaborating their earlier work on cooperative enquiry and action research, and now articulate their methods as expression of a participatory paradigm. They describe a participative paradigm: "the mind's conceptual articulation of the world is grounded in its experiential participation in what is present, in what there is."[37(p277)] Critical subjectivity extends to critical intersubjectivity. To elaborate the participatory nature of knowledge, they added axiology to ontology, epistemology, and methodology. Axiology makes explicit the ethics of knowledge development in the question: "What sort of knowledge is intrinsically valuable in human life?"[37(p277)] Ethics is now inherent in the whole process.

Reason and Bradbury present their edited book on "participatory inquiry and practice" as part of what they describe as the revolutionary transition in worldview "emerging at this historical moment."[38(p1)] In their introduction, they too trace the roots historically—from the reinvention of humanism in the 1950s through the cognitive and linguistic turns of the postmodern era that alerted us to the relationship between power and language, and so to the participatory worldview of today that draws on and takes us into a socially constructed world. They connect to Bohm, Abram, and Skolimowski among many other contemporary sages to elaborate an action science that "continually enquires into the meaning and purpose of our practice,"[38(p7)] relational and concerned with the betterment of the world and life in it. We *attend to* what we have come to know through an instrumental paradigm "to draw on techniques and knowledge of positivist science and to frame these within a human context."[38(p7)] They too emphasize the linguistic nature of things: "As soon as we attempt to articulate ('real' reality) we enter a world of human language and cultural expression."[38(p7)] They talk of knowledge as a verb rather than a noun in dialogue evoking attention to the ethical and political. Knowledge is "a living, evolving process of coming to know rooted in everyday experience."[38(p2)] In their view, inquiry is about the healing of the splits and alienation in contemporary experience.

Our consciousness of the trend in thought about the nature of human knowledge has given us (authors) a new lens on the discipline to see how the once-separated discipline and activities of nurses are one as process. After Reason and Bradbury[38] and Geering,[26] let us consider the discipline of nursing as a verb inviting the syntax to express culture and stories that convey nuances; it is the process of practice in context and informed in dialogue. Dialogue brings nursing theoretical insights and the schools of knowledge into the complexity of healthcare provision.[11] In nursing communities, our attention is drawn to the language, texts, and discourses that have confused and divided us and alienated many. Our professional responsibility is to participate in open, inclusive dialogue.

But this meaning of discipline begs a focus that orients practice to the social relevance of nursing: a nursing take on "the common good" to draw us into dialogue. Reason and Bradbury stated their moral purpose for inquiry, using terms appropriated from the literature through the ages: "The flourishing of life, the life of human persons, of human communities, and increasingly of the more-than-human world of which we are a part."[38(p10)] We can agree with this too, but want a focus that enables us to participate in a *nursing* community about nursing practice. For this, we have looked to our discipline's history.

The Focus of the Discipline

Each theorist proposed a focus for nursing—the theory—as she or he had conceptualized it. For other scholars it has been implicit. Also, there have been many threads of nurses' work and roles developing worldwide, in health systems without a specifically nursing purpose. We see the elaboration of advanced practice nursing happening within specialty fields and practices, the focus closely aligned with medical science concerning assessment-diagnosis-prescription or defined by the mission of employing organizations. As educators, we have observed students searching for a nursing purpose to anchor their theses, often reaching into other disciplines for ideas of social relevance.

Newman with Sime and Corcoran-Perry,[39] in describing their framework of 3 research paradigms, recognized the need for a focus statement to convey the social mandate of nursing. Noting the predominance of caring and health as integrative concepts in the nursing literature, they proposed the phrase "caring in the human health experience." Newman explained: "Caring designates the nature of the nursing practice participation … the experiential dimension characterizes the phenomenon (of human health) as something beyond the traditional objective-subjective perspective."[40(p48)] The phrase as a whole was the focus of the discipline. This statement has been important in drawing attention to the social relevance of our research efforts. In a phrase, the concepts of caring and health had more meaning for nursing than when considered separately; there is deeper meaning in expression of culture and history.

As students, our (authors') beginning research was underway at this time. We explored what the focus statement might mean as we studied the nature of practice. This led to the explication of a research-as-if-practice process.[41-44] But separateness still bothered us; a researcher is not a practitioner in the sense of having a work role and status within the health service organization. We must be able to state the social relevance of our practice, given our paradigm of a participatory, always-evolving-in-the-moment idea of knowledge. It must have meaning for the practice of all other nurses and for health service and policy trends.

In retrospect, we can see the 1991 focus statement representing its era and cultural context. The relational caring/experiential aspect of nursing was growing as a counterbalance to the expanding challenges of technological advances and fiscally driven health service reforms. We can see the strong influence of phenomenology, grounded theory, and hermeneutics on nurses' studies of "the lived experience" of people as patients and clients. Hence, the focus on experience privileges these methodologies and their parent disciplines—primary attention to individuals. Although, it acknowledges the moral relational core, the phrase separates "what is important" to be attended to from the action that addresses it. It is difficult to see how it focuses knowledge development for much of the work of nurses in established roles and career pathways.

Through our research projects in our respective countries and writing together to explore the nature of nursing practice in context, we have sought a broader statement: a cohesive statement that is more inclusive of the different forms of knowledge, and that resolves the current splitting of the relational and the technical. For this, we have turned our attention now to *humanness*.

This tunes us into the 1991 focus statement[39] and recent writing such as the *Consensus Statement on Emerging Nursing Knowledge* orchestrated by the Boston Group.[24] But, in replacing the action concept (caring), we are opening to all paradigms of action, whatever the nature of change and whatever part the nurse plays in change. Furthermore, while we (authors) agree that attention to people's experience is vital in nursing, we are now lifting our sights to more broadly attend to the *health circumstance*. For us, the discipline focus is *the humanness of the health circumstance*.

With this focus, we look beyond the separateness of human beings as nurse and patient in engagements, to being human whatever the health predicament, whoever is implicated in it, and however located in time and place. It contrasts with, but is essentially complementary to, the medical discipline focus on the incidence of disease, differential diagnosis, and treatment to date framed within a deterministic paradigm.

The phrase expresses social relevance. The public looks to nurses for a human face in the technically and fiscally oriented world; our understanding of health circumstance is what enables us to advocate the humanness of people's experience in the strategizing for service development and in community development. It gives a common focus to research framed within the extant theoretical orientations, research addressing the practicalities of specific activities expected of nurses, and research on issues of workforce and service management. It calls forth the examination of the ethics of nursing.

In Action

The lens of a participatory paradigm makes everything look different: practice, research, management, education, service design, and policy development. Our understanding of the paradigm has evolved through our research endeavors, as we sought to address the vacuum for a contextualized practice discipline. It has opened our thinking not only to an alternative form of nursing practice but also to the form of leadership through which policy, service development, and management can be constructed to support the healthcare provided by all nurses, whatever the paradigms for their activities. We can think now of an integrative people-pivotal paradigm for healthcare provision.[45] The following is a glimpse of our growing consciousness of the significance of nursing practice for healthcare and possibilities for action. In this we are not "proving" or "demonstrating" our thesis, we just want to illustrate a way of seeing and talking about nursing in context.

Importantly, our research starting point was the process of practice. We knew that to explore the relational nature of nursing we had to be practicing. We awoke to a general trend in thinking about our humanness and connected into the discourses referring to a "participatory paradigm."[41-44] Initially undertaken according to academic requirements, the research was not integral to the sanctioned, pressured yet seductive health service design, workforce, and professional structures. But it was *as if* practice; it was as close to the reality of practice as possible without being swallowed into the system.

The process we described was of partnership with people as patients/client (considered as collective) such that, through our conversations extending in time (multiple meetings), we made sense of what was happening for them. Holding the humanness of the circumstance as our orientation, *everything* happening and talked about, place and time, had relevance, as far as our minds allowed us: outsideless.[25] There was insight into how the predicament had come about and what it meant in life ahead for family, work, and play; meaning was actualized in the statements of action that each could, and would, take in the moment. In action, people as families and groups with really complex health circumstances managed tangled difficult times,[44] accessed services discerningly, made the best of healthcare available conscious of scarce resources, and addressed health matters that would have implications for later years or for following generations.[45]

The insights alerted us in our practitioner role to our responsibilities around the personal predicament as well as community life, collaboration among healthcare workers to orchestrate healthcare, health service management, and policy development. Hence, action was more than a set of activities, it was coherence in action around whatever was needed for everyone to get on with life as patients/clients, family and community members, citizens, and as nurses in their professional world. It included—but not necessarily—the *conventions* of healthcare. Knowledge was participatory in process for all; it was practice wisdom. As researchers, we developed narratives that presented the humanness of the health circumstance and these were used for influence in the various forums where policy and funding decisions are made.

Our interest turned to nurse roles, new and traditional, and how they might be complementary in contributing to the expected "health outcomes" of contracted services and the organization's mission. Projects were funded as practice and service innovation.[44,45] Education looked different; roles of teacher and learner had changed. As educators-researchers, we took one step back from the practitioner role—to mentorship with practitioners. Learning was integral to the dialogue of practice; roundtable forums were the medium.

As mentors-researchers, we came with our novice experience. We could see in our participation the expression of our own respective culturally and historically grounded education and wise mentorship from our earlier professional lives that had shaped our values, viewpoints, as well as hang-ups. The practitioners took their own lead in developing their practice in relation to each other. Together, we challenged our different languages, constantly reexamining viewpoints as a process of theorizing, each with our own take on the task to articulate practice, what it achieves, and the service model to support it. There was work to be done to create a practice, personally and culturally expressive and responsive within health service environments. It was intense work, but it evoked new vitality in its creativity and was deeply appreciated by all participants. One nurse said, she had "come home to nursing."[46]

Research, practice, service development, management, and education began to collapse into the dialogic process, with the patient/client and nurse partnership being pivotal.[45] Healthcare can become a dynamic collaborative endeavor. Now the new practice role is influencing reconfiguration in service delivery, integrative in the traditional silo structure of primary, secondary, and tertiary sectors and specialist divisions. In a participatory paradigm, nursing practice is collective. Nurses work in different paradigms, their activities given coherence in the core dialogue centered on and reaching out from partnerships with patients/clients. Professional forums are essential where the ethics of practice can take form for each nurse and standards continually examined. There is more work to be done.

Hence, with this eversion in healthcare provision, discipline development is in practice, leadership comes from practice, and attention primarily focused on the humanness of the health circumstance. Service models are shaped by and around practice. The roundtable forums expand and contract to dynamically address the current issues and challenges. They take account of the diversity of community life, other healthcare workers, service and policy developers, funders, health economists, and politicians. It is not all easy and smooth but the possibilities are open. There is even more work to be done.

 ## Conclusion

This discussion is intended as a contribution to the dialogue around the discipline, not a proposal of "how to" or theory. The separation of knowledge development in the academy from the activities of nurses-as-workforce has created a vacuum for a practice discipline that would enable nurses to articulate the significance of nursing, so essential in contemporary healthcare provision. We have tuned into the trend in thought around the human condition represented in the emergence of a participatory paradigm, and explored its meaning for nursing in the context of health service delivery, to have social relevance today. Turning our focus to the humanness of the health circumstance, our research has brought us to an understanding of the discipline as relational and evolving in the process of nursing practice in context. The discipline is here and now, alive and creative in forums for dialogue. Each one of us has responsibility in participation.

REFERENCES

1. Cowling R, Chinn PL, Hagedorn S. *A Nursing Manifesto: A Call to Conscience and Action.* http://www.nursemanifest.com/manifesto.htm. Published 2000. Accessed July 29, 2007.

2. Donaldson S, Crowley D. The discipline of nursing. In: Nicoll L, ed. *Perspectives on Nursing Theory.* Boston: Little Brown & Co; 1986:241–251.

3. Mitchell GJ, Bournes DA. Challenging the atheoretical production of nursing knowledge: a response to Reed and Rolfe's column. *Nurs Sci Q.* 2006;19(2):116–119.

4. Reed PG. The practice turn in nursing epistemology. *Nurs Sci Q.* 2006;19(1):36–38.

5. Reed PG, Rolfe G. Nursing knowledge and nurses' knowledge: a reply to Mitchell and Bournes. *Nurs Sci Q.* 2006; 19(2):120–122.

6. Rolfe G. Nursing praxis and the science of the unique. *Nurs Sci Q.* 2006;19(1):39–43.

7. Weinberg DB. When little things are big things. In: Nelson S, Gordon S, eds. *The Complexities of Care: Nursing Reconsidered.* Ithaca, New York: ILR/Cornell University Press; 2006: 30–43.

8. Besner J, Doran D, Hall LM, et al. *A Systematic Approach to Maximizing Nursing Scopes of Practice.* Canadian Health Services Research Foundation. http://wwwchsrf.ca/finaL-research/ogc/besner_e. php Published September 2005 Accessed July 29, 2007.

9. Thorne S, Kirkham SR, MacDonald-Emes J. Interpretive description: a noncategorical qualitative alternative for developing nursing knowledge. *Res Nurs Health.* 1997; 20:169–177.

10. Connor MJ. The practical discourse in philosophy and nursing: an exploration of linkages and shifts in the evolution of praxis. *Nurs Philos.* 2004;5:54–66

11. Doane GH, Varcoe C. Toward compassionate action: pragmatism and the inseparability of theory/practice. *Adv NursSci.* 2005;28(1):81–90.

12. Liaschenko J, Peter E. Nursing ethics and conceptualizations of nursing: profession, practice and work. *J Adv Nurs.* 2004;46(5):488–495.

13. Torres G, Yura H. *Today's Conceptual Framework: Its Relationship to the Curriculum Development Process.* New York: National League for Nursing; 1974.

14. Meleis AI. *Theoretical Nursing: Development and Progress.* 3rd ed. Philadelphia: Lippincott; 1997.

15. Newman MA. The continuing revolution: a history of nursing science. In Chaska NL, ed. *The Nursing Profession: A Time to Speak.* New York: McGraw-Hill; 1983: 385–393.

16. Parse RR. *The Human Becoming School of Thought: A Perspective For Nurses And Other Health Professionals.* Thousand Oaks, CA: Sage; 1998.

17. Newman MA. *Health as Expanding Consciousness.* 2nd ed. New York: National League for Nursing; 1994.

18. Newman MA. The research-practice relationship. *Nurs SciQ.* 1991;4(3):100–101.

19. Picard C, Jones D, eds. *Giving Voice To What We Know: Margaret Newman's Theory Of Health As Expanding Consciousness In Nursing Practice, Research And Education.* Boston: Jones & Bartlett; 2005.

20. Benner P. The roles of embodiment, emotion and life-world for rationality and agency in nursing practice. *Nurs Philos.* 2000;1:5–19.

21. Boyd CO. Toward a nursing practice research method. *Adv Nurs Sci.* 1993:16(2):9–25.

22. Connor MJ. *Courage and Complexity in Chronic Illness: Reflective Practice in Nursing.* Wellington, NZ: Daphne Brasell Press/Whitireia Publishing; 2004.

23. Roy C, Jones DA, eds. *Nursing Knowledge Development and Clinical Practice.* New York: Springer; 2007.

24. Armstrong K. *A History of God.* London: William Heinemann; 1993.

25. Cupitt D. *The Revelation of Being.* London: SCM Press; 1998.

26. Geering L. *Tomorrow's God: How We Create Our Worlds.* Wellington, New Zealand: Bridget Williams Books; 1994.

27. Bohm D. *Unfolding Meaning: A Weekend of Dialogue with David Bohm.* London: Routledge; 1985.

28. Maturana HR, Varela FJ. *The Tree of Knowledge: The Biological Roots of Human Understanding.* Revised ed. Boston: Shambhala; 1992.

29. Margulis L, Sagan D. *Acquiring Genomes: A Theory of the Origins of the Species.* New York: Basic Books; 2002.

30. Margulis L, Sagan D. *What is Life?* New York: Simon & Schuster; 1995.

31. Escher MC. *Exploring the Infinite: Escher on Escher.* van Hoorn WJ, Wierda F, compiler; Oneindige H, trans. New York: Harry N Abrams; 1989.

32. Skolimowski H. *The Participatory Mind. A New Theory of Knowledge and of the Universe.* England: Penguin books; 1994.

33. Abram D. *The Spell of the Sensuous: Perception and Language in a More-Than-Human World.* New York: Vintage Books; 1996.

34. Wheeler CE, Chinn PL. *Peace and Power: A Handbook of Feminist Process.* 3rd ed. New York: National League for Nursing; 1991.

35. Wheatley MJ. *Leadership and the New Science: Learning About Organization From an Orderly Universe.* San Francisco: Berrett-Koehler; 1992.

36. Zohar D, Marshall IN. *Spiritual Capital: Wealth We Can Live By.* San Francisco: Berrett-Koehler; 2004.

37. Heron J, Reason P. A participatory inquiry paradigm. *Qual lnq.* 1997;3(3):274–294.

38. Reason P, Bradbury H. Introduction: inquiry and participation in search of a world worthy of human aspiration. In: Reason P, Bradbury H, eds. *Handbook of Action Research: Participative Inquiry and Practice.* London: Sage; 2001:1–14.

39. Newman MA, Sime AM, Corcoran-Perry SA. The focus of the discipline of nursing. In: Newman MA, ed. *A Developing Discipline: Selected Works of Margaret Newman.* New York: National League for Nursing; 1995:33–42.

40. Newman MA. Prevailing paradigms in nursing. In: Newman MA, ed. *A Developing Discipline: Selected Works of Margaret Newman.* New York: National League for Nursing; 1995:43–54.

41. Litchfield MC. Practice wisdom. *Adv Nurs Sci.* 1999;22(2): 62–73.

42. Pharris MD. Coming to know ourselves as community through a nursing partnership with adolescents convicted of murder. *Adv Nurs Sci.* 2002;24(3):21–42.

43. Jonsdottir H, Litchfield MC, Pharris MD. The relational core of nursing: practice as it unfolds. *J Adv Nurs.* 2004;47(3):241–250.

44. Jonsdottir H. Research-as-if-practice: a study of family nursing partnership with couples experiencing severe breathing difficulties. *J Fam Nurs.* 2007;13(4):443–460.

45. Litchfield MC. *Towards a People-Pivotal Paradigm for Healthcare: Report of the Turangi Primary Health Care Nursing Innovation 2003–2006.* New Zealand Ministry of Health. http://www.moh.govt.nz/publicationpending.

46. Litchfield M, Laws M. Achieving family health and cost containment outcomes: innovation in the New Zealand health sector reforms. In: Cohen E, De Back V, eds. *The Outcomes Mandate: Case Management in Health Care Today.* St Louis: Mosby; 1999:306–316.

THE AUTHORS COMMENT | A Practice Discipline That's Here and Now

We have collaborated for many years in exploring the potential for development of nursing practice in our respective countries of Iceland and New Zealand, with our quite different cultures, histories, and health system contexts. We wanted to articulate the significance of nursing practice for health, each in our own way, to be able to contribute to health policy and construct models of service delivery that would assure a human face in the provision of healthcare. As students at the University of Minnesota, we had both participated in the academic dialogue as Margaret Newman elucidated her theory of health as expanding consciousness and had been inspired by her differentiation of a paradigm that would render nursing a distinct discipline. As we explored paradigms of theories, research, and practice through our projects, we realized the discipline of nursing must be dialogic in nature with nursing knowledge evolving personally and culturally in order to accommodate the diversity of perspectives around the world—and we needed to be participants in it. Therefore, we situated our exploration historically and, looking beyond the current theoretical and practice divisions in nursing and healthcare, we wanted to contribute a contemporary perspective of the discipline of nursing as the theorizing of each nurse within practice, and evolving through the dialogue of nurse forums.

MERIAN C. LITCHFIELD
HELGA JÓNSDÓTTIR

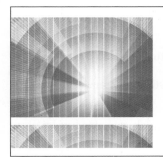

Author Index

A

Algase, Donna L.
An Ontological View of Advanced Practice
Nursing, 373
Anderson, Joan M.
The Advocate-Analyst Dialectic in Critical and
Postcolonial Feminist Research: Reconciling
Tensions Around Scientific Integrity, 163
Knowledge Development and Evidence-Based
Practice: Insights and Opportunities From
a Postcolonial Feminist Perspective for
Transformative Nursing Practice, 245
Arslanian-Engoren, Cynthia
An Ontological View of Advanced Practice
Nursing, 373

B

Baumbusch, Jennifer L.
Knowledge Development and Evidence-Based
Practice: Insights and Opportunities From a
Postcolonial Feminist Perspective for
Transformative Nursing Practice, 245
Bekhet, Abir K.
Theoretical Substruction Illustrated by the Theory of
Learned Resourcefulness, 330

C

Canam, Connie J.
The Link Between Nursing Discourses and Nurses'
Silence: Implications for a Knowledge-Based
Discourse for Nursing Practice, 65
Carper, Barbara A.
Fundamental Patterns of Knowing in Nursing, 201
Clark, Alexander M.
Complex Critical Realism: Tenets and Application in
Nursing Research, 135
Cody, William K.
Nursing Theory as a Guide to Practice, 94
Cowling, W. Richard III
The Power of Wholeness, Consciousness, and Caring:
A Dialogue on Nursing Science, Art, and
Healing, 384
Unitary Appreciative Inquiry: Evolution and
Refinement, 122

D

Davis, Caroline
Complex Critical Realism: Tenets and Application
in Nursing Research, 135
DeGroot, Holly A.
Scientific Inquiry in Nursing: A Model for
a New Age, 186
Dickoff, James
A Theory of Theories: A Position Paper, 337
Doane, Gweneth Hartrick
Knowledge Translation in Everyday Nursing: From
Evidence-Based to Inquiry-Based Practice, 83
Toward Compassionate Action: Pragmatism and the
Inseparability of Theory/Practice, 49
Transcending the Limits of Method: Cultivating
Creativity in Nursing, 74
Dodgson, Joan E.
The Cocreating Environment: A Nexus Between Classi-
cal Chinese and Current Nursing Philosophies, 179

E

Ellis, Rosemary
The Practitioner as Theorist, 57
Engebretson, Joan C.
A Multiparadigm Approach to Nursing, 393

F

Fawcett, Jacqueline
Criteria for Evaluation of Theory, 353
On Nursing Theories and Evidence, 24
Ferguson, Linda M.
From Practice to Midrange Theory and Back Again:
Beck's Theory of Postpartum Depression, 322
Fitzpatrick, Joyce J.
On Nursing Theories and Evidence, 25

G

Giuliano, Karen K.
Unity of Knowledge in the Advancement of Nursing
Knowledge, 431
Grace, Pamela J.
A Central Unifying Focus for the Discipline: Facilitat-
ing Humanization, Meaning, Choice, Quality of
Life, and Healing in Living and Dying, 403

H

Hardy, Margaret E.
Perspectives on Nursing Theory, 344
Theories: Components, Development, Evaluation, 313
Hartrick, Gweneth A.
Transcending the Limits of Method: Cultivating Creativity in Nursing, 74
Hicks, Frank D.
An Ontological View of Advanced Practice Nursing, 373
Higgins, Patricia A.
Levels of Theoretical Thinking in Nursing, 283
Holmes, Dave
The Use of Postcolonialism in the Nursing Domain: Colonial Patronage, Conversion, and Resistance, 258
Hupcey, Judith E.
Concept Analysis: Examining the State of the Science, 267

I

Im, Eun-Ok
Development of Situation-Specific Theories: An Integrative Approach, 290
The Situation-Specific Theory of Pain Experience for Asian American Cancer Patients, 102

J

James, Patricia
A Theory of Theories: A Position Paper, 337
Jones, Dorothy
The Focus of the Discipline Revisited, 363
Jónsdóttir, Helga
A Practice Discipline That's Here and Now, 438

K

Kagan, Paula N.
Historical Voices of Resistance: Crossing Boundaries to Praxis Through Documentary Filmmaking for the Public, 420
Koro-Ljungberg, Mirka
Validity and Validation in the Making in the Context of Qualitative Research, 172

L

Lasiuk, Gerri C.
From Practice to Midrange Theory and Back Again: Beck's Theory of Postpartum Depression, 322
Liehr, Patricia
Middle Range Theory: Spinning Research and Practice to Create Knowledge for the New Millennium, 302
Lissel, Sue L.
Complex Critical Realism: Tenets and Application in Nursing Research, 135

Litchfield, Merian C.
A Practice Discipline That's Here and Now, 438
Lopez, Ruth Palan
Unity of Knowledge in the Advancement of Nursing Knowledge, 431
Lowry, Lois W.
Nursing Theory and Practice: Connecting the Dots, 3

M

Marrs, Jo-Ann
Nursing Theory and Practice: Connecting the Dots, 3
Meleis, Afaf I.
Nursing Epistemology: Traditions, Insights, Questions, 228
Moore, Shirley M.
Levels of Theoretical Thinking in Nursing, 283

N

Neuman, Betty
On Nursing Theories and Evidence, 24
Newman, Margaret A.
The Focus of the Discipline Revisited, 363

P

Parse, Rosemarie Rizzo
Parse's Criteria for Evaluation of Theory With a Comparison of Fawcett's and Parse's Approaches, 358
Penrod, Janice
Concept Analysis: Examining the State of the Science, 267
Perron, Amélie
The Use of Postcolonialism in the Nursing Domain: Colonial Patronage, Conversion, and Resistance, 258
Pharris, Margaret Dexheimer
The Focus of the Discipline Revisited, 363
Porter, Sam
Fundamental Patterns of Knowing in Nursing, 236

R

Reed, Pamela G.
Nursing Reformation: Historical Reflections and Philosophic Foundations, 414
Nursing: The Ontology of the Discipline, 379
A Treatise on Nursing Knowledge Development for the 21st Century: Beyond Postmodernism, 38
Reimer-Kirkham, Sheryl
The Advocate-Analyst Dialectic in Critical and Postcolonial Feminist Research: Reconciling Tensions Around Scientific Integrity, 163
Knowledge Development and Evidence-Based Practice: Insights and Opportunities From a Postcolonial Feminist Perspective for Transformative Nursing Practice, 245

Repede, Elizabeth
    Unitary Appreciative Inquiry: Evolution and
        Refinement, 122
Risjord, Mark
    Rethinking Concept Analysis, 275
Rothbart, Daniel
    An Analysis of Changing Trends in Philosophies of
        Science on Nursing Theory Development and
        Testing, 154
Roy, Bernard
    The Use of Postcolonialism in the Nursing Domain:
        Colonial Patronage, Conversion, and
        Resistance, 258
Roy, Callista L.
    A Central Unifying Focus for the Discipline:
        Facilitating Humanization, Meaning, Choice,
        Quality of Life, and Healing in Living and
        Dying, 403
Rycroft-Malone, Jo
    Theory and Knowledge Translation: Setting Some
        Coordinates, 112

S

Schroeder, Carole A.
    Bridging the Gulf Between Science and Action: The
        "New Fuzzies" of Neopragmatism, 146
Schultz, Annette S. H.
    Knowledge Development and Evidence-Based Prac-
        tice: Insights and Opportunities From a Postco-
        lonial Feminist Perspective for Transformative
        Nursing Practice, 245
Schultz, Phyllis R.
    Nursing Epistemology: Traditions, Insights,
        Questions, 228
Silva, Mary Cipriano
    An Analysis of Changing Trends in Philosophies of
        Science on Nursing Theory Development and
        Testing, 154
    Philosophy, Science, Theory: Interrelationships and
        Implications for Nursing Research, 18
Smith, Marlaine C.
    The Focus of the Discipline Revisited, 363
    The Power of Wholeness, Consciousness, and Caring:
        A Dialogue on Nursing Science, Art, and
        Healing, 384
Smith, Mary Jane
    Middle Range Theory: Spinning Research and
        Practice to Create Knowledge for the New
        Millennium, 302

T

Tarlier, Denise
    Mediating the Meaning of Evidence Through
        Epistemological Diversity, 218
Tyer-Viola, Lynda
    Unity of Knowledge in the Advancement of Nursing
        Knowledge, 431

V

Varcoe, Colleen
    Knowledge Translation in Everyday Nursing: From
        Evidence-Based to Inquiry-Based Practice, 83
    Toward Compassionate Action: Pragmatism and the
        Inseparability of Theory/Practice, 49

W

Walker, Patricia H.
    On Nursing Theories and Evidence, 24–25
Warms, Catherine A.
    Bridging the Gulf Between Science and Action: The
        "New Fuzzies" of Neopragmatism, 146
Watson, Jean
    On Nursing Theories and Evidence, 24
    The Power of Wholeness, Consciousness, and Car-
        ing: A Dialogue on Nursing Science, Art, and
        Healing, 384
Webber, Pamela B.
    Yes, Virginia, Nursing Does Have Laws, 11
Whall, Ann L.
    An Ontological View of Advanced Practice Nursing, 373
    "Lest We Forget": An Issue Concerning the Doctorate
        in Nursing Practice (DNP), 63
White, Jill
    Patterns of Knowing: Review, Critique, and Update, 208
Willis, Danny G.
    A Central Unifying Focus for the Discipline:
        Facilitating Humanization, Meaning, Choice,
        Quality of Life, and Healing in Living and
        Dying, 403

Y

Yeo, Michael
    Integration of Nursing Theory and Nursing Ethics, 31

Z

Zauszniewski, Jaclene A.
    Theoretical Substruction Illustrated by the Theory of
        Learned Resourcefulness, 330

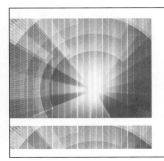

Subject Index

Note: Page numbers in *italics* denote figures; those followed by a t denote tables.

A

Abductive reasoning, 39
Academic discipline, 284, 286. *See also* Discipline(s)
Academic nurse, 97, 98
Accommodative cognitive style, 191
Action research, 71, 118, 150, 164, 295, 443
Addams, Jane, 147
Adult learning theory, 116
Advanced practice nursing
    application to, 375–376
    education, 375–376
    knowledge development and, 373–374
    ontological view of, 372–376
    practice, 376
    research, 376
Advocacy, 162–168
Advocate-analyst dialectic, in feminist research
    critical discourses, 163–164
    critical inquiry, 164, 166, 167
    postcolonial, central tenets, 164
    research methodology, 164, 166–167
    researcher positionality and influence on, 165–166
    rigor, 166
    scientific integrity, 166–167
    social justice, 162, 164, 167–168
    stakeholder agendas, 166
Aesthetic knowledge, 25t, 26–27
    unitary appreciative inquiry (UAI), 130
Alternative and complementary medicine, in multi-paradigm model, 394–396
Ambiguous state, nursing, 364
Analog model, 317
Analogy, 317
Applied science, 56, 358
Appreciating pattern, 388
Appreciative knowing, 126
Aristotelian analysis, evolution of meanings of law, 10
Aristotle, 39, 432, 434
Art of nursing, 26, 27, 201–202, 212–214, 220, 423
    esthetics, 201–202, 212–214, 239
Asian American cancer patients, pain experience for. *See* Situation-specific theory of pain experience for Asian American cancer patients (SPEAC)

B

Baccalaureate nursing program, 85
Balance, in multiparadigm model, 395
Barrett, Rogerian perspective and, 123
Bathing, 397, *397*
Beck, Cheryl Tatano, 321–327
    background of, 324
    empirical adequacy, 327
    internal consistency, 326–327
    life influences of, 324
    philosophical foundations, 325
    testing, 327
    theory origins of, 324–325
    theory scope, 325–326
Beck Depression Inventory (BDI), 325
Behavioral interventions, 140
Benner, Patricia, 404
Bernstein, Richard, 146–148
Bias
    investigator, 130
    in nursing research, 40
Binary thinking, 67, 70
Biomedicine, 261
Biopsychosocial pathways, integrative programs, 142–143

C

Care for self, 13–15, *14*
Caring
    as central nursing concept, 365, 385, 387
    discourse, 67–69
Carper's nursing knowledge model, 23, 26, 200–205
    critiques of, 207–215
Cash-value, 147
Cassandra Radical Feminist Nurses Network, 426–428
    historical and social context, 427
    objective, 426–427
    praxis in, 427–428
Causality, pragmatic view of, 149

Assimilative cognitive style, 191
Autopoiesis, 441
Axioms, 316, 317

The Center for Nursing Advocacy, 421
Change, in developmental-contextual worldview, 41
Charlotte Rainbow PRISM Model, 98
Chinese perspective, cocreating environment, 178–183
Chinn-Jacobs-Kramer model, 32, 167, 207–215, 218
Circumscribed theory, 346
Classism, evidence-based practice and, 251
Clinical knowledge, 231
Clinical nurse specialists' (CNSs'), 64, 69
    data analysis, 64
    interpretive analysis, 65
    nurses' silence, 65, 66
    study findings of, 65
Cocreating environment
    Chinese and Western conceptions of, 178
    comparative analysis, 180
    Daoist and Confucian philosophies, 178
    holistic nature of
        definitions, 180
        focus-field, 180–181
        unitary-transformative paradigm, 180
    nature of self, 181–182
    nexus, 183
    paradigmatic perspectives
        interactive-integrative, 179
        particulate-determinist, 179
        unitary-transformative, 179–180
    person–environment relationship, nature of
        Chinese perspective, 182–183
        unitary-transformative perspective, 182
Cognitive appraisal, 331
Cognitive style, of researcher, 191–192, 195–196
Coherence, 360
Collectivism, 433
Common sense, 93–94
Communication
    neopragmatist view of, 149, 150
    scientific inquiry, in nursing, 188
Community-oriented nurses, 98
Compassion, 51
Complementary contribution, in family diversity, 53–54
Complex systems, human as, 380
Concept advancement, 266, 269, 272
Concept analysis
    character of, 274
    colloquial, 279–280
    data sources, 275
    emergent perspectives on, 271
    epistemological foundation of, 277
    funding, 280
    mixed analyses, 280
    ontological consequences of contextualism, 277–278
    philosophical questions, 275
    principle-based, 271–272
    purpose of, 271
    science, state of, 266–272

theoretical, 279
traditional approaches to, 269–270
types of, 266–267
Walker and Avant's transformation, 276–277
Wilson's method, 275–276
Concepts. *See also* Conceptual frameworks
    abstract, 314–315
    definition
        operational, 314, 319
        theoretical, 314
    necessary, 315
    nonvariable, 313–314
    relationships between, *315,* 315–319, *316*
    sign rule for, 315–316
    sufficient, 315
    theoretical, 312–317
    time-ordered, 315
    variable, 314
Concepts-theory linkages, 267–268
Concept-truth linkages, 268–269
Conceptual definition, of study variables, 332t
Conceptual frameworks. *See also* Model(s)
    evaluation of, 312–320
    in theory development, 157–159
Conceptual knowledge, 231–232
Conceptual models, 44
Conceptual-theoretical-empirical (CTE) structures, 5–7
    definitions of, 6t
Confession, 397
Consciousness, as central nursing concepts, 365–366, 385
Consequences, in family diversity, 51–53
Constructed knowledge, 230
Constructivism, 134, 180, 258
Context stripping, 247
Contraindications, in family diversity, 53–54
Convergent thinking, 191–192
Correspondence, 360
CR. *See* Critical/complex realism
Creativity
    nursing. *See* Nursing creativity
    scientific, 185–186, 195
Critical appraisal, 232, 358
Critical emancipatory, 431
Critical reflection, 111, 130, 166, 251, 254
Critical social theory, 164, 289
Critical theory, 259
Critical thinking, 195, 196, 269
Critical/complex realism (CR)
    agency and structure interactions, 138
    history, 134
    methodological eclecticism and postdisciplinary
        study, 138
    open systems, 137–138
    physical and social entities, independent existence,
        135–136
    positivism, 134, 135

Critical/complex realism (CR) (*Continued*)
  relativism, 134, 135
  research process
    biopsychosocial pathways, integrative programs
      of, 142–143
    health outcomes, 139, 140t
    interventions, 140–142, 141t
  stratified emergent generative ontology
    causation, 137
    emergence, 136
    transfactuality, 136
CTE. *See* Conceptual-theoretical-empirical structures
Cultural safety, 165
  reframing, 253–254
Cultural sensitivity, 52
Culturally congruent care, law of, 15, *15*
Culture, definition, 101–102
Cycles of reflection and action, 125

D

Data analysis, 188
Data collection, 188, 191
Data generation, in unitary appreciative inquiry,
  128–129
Data synopsis, in unitary appreciative inquiry, 129
Decision-support computer program study (DSCP),
  104, 107
Deconstructionalism, 38. *See also* Postmodernism
Deductive reasoning, 38, 39
Deductive system, science as, 154
Definitions, 19
  cognitive appraisal, 331
  conceptual and operational, of study
    variables, 332t
  constructs, 330
  healing, 408
  health, 408
  humanization, 406–407
  meaning, 407–408
  of model components, 330–333
  nursing, 406
  operational, 314, 319, 332t
  positive cognitions, 332
  process regulating cognitions (PRC), 330
  theoretical, 314
  variables, 332
Demonstration projects, 98
Depressive Cognition Scale (DCS), 333
Developmental-contextual worldview, 41
Dewey's pragmatic theory, 147, 149
Diagnosis-intervention linkages, 5
Diagramming, linkage, 347, *347, 348*
Dialectics. *See* Advocate-analyst dialectic, in feminist
  research
Dickoff–James theory, 157
Disciplinary research norms, 193

Discipline(s)
  academic, 192, 286
  focus of, 443–444
  orthogonal subspaces of, 38
  professional, 337
  substantive focus of, 378
Discipline of nursing, 2, 3, 217, 362–369, 402–410
  central unifying focus of
    basic assumptions, 402–403
    future perspective, 409–410
    information and reasons for, 404–406
    inquiry process, 403–404
    linkages, 408–409
  contributions of, 97
  focus of, 362–369, 378–381
  multiparadigmatic, 394–396, *395*
  ontology of, 378–381
Discursive *vs.* nondiscursive experience, 416
Disease model. *See* Medical model
Divergent thinking, 191, 192
Doctorate in Nursing Practice (DNP), 62
Documentary filmmaking, 419–428
Donaldson theory, 149, 364
Dualism
  mind-body, 416
    multiparadigm model and, 395
  qualitative research, 174, 175

E

Eastern healing system, 395
EBP. *See* Evidence-based practice
Eclecticism and postdisciplinary study, 138
Education. *See* Nursing education
Emancipation, unitary appreciative inquiry, 127
Emancipatory inquiry, 425–426
Emancipatory knowing, 164
Embodiment, 88, 416
  of theory/evidence/practice, 89–90
Emergence, 136
Emergent ontology, complex realism (CR), 142
Empathy, 202, 212–213
Empirical adequacy, 355
Empirical generalizations, *vs.* hypothesis, 316–317
Empirical indicators, 7, 333
Empirical knowledge, 23, 25t, 39, 200, 208–209, 232–233
Empirical system, theoretical system and, 283
Empirical testing, 39
Empirical validity, 347–349
  nursing laws, 11–12
Empiricism, 37, 432
  postmodernism and, 39, 40
Empirics, 208–209, 210t, 232
  definition, 236
  dominance of, 235–236, 238
  as evidence-based practice, 236–237
Empowerment, 167, 168, 296

Epistemic relativism, 134
Epistemology, 416, 417
    definition, 227
    diversity, meaning of evidence through, 217–224
    knowledge translation, in nursing, 83–84
    knowledge *vs.* knowing and, 227–229
    nontranscendental, 172
    nursing, 227–233
    in nursing research, 20
    patterns of knowing and, 200–205, 229–231
    relational, 172
    transcendental, 172
    validation in, 173–174
Equifinality, 189
Essentialism, unitary appreciative inquiry and, 126
Esthetic knowledge, 208t, 212–214, 213t
Esthetics, 201–203, 239–240
    art of nursing, 201–202
    order and nursing practice, 43
    pattern of knowing, 202–203
    vs. scientific meaning, 202
Ethic of care, 34, 35
Ethical knowledge, 25t, 26, 204, 208t, 209–210, 211t
    as theory, 27
Ethical theory approach, 33–34
Ethics, 204, 241–242
    formula, 33
    medical, 33
Ethnic identity, 102
Ethnicity, 102, 106–107
Eurocentric thinking, 52
Events, in matrix process, 8
Evidence
    issues of, 220–221
    knowledge and, 221–223
    meaning of, through epistemological diversity, 217–224
Evidence-based health-care, ideology of, 223
Evidence-based medical practice, 5
Evidence-based medicine (EBM), 220, 223
Evidence-based nursing, 321
Evidence-based practice (EBP), 23–28, 88–89, 244–254
    critiques of, 237–238
    definition of, 28
    empirics
        definition, 236
        dominance of, 235–236, 238
    ethics, 241–242
    evolution of, 246–347
    patterns of knowing, 239
    philistine critique of esthetics, 239–240
    postcolonial feminist reading of, 247–251
        application standardization, 250–251
        classism, 251
        incomplete epistemologies, 248–250

    racism, 251
    sexism, 251
    theory-guided, 27–28
    unbearable lightness, 240–241
Evolutionary view, 270
Exemplar paradigm, 344
Experiential learning, 191
Expert practice, 94
Explicit knowledge, 229

F
Factor-isolating, 3
Factor-isolating theory, 50
Factor-relating, 3
Factor-relating theory, 50
Family diversity, pragmatism and, 51–54
    complementary contribution, 53–54
    consequences, 51–53
    contraindications, 53–54
    remake theory/reality, 54
    theory/practice integrity, 54
Family nursing, creativity and, 76–77
Fawcett's criteria, 358–360, 359t
    for nursing theory evaluation, 354t
Feminism, 98
    postcolonial, 244–254
        evidence-based practice, reading of, 247–251
    pragmatics and, 150
    transformative nursing practice and, 244–254
Feminist research, 162–168. *See also* Advocate-analyst dialectic, in feminist research
Flexner Report, 414
Formula ethics, 33
Foundational elements, 358
Funded research, 97

G
Gender issues. *See* Feminism; Women
Gilligan's moral development theory, 34
Goals, *vs.* values, 204
Grand theories, 5, 8, *284,* 284–286, 289, 323, 346
    deconstruction of, 38
    middle range theories and, 307
    nursing, *284,* 284–285
Grounded theory, 209, 229, 325

H
Hand washing, 388
Healing, 408
    context of, 43
    multiparadigm model of, 394–396, *395*
    neomodern view of, 44
Health, 408
    as central nursing concepts, 364–365
    circumstance, 444
    and disease status, SPEAC, 107

Health (*Continued*)
  and illness transition, 105
  outcomes, critical/complex realism
    application to areas of, 139, 140t
    deeper causation levels, *140*
    epidemiological studies, 139
Health experience, 364–365
Healthcare
  approach to, 98
  language of power in, 66
  system, 65, 223
Helicy, 380
Hermeneutic phenomenology, 53
Hermeneutics, 84, 87, 90
Heuristic potential, 360
Historical evolution, 358
Historicism, 432
  vs. logical positivism, 153–155, 154t
  in theory development, 159
HIV. *See* Human immunodeficiency virus
Holarchy, 2
Holism, 32, 392–394, 415–416
  cocreating environment, 180–181
  conceptual limitations of, 393–394, 415–416
  in nursing research, 21
  psychosocial/caring discourse, 67
Human becoming theory, 5
Human health experience, 404
Human immunodeficiency virus (HIV), 251
Human living, 404
Human Response Patterns, 4
Humanities, sciences and, 423
Humanization, 406–407
Humanness, 444
Humans, as systems, 379
Humeral healing system, 395
Humors, 4
Hybrid Model, 270
Hypotheses, 19, 316–317, 333
  vs. empirical generalizations, 316
  formulation of, 187
  vs. law, 317
  peeled-out, 43
  testing of, 319
  working, 285
Hypothetic-deductive logic, 39

I

Iconic model, 317–318
Inductive reasoning, 39
Inquiry-based practice, 88–89
Integrated systems, humans as, 380
Integrative approach, 289–290, *292,* 292–299, *296–297*
  assumption check, *292,* 292–294
  multiple source exploration, *292,* 294–295
  reporting in, 298–299

sharing in, 298–299
SPEAC, 102
theorizing, *292,* 295–298, *296–297*
validating in, 298–299
Intentionality, nursing laws, 14
Interactive-integrative paradigm, 367, 432, 433
Internal consistency, 352–353
International Classification of Diseases and Causes of
    Death, 4
International Classification of Injuries, Disabilities, and
    Handicaps, 4
Interpretive, 431
Intersubjectivity, 40, 315, 440
Introspection, 20
Intuitive knowledge, 20, 212
  in research, 195
Investigator bias, 40, 130
Ironist researcher, 76

J

Jacobs-Kramer-Chinn model, 32, 167, 207–215, 218
James, William, 49, 145–147

K

King's theory, 32
Knowledge, 166. *See also* Nursing knowledge; Scientific
    knowledge
  aesthetic, 25t, 26–27
  appreciative, 126
  development, 244–254, 362–364
    framework for, 38–39
    nursing philosophy, metanarratives for,
      41–42
  discourse, for nursing practice, 69–70
    advantage of, 70
    children in, 69
    CNSs, 69
    implications of, 70–71
    language of, 69
  empirical, 23, 25t, 208–209, 210t, 232–233
  esthetic, 201–203, 208t, 212–214, 213t
  ethical, 25t, 26, 208t, 209–210, 211t
  evidence and, 221–223
  explicit, 229
  intuitive, 20, 212
    in research, 195
  objective/empirical, 67
  patterns of, 204–205
  personal, 25t, 26, 203, 208t, 210–212, 229, 212t
  as process, in qualitative research, 175
  scientific, 431
  subjective/experiential, 67
  typology, 13, *13*
Knowledge translation
  critiques of
    epistemology, 83–84

ontology, 84
  theory-practice gap, 83
embodiment, 88
  of theory/evidence/practice, 89–90
epistemology, 82
and ideology, remaking of, 89
inquiry-based practice, 88–89
interconnection of theory, 82
ontology
  autonomization, 86
  deconstructive hermeneutics, 86
  in everyday nursing action, 85–87
  gap, 84–85
  ideology, 87
  inquiry, 87–88
  of knowing-in-action, 86–87
theory and, 111–119. *See also* Theory, and knowledge
      translation
Knowledge utilization, 321
Kohlberg's moral development theory, 34, 209
Kuhnian paradigms, *343,* 343–345

L
Language
  of nursing theory, 48
  of power in healthcare, 66
Law(s)
  of culturally congruent care, 15
  empirical validation, 11–12
  evolution of meanings of, 10–11
  logical adequacy, 12
  redefining, 12–13
  scientific, 345
    vs. hypothesis, 317
  self-care, 13–15, *14*
  transition thinking, 13
Learning, experimental, 191
Leininger's culture care theory, 15
Leininger's nursing theory, 285
Life patterning, 122–130
Linkage diagram, *347, 348*
Logic
  adequacy, nursing laws, 12
  hypothetico-deductive, 39
  in nursing research, 19
Logical positivism, 190, 431
  vs. historicism, 153–155, 154t
  in theory development, 158, 159
Logical probability, 21

M
Manifesting intention, 388
Maternity blues, 325
Matrix, 7, *7,* 8
Meaning, 407–408
  as central nursing concepts, 368–369

Mechanistic worldview, 41, 395
Medical ethics, 33
Medical model, 33, 393
  dominance of, 394
  historical context of, 394
  in multiparadigm model, 394–396, 395t
Medicine, paradigm shifts in, 41
Mental model, 7, 8
Merton's examination, of middle-range theory,
      301, 302, 307, 323, 324
Metanarratives
  diversity of, 41–42
  in knowledge development, 42–43
Metaparadigms, 41, 343–344, 381
  definition of, 343
  diversity of, 42
  nursing as, 381
Metaphysics, in nursing research, 20
Metatheory, 157, 283–284, *284, 286,* 323
Methodism, 228
Methodological knowledge and skill, 193
Methodological norms, 193, 196
Methodology, research, 187
Micro-range theory, 283, 285–286
Microtheories, 323
Middle range theory, 5, 285, 286, 289–292, *290,*
      301–308, 303–304t, 323–324
  analysis of, 305–306, 306t
  central tenets of, 302
  characterizations of, 302
  classification of, 306–307
  conceptual content of, 305–306
  critiques of, 307
  current status of, 302–305
  disciplinary themes in, 307–308, 308t
  evaluation of, 324
  examples of, 303t–304t
  generation of, 306–307
  grand theory and, 307
  historical context of, 301–302
  level of abstraction in, 306, 306t
  names of, 303–305, 306t
Midrange transition theory, 103–104
  concepts of, 103
  outcome indicators, 104
Mind-body dichotomy, 416
  multiparadigm model and, 395
Model(s), 317–318. *See also* Conceptual frameworks;
      Medical model; Nursing theory
  analog, 317
  conceptual, 44
  definition of, 317
  iconic, 317–318
  mental, 7, 8
  nursing theory and, 317–318
  scientific inquiry in, *188,* 188–194, 189t

Model(s) (*Continued*)
  symbolic, 318
  theoretical, 44
  use of, 318
Moderate realism, 268, 269, 277, 278
Modernism
  definition, 37
  neomodernism, 40–42, 44
  postmodernism and, 37–45
Moral development, 209
  Gilligan's theory of, 34
  Kohlberg's theory of, 34, 209
  nursing ethics and, 34
Moral knowledge, 204, 209–210
Morality. *See* Ethics; Values
Multiparadigm model, 394–396, *395*
Mutual process, as central nursing concepts, 366
Myth of methodology, 193

N

NANDA (North American Nursing Diagnosis
        Association), 4, 5
Narrative, in neopragmatism, 148, 149
National Institute for Nursing Research (NINR), 97, 98
Natural law. *See* Logical positivism; Received view
Neomodernism, 40–42, 44
Neopragmatism, 145–151
Neuman's systems model nurses, 367
Newman's theory, 8, 40, 43, 158, 364, 367, 369, 385, 386,
        405, 440, 443
NIC. *See* Nursing interventions classification
Nightingale, Florence, 2, 97, 164, 285, 321, 379, 413
NINR. *See* National Institute for Nursing Research
NOC. *See* Nursing outcomes classification
Nomad science, 262
Nomadology, 262
Nomenclature systems, 4
Nondiscursive experience, 416
Normative judgment, 204
Normative theory, 89, 393
Norms
  research, 193, 196
  scientific, 346
North American Nursing Diagnosis Association
        (NANDA), 4, 5
Notes on Nursing (Nightingale), 285
Nurse(s)
  academic, 97, 98
  as filmmakers, 420–423
  Cassandra Radical Feminist Network of, 426–428
  community-oriented, 98
  in documentary filmmaking, 419–428
  on film, 420–423
  historical narratives of resistance, 424
  knowledge
    and doctors, relationship between, 70
    social context of, 66–70
  professional, 416, 421
  sciences and humanities, 423
  as theorists, 56–60
  unitary appreciative inquiry, 125
Nurse filmmakers, 421–423
Nurse pragmatist, 149
Nurse Scientist program, 96
Nurse-initiated treatments, 5
Nursing. *See also* Art of nursing; Discipline of nursing;
        Medical model; Metaparadigms; Nursing prac-
        tice; Postmodernism; Praxis
  activities and interventions, 397, *397*
  as art, 201–202, 212–214, 423–424
  central concepts of, 364–369, 381
  central unifying focus
    basic assumptions, 402–403
    for discipline of nursing, 406
    future perspective, 409–410
    information and reasons for, 404–406
    inquiry process, 403–404
    linkages, 408–409
  conceptual models of, 44
  definitions of, 406, 415
  discipline of, 2, 3, 205, 217, 362–369, 402–410
    contributions of, 97
  Doctorate in Nursing Practice (DNP), 62
  family, 76–77
  history of, 413–414
  medical model and, 33, 393
  as metaparadigm, 381
  neomodern, 40–41, 44
  ontology of, 378–381
  pluralism in, 433
  postcolonialism in, 257–263
  postcritical discipline, 44–45
  as practice discipline, 437–445
  praxis in, 417
  as preparadigm science, 344–345
  as process, 415
  as process of well-being, 378–381
  as profession, 30, 414
  spirituality and, 396, 417
  true voice of, 35
  in worldview, 440–441
Nursing creativity
  authority
    of method, 75
    shift in, 75–76
  cultivating, 73–78
  and family nursing, 76–77
  ironism, 76
  mental theme parks, 75
  method, 73–74
  problem of theory, 77–78
  theoretically based methods, 73
Nursing Diagnosis: Definitions and Classifications
        (2001–2002), 4

Nursing discourses, 64–71
  clinical nurse specialists' (CNSs')
    data analysis, 64
    interpretive analysis, 65
    nurses' silence, 65, 66
    study findings of, 65
  and nurses' silence, 64–71
  social context, of nurses' knowledge and practice,
    69–70
    implications of, 70–71
    language of power, in healthcare, 66
    psychosocial/caring discourse, 67–69
    technical/rationalist discourse, 67
Nursing education
  critical studies, 425, 426
  documentaries in, 419
  history of, 414
  praxis in, 426
Nursing epistemology, 227–233
  definition, 227
  knowledge *vs.* knowing and, 227–229
  patterns of knowing and, 200–205, 229–231
  in research, 20
Nursing ethics, 204
  ethical theory approach, 33–34
  formula ethics and, 33
  medical ethics and, 33
  moral development approach to, 34
  in nursing knowledge, 25t, 26, 208t, 209–210, 211t
  nursing theory and, 27, 30–35
  in research, 20
Nursing history, 413–414, 419–428
Nursing image, 421, 422
Nursing interventions classification (NIC),
  5, 397, *397*
Nursing knowledge, 25
  advancement of, 430–435
  bottom-up approach to, 416–417
  Carper's model of, 23, 26, 200–205
    critiques of, 207–215
  clinical, 231
  conceptual, 231–232
  constructed, 230
  criteria of credibility for, 231–233
  development of, 433–434
    metanarratives for, 41–42
    modernism and, 37–45
  emancipatory, 127, 425–426
  empirical, 23, 25t, 39, 200, 208–209, 210t
  ethical, 25t, 26, 204, 208t, 209–210, 211t
  expanded hierarchy of, 6t
  explicit, 229
  framework of, 38–39, 113–114
  intuitive, 20, 195
  Jacobs-Kramer-Chinn model, 207–215, 218
  vs. knowing, 227–229
  Kramer-Chinn model of, 23, 26, 27

  methodologies for, 439
  model of, 208t
  neomodernism and, 40–41
  nondiscursive experience and, 416
  nonempirical, 40
  ontology, 84
  paradigms and, 430–433
  patterns of, 200–205, 207–215, 229–231, 367
    critique of, 207–215
    as theories, 23, 26–27
  Peplau's theory and, 39, 43
  personal, 25t, 26, 203, 208t, 210–212,
    212t, 229
  postmodernism and, 37–45
  from practice knowledge, 251–254
  pragmatic approach to, 417
  procedural, 230
  qualitative *vs.* quantitative, 159
  received, 230
  Roy's perspective on, 434–435
    diversity, 434
    unity, 434
    universal truths, 434–435
  from scientific knowledge, 416–417
  silent, 230
  social, 66–70
  sociopolitical, 214–215, 215t
  sources of, 19–21
  subjective, 230
  tacit, 229
  theoretical *vs.* practical, 229
  as theory, 23–27, 25t
  values and, 204
Nursing laws
  culturally congruent care, 15
  definition, 11
  empirical validation, 11–12
  evolution of meanings of, 10–11
  logical adequacy, 12
  redefining, 12–13
  self-care, 13–15, *14*
  transition thinking, 13
Nursing models. *See also* Model(s)
  medical, 392–393
  nursing theory and, 317–318
Nursing outcomes classification (NOC), 5
Nursing paradigms, 432–433
Nursing philosophy. *See* Philosophy of nursing
Nursing practice. *See also* Nursing
  in action, 444–445
  autonomous, 99
  classification system for, 4
  creativity in, 73–78, 195
  evidence-based, 23–28
    definition, 28
    theory-guided, 26–28
  feminism and, 244–254

Nursing practice (*Continued*)
    humanization, 406–409
    implications, of knowledge discourse, 70–71
    knowledge-based discourse for, 69–70
    as metanarrative for knowledge development, 41
    nursing theory and, 56–60, 99, 345
    paradigms, 432–433
    vs. process, 417
    theory-guided, 93–99
        education for, 95
        Parse's theory, 99
Nursing practice theory, 56–60, 286. *See also* Nursing
        theory
    development of, 59
    explicit, 59, 60
    need for, 58–59
    nursing knowledge and, 251–254
    usefulness of, 349
Nursing praxis, 219–220
    evidence, meaning of, 223–224
Nursing processes, 374–375, 378–381
    centrality of, 415
    complexity of, 380
    example of, 380–381
    inherent, 378–381
Nursing research. *See also* Nursing science; Research;
        Scientific research
    action, 71, 150
    bias in, 40
    cognitive style and, 191–192, 195–196
    creativity in, 185, 186
    critical/complex realism (CR)
        biopsychosocial pathways, integrative programs of,
            142–143
        health outcomes, 139, 140t
        interventions, 140–142, 141t
    extrapersonal factors in, 193–194
    holistic approach in, 21
    individual influences in, 193
    institutional influences in, 193
    intrapersonal factors in, 189–193
    intuition in, 195
    methodological knowledge and skill in, 193
    methodological norms in, 193, 196
    personal experience and, 192
    phases of, 187–188
    philosophical basis of, 19–21
    pragmatic, 149, 150
    as praxis, 43
    qualitative *vs.* quantitative, 159
    sociohistorical context for, 194
    subjectivity in, 187, 188
    systems/process model for, *188,* 188–194, 189t
Nursing scholars
    on central unifying focus of discipline, 404
    in knowledge development, 362–364

    philosophical positions of, 293
    theological, 441
Nursing science, 97–98. *See also* Nursing research
    caring, 385
    consciousness, 385
    current status of, 201
    development of, 200
    focus of, 362–369
    history of, 39
    as human *vs.* natural science, 191
    meaning, 386
    medical model and, 393
    modernism and, 39–40
    normative, 32
    nursing knowledge, 386
    vs. nursing philosophy, 30–32
    pattern, 385
    as pattern of knowing, 200
    perspectives and syntheses, 383–386
    postmodern, 39–40
    pragmatic, 149, 150
    received view in, 190
    relationship, 386
    researcher's beliefs about, 190
    transformation and transcendence, 385–386
    unitary appreciative inquiry (UAI), 121, 125, 127
    wholeness, 384–385
    worldview and, 374
Nursing syntax, in theory development, 313, 315, 316
Nursing theory, 2–8, 30–35, 93–99, 157–160
    aesthetic, 25–27
    conceptual basis of, 312–317
    definitions, 26
    development of, 153–160, 345–346
        conceptual frameworks in, 157–159
        history of, 157–159
        logical positivism in, 158, 159
        models in, 317–318
        ontological view of, 208
        philosophy, 19–20
        trends in, 157–159
        trends in science philosophy and, 153–160
    diagramming of, *347, 348*
    empirical, 23, 25t, 347–349
    evaluation of, 32–33, 349
        criteria for, 318–320, 347–349
    evidence-based practice and, 23–28
    Fawcett's criteria for evaluation of, 354t
    grand, *284,* 284–286
    language of, 48
    of learned resourcefulness, 329–334
    Leininger's, 285
    levels of, 283–286
    logical adequacy of, 318–319, 347
    metatheory, 283–284, *284,* 286
    micro-range, 283, 285–286

middle-range, 285, 286, 301–308, 303–304t
novelty and viability, 341–342
nursing ethics, 25t, 26, 30–35
nursing models and, 317–318
nursing philosophy and, 17–21, 153–157
nursing practice and, 56–60, 99, 345
nursing research and, 19–21
nursing science and, 30
operational system, 333–334
Parse's, 43
peeled-out, 43
Peplau's, 39, 42, 43
personal, 25t, 26
philosophy, 19–20
practice guides, 93–99
practice-derived, 251–254
Rogers', 380
Roy's, 30–32
semantics of, 313, 315
as situation-producing theory, 339–341
statements of, 316–317
structure of, 340–341
syntax of, 313, 315
testability of, evaluation of, 315, 347–348
theoretical substruction, 329–334
values in, 31–33
Watson's, 285
Nursing theory movement, 98
Nursing theory-guided practice, 98
Nursology, 43, 381

O
Objective knowledge, 67
Omaha classification system, 6
Ontological competencies, 387–388
Ontological realism, 208–209
Ontology, knowledge translation
    autonomization, 86
    deconstructive hermeneutics, 86
    in everyday nursing action, 85–87
    gap, 84–85
    ideology, 87
    inquiry, 87–88
    of knowing-in-action, 86–87
        inquiry, 87–88
Open philosophy, 39, 45
Open systems
    in complex world, 137–138
    humans as, 380
    in Rogers' theory, 380
Operational definitions, 314, 319, 332
Operational system, 333–334
Oppression, 167, 168
Organismic worldview, 41
Orthogenetic principle, 380
Orthogonal subspaces, of disciplines, 38

P
Pain experience, for Asian American cancer patients.
    See Situation-specific theory of pain
    experience for Asian American cancer
    patients (SPEAC)
Paniculate-deterministic paradigms, 432
Paradigm(s). See also Metaparadigms; Rogers'
    science of unitary human beings;
    Worldview(s)
    critical, 149, 150
    diversity of, 42
    exemplar, 344
    explanatory, 395t
    interactive-integrative, 367, 432, 433
    Kuhnian, 343, 343–345
    metaparadigms and, 343–344
    multiple, 394–396
    nursing, 432–433
    paniculate-deterministic, 432
    participatory, 440–443
    postpositivist, 179, 262
    preparadigms and, 343–345
    search for, 431–432
    simultaneity, 432
    totality, 432
    unitary, 123, 365
    unitary-transformative, 432
    worldviews and, 430–431
Paradigm shifts, 394
    in medicine, 41
Parse's criteria, in evaluation of theories,
    358–360, 359t
Parse's nursing theory, 43, 99
Parsimony, 353
Participatory paradigm, 440–443
Particularism, 229
Particulate-deterministic paradigm, 179, 433
Paternalism, in Roy's adaptation model,
    31, 32
Patronage, 261–262
Pattern(s)
    as central nursing concept, 385
    in matrix process, 7, 7, 8
    of response, SPEAC, 108–109
Patterns of Unitary Man, 4
PCF. See Postcolonial feminism
PDSS. See Postpartum Screening Scale
Peeling out, 43
Peplau's theory, 39, 42, 43
Personal knowledge, 25t, 26, 203, 208t, 210–212,
    212t, 229
Person-environment relationship, nature of
    Chinese perspective, 182–183
    unitary-transformative perspective, 182
Phenomenology, hermeneutic, 53
Philosophic inquiry, 283, 284

Philosophy
    development of, 179
    discursive *vs.* nondiscursive, 416
    in nursing research, 19–20
    in nursing theory, 19–20
    science and, 17–18
    worldview and, 374
Philosophy of nursing, 41–42. *See also* Positivism
    definition, 41
    discursive *vs.* nondiscursive, 416
    integrative, 414–417
    metanarratives for knowledge development,
        41–42
Philosophy of science
    changes in, effects of on nursing theory, 153–160
    goal of, 156–157
    historicism in, 153–156, 159
    integration, 156, *156*
    received view in, 153–160, 190
    reductionism in, 156
    in theory development, 157–159
    trends in, 157–159
Physician-initiated treatments, 5
Pierce, Charles Sanders, 48, 146
Pluralism, in nursing, 433
Plurality, in neopragmatism, 148
Political knowledge, 214
Positive cognitions, 332
Positivism, 134, 135, 190. *See also* Received view
    acontextual nature of, 30–31
    critiques of, 157–159
    vs. historicism, 153–155
    limitations of, 157–159
    logical, 190, 395, 431
    nursing syntax and, 292–299
    in nursing theory, 292–299
    in theory development, 158, 159
Possibilities, 95–96
Postcolonial feminism (PCF), 244–254
    evidence-based practice, reading of, 247–251
        application standardization, 250–251
        classism, 251
        incomplete epistemologies, 248–250
        racism, 251
        sexism, 251
    transforming practice and, 251–254
Postcolonial feminist research, 164
Postcolonial feminist theory, 248
Postcolonialism
    biomedicine, 261
    colonial patronage, resistance to, 261–262
    conversion of nursing, 261
    critique of, 259–260
    definition, 258–260
    evidence-based medicine, 257
    expanding, 258–260

knowledge hierarchization, 262–263
    nursing, 260–261
Postdisciplinary study, eclecticism and, 138
Postmodernism
    central tenets of, 38
    context in, 43
    deconstructionalism and, 38
    definition, 37
    empiricism and, 37, 40
    history of, 37–38
    locus of meaning in, 43
    modernism and, 37–45
    neomodernism and, 40–41
    nursing knowledge and, 37–45
    nursing practice and, 43
    nursing science and, 39–40
Postpartum depression (PPD), 142, 322, 325
Postpartum Depression Predictors Inventory
        (PDPI), 327
Postpartum psychosis, 325
Postpartum Screening Scale (PDSS), 327
Postpositivism, 190, 431
Posttraumatic stress disorder (PTSD), 422
Postulates, 18–19
Power
    of autonomous nursing practice, 99
    emancipatory inquiry and, 425–426
    language of, in healthcare, 66
    praxis and, 127
    of wholeness and caring, 383–390
Practical consequences, 53
Practical knowledge, 126, 127, 232
Practice
    reflections on, 93
    theory guides, 93
Practice theories, 7, 289–292, *290*
Practice-minded theory, 50
Practice-oriented theory, 3
Pragmatic adequacy, 355–356
Pragmatic, definition of, 145–146
Pragmatism, 48–50, 145–151, 148t, 360
    definition of, 48, 145–146
    family diversity and
        complementary contribution, 53–54
        consequences, 51–52
        contraindications, 53–54
        remake theory/reality, 54
        theory/practice integrity, 54
    feminism, 150
    history of, 146–147
    implications in, 54–55
    as new fuzziness, 147
    nursing and, 149–150
    principles of, 146
    revival of, 147–149
    theory development through, 49–50

Pragmatists, 76
Praxis, 54, 381, 427–428
  advocate-analyst dialectic, 164
  in documentary filmmaking, 425
  nursing as, 219–220
    evidence, meaning of, 223–224
  in nursing education, 426
  nursing research as, 43
  for resistance and social activism, 424–426
  unitary appreciative inquiry, 122, 125–126
Predictive theory, 50
Pressure to Move Scale (PMS), 333
Primitive terms, 19
Principle of equifinality, 189
Problem of theory, 77–78
Problem-solving, 93–94
  cognitive style and, 191
  creative, 186, 187
  phases of, 187
Procedural knowledge, 230
Process regulating cognitions (PRC), 330
Profession, nursing as, 30, 414
Professional nurses, 416–417, 421
Professional organization productions, 421
Promoting Action on Research Implementation in
    Health Services (PARIHS), 114
Promoting/inhibiting theory, 50
Propositional knowing, 127, 130
Psychoneuroimmunology theory, 41, 396
Psychosocial/caring discourse
  arbitrary dichotomy, 68
  biomedical/technical discourse, 68
  holism, 67
  nurse-patient relationship, 67
  nursing practice, 67
Purification, in multiparadigm model, 395
Putnam, Hilary, 146

Q
Qualitative research
  assumptions
    knowledge, as process, 175
    pluralism, 175
    reality and subjects, interconnectedness, 174–175
  epistemology
    nontranscendental, 172
    relational, 172
    transcendental, 172
  (e)pistemological validation in, 173–174
  reductionist views
    Anderson and Herr's concepts of, 173
    audit trail, 172
    epistemological-methodological, 173
    rigor of, 172
    theoretical perspective, 173
    triangulation, 172

unthinkability, 176
  validity and validation, definition of, 171
Quality of life, 408
Quality of research, 129, 130

R
Racism, evidence-based practice and, 251
Random clinical trials, 246
Rationalism, 20, 432
Realism, scientific, 149
Reasoning
  abductive, 39
  deductive, 38, 39
  inductive, 39
Received knowledge, 230
Received view, 190, 432
Reciprocal-interaction, 433
Reciprocity, 211
Reductionism in, 156
Reflective thinking, 186, 195
Relational statements, 358
Relocation adjustment, 332
Relocation controllability, 332
Remake theory/reality, in family diversity, 54
Repression, 94–95
Research
  experience, 192
  findings, communication of, 188
  methodology, 187
  unitary appreciative inquiry (UAI), 123–125
Responsive action, 49
Risk taking, knowledge development and, 51
Rogers' science of unitary human beings, 380
Rogers unitary appreciative inquiry, 121, 123
Rorty, Richard, 146, 147
Rosenbaum's resourcefulness theory, 329–334
Roy's adaptation model, 30–32, 367
Roy's perspective, on nursing knowledge, 434–435
  diversity, 434
  unity, 434
  universal truths, 434–435

S
Science, 62
  components of, 154–155, 154t
  domains of, 155
  and humanities, 423
  introspection in, 20
  intuition in, 20
  logical positivist vs. historicist view of,
      153–155, 154t
  nature of, 185–187
  objectivity of, 31
  philosophy and, 17–18
  as product vs. process, 154, 154t, 155
  royal, 262

Science (*Continued*)
state of, 262
concept analysis, 266–272
theory and, 18–19
of unitary human beings, 121, 127
worldview and, 374
Scientific creativity, 186, 187
Scientific integrity, in advocate-analyst dialectic,
166–167
broad interpretation of, 166
methodological principles, 166–167
Scientific knowledge, 431. *See also* Positivism; Received
view
development of
metaparadigm stage of, 344
preparadigm stage of, 343–345
transformed into nursing knowledge, 416–417
Scientific laws, 11–12, 345
vs. hypotheses, 317
Scientific method, 21
Scientific norms, 346
Scientific principles, 18
Scientific progress, assessment of, 156, *156*
Scientific realism, 149
Scientific research
bias in, 40
creativity in, 185–186, 195
data collection and analysis in, 188
evaluation of, 348–249
historicist view of, 155–157
intuition in, 195
methodological norms in, 193, 196
stages of, 187–188
study design in, 187
systems/process model for, *188,* 188–194, 189t
traditions of, 155–156
Self-care, law of, 13–15, *14*
Self-Control Schedule (SCS), 333
Self-knowledge, 195, 210–212, 229. *See also* Personal
knowledge
Semantic integrity, 360
Semantics, of nursing theory, 313, 315
Sets, 18–19
Sexism, evidence-based practice and, 251
Sign rule, 314–315
Silent knowing, 230
Simplicity, 360
Simultaneity paradigms, 432
Situation-producing, 3
Situation-producing theory, 50, 54, 339–341
ingredients of, 340
nursing theory as, 339–341
Situation-related theory, 50
Situation-relating, 3
Situation-specific theory, 289–292,
290, 323

Situation-specific theory of pain experience for Asian
American cancer patients (SPEAC), *102*
assumptions, 102–103
concepts in, 104–105
culture, 101–102
ethnic identity, 102
ethnicity, 102
integrative approach, 102
nature of transition
critical points, changes, and awareness, 105–106
health/illness transition, 105
single/multiple transitions, 105
pain management methods, 101
patterns of response
mind control, 108–109
natural, 108
normal, 108
tolerance, 108
sources for
concepts, 104–105
decision-support computer program study, 104
literature review, 104
midrange transition theory, 103–104
transition conditions
demographic factors, 106
ethnicity-related factors, 106–107
health/disease status, 107
need for help, 107–108
social support, 107
Skepticism, 228
Social context, of nurses' knowledge and practice
discourse, 69–70
implications of, 70–71
language of power, in healthcare, 66
psychosocial/caring discourse, 67–69
technical/rationalist discourse, 67
Social entities, complex realism, 135–136
Social equity, 167
Social justice, advocate-analyst dialectic, 162, 164,
167–168
Social support, transition conditions, 107
Sociopolitical knowledge, 214–215, 215t
Spirituality, 417
in multiparadigm model, 396
Stakeholder agendas, in feminist research, 166
Standard Diagnostic and Statistical Manual of Mental
Disorders, 4
Standard Nomenclature of Disease and Operations, 4
Static doctrines, 51
Structuration theory, 116
Study design, 187
Subjective knowledge, 230
Subjectivity, in research, 187, 188
Substruction, 329
Supranormal, in multiparadigm model, 395, 397,
397t, 398

Symbolic model, 318
Syntax of nursing, in theory development, 313, 315, 316
Systematized Nomenclature of Medicine, 4
Systematized Nomenclature of Pathology, 4
Systemic structure, in matrix process, 8

T

Tacit knowledge, 229
Technical/rationalist discourse, 67
Teetering on the Edge, 325–326, *326*
Terms
    key, 19
    primitive, 19
Testability, 353
Theoretical congruence, 189
Theoretical experience, 192
Theoretical models, 44
Theoretical reduction, 156
Theoretical substruction, 329–334
    research example, 329–334, *331*
Theoretical system, empirical system and, 283
Theoretical terms, 19
Theoretical thinking, 282–287
    evidence of, 286
    for knowledge development, 286–287
    levels of, 283–286, *284*
Theorizing, 94, *292*, 295–298, *296–297*
Theory, 13, 164, 322–323, 336–337. *See also* Hypotheses; Middle range theory; Model(s); Nursing theory; Postmodernism
    cash-value of, 147
    circumscribed, 346
    components of, 18
    conceptual content of, 305–306, 312–317
    cultural care diversity, 367
    deconstruction of, 38, 282
    definitions of, 26, 306, 345
    development of, 345–346
    empirical adequacy of, 319, 347–349
    evaluation of, 347–349
        criteria for, 347–349, 352–356
    generality of, 319
    grand, 323, 346
        deconstruction, 38
    grounded, 325
    hypotheses and, 19
    interconnection of, 82, 84
    and knowledge translation, 111
        adult learning theory, 116
        coherent overarching framework, 113–114
        conceptual, development of, 113
        context (doubt), 115
        definition, 113
        evaluation of, 112–113
        facilitation, 115
        implementation research, 112, 117, 118

individual, group, and organization levels, findings, 116, 117, 117t
        interventions, 112
        outcomes, measures, and variables, identification of, 112
        PARIHS framework, 114
        research agenda, 117–118
        selection of, 115–117, 115t
        structuration theory, 116
        world views, 113
    of learned resourcefulness, 329–334, *331*
    levels of, 50
    logical adequacy of, 318–319, 347, *347*
    metatheory, 283–284, *284,* 286, 323
    micro-range, 283, 285–286
    microtheories, 323
    middle-range, 285, 286, 301–308, 303–304t, 323–324
    models and, 317–318
    novelty and viability, 341–342
    operational definitions in, 314, 319
    postcolonial feminist, 164
    postmodern view of, 39
    pragmatic adequacy of, 319–320
    pragmatism, 49–50
    predictability of, 319
    problem of, 77–78
    for professional purpose, 337
    science and, 18–19
    situation-producing, 338
    situation-specific, 323
    situation-specific theory of, 101–109
    statements of, 316–317
    tentative nature of, 320
    testability of, 155, 319
    theoretical definitions in, 314
    of theories, 336–342
    of translation, 82–90
    types of, 323
    universality, 367
    usefulness of, 319–320
Theory development, 50–51, 54
Theory guides practice, 93
Theory of health as expanding consciousness, 5
Theory/practice integrity, in family diversity, 54
Tolerance
    in neopragmatism, 148, 150
    SPEAC, 108
Totality paradigms, 432
Totality-simultaneity paradigms, 432
Transformative paradigm, 432
Transition, in SPEAC
    conditions
        demographic factors, 106
        ethnicity-related factors, 106–107
        health/disease status, 107

Transition, in SPEAC (*Continued*)
    need for help, 107–108
    social support, 107
  nature of
    critical points, changes, and awareness, 105–106
    health/illness transition, 105
    single/multiple transitions, 105
Transition thinking, 13
Truth, 162
  correspondence norms of, 190
  logical positivist view of, 190
  postpositivist view of, 190
  practical effects of, 146
  pragmatic view of, 146, 147, 149

U

Understanding, 95
Unitary appreciative inquiry (UAI)
  conceptual development, 121
  expanding potentials, 130–131
  history, 121–123
  human wholeness, 123–131
  methodology, 124, 125
  praxis, 122
  process of
    appreciation, 126
    emancipation, 127
    participation, 126–127
    praxis, 125–126
    reflection and action, 125
  refinements
    assumptions and conceptual underpinnings, 127–128
    credibility and legitimacy, 129–130
    data generation, 128–129
    data synopsis, 129
    research, 122–123
  research
    community assessment project, 125
    data collection process, 123
    life situations, 123
    participatory dreaming, 124
    patterning profile, 124
    unitary healing praxis model for, 124
    women in despair, 123, 124
Unitary paradigms, 432
Unitary science, 127, 128
Unitary-transformative paradigm, 362, 432
  cocreating environment, 182

Universal truths, 434–435
Utility, pragmatic view of, 145, 149

V

Validity
  empirical, 347–349
  qualitative research, context of, 171–176
Values. *See also* Ethics; Spirituality
  vs. goals, 204
  in nursing theory, 31–33
  Roy's adaptation model, 31–32
Variables, 313–314, 332
Vision, in matrix process, 7
Vulnerability, 165

W

Wald, Lillian, 98
Walker and Avant's transformation, 276–277
Watson's nursing theory, 285
Well-being, process of, 378–381
Werner's orthogenetic principle, 380
Wholeness, power of, 384–385
Wilson's method, 275–276
Women
  in despair, unitary appreciative inquiry, 123, 124
  moral development in, 34
  silent knowledge of, 230
Working hypotheses, 285
Worldview(s), 41–42
  development of, 374
  developmental-contextual, 41
  diversity of, 42
  holistic, 180–181
    of environment, 180–181
  mechanistic, 41, 395
  in nursing, 440–441
  nursing science, 374
  organismic, 41
  paradigms and, 430–431
  participatory, 442, 443
  particulate-deterministic, 433
  philosophical, 374, 432
  of researcher, 189–191
  science, 374
  shifting, 441–443
  simultaneous action, 41
  theory and knowledge translation, 113
  unitary-transformative, 41